The Ultimate UCAT Collection

UniAdmissions

Subsequent Editions: 2019, 2018

ISBN 978-1-912557-57-8

Published by *RAR Medical Services Limited, trading as* **Infinity Books.**

www.uniadmissions.co.uk / info@uniadmissions.co.uk
www.uniadmissions.com.au / www.uniadmissions.co.nz
info@uniadmissions.com.au / info@uniadmissions.co.nz

Tel: +64 9801 2607 / +61 7391 11767
Tel: +44 (0) 208 068 0438

The Ultimate UCAT Collection

Three Books in One

Dr. Wiraaj Agnihotri
Dr. Rohan Agarwal

UniAdmissions

About the Authors

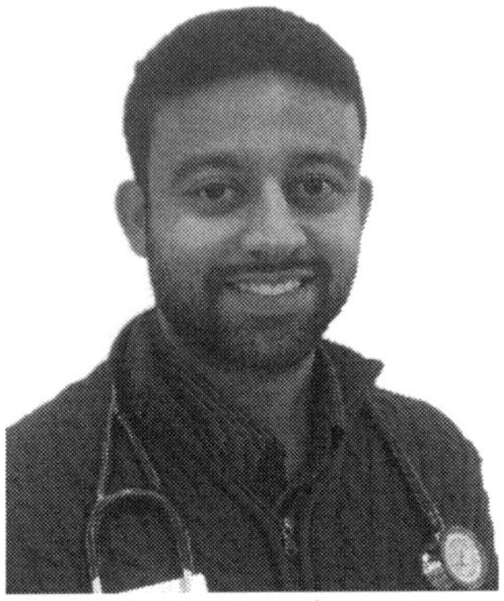

Wiraaj graduated in 2012 with an honours degree in Natural Sciences from Pembroke College, Cambridge where he was selected to receive annual scholarship funding from the Cambridge Trusts. In his final year at Cambridge he specialised in the rigorous Mechanisms of Disease option during which he wrote an independent research dissertation on autoimmune thyroid disease.

Wiraaj subsequently completed graduate medical studies (MBBS) at the University of Sydney in 2016. He is currently a resident medical officer in Sydney where he plans to pursue further clinical specialisation as an internal medicine physician.

With a longstanding passion for teaching, Wiraaj has been heavily involved in tutoring students at various stages of their education. Over the years Wiraaj has successfully coached a great number of students into Medical Schools globally. Outside of medicine and education, Wiraaj enjoys playing jazz guitar and football

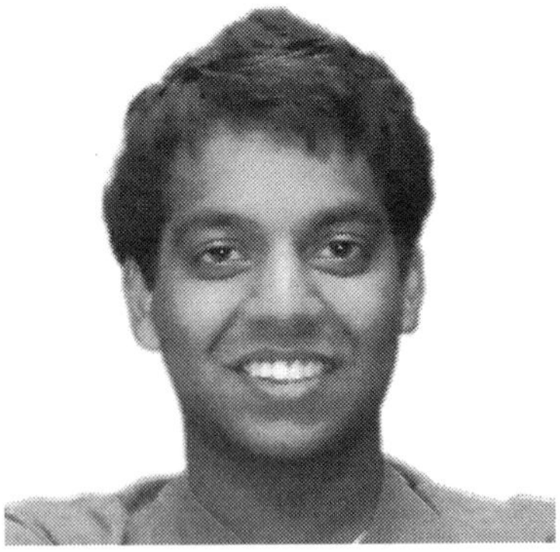

Rohan is **Director of Operations** at *UniAdmissions* and is responsible for its technical and commercial arms. He graduated from Gonville and Caius College, Cambridge, and is now a doctor in Leicester. Over the last five years, he has tutored hundreds of successful Oxbridge and Medical applicants. He has authored twenty books on admissions tests and interviews.

He has taught physiology to undergraduates and interviewed medical school applicants for Cambridge. He has also published research on bone physiology and writes education articles for the Independent and Huffington Post. In his spare time, Rohan enjoys playing the piano and table tennis.

How to use this Book

Congratulations on taking the first step to your UCAT preparation! First used in 2008, the UCAT is a difficult exam and you'll need to prepare thoroughly in order to make sure you get that dream university place.

The *Ultimate UCAT Collection* is the most comprehensive UCAT book available – it's the culmination of three top-selling UCAT books:

- *The Ultimate UCAT Guide*
- *UCAT Practice Papers: Volume 1*
- *UCAT Practice Papers: Volume 2*

Whilst it might be tempting to dive straight in with mock papers, this is not a sound strategy. Instead, you should approach the UCAT in the three steps shown below. Firstly, start off by understanding the structure, syllabus and theory behind the test. Once you're satisfied with this, move onto doing the 1250 practice questions found in *The Ultimate UCAT Guide* (not timed!). Then, once you feel ready for a challenge go through the 6 UCAT Mock Papers found in *UCAT Practice Papers* – these are a final boost to your preparation.

As you've probably realised by now, there are well over 2,500 questions to tackle meaning that this isn't a test that you can prepare for in a single week. From our experience, the best students will prepare anywhere between four to eight weeks (although there are some notable exceptions!).

Remember that the route to a high score is your approach and practice. Don't fall into the trap that "you can't prepare for the UCAT"– this could not be further from the truth. With knowledge of the test, some useful time-saving techniques and plenty of practice you can dramatically boost your score.

Work hard, never give up and do yourself justice. Good luck!

The Ultimate UCAT Guide

The Basics

What is the UCAT?

The University Clinical Aptitude Test (UCAT) is a newly introduced two hour computer based exam that is taken by applicants to Australian + New Zealand medical and dental schools. The questions are randomly selected from a huge question bank. Since every UCAT test is unique, candidates can sit the UCAT at different times. You sit the test on a date of your choosing in July. **The UCAT replaces the UMAT from 2019. However, the UCAT is virtually identical to the UKCAT which has been used since 2006 in the United Kingdom.** You register to sit the test online and book a time slot. On the day, bring along a printout of your test booking confirmation and arrive in good time. Your identity will be checked against a photographic ID that you'll need to bring. You then leave your personal belongings in a locker and enter the test room. Make sure you go to the toilet and have a drink before going in, to save wasting time during the test.

Test Structure:

Section	What does it test?	Questions	TIME
ONE	**Verbal Reasoning**: Essentially a reading comprehension test, with questions based on passages. This is a test of accuracy and speed of reading.	44	22 minutes
TWO	**Decision Making:** Tests your application of logic and approach to problem solving. Developing a structured approach will help you succeed.	29	32 minutes
THREE	**Quantitative Reasoning**: The maths is usually intellectually straightforward but can involve complex or multi stage calculations against the clock. Assesses your understanding of numbers.	36	25 minutes
FOUR	**Abstract Reasoning**: Matching shapes to which set they belong in. This tests your pattern recognition skills and rewards those who have clear and logical organisation of thought.	55	14 minutes
FIVE	**Situational Judgement**: This tests your ability to make decisions in a clinical environment. To perform well, you must understand the role and responsibilities of a medical student.	69	27 minutes

Why is the UCAT used?

For medical schools, choosing the best applicants is hard. Every year, medical schools are flooded with talented applicants, all of whom have top grades and great personal statements. They felt they needed extra information to help them find the very best from the pool of very talented applicants they always had. That's why admissions tests were created.

The UCAT was first introduced in 2006 to help medical schools make their choices. The test examines skills in different areas, all of which are related to critical thinking and decision making. The idea was to create a pure aptitude test, something which cannot be prepared for. However this is certainly not the case with the UCAT, and this is even acknowledged by UCAT itself based on their research. In our experience, you can improve your UCAT score with only a small amount of work, and with proper organised preparation the results can be fantastic.

Who has to sit the UCAT?

You have to sit UCAT if you are applying for any of the universities that ask for it in the current application cycle. You are strongly advised to check this list in May to see if the universities you are considering require it.

When do I sit the UCAT?

When you register to sit UCAT online, you choose your date and time slot and also the test centre. The UCAT can be sat from 1st July through to 31st July. Registration for the test opens on March 1st – we recommend you book your test early so you have the best choice of possible dates.

Many students find it helpful to sit UCAT towards the end of the exam window – this gives you maximum time to prepare, but gets the test complete before you go back to school, so you have one less thing to worry about at that busy time. Remember that you may want to modify your university choices based on your UCAT score to maximise your chances of success.

Registration Opens 1 March 2019 → **Testing Begins** 1 July 2019 → **Registration Closes** 16 May 2019 → **Testing Finishes** 31 July 2019

How much does it cost?

As the UCAT has only newly been introduced, test fees have yet to be confirmed. However you can keep up to date with any new information that is released online at: www.ucatofficial.com/ucat-anz/dates-and-fees/.

Some candidates who might struggle to fund the UCAT fee are eligible to apply for the UCAT ANZ Concessions Scheme. Candidates who hold a valid and current Health Care Card or Pensioner Concession Card (both of which are issued by Centrelink) may apply for the reduced test fee. If eligible to apply, you need to apply with supporting evidence by the deadline of 10th May 2019.

Can I re-sit the UCAT?

You cannot re-sit UCAT in the same application cycle – whatever score you get is with you for the year. That's why it's so important to make sure you're well prepared and ready to perform at your very best on test day.

If I reapply, do I have to resit the UCAT?

If you choose to re-apply the following year, you need to sit UCAT again. You take your new score with you for the new applications cycle. UCAT scores are only valid for one year from the test date.

When do I get my results?

Because the test is computerised, results are generated immediately and you will be given your score on the day of the test. You will be given a printed sheet with your details and your score to take away. Knowing your score is useful as it can help you choose your universities tactically to maximise your chances of success. Note that you don't put your UCAT score anywhere on your UCAS form, nor do you contact any universities to inform them. Universities that request UCAT are sent your scores directly by UCAT, so you don't need to do anything besides apply through UCAS.

Where do I sit the UCAT?

UCAT is a computerised exam and is sat at Pearson VUE test centres. When you book the test, you choose the most convenient test centre to sit it at.

How is the UCAT Scored?

When you finish the test, the computer works out your raw score by adding up your correct responses. There are no mark deductions for incomplete or incorrect answers, so it's a good idea to answer every question even if it's a guess. For the four cognitive sections, this is then scaled onto a scale from 300 – 900. The totals from each of these sections are added together to give your overall score out of 3,600. The new decision making section is now fully introduced into the test, and is scored as normal.

For section 5 (the situational judgement test, SJT) the scoring is slightly different. Here the appropriateness of your responses is used to generate a banding, from band 1 (being the best) to band 4 (being the worst). This is presented separately to the numerical score, such that every candidate's score contains a numerical score out of 3,600 and an SJT banding.

How does my score compare?

2019 will be the first year that the UCAT runs –this means that there is not historical data for the UCAT although we can use the UCKAT scores as a guide as it has been around for much longer. In the UKCAT, the scaling is such that around 600 represents the average score in any section, with the majority of candidates scoring between 500 and 700. Thus, a score higher than 700 is very good and a score less than 500 is very weak.

For reference, in the 2017 entry cycle the UKCAT mean scores at the end of testing were 570, 647, 695, 629 for the first four sections, giving an overall score of 2485 or 622 per section.

How is the UCAT used?

Universities haven't yet declared how they will use the UCAT but it's highly likely that different universities will use your UCAT score in different ways. Firstly, universities that do not explicitly subscribe to UCAT cannot see your UCAT score and are unaware whether or not you sat UCAT. Universities that use UCAT can use it in a variety of ways – some universities use it as a major component of the assessment such as selecting candidates for interview based upon the score. Others use it as a smaller component, for example to settle tie-breaks between similar candidates. Each university publishes guidance on how they use the UCAT, so you should check this out for the universities you are considering.

It's important to know how UCAT is used in order to maximise your chances. If you score highly in UCAT, you might decide to choose universities that select for interview based on a high UCAT score cut-off. That way, you help to stack the odds in your favour – you might, for instance, convert a one in eight chance to a one in three chance. If your score isn't so good, consider choosing universities that don't use UCAT in that way, otherwise you risk falling at the first hurdle and never getting the chance to show them how great you actually are.

By this logic, **it makes sense for all medical applicants to sit UCAT** – if you score well it opens doors, and if you don't you don't even have to apply to UCAT universities. It makes sense not to place all your eggs in one basket. If you were to, for example, apply to only BMAT universities, you risk jeopardising your entire application if you are unlucky on test day.

Can I qualify for extra time?

Yes – some people qualify for extra time in the UCAT, sitting what is known as UCAT SEN. If you usually have extra time in public exams at school, you are likely to be eligible to sit the UCAT SEN. The overall time extension is 30 minutes, bringing the total test time up from 120 to 150 minutes; this is allocated proportionately across the different sections. If you have any medical condition or disability that may affect the test, requiring any special provision, or requiring you to take any medical equipment or medication into the test you should contact customer services to discuss how to best proceed.

General Advice

Practice

Preparing for the UCAT will almost certainly improve your UCAT score. You are unlikely to be familiar with the style of questions in sections 3, 4 and 5 of the UCAT when you first encounter them. With practice, you'll become much quicker at interpreting the data and your speed will increase greatly. Practising questions will put you at ease and make you more comfortable with the exam format, and you will learn and hone techniques to improve your accuracy. This will make you calm and composed on test day, allowing you to perform at your best.

Initially, **work through the questions at your own pace**, and spend time carefully reading the questions and looking at the additional data. The purpose of this is to gain familiarity with the question styles and to start to learn good techniques for solving them. Then closer to test day, make sure you practice the questions under exam conditions and at the correct pace.

Start Early

It is much easier to prepare if you practice little and often. Start your preparation well in advance, ideally by early July but you are advised to start no later than early August. This way, you will have plenty of time to work through practice questions, to build up your speed and to incorporate time-saving techniques into your approach. How to start – well by reading this you're obviously on track!

How to Work

Although this obviously depends on your learning style, it can be helpful to split your preparation into two stages. Early on, it's often best to focus on only one section per day. Firstly read about the section, then maybe follow through a fully worked example, then try some practice questions, stop and mark them and work out anywhere you've gone wrong. By working on only one section per day, you focus your thoughts and allow yourself to get deeper into understanding the question type you're working on. The aim of early preparation is to *learn* about the test and the question styles. Don't worry so much about timing as you do about accuracy and technique. It is a good idea to start on the verbal reasoning and quantitative reasoning as these take the greatest amount of time to improve.

Nearer to test day, you'll need to work on multiple sections per day to help train your thinking to switch quickly from one mode to another. Start to attempt questions with strict timing. The aim now is that you're comfortable in answering the questions, so the next step is to work on exam technique to ensure you know what to expect on the day. Attempt the online UCAT practice questions – although there are not very many of these, they are set out as the computer will be on the day with the official UCAT calculator, so getting familiar with this is important.

Repeat Tough Questions

When checking through answers, pay particular attention to questions you have got wrong. Look closely through the worked answers in this book until you're confident you understand the reasoning- then repeat the question later without help to check you can now do it. If you use other resources where only the answer is given, have another look at the question and consider showing it to a friend or teacher for their opinion.

Statistics show that without consolidating and reviewing your mistakes, you're likely to make the same mistakes again. Don't be a statistic. Look back over your mistakes and address the cause to make sure you don't make similar mistakes when it comes to the test. You should avoid guessing in early practice. Highlight any questions you struggled with so you can go back and improve.

Positive Marking

When it comes to the test, the marking scheme is only positive – you won't lose points for wrong answers. You gain a mark for each correct answer and do not gain one for each wrong or unanswered one. Therefore if you aren't able to answer a question fully, you should guess. Since each question provides you with 3 to 5 possible answers, you have a 33% to 20% chance of guessing correctly – something which is likely to translate to a number of points across the test as a whole.

If you do need to guess, try to make it an educated one. By giving the question a moment's thought or making a basic estimation, you may be able to eliminate a couple of options, greatly increasing your chances of a successful guess. This is discussed more fully in the subsections.

Mock Papers

There are 2 full UCAT papers freely available online at **www.UCAT.ac.uk** and once you've worked your way through the questions in this book, you are highly advised to attempt both of them and check your answers afterwards. There are also a further 2 full mock papers available at **www.uniadmissions.co.uk/UCAT-mock-papers**.

Prioritising Sections

Many students find sections 3 and 4 the easiest to improve on. Initially, section 4 can often be the hardest section, but because you start form a lower point with a bit of familiarity and practice your score can increase greatly. Likewise you can achieve good gains with section 3. Although the subject matter of the questions is not new, with practice you gain familiarity with the style of UCAT questions and with using the calculator. This familiarity can give you a useful speed boost, increasing your score. If you start your preparation late, it would be wise to concentrate most on these sections in order to achieve the best gains.

A word on timing...

"If you had all day to do your UCAT, you would get 100%, 3600 points. But you don't."

Whilst this isn't completely true, it illustrates a very important point. Once you've practiced and know how to answer the questions, the clock is your biggest enemy. This seemingly obvious statement has one very important consequence. **The way to improve your UCAT score is to improve your speed.** There is no magic bullet. But there are a great number of techniques that, with practice, will give you significant time gains, allowing you to answer more questions and score more marks.

Timing is tight throughout the UCAT – mastering timing is the first key to success. Some candidates choose to work as quickly as possible to save up time at the end to check back, but this is generally not the best way to do it. UCAT questions have a lot of information in them – each time you start answering a question it takes time to get familiar with the instructions and information. By splitting the question into two sessions (the first run-through and the return-to-check) you double the amount of time you spend on familiarising yourself with the data, as you have to do it twice instead of only once. This costs valuable time. In addition, candidates who do check back may spend 2–3 minutes doing so and yet not make any actual changes. Whilst this can be reassuring, it is a false reassurance as it has no effect on your actual score. Therefore it is usually best to pace yourself very steadily, aiming to spend the same amount of time on each question and finish the final question in a section just as time runs out. This reduces the time spent on re-familiarising with questions and maximises the time spent on the first attempt, gaining more marks.

There is an option to flag questions for review, making it easier to check back if you have time at the end of the section. There is absolutely no disadvantage to using this. If you've guessed a question then it makes sense to mark it, so you know where to best spend your spare time if you do finish the section early. Always select an answer first time round (even if it's a guess), as there is no negative marking – you may not have time to turn back later on.

It is essential that you don't get stuck with the hardest questions – no doubt there will be some. In the time spent answering only one of these you may miss out on answering three easier questions. If a question is taking too long, choose a sensible answer and move on. Never see this as giving up or in any way failing, rather it is the smart way to approach a test with a tight time limit. With practice and discipline, you can get very good at this and learn to maximise your efficiency. It is not about being a hero and aiming for full marks – this is essentially impossible and in any case completely unnecessary. It is about maximising your efficiency and gaining the maximum possible number of marks within the time you have.

Verbal Reasoning

The Basics

Section 1 of the UCAT is the verbal reasoning subtest. It tests your ability to quickly read a passage, find information that is relevant and then analyse statements related to the passage. There are 44 questions to answer and in 21 minutes, so you have just under 30 seconds per question. As with all UCAT sections, you have one minute to read the instructions. The idea is that this tests both your language ability and your ability to make decisions, traits which are important in a good doctor.

You are presented with a passage, upon which you answer questions. Typically, there are 11 separate passages, each with 4 questions about it. There are two styles of question in section 1, and each requires a slightly different approach. All questions start with a statement relating to something in the passage.

In the first type of question, you are asked if the statement is true or false based on the passage. There is also the option to answer "cannot tell". Choose "true" if the statement either matches the passage or can be directly inferred from it. Choose "false" if the statement either contradicts the passage or exaggerates a claim the passage makes to an extent that it becomes untrue.

Choosing the "cannot tell" option can be harder. Remember that you are answering based *ONLY* on the passage and not on any of your own knowledge – so you choose the "cannot tell" option if there is not enough information to make up your mind one way or the other. Try to choose this option actively. "Cannot tell" isn't something to conclude too quickly, it can often be the hardest answer to select. Choose it when you're actively looking for a certain piece of information to help you answer a question, and you cannot find it.

In the other type of question, you are given a stem and have to select the most appropriate response based on the question. There is only one right answer – if more than one answer seems appropriate, the task is to choose the *best* response. Remember that there is no negative marking in the UCAT. There will be questions where you aren't certain. If that is the case, then choose an option that seems sensible to you and move on. A clear thought process is key to doing well in section 1 – you will have the opportunity to build that up through the worked examples and practice questions until you're answering like a pro!

This is the first section of the UCAT, so you're bound to have some nerves. Ensure that you have been to the toilet because once the exam starts you can't pause and go. Take a few deep breaths and calm yourself down. Try to shut out distractions and get yourself into your exam mindset. If you're well prepared, you can remind yourself of that to help keep calm. See it as a job to do and look at the test as an opportunity. If you perform well it will boost your chances of getting into good medical schools. If the worst happens, there are plenty of good medical schools that do not use UCAT, so all is not lost.

How to Approach This Section

Time pressure is a recurring theme throughout the UCAT, but it is especially important in Section 1, where you have only 30 seconds per question and a lot of information to take in.

You should look carefully to see what the question is asking. Often it's best to read the question before reading the passage. Then when reading the passage you're likely to find the information you need much more quickly. Sometimes the question will simply need you to find a phrase in the text. In other instances, your critical thinking skills will be needed and you'll have to carefully analyse the information presented to you.

Extreme Words

Words like "extremely", "always" and "never" can give you useful clues for your answer. Statements which make particularly bold claims are less likely to be true, but remember you need a direct contradiction to be able to conclude that they are false. To answer an "always" question, you're looking for a definition. Always be a bit suspicious of "never" – make sure you're certain before saying true, as most things are possible.

Prioritise

With UCAT, you can leave and come back to any question. **By flagging for review**, you make this easier. Since time is tight, you don't want to waste time on long passages when you could be scoring easier marks. Score the easy marks first, then come back to the harder ones if time allows. If time runs too short, at least take enough time to guess the answers as there's a good chance you could pick up some marks anyway.

Be a Lawyer

Put on your most critical and analytical hat for section A! Carefully analyse the statements like you're in a court room. Then look for the evidence! **Examine the passage closely, looking for evidence** that either supports or contradicts the statement. Remember **you're making decisions based on ONLY the passage**, not using any prior knowledge. Does the passage agree or disagree? If there isn't enough evidence to decide, don't be afraid to say "cannot tell".

Read the Question First

Follow our top tip and read the question before the passage. There is simply not enough time to read all the passages thoroughly and still have time to complete everything in 22 minutes. By reading the statement or question first, you can understand what it is that is required of you and can then pick out the appropriate area in the passage. Do not fall into the trap of trying to read all of the passage, you will not score highly enough if you do this.

When skim reading through the passage, it is inevitable that you will lose accuracy. However you can reduce this effect by doing plenty of practice so your ability to glean what you need improves. A good tip is to practice reading short sections of complicated texts, such as quality newspapers or novels, at high pace.

Find the Keywords

The keyword is the most important word to help you relate the question to the passage; sometimes there might be two keywords in a question. When you read the passage, focus in on the keywords straight away. This gives you something to look for in the passage to identify the right place to work from. It is usually easy to find the keyword/s, and you'll become even better with practice. When you find it, go back a line and read from the line before through the keyword to the end of the line after. Usually, this contains enough relevant information to give you the answer.

If this is not successful, you need to consider your next steps. Time is very tight in the UCAT and especially so in section 1. There are other passages that need your attention, and there may be much easier marks waiting for you. If reading around the keyword has not given you the right answer it may well be time to move on. It might be that there is a more subtle reference somewhere else, that you need to read the whole passage to reach the answer or indeed that the answer cannot be deduced from the passage. Either way, if it's difficult to find your time could be better spent gaining marks elsewhere. Make a sensible guess and move on.

Use only the Passage

Your answer ***must*** only be based on the information available in the passage. Do not try and guess the answer based on your general knowledge as this can be a trap. For example, if the question asks who the first person was to walk on the moon, then states "the three crew members of the first lunar mission were Edwin Aldrin, Neil Armstrong and Michael Collins". The correct answer is "cannot tell" – even though you know it was Neil Armstrong and see his name, the passage itself does not tell you who left the landing craft first. Likewise if there is a quotation or an extract from a book which is factually inaccurate, you should answer based on the information available to you rather than what you know to be true.

If you have not been able to select the correct answer, eliminate as many of the statements as possible and guess – you have a 25 – 33% chance of guessing correctly in this section even without eliminating any answers, and if you've read around some keywords in the text you may well have at least some idea as to what the answer is. These odds can add a few easy marks onto your score.

Flagging for Review

There is an additional option to flag a question for review. All it does is mark the question in an easy way for it to be revisited if you have time later in the section. Once the section is complete, you cannot return to any questions, flagged or unflagged. But be warned coming back to questions can be inefficient – you have to read the instructions and data each time you work on the question, so by coming back again you double the amount of time spent on doing this, leaving less time for actually answering questions. We feel the best strategy is to work steadily through the questions at a consistent and even pace.

That said, flagging for review has one great utility in Section 1. If you come across a long or technical passage, you may want to flag for review immediately and skip on to the next passage. By coming back to the passage at the end, you allow yourself the remaining time on the hardest question. This has an advantage in each of two scenarios. If you're really tight for time, at least you maximised the time you did have answering the easier questions, thereby maximising your marks. If it turns out you have extra time to spare, you can spend it on the hardest question, allowing you a better chance to get marks you otherwise would have struggled to obtain.

Remember to find the right balance: if you flag too many questions you will be overloaded and won't have time to focus on them all; if you flag too few, you risk under-utilising this valuable resource. You should flag only a few questions per section to allow you to properly focus on them if you have spare time.

Verbal Reasoning Questions

For questions 1 – 106 decide if each of the statements is true, false or can't tell:

SET 1

The Kyoto Protocol is an international agreement written by the United Nations in order to reduce the effects of climate change. This agreement sets targets for countries in order for them to reduce their greenhouse gas emissions. These gases are believed to be responsible for causing global warming as a result of recent industrialisation.

The Protocol was written in 1997 and each country that signed the protocol agreed to reduce their emissions to their own specific target. This agreement could only become legally binding when two conditions had been fulfilled: When 55 countries agreed to be legally bound by the agreement and when 55% of emissions from industrialised countries had been accounted for.

The first condition was met in 2002 however countries such as Australia and the United States refused to be bound by the agreement so the minimum of 55% of emissions from industrialised countries was not met. It was only after Russia joined in 2004 that allowed the protocol to come into force in 2005.
Some climate scientists have argued that the target combined reduction of 5.2% emissions from industrialised nations would not be enough to avoid the worst consequences of global warming. In order to have a significant impact, we would need to aim at reducing emissions by 60% and to get larger countries such as the US to support the agreement.

1. The Kyoto Protocol is legally binding in all industrialised countries.
2. The greenhouse gas emissions from Australia and the United States represent 45% of emissions from industrialised countries.
3. Each country chose the amount by which they would reduce their own emissions.
4. The global emission of greenhouse gases has reduced since 2005.
5. The harmful effects of climate change would be avoided if all countries reduced their emissions by 60%.

SET 2

The space race was a competition between the Soviet Union and the United States to show off their technological superiority and economic power. It took place during the Cold War when there was a tense relationship between these nations. As the technology used in space exploration could also have military applications, both nations had many scientists and technicians involved.

In 1957, the USSR launched the first artificial satellite into the Earth's orbit, named Sputnik. The launch of this satellite was one of the first steps towards space exploration. The Americans were worried that the Soviets could use similar technology to launch nuclear warheads. This prompted urgency within the Americans, leading President Eisenhower to found NASA, and so began the space race.

The Soviets took another step forward in April 1961 when they sent the first person into space, a cosmonaut named Yuri Gagarin. This prompted President John F. Kennedy to make the unexpected claim that the US would beat the Soviets to land a man on the moon and that they would do so before the end of the decade. This led to the foundation of Project Apollo, a programme designed to do this.

In 1969, Neil Armstrong and Buzz Aldrin set off for the moon on the Apollo 11 space mission and became the first astronauts to walk on the moon. Neil Armstrong famously said "one small step for man, one giant leap for mankind." This lunar landing led the US to win the space race that started with Sputnik's launch in 1957.

6. The Soviet Union were mainly concerned with launching satellites into space for a military advantage over the United States.
7. Project Apollo was founded in order for the United States to defeat the Soviet Union in the Cold War.
8. Yuri Gagarin did not become the first man on the moon because the Soviet technology could not handle the conditions on the moon.
9. The United States began their attempts at space exploration when the Soviets launched Sputnik.
10. The United States were losing the space race when John F. Kennedy said they would land a man on the moon.

SET 3

A marathon is a long distance running event that is 26.2 miles long. This race was named after the famous Battle of Marathon. The first Persian invasion of Greece took place in 490 BC. The Greek soldiers did not expect to defeat the Persian army, which had greater numbers and superior cavalry. The Greek commander utilised a tactical flank to defeat the Persians forcing them to retreat back to Asia. According to legend, the fastest Greek runner, Pheidippides, was ordered to run from Marathon to Athens to announce the Greek victory over the Persians, but then collapsed and died of exhaustion. This legendary 25 mile journey from Marathon to Athens is the basis for modern marathons.

The initial organisers of the Olympic Games in 1896 wanted an event that would celebrate the glory of Ancient Greece. They therefore chose to use the same course that Pheidippides ran. In subsequent Olympic Games, the exact length of the route depended on the location but was roughly similar to the 25 mile distance. The current standardised distance of 26.2 miles has been chosen by the IAAF and used since 1921, and has been taken from the distance used at the 1908 Olympics in London. Nowadays, more than 500 marathons are organised each year.

11. Pheidippides was chosen as he was the only Greek runner determined enough to make the journey to Athens
12. Marathon distances have been standardised since the 1908 Olympics
13. The Persian commander believed he would defeat the Greeks in the Battle of Marathon.
14. The original route from Marathon to Athens is used for IAAF marathons today.
15. The Persian soldiers were trained better than the Greek soldiers.

SET 4

Many species of bird migrate northwards in the spring to take advantage of the abundance of nesting locations and insects to eat. As the availability of food resources decreases during the winter to the point where the birds cannot survive, the birds migrate south again. Some species are capable of flying all the way around the earth.
The act of migration itself can be risky for birds due to the amount of energy required to sustain flight over these long distances. Many juvenile birds can die from exhaustion during their first migration. Due to this inherent risk of migration, many species of birds have acquired different adaptations to increase the efficiency of flight. Flying with other birds in certain formations can allow their flight patterns to be more energy efficient.

The Northern bald ibis migrates from Austria to Italy. The behaviour of these birds is such that they migrate together within a flock and each individual bird continuously changes its position within the flock. Each individual bird benefits by spending some time flying in the updraft produced by the leading birds and a proportional amount of time leading the formation. Although it would theoretically be possible for an individual bird to take advantage of this energy-efficient flight without leading the formation itself, no Northern bald ibis has been shown to do this.

16. As migration is risky and dangerous, it would be better for birds not to migrate.
17. All migrating birds do so in flocks to increase their efficiency
18. All the birds within a flock of Northern bald ibis benefit from flocking behaviour
19. A bird within a Northern bald ibis flock that does not lead will be forbidden from flying with the rest of the flock
20. The migration timing depends on different seasons

SET 5

The dramatic decline of the bee population in the UK has been attributed to a number of causes such as the loss of wild flowers in the countryside. Bees require these wildflowers for food and it has been estimated that 97% of the flower-rich grassland has been lost since the 1930s. Other causes include climate change and pesticides that are toxic to bees. This is particularly problematic in the UK, which has had a 50% reduction in the honey bee population between 1985 and 2005 whilst the rest of Europe has only averaged a 20% reduction during the same time period.

This loss of flowers from the British countryside has been caused by agricultural pressures. In order to increase food production, traditional farming methods have been abandoned in favour of techniques that increase productivity. These techniques, however, involve the reduction of wild flowers.

Bumblebees are required to pollinate wildflowers and commercial crops. A reduction of wildflower pollination will result in their decline, which will ultimately affect other wildlife as they can be involved in a complex food chain. The commercial crops will need to be pollinated artificially using expensive methods that will ultimately drive up the price of fruits and vegetables. The global economic value of pollination from bees has been estimated at €265 billion annually.

21. The bee population in the UK has decreased by 97% since the 1930s.
22. The UK is the country with the largest decline in bee population
23. Reverting back to traditional farming methods will decrease the overall production of food
24. Artificial pollination will be capable of replacing bees if it becomes cheap enough
25. Increasing pesticide-free fruit and vegetable growth will slow the decline in bee population

SET 6

Driving in snowy and icy conditions can be dangerous as it increases stopping distances. The stopping distance represents how far a car will travel before slowing down to a halt. It is made up of the thinking distance, which is how long it takes for a driver to react, and the braking distance, which represents the time taken for the brakes to fully stop the car.

It is advised to fit winter tyres during the winter season as these have much better grip on snow and ice. These tyres are made out of a softer material than regular tyres, allowing them to have more traction at colder temperatures. This ultimately reduces the braking distance.

As the brakes are not very effective at stopping a vehicle on icy roads, it is recommended to steer out of trouble if possible rather than applying the brakes. It is therefore important to be travelling at slower speeds to avoid the need to suddenly brake.

If the car is stuck and cannot move, the driver can stay warm by running the engine to generate heat. However, if the exhaust pipe becomes blocked by snow and the fumes cannot escape then the engine must be turned off. This is because the engine produces carbon monoxide, which is extremely toxic and odourless.

26. Driving whilst tired increases the braking distance.
27. Regular tyres are more dangerous than winter tyres in cold conditions as they are harder
28. It is always safe to run the engine for heat in cold conditions
29. It is dangerous to use winter tyres in hot summer conditions.
30. To avoid a collision on icy surfaces, it is important to gently apply the brakes.

SET 7

The Socratic method is a form of philosophical questioning named after the Greek philosopher Socrates. It takes place as a dialogue between Socrates and another individual and attempts to investigate difficult concepts such as justice and ethics. In this dialogue, Socrates' partner puts forward an opinion or a thesis. Socrates then proposes extra premises that will attempt to disprove the original thesis. If there is an opposition, this shows that the original thesis is false and that the opposite is true.

In this dialogue, Socrates often showed other philosophers and thinkers how their reasoning was wrong. Some respected him for doing so as he was aware of the fact that his knowledge was limited and that he was merely questioning everything critically. However, many people were angered by him asking questions without providing any answers to these difficult questions himself. This led to him making a number of enemies in Greece.

In 399 BC, Socrates was accused of heresy and corruption of the youth by three of his enemies. He was then trialled and found guilty by the jury and so sentenced to death by drinking the poison hemlock. One of his friends, Crito, bribed the guards to allow Socrates to escape; however he chose not to flee away. Many have referred to him as a martyr as he chose to die standing for knowledge and wisdom.

31. Socrates was the first person to use this method of questioning.
32. The Socratic method questions the wisdom of the person forming the opinions.
33. As described in the passage, the Socratic method involved corrupting the youth and heresy.
34. Socrates chose not to escape from prison because he was afraid his enemies would find him again.
35. Socrates was able to define concepts such as justice and ethics himself.

SET 8

The Anglo-Saxons were the group of people who lived in England between the 5th Century and the Norman conquest in 1066 AD. When the Germanic tribes of the Saxons, Angles and Jutes came to Britain in 449 AD, they pushed the Celtic Britons who were there before them up into Wales. The combination of the Germanic dialects of these different tribes became Anglo-Saxon or Old English.

Old English is very different from Modern English and uses more Germanic words and its grammar is closer to Old German. If English speakers were to read a passage of Old English, they would struggle to understand any more than a few words. It is thought that this Old English is most similar to the Dutch dialect spoken in Friesland, a province in the north of the Netherlands. One of the famous literary works written in Old English was the poem Beowulf. It is not known who wrote this poem and only one original manuscript of the poem still exists today. The story involves the hero Beowulf who fights and kills the giant Grendel. All the people celebrate the death of Grendel however Grendel's mother comes to the town and attempts to kill as many people for revenge. Beowulf then fights Grendel's mother and kills her as well.

36. The Jute tribe did not contribute to the Anglo-Saxon language.
37. German speakers would be able to read Beowulf in its original language.
38. Beowulf was the strongest warrior at that time.
39. A dialect of Old English is currently spoken in the Netherlands.
40. The Celts lived in England in 449 AD

SET 9

A constellation is a group of stars that are often visible forming a pattern in the sky. The constellation's visibility depends on a number of factors. The biggest factor is your position on the Earth, for example the constellation Cassiopeia is only visible in the northern hemisphere. As the Earth orbits the Sun, another significant factor affecting constellation visibility is the season on Earth.

As the Earth rotates on its own axis, certain stars and constellations can appear to rise and fall in the night sky. Constellations that do not move in this manner are called circumpolar. This factor can allow people to navigate on the Earth using the positioning of the stars. This is especially useful during marine navigation as there are no visible landmarks. The most commonly used star for navigation is the North Star Polaris, as its position is constant within the night sky.

There are 12 constellations that take the form of animals or humans known as the zodiac signs. This is the basis for the origin of star signs in astrology, which suggests that human behaviour is influenced by the celestial phenomena. The star sign of a person represents the position of the sun at the moment of their birth. The zodiac sign which shares the same position as the sun in the sky becomes their star sign.

41. Certain stars are not visible from the southern hemisphere
42. The constellation Cassiopeia is circumpolar
43. Star signs are chosen by the constellations visible at birth
44. Polaris is used for navigation as it is the brightest star in the sky
45. Different constellations are visible from London and Sydney.

SET 10

Maple syrup is a sweet syrup made from maple trees. The sap from the trees is harvested during March. It is then boiled to evaporate water, making it denser and sweeter. It takes roughly 40 litres of maple sap to produce 1 litre of maple syrup. This current process is very similar to that used by the Native Americans except it uses more advanced equipment.

According to American Indian legend, the maple trees originally made life free from hardship. They produced a thick syrup all year round which the people would drink. A mythological creature named Glooskap saw that the people of a village were strangely silent. The men were not getting ready to hunt and the women were not minding the fires. He found the villagers sitting near the maple trees letting its syrup drip into their mouth.

Glooskap was angered by their laziness and used his powers to fill the trees with water so that they would only produce a dilute, watery sap. This meant that the people had to boil the sap to produce the sweet syrup. Although it wasn't very difficult to do this, it meant that they had to look after their fires and gather firewood. Furthermore, it meant that the trees were not able to produce enough sap to sustain the people all year so they would be forced to hunt and forage during the spring and summer.

46. Sweet syrup can be made from the sap from other trees.
47. Glooskap was angered because there was no syrup left for him to drink.
48. The technique for making maple syrup is similar to that used in the time of the American Indian legends.
49. Sap is only harvested from maple trees for one month a year.
50. Hunting animals was more difficult than drinking maple syrup.

SET 11

Stockholm syndrome is an interesting phenomenon that sometimes happens to people who have been kidnapped or held hostage. They may feel some loyalty or attraction towards the person that has kidnapped them.

This phenomenon was named after a bank robbery in Stockholm, Sweden in 1973. Four bank workers were kept hostage by two criminals who wanted to rob the bank. After being held against their will for six days, they showed that they had formed a positive relationship with their captors. The hostages were seen to be hugging and kissing the men who had kidnapped them.

It can be hard to explain why this might be the case as it involves the captor putting the hostage in a terrifying situation. In the mind of the hostage it is this person who can ultimately decide if the hostage is going to die. As a result of this fear of death, any small act of kindness prompts them to be thankful for the gift of life. This can ultimately lead to them developing Stockholm syndrome.

It is important to understand the interaction between victims and captors in cases of Stockholm syndrome as this knowledge can improve the chances of hostage survival. As such, the FBI is willing to devote resources in order to improve crisis negotiation.

51. People who get kidnapped will eventually develop positive emotions towards their kidnapper.
52. The bank workers hugged and kissed their kidnappers because the criminals forced them to.
53. Stockholm syndrome is useful to understand for crisis negotiation.
54. According to the passage, it is the victims that fear for their life that tend to develop Stockholm Syndrome.
55. The bank robbery in 1973 was the first recorded instance of a positive relationship developing between captors and hostages.

SET 12

Clownfish are a type of fish that live in salt water. They are orange fish that have white stripes. They are capable of growing up to 10-18 cm. They have also been called anemone fish as they have a symbiotic relationship with certain sea anemones.

The tentacles of sea anemone are capable of stinging fish that come near them, which the anemone then eat. The clownfish have a special mucous covering that protects them from this sting. As a result of this, clownfish that live inside sea anemone are safe from other predators but do not get stung themselves. The sea anemone benefit from the clownfish as the clownfish eat the algae that grows on the anemone. The bright colour of the clownfish lures in small fish to the anemone which ultimately get stung. They also receive better water circulation from the action of the clownfish fins.

Many people like keeping clownfish in aquariums because of their bright orange colour and how easy they are to look after. This can be dangerous as the clownfish lifespan is greatly increased by living within an anemone. Even if an anemone is added to the aquarium, only certain species of clownfish are capable of living within certain species of anemone.

56. A clownfish that loses its mucous layer can live inside sea anemone.
57. Clownfish help sea anemone to eat fish.
58. Clownfish will die if they do not have an anemone to live in.
59. Clownfish have a mutually beneficial relationship with all anemone.
60. Anemone protect clownfish from predators.

SET 13

The guillotine was a machine used to kill people by chopping off their head. It consists of a heavy blade attached to a frame. When the blade was released, it would fall down under its own weight and chop off the victim's head, killing them instantly. It was commonly used in France during the French Revolution as it was the only legal method of execution in order to enact the death penalty.

The guillotine was named after a French doctor called Joseph Guillotin. He decided that a more humane way of executing someone was needed as he realised he was unable to get rid of the death penalty. He decided that using an automatic mechanical device for decapitation would be more humane than by a person with an axe. The first guillotine built was then tested on animals to see if the axe would have enough force to decapitate its victim.

Before the guillotine was used in execution, the criminal would be hanged. This was seen to be less humane as the victim was supposed to die from the impact of the rope snapping their necks, however this did not happen all the time. The victim could be in agony for up to forty minutes before eventually dying from asphyxiation.

61. Joseph Guillotin agreed with the death penalty.
62. According to the passage, the guillotine was used for execution before the French Revolution.
63. Hanging usually causes death by asphyxiation.
64. The guillotine was seen as being more humane as it was automatic with the blade falling through its own weight.
65. During the French Revolution, hanging was the common form of execution.

SET 14

"The Gherkin" is a building in the City of London named after and famous for its distinctive shape. Its modern architecture was designed by Norman Foster and was built between 2001 and 2003. Norman Foster is famous for utilising the laws of physics in designing many of his buildings. The walls of the Gherkin would allow air to enter the building for passive cooling. As this air warms up, it rises and is then let out of the building.

The site where the Gherkin is built used to belong to the Baltic Exchange, the headquarters of the global marketplace for ship sales. In 1992, the site was damaged by bombs placed by the Provisional IRA. As there were many historic buildings in the area and only a few were damaged, the City of London governing body was insistent that any redevelopment must restore the old historic look. They later discovered that the amount of damage caused was too severe and so removed this restriction.

The building was sold in 2007 for a sum of £630 million, making it the most expensive office building in the UK. The building was then put up for sale in 2014, initially at a lower price as its owners could not afford to pay loan repayments due to high interest rates and the devaluing of the British pound. It was bought by a Brazilian billionaire for £700 million.

66. According to the passage, The Gherkin is famous because of its passive cooling system.
67. The Baltic Exchange was built with a modern architectural design.
68. The Gherkin was sold in 2014 at a loss.
69. The Provisional IRA intended to destroy the Baltic Exchange.
70. Norman Foster has designed many buildings that incorporated physics in their design.

SET 15

The living wage represents the minimum hourly rate for employment which allows an individual to cover their basic costs of living. This wage is set at £9.15 per hour in London and £7.85 per hour in the rest of the UK. This difference in living wage between London and the rest of the UK is explained by the significant costs associated with living in London.

The minimum wage is currently £6.50 for employees aged over 21 and £5.13 for employees aged between 18 and 20. This is lower than the living wage values quoted above and represents the legal minimum wage. It would be illegal for an employer to pay less than these values. Although many employers have agreed to pay a living wage, they are not legally obliged to do so.

The introduction of the living wage in companies has been argued to be beneficial for these companies. Many employers found that employees who were paid the living wage were able to work harder with better quality. It has also improved the quality of life for the families of employees as it has allowed those who are parents to spend more time with their children. However, some employers have argued that the introduction of the living wage would force them to fire some workers, forcing others to work harder.

71. The living cost across UK cities is approximately equal.
72. Companies introduce the living wage to avoid the legal complications of underpaying their employees.
73. A 24 year old working at minimum wage would be able to live comfortably in Manchester
74. Introducing a living wage would be beneficial for all employees.
75. Paying someone a living wage will only benefit that individual

SET 16

The ecological footprint is a simple way to look at how sustainable people are being. It is based on the idea that all the resources taken from the Earth are finite. It is defined by how much land and water would be required to produce the resources that the population consumes within a year. It has been calculated that there are currently 11.2 billion bio-productive hectares available on the Earth.

A study in 2004 has suggested that our ecological footprint is 13.5 billion hectares, meaning that we are using the Earth's resources 20% faster than they are being renewed. This will ultimately result in the loss of all the Earth's resources.

Individual countries can look at their own ecological footprint and compare it to the size of their bio-productive capacity. Some countries are in an ecological deficit - they require more land than their bio-productive capacity to sustain them. Other countries have an ecological reserve, meaning that their bio-productive capacity is greater than their footprint.

It can be difficult for individual countries to reduce their ecological footprint. This can either be performed by reducing that countries reliance on unsustainable resources or by increasing the amount of bio-productive land available. It is important, however, that a global effort is made to increase our sustainability.

76. The ecological footprint of a country directly depends on its population.
77. The combined area of the Earth's land and water mass is 11.2 billion hectares
78. The ecological footprint can be reduced by using sustainable resources.
79. Only the countries with an ecological deficit are able to tackle the global problem of sustainability.
80. The bio-productive capacity of the Earth is fixed.

SET 17

English punk rock band The Sex Pistols formed in 1975, and sparked off the British punk movement, leading to the subsequent creation of multiple punk and alternative rock acts. They produced only one album - 'Never Mind the Bollocks, Here's the Sex Pistols' – in their brief existence. However, despite these, some state The Sex Pistols are one of the most important bands in the history of popular music.

Originally, the band was made up of Johnny Rotten (the singer), Paul Cook (the drummer) and Glen Matlock (the bassist), however the latter was subsequently replaced by Sid Vicious. The band was involved in numerous controversies, due to their lyrics, performances and public appearances. One may argue the band was asking for trouble when they created songs attacking the music industry (such 'EMI') and commenting on controversial topics like consumerism, the Berlin wall, the Holocaust and abortion ('Bodies'). The band did not take kindly to local figureheads, as demonstrated with the release of 'God Save the Queen' in 1977, which was an attack on both conforming to societal norms and also blindly accepting the royalty as an authority.

81. It is believed by some that pop music's most influential act is The Sex Pistols.
82. The Sex Pistols kick-started the punk movement.
83. The Sex Pistols' lyrics denounced abortion.
84. The Sex Pistols controversially equated the music industry with the Holocaust.
85. The Sex Pistols' songs showed they were staunch royalists.
86. The Sex Pistols had two bassists.

SET 18

Cancer is a disease of the tissues of the body which occurs when cells begin to grow and replicate rapidly. These cells are capable of becoming masses called tumours which can obstruct the parts of the body in which they are found. Some of these tumours are also able to spread to other parts of the body in a process known as metastasis.

The incidence of cancer has significantly increased recently in the Western developed world. The most common form of cancer in the UK is breast cancer, even though it very rarely affects men. Most cancers seem to have no obvious cause whilst a few are known to have a specific cause. Mesothelioma, for example, is a type of lung cancer that is caused by exposure to asbestos. People who have worked with asbestos without adequate protection in the past are eligible for compensation from the government.

Before the 19th century, the only way to treat a cancer was to physically remove the tumour from the body. This usually involved amputation or removing a lot of tissue. It was only in the 19th century when improvements in surgical hygiene enhanced the success rates of tumour removal. At this time, Marie and Pierre Curie discovered the first non-surgical treatment, which involved irradiating the tumour.

87. Everyone exposed to asbestos will eventually suffer from mesothelioma.
88. Breast cancer is the most common type of cancer in British women.
89. The surgical success rate for tumour removal in the 19th century was improved by irradiating the tumour.
90. Irradiation is more effective than surgery in removing tumours.
91. Only cells that are capable of spreading cause tumours.

SET 19

The indigenous Australians are the native people of Australia, also known as the Aborigines. It is believed that they arrived in Australia 50,000 years ago from South-east Asia. They lived a traditional life, which involved living in wooded areas and hunting animals with spears and boomerangs. This lifestyle would not harm the environment of Australia as they believe that the land, with all of its animals and plants, is sacred.

When the British people came to Australia in 1788, there were not many people living in Australia. According to British law, any land could be claimed for the monarchy if they believed that nobody owned it and so they claimed all of the land. It was later agreed by the Australian government in 1976 that the aboriginal people would have the rights to the land where they were originally located if they could prove that they have been living there.

Nowadays, many of the 517,000 aboriginal people in Australia have chosen to integrate with the modern ways of life. They live in cities and towns and some of them have acquired professional jobs. Others have decided to maintain their traditional aboriginal way of living. Few have been unfortunate in that they haven't been educated enough to benefit from Australian society but have also lost their traditional aboriginal ways.

92. The British people claimed the Australian land because the Aborigines only lived in the wooded areas.
93. There are 517,000 Aborigines currently living in the cities and towns of Australia.
94. The aboriginal people were able to reclaim all their land in 1976.
95. Most Aborigines have received enough education to integrate with Australian culture.
96. The Aborigine lifestyle is similar to that of the south-east Asians from 50,000 years ago.

SET 20

Chilli peppers are a type of fruit grown all over the world. Most of these peppers are spicy and used in cooking. These peppers are believed to initially originate from Bolivia. As they spread throughout Europe, it was found that their spiciness had a similar taste to black peppercorns, which were incredibly valuable in the 15th century. As such, many people began to grow chilli peppers, which spread rapidly to India and China.

These chilli peppers began to be incorporated into the cooking of different cultures, being used more commonly in hotter countries. There are a number of reasons suggested for why these countries would prefer spicy food. One suggestion is that spicy food would help people to sweat in hot conditions, allowing them to cool down. This however, is unlikely to explain the prevalence of chilli peppers as it is possible to sweat without eating them. Adding spice to food was also found to be a convenient method of preserving food as it discouraged the growth of bacteria.

The peppers are spicy because they produce the chemical capsaicin. This chemical binds to receptors in the mouth and throat and cause the sensation of heat. This receptor is also capable of responding to heat directly. This is an example of labelled line coding which suggests that the perception of a stimulus is determined by which receptor it activates, not the nature of the stimulus itself.

97. Chilli peppers became more valuable in the 15th century.
98. Eating chilli peppers in hot conditions causes sweating.
99. All chilli peppers are spicy.
100. An individual lacking the capsaicin receptor would be able to eat the spiciest chillies without any pain.
101. Different methods of activating the capsaicin receptor (TRPV1) cause different sensations.

SET 21

The social determinants of health are factors in which people are born, grow, live, work and age. These factors depend on the social distribution of resources and can affect the life expectancy and quality of life that people have. These factors refer to the social context that people live in and include characteristics such as level of education, culture, stress and socioeconomic conditions as well as many others. It can be difficult to see how some of these factors may affect somebody's health but it is likely to involve a combination of multiple factors.

A number of mechanisms acting together have been described to explain why someone with a poor diet would have a lower life expectancy. One such mechanism is as follows: This individual would be more likely to be malnourished which would weaken their immune system. This would ultimately increase their likelihood of suffering from infections. Recurrent infections would place strain on the body, which could eventually result in organ failure. On average, the life expectancy in the most deprived areas can be up to 10 years lower than in the least deprived areas.

Many of these health inequalities are avoidable. Understanding how these social determinants affect the health of a population will allow us to improve its care. Knowledge of how social policies impact health can better allow us to monitor changes in health care, and is allowing us to reduce the gaps between those with a more disadvantaged social background from those with a privileged background.

102. Dropping out of school can have an effect on an individual's health.
103. The effects of the social determinants of health are principally measured by life expectancy.
104. The health impact of poor diet can be avoided completely by using multivitamins that supplement the immune system.
105. Nothing can be done to improve the health care of the poor in comparison to the rich.
106. Alan lives in a less deprived area than Henry so Alan will live longer than Henry.

SET 22

J.S. Mill describes his ethical theory and the reception of this in his book, 'Utilitarianism', and states:

'The creed which accepts as the foundation of morals, Utility, or the Greatest Happiness Principle, holds that actions are right in proportion as they tend to promote happiness, wrong as they tend to produce the reverse of happiness. By happiness is intended pleasure, and the absence of pain; by unhappiness, pain, and the privation of pleasure. To give a clear view of the moral standard set up by the theory, much more requires to be said; in particular, what things it includes in the ideas of pain and pleasure; and to what extent this is left an open question. But these supplementary explanations do not affect the theory of life on which this theory of morality is grounded—namely, that pleasure, and freedom from pain, are the only things desirable as ends; and that all desirable things are desirable either for the pleasure inherent in themselves, or as means to the promotion of pleasure and the prevention of pain.

Now, such a theory of life provokes in many minds, and among them in some of the most estimable in feeling and purpose, dislike. To suppose that life has (as they express it) no higher end than pleasure—no better and nobler object of desire and pursuit—they designate as utterly mean and grovelling; as a doctrine worthy only of swine, to whom the followers of Epicurus were, at a very early period, contemptuously likened; and modern holders of the doctrine are occasionally made the subject of equally polite comparisons by its German, French, and English assailants.

When thus attacked, the Epicureans have always answered, that it is not they, but their accusers, who represent human nature in a degrading light; since the accusation supposes human beings to be capable of no pleasures except those of which swine are capable.'

107. How do the Epicureans answer their critics?
A. By claiming the critics are miserable, in their refusal to embrace pleasure.
B. That the critics do not understand the multiplicity of things contained in the word 'pleasure'.
C. By calling their critics degraded.
D. By suggesting their critics are more susceptible to animalistic pleasures than they.

108. Which of the following actions are NOT in keeping with the theory of utility?
A. Providing a crash mat for a gymnast, to prevent him or her hurting him or herself.
B. Getting a crash mat for yourself, to prevent hurting yourself when performing gymnastics.
C. Not eating a chocolate bar because social pressures deem it wrong.
D. Eating a chocolate bar because it is delicious.

109. Which of the following does the passage suggest about critics of utilitarianism?
A. They are Christians.
B. They are European.
C. They are unintelligent.
D. They are reactionary.

110. Utilitarianism is only concerned with ends.
A. True
B. False
C. Can't tell

111. The above passage defines:

A. What is included by the term pleasure
B. What is included by the term pain
C. What is meant by Epicureanism
D. What is meant by utility

SET 23

Geology deals with the rocks of the earth's crust. It learns from their composition and structure how the rocks were made and how they have been modified. It ascertains how they have been brought to their present places and wrought to their various topographic forms, such as hills and valleys, plains and mountains. It studies the vestiges, which the rocks preserve, of ancient organisms that once inhabited our planet. Geology is the history of the earth and its inhabitants, as read in the rocks of the earth's crust.

To obtain a general idea of the nature and method of our science before beginning its study in detail, we may visit some valley, on whose sides are rocky ledges. Here the rocks lie in horizontal layers. Although only their edges are exposed, we may infer that these layers run into the upland on either side and underlie the entire district; they are part of the foundation of solid rock found beneath the loose materials of the surface everywhere.

Take the sandstones ledge of a valley. Looking closely at the rock we see that it is composed of myriads of grains of sand cemented together. These grains have been worn and rounded. They are sorted also, those of each layer being about of a size. By some means they have been brought hither from some more ancient source. Surely these grains have had a history before they here found a resting place—a history which we are to learn to read.
The successive layers of the rock suggest that they were built one after another from the bottom upward. We may be as sure that each layer was formed before those above it as that the bottom courses of stone in a wall were laid before the courses which rest upon them.

112. Based on the passage, each of these statements can be verified, EXCEPT?
A. We can learn about earth's inhabitants through its crust.
B. Individual layers of sandstone form one after another.
C. Rocks are made of sand.
D. Geology does not always demand explicit evidence.

113. Wall-building is used in this passage to help us understand:
A. Mountains
B. Valleys
C. Hills
D. Plains

114. The sand mentioned in the passage comes from:
A. An ancient beach
B. The sea
C. The earth's crust
D. It is undisclosed

115. A foundation of rock is **NOT** found underneath:
A. Upland
B. Lowland
C. Nowhere
D. Water

116. Grains of sand' are described as sorted by:
A. Shape
B. Texture
C. Age
D. Measurements

SET 24

The genus of plants called Narcissus, many of the species of which are highly esteemed by the floriculturist and lover of cultivated plants, belongs to the Amaryllis family (Amaryllidaceæ.) This family includes about seventy genera and over eight hundred species that are mostly native in tropical or semi-tropical countries, though a few are found in temperate climates.

Many of the species are sought for ornamental purposes and, on account of their beauty and remarkable odour, they are more prized by many than are the species of the Lily family. In this group is classed the American Aloe (Agave Americana) valued not only for cultivation, but also by the Mexicans on account of the sweet fluid which is yielded by its central bud. This liquid, after fermentation, forms an intoxicating liquor known as pulque. By distillation, this yields a liquid, very similar to rum, called by the Mexicans mescal. The leaves furnish a strong fibre, known as vegetable silk, from which, since remote times, paper has been manufactured.
The popular opinion is that this plant flowers but once in a century; hence the name 'Century Plant' is often applied to it, though under proper culture it will blossom more frequently.

117. Which of the following are **NOT** mentioned as potential uses for a narcissus plant:

A. Perfume production
B. Alcohol production
C. Visual decoration
D. Stationary production

118. Why is the plant known as 'the century plant'?

A. It is sown only once every hundred years.
B. It can only able to be fertilised once a century.
C. It is perceived as blooming centennially.
D. It can only able to flower once within a hundred years.

119. Which of the following statements is most supported by the above passage:

A. Lilies are generally valued less than members of the Narcissus genus.
B. Lilies are famously not as attractive as members of the Narcissus genus.
C. A number are people prefer members of the Narcissus genus over Lilies.
D. Members of the Narcissus genus are a welcome addition to any household.

120. Which of the following statements is NOT true:

A. American Aloe can be used to make rum.
B. The Amaryllis family contains more than six hundred species of Narcissus.
C. Members of the Narcissus genus can be found in all climates.
D. The members of the Narcissus genus have a distinctive smell.

121. Which of the following statements can be verified by the passage:

A. The 'Narcissus' genus is named after the mythical character, famed for his beauty.
B. Agave syrup can be collected by American Aloe.
C. A genus belongs to a family.
D. Members of the Narcissus genus are used for their soothing properties.

SET 25

The following passage is found in a book on nature published in 1899:

Five women out of every ten who walk the streets of Chicago and other Illinois cities, says a prominent journal, by wearing dead birds upon their hats proclaim themselves as lawbreakers. For the first time in the history of Illinois laws it has been made an offense punishable by fine and imprisonment, or both, to have in possession any dead, harmless bird except game birds, which may be possessed in their proper season. The wearing of a tern, or a gull, a woodpecker, or a jay is an offense against the law's majesty, and any policeman with a mind rigidly bent upon enforcing the law could round up, without a written warrant, a wagon load of the offenders any hour in the day, and carry them off to the lockup. What moral suasion cannot do, a crusade of this sort undoubtedly would.

Thanks to the personal influence of the Princess of Wales, the osprey plume, so long a feature of the uniforms of a number of the cavalry regiments of the British army, has been abolished. After Dec. 31, 1899, the osprey plume, by order of Field Marshal Lord Wolseley, is to be replaced by one of ostrich feathers. It was the wearing of these plumes by the officers of all the hussar and rifle regiments, as well as of the Royal Horse Artillery, which so sadly interfered with the crusade inaugurated by the Princess against the use of osprey plumes. The fact that these plumes, to be of any marketable value, have to be torn from the living bird during the nesting season induced the Queen, the Princess of Wales, and other ladies of the royal family to set their faces against the use of both the osprey plume and the aigrette as articles of fashionable wear.

122. In 1899:
A. Women across the USA could be prosecuted for owning ornamental dead birds.
B. There was a significant rise of female arrests in America.
C. Possession of a dead gull could lead to trouble.
D. Americans responded to law by citing the use of jays as ornamentation unfashionable.

123. Ostrich feathers were seen as preferable to osprey plums because:
A. Ostriches are less intelligent birds.
B. Ostriches are killed for their meat, so one might as well use their feathers.
C. Queen Elizabeth has an especial love of ospreys.
D. Harvesting osprey feathers was seen as an inhumane process.

124. Games birds could be possessed by citizens of Illinois all year round.
A. True
B. False
C. Can't tell

125. Banning Osprey feathers in the UK's army was difficult because:
A. Many uniforms required them.
B. The Princess did not have the authority to implement the ban.
C. Her ultimate support was predominately female, and thus their concerns seemed to have no relevance from the male domain of the army.
D. It would be hard to differentiate between other regiments within the army, who were already wearing ostrich feathers.

126. Which of the following could NOT be legally owned in Illinois, according to the passage:
A. A live bird intended for personal ornamentation.
B. A dead bird of prey that had violently attacked you.
C. Feathered garments.
D. None of the above.

SET 26

Indie game developer Lucas Pope created 'Papers Please', a video game where the player is an immigration officer processing people attempting to enter Arstotzka, a fictional dystopia. Released in 2013, the game was originally made for Microsoft Windows and OS X platforms. It was subsequently released for Linux and the iPad in 2014.

The game is set in 1982, and gameplay involves the player processing large numbers of applicants attempting to enter the country, through checking various pieces of paperwork. This is intended to keep criminals out, whether they are terrorists or drug smugglers. When looking through the applicant's 'papers', discrepancies may be discovered: the player must then enquire about these and may go on to use other tools, such as a body scanner and finger printing to discover the truth of the candidate's motives. Applicants may attempt to bribe the officer in order to get through. Ultimately, the game player must stamp candidates passports, either accepting into or rejecting them from the country. Their work is being monitored, however: after two false acceptances/rejections, the player will be pecuniarily punished, with their day's wages being decreased in response to their administrative sloppiness. They have a limited amount of time, representing each 'day', to work, during which they will be paid in accordance to the number of people processed.

127. Which of the following statements is best supported by the above passage:

A. Lucas Pope created the Papers Please for a small games company.
B. Papers Please is a multi-platform game.
C. Arstotzka is a fictionalised version of an ex-Soviet block state.
D. The game gained significant media attention in 2014.

128. Which of the following statements best sums up the official job of the player's character:

A. To accept as many applicants into Artstotzka as possible.
B. To reject as many new applicants entering Arstotzka as possible.
C. To avoid making mistakes in processing people.
D. To stamp passports.

129. Discrepancies in information provided by applicants lead to the player:

A. Interrogating and performing a fingerprint check on the suspicious individual.
B. Interrogating and performing a full body scan on the suspicious individual.
C. Asking the suspicious individual for further information.
D. Performing one or multiple physical assessments of the individual.

130. Which of the following statements is true:

A. The game-player solely makes money through processing applicants.
B. The game-player will ultimately be responsible for multiple arrests.
C. The game-player will not be forgiven for their mistakes.
D. The game-player may be subject to fiscal penalisation.

SET 27

Emerging in 1970s USA, Blaxploitation, or 'blacksploitation', gives homage to many other genres: within it, there are western, martial arts films, musicals, coming-of-age dramas and comedies, and the genre has even parodied itself with films like 'Black Dynamite'. Blaxploitation movies may take place in the South, and focus on issues like slavery, or be set in the poor neighbourhoods of the Northeast or West coast, but in any case they will feature a predominately black cast. It is also known to feature soundtracks comprised of soul and funk music, and the common feature of character's using the words 'honky', 'cracker' and other slurs against white people.

Originally, the genre's exports were aimed at city-dwelling black Americans, but their appeal has since grown and is not exclusive to any race. Despite the negative sound of the title 'blaxploitation', the term was coined by ex-film publicist Junius Griffin, the then head of LA's NAACP, National Association for the Advancement of Coloured People. He came up with the name through a play on the word 'sexploitation' describing films which featured pornographic scenes.

The film 'Shaft' and 'Sweet Sweetback's Baadasssss Song' are two of the forerunners of this genre, both released in 1971. The latter has been said, by Variety, to have created the genre

131. Which of the following statements is supported by the information in the above passage:

A. 'Blaxploitation' was a term coined by porn directors moving into a new genre.
B. 'Blaxploitation' was a term made popular by black audiences.
C. 'Blaxploitation' was a term coined by a civil rights activist.
D. 'Blaxploitation' was a term criticised by white sympathisers.

132. Which of the following statements best describes the most common element of a Blaxploitation film:

A. Characters performing funk songs.
B. Characters coming to terms with the legacy of slavery.
C. Characters performing martial arts.
D. Characters using racial slurs.

133. Which of these statements best describes casting in Blaxploitation films:

A. Primarily white
B. Primarily black
C. Exclusively white
D. Exclusively black

134. Which of the following best describes the audiences of Blaxploitation films:

A. Originally for all middle-class African-Americans.
B. Originally for all urban-dwellers.
C. Multi-ethnic.
D. Shrinking since the mid-1970s.

135. The legacy of films including soft-core porn is knowingly acknowledged in the name of two Blaxploitation titles, 'Shaft' and 'Sweet Sweetback's Baadasssss song', both of which suggest body parts associated with sex films.

A. True
B. False
C. Can't tell

SET 28

When discussing his famous character Rorschach, the antihero of 'Watchmen', Moore explains, 'I originally intended Rorschach to be a warning about the possible outcome of vigilante thinking. But an awful lot of comic readers felt his remorseless, frightening, psychotic toughness was his most appealing characteristic – not quite what I was going for.' Moore misunderstands his own hero's appeal within this quotation: it is not that Rorschach is willing to break little fingers to extract information, or that he is happy to use violence, that makes him laudable. The Comedian, another 'superhero' within the alternative world of Watchmen, is a thug who has won no great fan base; his remorselessness (killing a pregnant Vietnamese woman), frightening (attempt at rape), psychotic toughness (one only has to look at the panels of him shooting out into a crowd to witness this) is repulsive, not winning. This is because The Comedian has no purpose: he is a nihilist, and as a nihilist, denies any potential meaning to his fellow man, and so to the comic's reader. Everything to him is a 'joke', including his self, and consequently his own death could be seen as just another gag.

Rorschach, on the other hand, does believe in something: he questions if his fight for justice 'is futile?' then instantly corrects himself, stating 'there is good and evil, and evil must be punished. Even in the face of Armageddon I shall not compromise in this.' Jacob Held, in his essay comparing Rorschach's motivation with Kantian ethics, put forward the postulation 'perhaps our dignity is found in acting as if the world were just, even when it is clearly not.' Rorschach then causes pain in others not because he is a sadist, but because he feels the need to punish wrong and to uphold the good, and though he cannot make the world just, he can act according to his sense of justice - through the use of violence.

136. Which of the following best describes 'Watchmen':

A. A book that contains only vicious characters.
B. An expression of despair when contemplating an imperfect world.
C. An example of how an author's intentions are not always realised.
D. A book that accidentally glamorises violence.

137. 'The Comedian' is a misnomer - the character that goes by this title should not, logically, be called this.

A. True
B. False
C. Can't tell

138. Which of the following best articulates the view put forward by Jacob Held?

A. We find dignity through just actions.
B. If one decides to behave as though the world is fair, this may lead to a discovery of self-worth.
C. It is shameful to view the world as corrupt.
D. Self-value can only be found in madness.

139. What does the passage above argue?

A. Rorschach breaking little fingers is preferable to the Comedian attempting rape somebody.
B. The Comedian's depressing sense of humour has made him unpopular.
C. Rorschach is not actually violent.
D. Rorschach is popular because his aggressive behaviour has a moral intent, and is not just violence.

140. What does the word 'nihilist' mean in the context of the passage?

A. Someone who believes there is no meaning to life.
B. Someone who is full of anger at the corruption of society.
C. Someone who is narcissistic.
D. Someone who hates other people.

SET 29

'The Bechdel Test', also known as the 'Mo Movie Measure' and 'The Bechdel Rule' is named after cartoonist Alison Bechdel, who in 1985 wrote a cartoon containing the original proposal of the 'test'. It depicts one woman telling another that she has 'a rule' that she will only see a film if it satisfies three basic requirements: that it contains at least two women, that they talk to each other and that their conversation is on something other than a man. The second woman states that this is 'pretty strict, but a good idea', to which the first responds the last film she saw that complied with this was 'Alien'. The original notion described in the strip has been attributed to Liz Wallace, and the test is sometimes referred to as the Bechdel/Wallace Test.

Following this, a website entitled 'The Bechdel Test Movie List' has formed an extensive list of cinematic output, showing movies that pass and do not pass the test. One may be surprised at the number of movies that would not be watched by first woman in the Bechdel comic: many blockbusters do not make the mark, and such titles as 'Godzilla', 'The Imitation Game' and 'Robocop' all feature on the list of 'failed' films.

141. According to The Bechdel Test, 'The Imitation Game' is a sexist film.

A. True
B. False
C. Can't tell

142. Which of the following films would pass the Bechdel test:

A. One where the only conversation between two women is on woman A's brother.
B. One where there are two conversations, one on woman A's son and another on woman B's boss, Mr Smith.
C. One where there are five women, in which at one point they all have a chat about how to lose weight and the best hair removal techniques.
D. One where there is one woman who chats about all manner of things with her male colleagues, including her USA presidential campaign.

143. 50% of horror films, according to the above extract, pass the Bechdel test.

A. True
B. False
C. Can't tell

144. Which of the following phrases best describes the reaction of the second woman within the comic strip:

A. Ecstatically approving
B. Condemning
C. Cautiously approving
D. Apathetic

145. The two women in the comic strip are manifestations of Bechdel and Wallace, with the piece of art being a recreation of their original conversation on this matter.

A. True
B. False
C. Can't tell

SET 30

There are many comic tropes a comedian or group of comedians may want to employ in their set or act, but for the purpose of this extract we shall focus on the device of the 'call-back'. A call-back is a reference made to a previous joke, in a different context: for example, a comedian may make the joke 'why did the chicken cross the road? To get to the other side' early on in his or her set, and then later on may reference this again by telling an anecdote and saying 'so then I crossed the road - oh, look, there's a chicken! Strange, I could have sworn he was over there a moment ago'. Though the call-back may appear to simply rely on the idea that repetition is inherently funny, it actually has several desirable effects. Firstly, it means that one joke can provide more than one laugh, as the memory of the previous joke encourages renewed chuckling, and so the original quip's comic potential is increased. It also builds up a relationship between comedian and audience, as it builds up a sense of familiarity with the speaker and his or her subject matter, and this bond also may encourage more laughter - the second joke creates the same feeling as an 'in-joke'. If used at the end of a set - as a call-back often is - it gives a sense of completion, and also may lead to the ending of the act culminating in the largest laugh.
In TV, a call-back often refers to a joke made in a previous episode.

146. Repetition is inherently funny.

A. True
B. False
C. Can't tell

147. Which of the following best explains how a call-back works:

A. Previous understanding of a subject makes it potentially more comic.
B. Doubling a joke makes it potentially twice as funny.
C. Making the audience feel comfortable is more likely to make them laugh.
D. We find people we have a relationship with funny.

148. For a call-back to work, the original joke has to be significantly funny.

A. True
B. False
C. Can't tell

149. A call-back cannot be used in an un-comic setting.

A. True
B. False
C. Can't tell

150. Which of the following statements is best supported by the above passage:

A. A call-back is used to create a sense of the circle having fully come to pass.
B. A call-back can be a useful addition to an individual comedian's set.
C. A call-back creates unity through disparate TV episodes.
D. A call-back is an especially important trope to consider.

SET 31

Harriet Beecher (Stowe) was born June 14, 1811, in the characteristic New England town of Litchfield, Connecticut. Her father was the Rev. Dr. Lyman Beecher, a distinguished Calvinistic divine, her mother Roxanna Foote, his first wife. Harriet Beecher was ushered into a household of happy, healthy children, and found five brothers and sisters awaiting her. The eldest was Catherine, born September 6, 1800. Following her were two sturdy boys, William and Edward; then came Mary, then George, and at last Harriet. Another little Harriet was actually born three years before, but died when aged only one month old; the fourth daughter, the subject of this passage, was named in memory of this sister Harriet Elizabeth. Just two years after Harriet was born, in the same month, another brother, Henry Ward, was welcomed to the family circle, and after him came Charles, the last of Roxanna Beecher's children.

The first memorable incident of Harriet's life was the death of her mother, which occurred when she was four years old, and which ever afterwards remained with her as the most tender, sad and sacred memory of her childhood. Mrs Stowe's recollections of her mother are found in a letter to her brother Charles, afterwards published in the 'Autobiography and Correspondence of Lyman Beecher.' She says: —

"I was between three and four years of age when our mother died, and my personal recollections of her are therefore but few. But the deep interest and veneration that she inspired in all who knew her were such that during all my childhood I was constantly hearing her spoken of, and from one friend or another some incident or anecdote of her life was constantly being impressed upon me.

151. Harriet, the main character in the article, was the third daughter of Roxanna Beecher:

A. True
B. False
C. Can't tell

152. Which of the following statements, according to the passage, are true:

A. Harriet Beecher had a religious father.
B. Harriet Beecher was born in the English town Litchfield.
C. Harriet Beecher was born in the 18th century.
D. Harriet Beecher was born in an average American town.

153. Roxanna Beecher was an admired woman.

A. True
B. False
C. Can't tell

154. Harriet Beecher Stowe's mother's death is described as:

A. Her saddest memory of her life.
B. The earliest significant event in her life.
C. Her most tender memory of her life.
D. All of the above.

155. Which of the following statements is supported by the above passage:

A. Harriet Beecher was between three and four when her mother died.
B. Harriet Beecher had five brothers waiting for her when she was born.
C. Harriet Beecher was a letter-writer.
D. Harriet Beecher was an autobiographer.

SET 32

Gutenberg's father was a man of good family. Very likely the boy was taught to read. But the books from which he learned were not like ours; they were written by hand. A better name for them than books is 'manuscripts,' which means handwritings.

While Gutenberg was growing up a new way of making books came into use, which was a great deal better than copying by hand. It was what is called block printing. The printer first cut a block of hard wood the size of the page that he was going to print. Then he cut out every word of the written page upon the smooth face of his block. This had to be very carefully done. When it was finished the printer had to cut away the wood from the sides of every letter. This left the letters raised, as the letters are in books now printed for the blind.
The block was now ready to be used. The letters were inked, paper was laid upon them and pressed down. With blocks the printer could make copies of a book a great deal faster than a man could write them by hand. But the making of the blocks took a long time, and each block would print only one page.

Gutenberg enjoyed reading the manuscripts and block books that his parents and their wealthy friends had; and he often said it was a pity that only rich people could own books. Finally he determined to contrive some easy and quick way of printing.

156. Which of the following reasons can be inferred from the above passage to explain Gutenberg's desire to create a new way of printing was:

A. It was a lucrative business to go into.
B. He wanted to make text more accessible.
C. He was tired of waiting for each book to be hand written or block pressed, and wanted quicker access to literature.
D. He found the current books too costly for him to continue his reading habit.

157. Which of the following of the following is **NOT** mentioned as a concern of block printing?

A. It exhausts the carver.
B. It is intricate and demands attention to detail.
C. It is a lengthy process.
D. An individual block has limited utility.

158. Which of the following statements is definitely true according to the above passage?

A. Gutenberg was taught to read as a boy.
B. Gutenberg's father belonged to the aristocracy.
C. Block printing was the predominant book manufacturing process whilst Gutenberg was growing up.
D. Gutenberg's family was somewhat sociable.

159. Printing with the block process was a simple task of inking up the prepared block and pressing it down on a piece of paper, to make one page of the text.

A. True
B. False
C. Can't tell

160. Which of the following statements are **NOT** supported by the above passage:

A. Manuscripts were beautifully crafted.
B. 'Manuscripts' is an appropriate name for what it describes.
C. Block printing is an appropriate name for what it describes.
D. Having well off friends was a good way to expand your reading.

SET 33

Cassandra may be considered an odd name to give your daughter, when you consider the mythical significance of it. Cassandra was a figure in ancient Greek mythology, a Trojan girl born to King Priam, who had been cursed: she had the gift of prophecy, but no one would believe in her words. She ultimately ends up taken from her homeland, as the sexual slave of Agamemnon. Agamemnon's wife then slaughters the girl, and one might wonder why any parent would name their daughter after such an ill-fated figure.

There are several stories that explain how Cassandra gained her gift and her curse. One narrative states that the god Apollo gave the girl the ability to tell the future, in an attempt to seduce her. When she refused him, he corrupted her gift. Another version tells us that Cassandra originally told Apollo she would have sex with him, in exchange for the gift of prophecy. When she subsequently refused him, having attained this power, he then spat in her mouth during a kiss, and this action made her ever after doomed to be disbelieved.

The figure of Cassandra has been presented in various pieces of classical literature, including Homer's epic poem 'The Iliad', Euripides' 'Trojan Women' and Aeschylus' 'The Agamemnon'. Although the presentation of her character alters in the different manifestation, the tragic fate of the woman is known within the different texts, as it would be known by the different authors and audiences of these works.

161. Throughout mythology, Apollo is always presented as the figure who gives Cassandra prophecy.

A. True
B. False
C. Can't tell

162. Which of the following statements is best supported by the passage:

A. Parents who call their daughter Cassandra must hate their children.
B. Cassandra prizes chastity higher than her personal comfort.
C. Cassandra had supernatural powers.
D. Cassandra is often seen as a home wrecker.

163. Which of the following statements is **NOT** supported by the passage:

A. Cassandra comes from a royal line.
B. Cassandra had a happy childhood before her horrible fate.
C. Cassandra has been written about for the stage.
D. Homer has been inspired by Cassandra.

164. Cassandra's personality is consistently presented in the different pieces of literature she is included in.

A. True
B. False
C. Can't tell

165. Which of the following is offered in the above passage to explain Apollo's ire:

A. Cassandra breaking her promise.
B. Cassandra not accepting his gift.
C. Cassandra demanding more gifts.
D. Cassandra not acknowledging his gifts.

SET 34

Despite the fact that some associate musicals with cheesy joy, the genre is not limited to gleeful stories, as can be demonstrated by the macabre musical, 'Sweeney Todd'. The original story of the murderous barber appears in a Victorian penny dreadful, 'The String of Pearls: A Romance'. The penny dreadful material was adapted for the 19th century stage, and in the 20th century was adapted into two separate melodramas, before the story was taken up by Stephen Sondheim and Hugh Wheeler. The pair turned it into a new musical, which has since been performed across the globe and been adapted into a film starring Johnny Depp.

Sondheim and Wheeler's drama tells a disturbing narrative: the protagonist, falsely accused of a crime by a crooked judge, escapes from Australia to be told that his wife was raped by that same man of the court. In response, she has committed suicide, and her daughter - Todd's daughter - has been made the ward of the judge. The eponymous figure ultimately goes on a killing spree, vowing vengeance for the people who have wronged him but also declaring 'we all deserve to die', and acting on this belief by killing many of his clients, men who come to his barbershop. His new partner in crime, Mrs Lovett, comes up with the idea of turning the bodies of his victims into the filling of pies, as a way of sourcing affordable meat - after all, she claims, 'times is hard'.

Cannibalism, vengeance, murder and corruption - these are all themes that demonstrate that this show does not conform to a happy-clappy preconception of its genre.

166. Which of the following statements are best supported by the above passage:

A. Sondheim is a brilliant musician and lyricist.
B. Most musicals deal with morbid themes.
C. Wheeler is an avid penny dreadful fan.
D. Generalisations can be misleading.

167. All the adjectives below are explicitly supported by the passage as ways of describing the crimes described within it, except:

A. Comic
B. Culinary
C. Vengeful
D. Sexual

168. Mrs Lovett and Sweeney Todd are in a romantic relationship.

A. True
B. False
C. Can't tell

169. The best way to describe the belief of Todd as mentioned in the above passage:

A. Bad people should die so good can live and prosper.
B. Good people should die because the bad have basically taken over.
C. All men should die.
D. All humans merit death.

170. Which of the following statements is best supported in the above passage:

A. There are four themes in 'Sweeney Todd'.
B. Legal corruption is the predominate theme of 'Sweeney Todd'.
C. Several 'Sweeney Todd' themes are morbid.
D. There is nothing positive in 'Sweeney Todd'.

SET 35

The United States released the following as part of a pamphlet titled 'If Your Baby Must Travel in Wartime', released during the Second World War:

'Have you been on a train lately? The railroads have a hard job to do these days, but one that they are doing well. But before you decide on a trip with a baby, you should realise what a wartime train is like. So let's look into one.
This train is crowded. At every stop more people get on—more and still more. Soldiers and sailors on furloughs, men on business trips, women — young and not so young — and babies, lots of them, mostly small.
The seats are full. People stand and jostle one another in the aisle. Mothers sit crowded into single seats with toddlers or with babies in their laps. Three sailors occupy space meant for two. A soldier sits on his tipped-up suitcase. A marine leans against the back of the seat. Some people stand in line for 2 hours waiting to get into the diner, some munch sandwiches obtained from the porter or taken out of a paper bag, and some go hungry. And those who get to the diner have had to push their way through five or six moving cars.

You will want to think twice before taking your baby into such a crowded, uncomfortable place as a train. And having thought twice, you'd better decide to stay home unless your trip is absolutely necessary.

But suppose you and your baby must travel. Well then, you will have to plan for the dozens of small but essential things incidental to travelling with a baby and equip yourself to handle them.'

171. First World War passenger trains were exceptionally crowded.
A. True
B. False
C. Can't tell

172. Which of the following phrases is described by the above passage:
A. A soldier responds to the situation by creating his own seat.
B. A sailor rest against a seat's back.
C. Many people queue for over an hour to get to the diner car.
D. Many go without eating for the duration of a train journey.

173. The pamphlet wishes to increase the number of passengers on trains.
True
A. False
B. Can't tell

174. Every station the described train passes through has passengers wanting to get onto the vehicle.
A. True
B. False
C. Can't tell

175. Which of the following does the above passage do:
A. Compliment the railroads.
B. Insult passengers who are mothers.
C. Insult passengers who work for the navy.
D. Compliment soldiers.

SET 36

The following extract is from 'Foods That Will Win the War', published in the USA during the First World War:
'A slice of bread seems an unimportant thing. Yet one good-sized slice of bread weighs an ounce. It contains almost three-fourths of an ounce of flour. If every one of the country's 20,000,000 homes wastes on the average only one such slice of bread a day, the country is throwing away daily over 14,000,000 ounces of flour—over 875,000 pounds, or enough flour for over a million one-pound loaves a day. For a full year at this rate there would be a waste of over 319,000,000 pounds of flour—1,500,000 barrels—enough flour to make 365,000,000 loaves.

As it takes four and one-half bushels of wheat to make a barrel of ordinary flour, this waste would represent the flour from over 7,000,000 bushels of wheat. Fourteen and nine-tenths bushels of wheat on the average are raised per acre. It would take the product of some 470,000 acres just to provide a single slice of bread to be wasted daily in every home.

But someone says, 'a full slice of bread is not wasted in every home.' Very well, make it a daily slice for every four or every ten or every thirty homes—make it a weekly or monthly slice in every home—or make the wasted slice thinner. The waste of flour involved is still appalling. These are figures compiled by government experts, and they should give pause to every housekeeper who permits a slice of bread to be wasted in her home.'

176. According to the above passage, a slice of bread:

A. Contains 1/6 lb. of flour
B. Contains a 1/4-ounce of air
C. Is 75% flour
D. Is one fourth salt, butter and yeast

177. The passage denies that 20,000,000 homes at the point of writing wasted at least a slice of bread a day.

A. True
B. False
C. Can't tell

178. If 20,000,000 homes wasted a slice of bread, this waste would be equal to:

A. One million loaves of bread a day.
B. Over 319,000,000 bushels of flour in 365 days
C. 1.5 million barrels per annum.
D. Over 365,000 loaves a year.

179. According to the above passage, a slice of bread is an unimportant thing.

A. True
B. False
C. Can't tell

180. Which of the following statements are supported by the above passage:

A. The writer has received much criticism for his views.
B. The government should do more to inform the public about waste.
C. The government has taken responsibility for public waste.
D. Responsibility lies with the person who keeps the house.

SET 37

At the election of President and Vice President of the United States, and members of Congress, in November, 1872, Susan B. Anthony, and several other women, offered their votes to the inspectors of election, claiming the right to vote, as among the privileges and immunities secured to them as citizens by the fourteenth amendment to the Constitution of the United States. The inspectors, Jones, Hall, and Marsh, by a majority, decided in favour of receiving the offered votes, against the dissent of Hall, and they were received and deposited in the ballot box. For this act, the women, fourteen in number, were arrested and held to bail, and indictments were found against them, under the 19th Section of the Act of Congress of May 30th, 1870, (16 St. at L. 144.) independently charging them with the offense of knowingly voting without having a lawful right to vote. The three inspectors were also arrested, but only two of them were held to bail, Hall having been discharged by the Commissioner on whose warrant they were arrested. All three, however were jointly indicted under the same statute—for having knowingly and wilfully received the votes of persons not entitled to vote.

Of the women voters, the case of Miss Anthony alone was brought to trial, a nolle prosequi having been entered upon the other indictments. Upon the trial of Miss Anthony before the U.S. Circuit Court for the Northern District of New York, at Canandaigua, in June, 1873, it was proved that before offering her vote she was advised by her counsel that she had a right to vote; and that she entertained no doubt, at the time of voting, that she was entitled to vote.

181. According to the above passage, how many people in total were arrested due to the group of women voting?

A. Fourteen
B. Three
C. Seventeen
D. Sixteen

182. Susan B. Anthony was the only person brought to trial because of the incident.

A. True
B. False
C. Can't tell

183. Which of the following best describes initial opinions of the election officers:

A. United by each member's personal support of the women's votes.
B. Divided in response to the women's actions.
C. Apathetic about the women's actions.
D. United by general disapproval of the women's actions.

184. Which defence for Susan B. Anthony is mentioned above?

A. She did not realise she was not allowed to vote.
B. That all people born in the USA should be able to vote for their president.
C. That gender should not prevent her vote.
D. The election officers accepted her vote, showing the responsibility is not with her.

185. The women were charged jointly under the same indictment.

A. True
B. False
C. Can't tell

SET 38

The following is taken from a book about Norway published in 1909:

'In a country like Norway, with its vast forests and waste moorlands, it is only natural to find a considerable variety of animals and birds. Some of these are peculiar to Scandinavia. Some, though only occasionally found in the British Isles, are not rare in Norway; whilst others (more especially among the birds) are equally common in both countries.
There was a time when the people of England lived in a state of fear and dread of the ravages of wolves and bears, and the Norwegians of the country districts even now have to guard their flocks and herds from these destroyers. Except in the forest tracts of the Far North, however, bears are not numerous, but in some parts, even in the South, they are sufficiently so to be a nuisance, and are ruthlessly hunted down by the farmers. As far as wolves are concerned civilization is, fortunately, driving them farther afield each year, and only in the most out-of-the-way parts are they ever encountered nowadays. Stories of packs of hungry wolves following in the wake of a sleigh are still told to the children in Norway, but they relate to bygone times—half a century or more ago, and such wild excitements no longer enter into the Norsemen's lives.'

186. Which of the following is best supported by the above passage:

A. The variety of birds and animals to be found in Norway is unique to that country.
B. The variety of birds and animals to be found in Norway is common to all European countries.
C. By having forests, a country is more likely to have a variety of birds and animals.
D. England and Norway have similar geographical features.

187. English people are described as:

A. Having been anxious of certain animals.
B. Sceptical of bears.
C. Living in fear of wolves.
D. Developmentally behind the Norwegians.

188. Bears are described as:

A. Hunting
B. Scavenging
C. Damaging
D. Man-eating

189. Bears are also:

A. Numerous in all forest tracts.
B. Numerous throughout the North.
C. Numerous throughout the South.
D. At risk in parts of Norway.

190. The passage suggests:

A. The movement of wolves to the out-of-reach parts of Norway is beneficial.
B. Wildlife currently threats Norwegian children.
C. Regret at the loss of adventures.
D. Norsemen particularly respect their natural surroundings.

SET 39

The following extract is taken from Freud's book 'Dream Psychology: Psychoanalysis for Beginners'

In what we may term pre-scientific days, people were in no uncertainty about the interpretation of dreams. When they were recalled after awakening they were regarded as either the friendly or hostile manifestation of some higher powers, demoniacal and divine. With the rise of scientific thought the whole of this expressive mythology was transferred to psychology; today there is but a small minority among educated persons who doubt that the dream is the dreamer's own psychical act.

But since the downfall of the mythological hypothesis an interpretation of the dream has been wanting. The conditions of its origin; its relationship to our psychical life when we are awake; its independence of disturbances which, during the state of sleep, seem to compel notice; its many peculiarities repugnant to our waking thought; the incongruence between its images and the feelings they engender; then the dream's evanescence, the way in which, on awakening, our thoughts thrust it aside as something bizarre, and our reminiscences mutilating or rejecting it—all these and many other problems have for many hundred years demanded answers which up till now could never have been satisfactory. Before all there is the question as to the meaning of the dream, a question that is in itself double-sided. There is, firstly, the psychical significance of the dream, its position with regard to the psychical processes, as to a possible biological function; secondly, has the dream a meaning—can sense be made of each single dream as of other mental syntheses?

191. Dreams used to be regarded as having a potentially religious quality.

A. True

B. False

C. Can't tell

192. According to the passage, at this point of time, amongst the educated:

A. A vocal majority believe that dreams come from somewhere outside the dreamer.

B. A small minority believes that dreams come from the dreamer alone.

C. The majority accepts that a dreamer's dream is his or her own psychical act.

D. A vocal minority believes dreams are the direct products of angels and devils.

193. With a dream:

A. Images seemingly logically dictate feelings.

B. Events happen which are pleasant to waking thought.

C. Only boring things occur that are often too dull to be remembered.

D. There are relationships between images and feelings that would appear illogical to the awake mind.

194. The passage wonders about the significance of individual dreams.

A. True

B. False

C. Can't tell

195. Which of the following statements is supported by the above passage:

A. There is a definite link between the waking and dreaming self.

B. Human society has never had a hypothesis to explain dreams that has satisfied them.

C. A memory of a dream may be untrustworthy.

D. The origin of the dream has been scientifically sourced.

SET 40

Most of the colonists who lived along the American seaboard in 1750 were the descendants of immigrants who had come in fully a century before; after the first settlements there had been much less fresh immigration than many latter-day writers have assumed. According to Prescott F. Hall, "the population of New England ... at the date of the Revolutionary War ... was produced out of an immigration of about 20,000 persons who arrived before 1640," and we have Franklin's authority for the statement that the total population of the colonies in 1751, then about 1,000,000, had been produced from an original immigration of less than 80,000. Even at that early day, indeed, the colonists had begun to feel that they were distinctly separated, in culture and customs, from the mother-country and there were signs of the rise of a new native aristocracy, entirely distinct from the older aristocracy of the royal governors' courts. The enormous difficulties of communication with England helped to foster this sense of separation. The round trip across the ocean occupied the better part of a year, and was hazardous and expensive; a colonist who had made it was a marked man—as Hawthorne said, "the petit maître of the colonies." Nor was there any very extensive exchange of ideas, for though most of the books read in the colonies came from England, the great majority of the colonists, down to the middle of the century, seem to have read little save the Bible and biblical commentaries, and in the native literature of the time one seldom comes upon any reference to the English authors who were glorifying the period of the Restoration and the reign of Anne.

196. Over half of the 1750 colonists that lived on the American seaboard had genetic links to immigrants who had arrived a century ago.

A. True
B. False
C. Can't tell

197. Which of the following statements is supported by the above passage:

A. According to Hall, America's population at the date of the Revolutionary war could be entirely traced back to 20,000 immigrants.
B. The population in the 1751 colonies was over ten times the original immigration that moved there.
C. According to Hall, in 1751 the population in the American colonies was one million.
D. According to Hall, 80,000 people led to a population of 1,000,000.

198. According to the passage, the new aristocracy that existed in the colonies was:

A. Similar to the England's.
B. Similar to European aristocratic systems in general.
C. Not based in royal governors' courts.
D. Not based on genetic lines.

199. Most of the books on board ships were Bibles and Biblical commentaries.

A. True
B. False
C. Can't tell

200. Which of these is **NOT** given as a reason for poor communications with England:

A. Travel between America and England was costly.
B. The English saw the early colonists as backwards.
C. Travel between America and England was slow.
D. Travel between America and England was dangerous.

SET 41

In discussing Russia's role in the past World War, it is customary to cite the losses sustained by the Russian Army, losses running into many millions. There is no doubt that Russia's sacrifices were great, and it is just as true that her losses were greater than those sustained by any of the other Allies. Nevertheless, these sacrifices are by far not the only standard of measurement of Russia's participation in this gigantic struggle. Russia's role must be gauged, first of all, by the efforts made by the Russian Army to blast the German war plans during the first years of the War, when neither America, nor Italy, nor Romania were among the belligerents, and the British Army was still in the process of formation.

[Secondly], and this is the main thing, the role played by the Russian Army must be considered also in this respect that the strenuous campaign waged by Russia, with her 180 millions of inhabitants, for three years against Germany, Austro-Hungary and Turkey, sapped the resources of the enemy and thereby made possible the delivery of the final blow. This weakening of the powers of the enemy by Russia was already bound at various stages of the War to facilitate correspondingly the various operations of the Allies. Therefore, at the end of the War, three years of effort on the part of Russia had devoured the enemy's forces, enabling the Allies to finally crush the enemy. The final catastrophe of the Central Powers was the direct consequence of the offensive of the Allies in 1918, but Russia made possible this collapse to a considerable degree, having effected, in common with the others, the weakening of Germany, and having consumed during the three years of strenuous fighting countless reserves, forces, and resources of the Central Powers.

Could Germany have won the War? A careful analysis of this question brings home the conviction that Germany was very close to victory, and that it required unusual straining of efforts on the part of France and Russia to prevent Germany from "winning out."

201. According to the passage, Russia's greatest contribution to the War was?
A. Contributing more sacrifices than any other ally.
B. Blasting the German war plans during the first years of the War.
C. Consuming countless reserves, forces and resources of the Germans.
D. Sapping the resources of Germany, Austro-Hungary and Turkey for 3 years.

202. How many countries were Russian allies?
A. 2. B. 3. C. 4. D. 5.
E.

203. Russia was the main country fighting against Germany in the early years of the War?
A. True. B. False. C. Can't tell.

204. The War was won by?
A. Germany running out of resources.
B. The offensive drive of the Allies.
C. The arrival of America.
D. Turkey and Austro-Hungary changing sides.

205. If it were not for Russia, Germany would have won the war?
A. True. B. False. C. Can't tell.

SET 42

We freeze some moments in time. Every culture has its' frozen moments, events so important and personal that they transcend the normal flow of news.

Americans of a certain age, for example, know precisely where they were and what they were doing when they learned that President Franklin D. Roosevelt had died. Another generation has absolute clarity of John F. Kennedy's assassination. And no one who was older than a baby on 11th September, 2001, will ever forget hearing about, or seeing, aeroplanes flying into skyscrapers.

In 1945, people gathered around radios for the immediate news and stayed with the radio to hear more about their fallen leader and about the man who took his place. Newspapers printed extra editions and filled their columns with detail for days and weeks afterward. Magazines stepped back from the breaking news and offered perspective.

11th September, 2001, followed a similarly grim pattern. We watched again and again the awful events. Consumers of news learned about the attacks, thanks to the television networks that showed the horror so graphically. Then we learned some of the how's and why's, as print publications and thoughtful broadcasters worked to bring depth to events that defied mere words. Journalists did some of their finest work and made me proud to be one of them.

But something else, something profound, was happening this time around: news was being produced by regular people who had something to say and show, and not solely by the "official" news organisations that had traditionally decided how the first draft of history would look. This time, the first draft of history was being written in part, by the former audience. It was possible, it was inevitable, because of new publishing tools available on the Internet.

206. The author of this passage is a journalist.

A. True.
B. False.
C. Can't tell.

207. Which media outlet tended to share a different point of view to the others?

A. Radios.
B. Newspapers.
C. Magazines.
D. Televisions.

208. Which media outlet had the biggest effect on changing the way news is spread?

A. The Internet.
B. Newspapers.
C. Magazines.
D. Televisions.

209. Which media outlet was mainly responsible for notifying consumers of the news that events had occurred in 1945?

A. Televisions.
B. Newspapers.
C. Radios.
D. Magazines.

210. What was the big news story in 1945?

A. President Franklin D. Roosevelt died.
B. John F. Kennedy was assassinated.
C. An aeroplane exploded into skyscrapers.
D. John. F Kennedy was elected.

SET 43

There is nothing in England today with which we can compare the life of a fully enfranchised borough of the fifteenth century. The town of those earlier days, in fact, governed itself after the fashion of a little principality. Within the bounds which the mayor and citizens defined with perpetual insistence in their formal perambulation year after year, it carried on its isolated self-dependent life.

The inhabitants defended their own territory, built and maintained their walls and towers, armed their own soldiers, trained them for service and held reviews of their forces at appointed times. They elected their own rulers and officials in whatever way they chose to adopt, and distributed among officers and councillors just such powers of legislation and administration as seemed good in their eyes. They drew up formal constitutions for the government of the community, and as time brought new problems and responsibilities, more were made, re-made and revised again; their ordinances with restless and fertile ingenuity, till they had made of their constitution a various medley of fundamental doctrines and general precepts and particular rules, somewhat after the fashion of an American state of modern times.

In all concerns of trade, they exercised the widest powers, and bargained and negotiated and made laws as nations do on a grander scale today. They could covenant and confederate, buy and sell, deal and traffic after their own will; they could draw up formal treaties with other boroughs, and could admit them to or shut them out from all the privileges of their commerce; they might pass laws of protection or try experiments in free trade. Often, their authority stretched out over a wide district, and surrounding villages gathered to their markets and obeyed their laws; it might even happen in the case of a staple town that their officers controlled the main foreign trade of whole provinces.

211. In the 15th century, towns drew up treaties to defend each other in times of attack.
A. True.
B. False.
C. Can't tell.

212. How were the leaders of boroughs brought into power?
A. Power was passed down the family.
B. Invaders conquered towns and become the rulers.
C. Inhabitants elected their own rulers.
D. There was a leader of the whole country, with majors in each borough.

213. Town life in the 15th century is more comparable to the American state of modern times than England in modern times.
A. True.
B. False.
C. Can't tell.

214. The authorities in the 15th century controlled who?
A. Their respective villages only.
B. Their respective towns only.
C. Their respective towns and surrounding villages.
D. The whole country.

215. How might disputes between boroughs have been settled in the 15th century?
A. By war.
B. By banning trading between boroughs.
C. With a treaty.
D. All of the above.

SET 44

Nowhere is the influence of sex more plainly manifested than in the formulation of religious conceptions and creeds. With the rise of male power and dominion, and the corresponding repression of the natural female instincts, the principles that originally constituted the God-idea gradually gave place to a Deity better suited to the peculiar bias that had been given to the male organism. An anthropomorphic God, like that of the Jews, whose chief attributes are power and virile, could have had its origin only under a system of masculine rule.

Religion is especially liable to reflect the vagaries and weaknesses of human nature; and, as the forms and habits of thought connected with worship take a firmer hold on the mental constitution than do those belonging to any other department of human experience. Religious conceptions should be subjected to frequent and careful examination in order to perceive, if possible, the extent to which we are holding on to ideas which are unsuited to existing conditions.

In an age when every branch of inquiry is being subjected to reasonable criticism, it would seem that the origin and growth of religion should be investigated from beneath the surface and that all the facts bearing upon it should be brought forward as a contribution to our fund of general information. As well might we hope to gain a complete knowledge of human history by studying only the present aspect of society, as to expect to reach reasonable conclusions respecting the prevailing God-idea by investigating the various creeds and dogmas of existing faiths.

216. Masculine rule has always occurred.
A. True.
B. False.
C. Can't tell.

217. Which god has attributes of power?
A. All gods.
B. The Jewish god.
C. The Christian god.
D. No gods.

218. Why is it a good idea to study the different Gods?
A. It provides an insight to societies of the past.
B. Because it is important to understand and respect other people's religion.
C. To find out which God is the most powerful.
D. To find out about the weaknesses of human nature.

219. Where is the influence of sex most clearly displayed?
A. In the formation of religion.
B. In the rules of religion.
C. By the lack of opposition against religion by women.
D. By the gods attributes.

220. The author is religious.
A. True.
B. False.
C. Can't tell.

SET 45

"What is a novel?" A novel is a marketable commodity, of the class collectively termed "luxuries," as not contributing directly to the support of life or the maintenance of health. The novel, therefore, is an intellectual artistic luxury in that it can be of no use to a man when he is at work, but may conduce to peace of mind and delectation during his hours of idleness.

Probably, no one denies that the first object of the novel is to amuse and interest the reader. But it is often said that the novel should instruct as well as afford amusement, and the "novel-with-a-purpose" is the realisation of this idea. The purpose-novel, then, proposes to serve two masters, besides procuring a reasonable amount of bread and butter for its writer and publisher, it proposes to escape from my definition of the novel in general and make itself an "intellectual moral lesson" instead of an "intellectual artistic luxury." It constitutes a violation of the unwritten contract tacitly existing between writer and reader. A man buys what purports to be a work of fiction, a romance, a novel, a story of adventure, pays his money, takes his book home, prepares to enjoy it at his ease, and discovers that he has paid a dollar for somebody's views on socialism, religion, or the divorce laws.

221. According to the author, a writer should write a novel with the sole purpose of amusement?

A. True.
B. False.
C. Can't tell.

222. Which of the following is the best use of a novel?

A. To be of use to a man when he is at work.
B. To spread the author's views on socialism, religion, or the divorce laws to those who otherwise would not listen to them.
C. To make moral lessons more interesting.
D. To pleasure a man during periods of idleness.

223. The writer of the passage regards a novel which has a strong view on socialism as their biggest hate.

A. True.
B. False.
C. Can't tell.

224. What is the unwritten contract between the author and reader?
A. A novel should provide an intellectual moral lesson.
B. A novel should have a purpose.
C. A novel should afford amusement.
D. A novel should be a work of fiction.

225. What is the most common opinion which the author does not share?
A. A novel should have a purpose.
B. A novel should instruct the reader.
C. A novel should conduce to peace of mind.
D. A novel should afford amusement.

SET 46

What is patriotism? Is it love of one's birthplace, the place of childhood's recollections and hopes, dreams and aspirations? Is it the place where, in child-like naivety, we would watch the fleeting clouds and wonder why we too could not run so swiftly? The place where we would count the milliard glittering stars, terror-stricken lest each one "an eye should be," piercing the very depths of our little souls? Is it the place where we would listen to the music of the birds and long to have wings to fly, even as they, to distant lands? Or the place where we would sit at mother's knee, enraptured by wonderful tales of great deeds and conquests? In short, is it love for the spot, every inch representing dear and precious recollections of a happy, joyous, and playful childhood?

If that were patriotism, few American men of today could be called upon to be patriotic, since the place of play has been turned into a factory, mill, and mine, while deafening sounds of machinery have replaced the music of the birds. Nor can we still hear the tales of great deeds, for the stories our mothers tell today are but those of sorrow, tears and grief. What, then, is patriotism? "Patriotism, sir, is the last resort of scoundrels," said Dr. Johnson. Leo Tolstoy, the greatest anti-patriot of our times, defines patriotism as the principle that will justify the training of wholesale murderers; a trade that requires better equipment for the exercise of man-killing than the making of such necessities of life as shoes, clothing, and houses; a trade that guarantees better returns and greater glory than that of the average workingman.

226. The author believes patriotism as being the love for the spot where one grew up and had many happy memories.

A. True. B. False. C. Can't tell.

227. According to the author, are few American's of today patriotic?

A. Yes, because where they grew up has been destroyed.
B. Yes, because the current generation didn't have anywhere where they could listen to the music of the birds when they were children as the sounds of machinery has replaced this.
C. Yes, because not many people do justify the training of wholesale murderers.
D. No, because the definition of patriotism has not been defined and so one cannot say whether few American's of today are patriotic.

228. What is a possible negative of being patriotic?

A. Justifying mass killing.
B. Being depressed when one's birthplace is replaced by factories, mills and mines.
C. Reducing production of necessities such as workplaces.
D. Encouraging migration to distant lands.

229. The most common stories of today when children sit at their mother's knee are what?

A. Wonderful tales of great deeds and conquests.
B. Stories to encourage dreams and aspirations.
C. Stories of sorrow, tears, and grief.
D. Tales of flying away to distant lands.

230. What might a young child wonder?

A. What distant lands are like?
B. Whether the conquests of their Mothers stories are true.
C. Whether their birthplace will one day be turned into a factory.
D. Why they cannot keep up with clouds.

SET 47

The law of benefits is a difficult channel, which requires careful sailing or rude boats. It is not the office of a man to receive gifts. How dare you give them? We wish to be self-sustained. We do not quite forgive a forgiver. The hand that feeds us is in some danger of being bitten. We can receive anything from love, for that is a way of receiving it from ourselves (hence the fitness of beautiful, not useful things for a gift); but not from anyone who assumes to bestow. We sometimes hate the meat that we eat, because there seems something of degrading dependence in living by it.

He is a good man, who can receive a gift well. We are either glad or sorry at a gift, and both emotions are unbecoming. Some violence, I think, is done, some degradation borne, when I rejoice or grieve at a gift. I am sorry when my independence is invaded, or when a gift comes from such as do not know my spirit, and so the act is not supported; and if the gift pleases me overmuch, then I should be ashamed that the donor should read my heart and see that I love his commodity, and not him.

This giving is flat usurpation, and therefore, when the beneficiary is ungrateful, as all beneficiaries hate all Timons, not at all considering the value of the gift, but looking back to the greater store it was taken from, I rather sympathize with the beneficiary than with the anger of my lord, Timon. For, the expectation of gratitude is mean and is continually punished by the total insensibility of the obliged person.

231. Who is described as a good man?
A. A man who can forgive a forgiver.
B. A man who can give a good gift.
C. A man who can take a gift well.
D. A man who can enjoy the meat he eats.

232. Why do some men not like to receive a gift?
A. Because men wish to maintain themselves by independent effort.
B. They do not wish to depend upon it.
C. They only like to receive gifts of love.
D. They prefer to pick their own gifts.

233. The author of this passage does not like to receive gifts.
A. True.
B. False.
C. Can't tell.

234. When is it most acceptable to give a gift?
A. When you can read someone's heart and present the perfect gift.
B. For those most in need.
C. Never.
D. When the receiver loves you.

235. What is the major negative of enjoying a gift?
A. You have to return the favour.
B. It is going against the desire to self-sustain.
C. Appreciating the item rather than the effort of the giver.
D. All of the above.

SET 48

English writers who have spoken of Goethe's "Doctrine of Colours," have generally confined their remarks to those parts of the work in which he has undertaken to account for the colours of the prismatic spectrum, and of refraction altogether, on principles different from the received theory of Newton. The less questionable merits of the treatise consisting of a well-arranged mass of observations and experiments, many of which are important and interesting, have thus been in a great measure overlooked. The translator, aware of the opposition which the theoretical views alluded to have met with, intended at first to make a selection of such of the experiments as seem more directly applicable to the theory and practice of painting. Finding, however that the alterations this would have involved would have been incompatible with a clear and connected view of the author's statements, he preferred giving the theory itself, reflecting, at the same time, that some scientific readers may be curious to hear the author speak for himself even on the points at issue.

In reviewing the history and progress of his opinions and research, Goethe tells us that he first submitted his views to the public in two short essays entitled "Contributions to Optics." Among the circumstances which he supposes were unfavourable to him on that occasion, he mentions the choice of his title, observing that by a reference to optics he must have appeared to make pretensions to a knowledge of mathematics, a science with which he admits he was very imperfectly acquainted.

236. Mathematics was Goethe's greatest science.
   A. True.
   B. False.
   C. Can't tell.

237. What was Goethe's most popular work?

A. His paper on 'Contribution to Optics'.
B. His paper on 'Doctrine of Colours'.
C. His ideas of refraction.
D. His ideas of mathematics.

238. What was the main problem the translator faced when writing the paper 'Doctrine of colours'?

A. He wanted to present the scientific evidence before the theory to the audience, while Goethe did not.
B. He wanted to present the theory and then back it up with scientific evidence to the audience, while Goethe did not.
C. He wanted to wait until there was more scientific evidence before publishing as he knew the opposition would believe Goethe's theory.
D. The translator did not believe Goethe's theory and didn't want to write a paper which may convince others it is true.

239. How many papers did Goethe publish, according to the article?
   A. 1
   B. 2
   C. 3
   D. 4

240. What is considered Goethe's most notable work?
   A. About colours of the prismatic spectrum and of refraction.
   B. His contribution to optics in general.
   C. Disproving Newton's theories.
   D. Changing the ways in which theories are presented.

SET49

That marriage is a failure none but the very stupid will deny. One has but to glance over the statistics of divorce to realize how bitter a failed marriage really is. Nor will the stereotyped Philistine argument that the laxity of divorce laws and the growing looseness of women account for the fact that: first, every twelfth marriage ends in divorce; second, that since 1870 divorces have increased from 28 to 73 for every hundred thousand population; third, that adultery, since 1867, as ground for divorce, has increased 270.8 percent; fourth, that desertion increased 369.8 percent.

Henrik Ibsen, the hater of all social shams, was probably the first to realize this great truth. Nora leaves her husband, not as the stupid critic would have it, because she is tired of her responsibilities or feels the need of woman's rights, but because she has come to know that for eight years she had lived with a stranger and borne him children. The moral lesson instilled in the girl is not whether the man has aroused her love, but rather is it, "How much?" The important and only God of practical American life: Can the man make a living? Can he support a wife? That is the only thing that justifies marriage. Gradually, this saturates every thought of the girl; her dreams are not of moonlight and kisses, of laughter and tears; she dreams of shopping tours and bargain counters. Can there be anything more humiliating, more degrading than a life-long proximity between two strangers? No need for the woman to know anything of the man, save his income. As to the knowledge of the woman—what is there to know except that she has a pleasing appearance?

241. According to the passage, most women get married for the sake of money.
   A. True.
   B. False.
   C. Can't tell.

242. The author believes that marriages end due to the "looseness" of women.
   A. True.
   B. False.
   C. Can't tell.

243. Nora did not want children.
   A. True.
   B. False.
   C. Can't tell.

244. In America, every twelfth marriage ends in divorce.
   A. True.
   B. False.
   C. Can't tell.

245. Women always end up dreaming of moonlight kisses later in marriage.
   A. True.
   B. False.
   C. Can't tell.

SET 50

During the 1960s and 70s, terrorism was a contemporary subject due to the conflict between the UK government and the IRA. 'The Troubles' (the name given to the violence) originated in the 1920s and eventually resulted in bombings on the streets of Northern Ireland and occasionally in England. The government felt that in order to prevent mayhem, their actions needed to be swift and decisive. Thus, a series of temporary measures were initiated; policemen and soldiers all over Ulster were given the right to stop, question, search and arrest members of the public.

In 2000, the Terrorism Act 2000 was passed as a definitive measure following twenty years of temporary measures. Policemen were given wider stop and search powers and enabled to detain suspects for up to 48 hours without charge. The Act was met with strong criticism as it outlawed certain Islamic fundamentalist groups and this was seen as a portrayal of Islam as a religion that fuels terrorism. This, in turn, made it likely that discrimination would occur in the form of the disproportionate stopping and searching of Asians who were thought to 'look Muslim'.

Although, prior to the September 2001 attacks on Washington D.C, government legislation in the UK had attempted to prevent the occurrence of terrorism; the counter-terrorism strategies had focused a lot of attention on the punishment of terrorists and the criminalisation of new offences following their occurrence. However, the Anti-Terrorism Crime and Security Act 2001 (ATCSA) marked a more firm move towards the 'management of anticipatory risk' (Piazza, Walsh, 2010) which was to characterize the counter-terrorism legislation of the 21st century.

246. In the 1960s, policemen and soldiers all over Ulster were given the right to stop, question, search and arrest members of the public.
    A. True.
    B. False.
    C. Can't tell.

247. The Terrorism Act 2000 is still implemented today.
    A. True.
    B. False.
    C. Can't tell.

248. The act in 2000 was passed in an effort to combat the threat of Islamic extremists.
    A. True.
    B. False.
    C. Can't tell.

249. The act targets preventing rather than punishing terrorism acts.
    A. True.
    B. False.
    C. Can't tell.

250. Terrorism management was a big problem between 1980 and 2000.
    A. True.
    B. False.
    C. Can't tell.

Decision Making

The Basics

The Decision Making section is **brand new** to the UCAT in 2017. It replaces an old section called Decision Analysis which involved deciphering the meaning of various coded phrases and is no longer tested.

The section lasts 31 minutes (with one additional minute to read the instructions), and there are 29 questions to be answered – so you need to work quickly and efficiently at a rate of about one question per minute. You will be presented with questions that may refer to text, charts, tables, graphs or diagrams. All of the questions are standalone and do not share data, so make sure to focus on each question independently.

This section was a component of the test last year, but was not scored. This year the section will be scored just like every other subsection, and the score from this section will contribute to your overall score and result.

The Questions

The idea behind this section is to assess how you use information and data to make decisions – a skill that is essential to working effectively as a doctor. The questions come in a variety of styles, but all are focussed on testing your decision making ability.

The questions making up the decision making section can be broken down into six main styles. All of the questions in this section will belong to one of these styles, so by familiarising yourself with the theory you will make it much easier to answer the questions. The six styles are:

1) **Logical Puzzles**
2) **Syllogisms**
3) **Interpreting Information**
4) **Recognising Assumptions**
5) **Venn Diagrams**
6) **Probabilistic Reasoning**

The questions may provide multiple pieces of information which build together to give the overall picture. Remember to consider each of these in turn and build up your understanding of the situation in pieces before bringing it all together.

The most important thing is to understand the premise of the question. There is often a clear chain of logic from the start of the question to the final answer, so the sooner you work this out, the sooner you can begin answering on the right track.

Strategy

As there are different styles of questions in this section, the best way to think about preparation is to subdivide the questions into their different styles and develop a clear approach to each

As a general principle, drawing diagrams can be helpful. If for example, the question has a number of people in it, write their names down on your whiteboard (or just the first initial to save space and time). If the question talks about compass directions, draw a simple map. If it talks about categories, a Venn diagram can help. If it involves a timetable or timed events, draw out a timeline to simplify your thought process. By using visual tools to complement the words, you make it easier to understand and solve the problem.

Logical Puzzles

The logical puzzle questions require you to make an inference based on the available information to get to the answer. Commonly, this will manifest in being presented with some background information (a general statement) and then some extra information (a specific statement), and both must be combined to make the conclusion and find the answer. Deductive reasoning can be used in either a positive way to prove something, or in a negative way to disprove something. By familiarising yourself with the structures, you will improve your ability to notice and use the relevant information.

An example of **positive inductive reasoning**:

1) All birds have wings
2) Ostriches are birds
3) Therefore the ostrich has wings

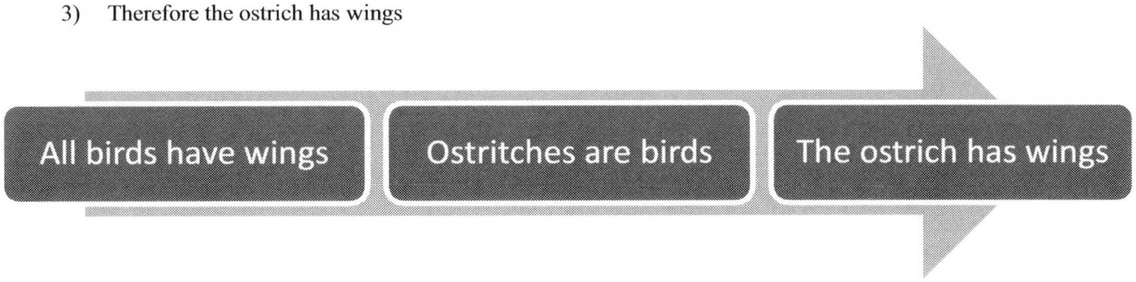

An example of **negative inductive reasoning**:

1) All birds have feathers
2) Elephants do not have feathers
3) Therefore elephants are not birds

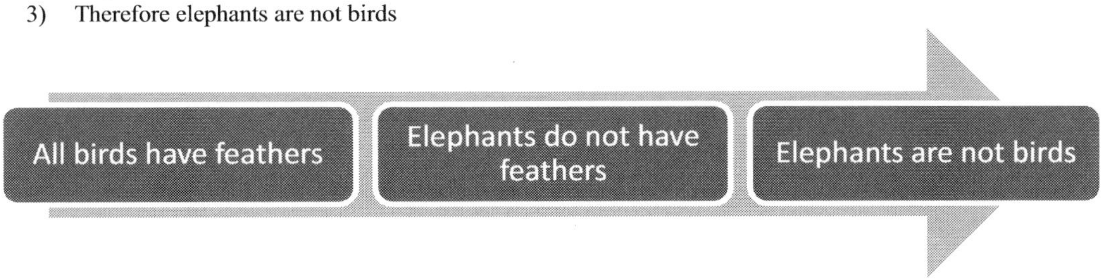

Syllogisms

Syllogisms are an additional application of deductive reasoning. In these questions, you will be presented with information that can be used to make certain conclusions, but which will also give and incomplete description of the situation. Then, the task is to determine which answer/answers is/are supported and which aren't. To do well in these questions, you have to be very clear about the limitations of the information available – if the statement cannot be deduced from the information in the questions, then it is not true.

Interpreting information

For the interpreting information questions, you will be presented with a more complex and less directly relevant set of information than in the logical deduction questions. This information may be in the form of a passage of text describing something, or alternatively it could be in the form of a table, chart or graph. You will then have to use the information source to extract the relevant information to answer the question. Don't be afraid to use rounding and estimations – if the differences are substantial, you may not need to calculate figures exactly.

To answer these questions effectively, look at the question before digesting the data. Once you understand the premise of the question, you can approach the data in a much more focussed way to gather the information you need and ignore the distracters designed to make the question more difficult. When analysing graphs and charts, always follow a systematic approach to ensure you grasp the key message as easily as possible, such as the method illustrated below.

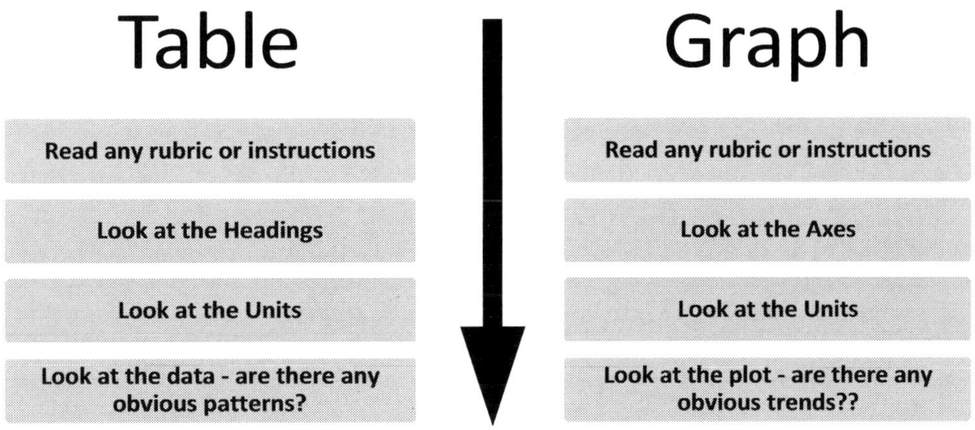

Recognising assumptions

Assumptions are an important component of decision making, and proper use of them is essential to being a good decision maker. Relying too heavily on assumptions leaves the decision at risk of being wrong, whereas reluctance to make assumptions can make the decision process extremely slow and laborious. The questions of this style aim to probe your understanding of assumption making as a component of the decision process.

Many of these questions will ask you to select the strongest argument for or against a statement. To help you select the best option, use the acronym **FREES**. Factual – the argument should be based on fact rather than opinion. Relevant – the argument should directly address the statement in the question. Entire – the argument should address the whole question, not only one aspect of it. Emotionless – the argument should avoid emotional pleas and derive strength from relevant evidence. Sensible – the argument should be a generally sensible and reasonable approach to take.

F	• Factual
R	• Relevant
E	• Entire
E	• Emotionless
S	• Sensible

Venn diagrams

The category of "Venn diagram" questions encompasses any that require the use of Venn diagrams within the question. Venn diagrams might be used in the question itself to present the data, they may be required as a part of the working to deduce the correct answer, or it may be that the answers are presented in the form of Venn diagrams, and you have to choose the most appropriate response.

Venn diagrams can take a number of forms. Some may look like the style of diagram you will have seen for many years, with two or three overlapping segments into which items are sorted. But they don't necessarily look like that. Provided the basic rules are followed – that to sort any item, it is placed into each and every circle that it belongs to – then any shape can be formed. The shape and structure of the diagrams has to be altered to allow all circles that need to overlap to be able to do so. To build your skills, practice drawing Venn diagrams to classify common objects – for example vehicles, kitchen utensils, farm animals or school subjects in different ways. Below are examples of Venn diagram structures that you may encounter in this section of the UCAT.

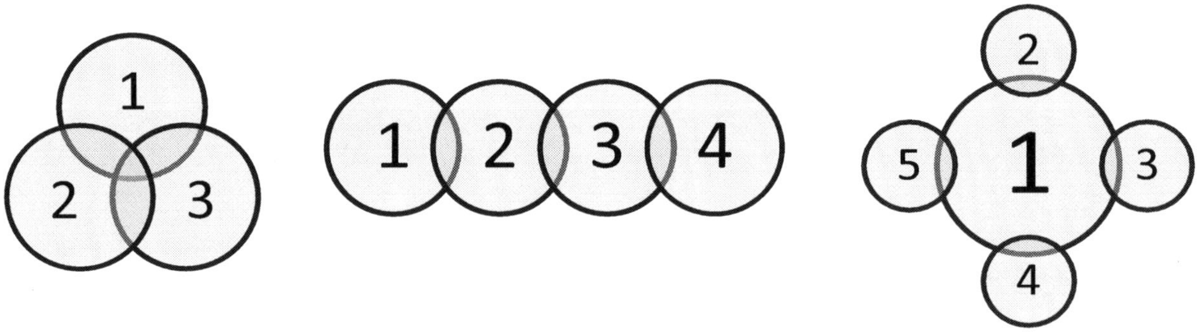

Probabilistic reasoning

These questions assess your ability to use probabilistic reasoning in the decision making process. You may be presented with probabilistic information in a variety of forms – fractions, decimals, percentages or odds – so do remind yourself of these different notations if you haven't seen them in a while. Whenever you see a probability, take the time to note exactly what occurrence the probability is representing, and whether it is the positive probability (of a thing happening) or a negative probability (of it not happening).

A good rule of thumb with probability is this. If you are asked the probability of something **or** something occurring, then the overall probability is higher than only one of them occurring so you add the probabilities. If you are asked the probability of something **and** something occurring, then the overall probability is lower than only one of them occurring, so you multiply the probabilities. For example, if asked about the probability of rain on two given consecutive days, when the probability of rain on any given day is 0.4, then it can be calculated as follows:

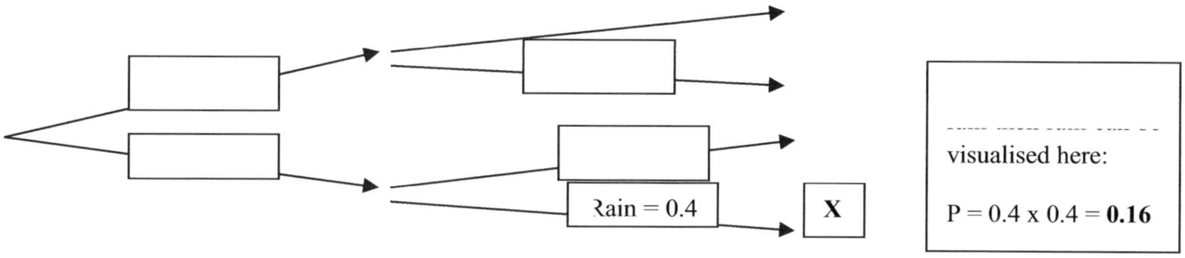

Worked example

A Surgeon is planning his surgery list for the next day. He has a total of 5 surgeries planned for the day.
Mrs Smith has an infected arm wound that needs to be cleaned and stitched. Due to the infection, the surgeon will operate on her last.

Start building up the order as information in gathered

Mr Hunt has a broken leg and will be operated on before Mr Pierce.
Mr Perry will be operated on first, his procedure will take 1hr.
Mr Dutch has his procedure 2hrs before Mr Hunt and 60mins after Mr Perry.

Mr Perry				

Which of the following statements is **TRUE**?

A. Mr Hunt's leg is infected
B. Mr Dutch will be operated on third
C. There are no women on the operating list
D. **Mr Pierce will be operated on after Mr Hunt**

Answer **D**: the only order that satisfies the information is Perry-Dutch-Hunt-Pierce-Smith

Top tip! Read the question before starting to interpret tables, charts or graphs. That way, you know information you need and what is there to distract you!

Decision Making Questions

Question 1:

Pilbury is south of Westside, which is south of Harrington. Twotown is north of Pilbury and Crewville but not further north than Westside. Crewville is:

A. South of Westside, Pilbury and Harrington but not necessarily Twotown.
B. North of Pilbury, and Westside.
C. South of Westside and Twotown, but north of Pilbury.
D. South of Westside, Harrington and Twotown but not necessarily Pilbury.
E. South of Harrington, Westside, Twotown and Pilbury.

Question 2:

The hospital coordinator is making the rota for the ward for next week; two of Drs Evans, James and Luca must be working on weekdays, none of them on Sundays and all of them on Saturdays. Dr Evans works 4 days a week including Mondays and Fridays. Dr Luca cannot work Monday or Thursday. Only Dr James can work 4 days consecutively, but he cannot do 5.

What days does Dr James work?

A. Saturday, Sunday and Monday.
B. Monday, Tuesday, Wednesday, Thursday and Saturday.
C. Monday, Thursday Friday and Saturday.
D. Tuesday, Wednesday, Friday and Saturday.
E. Monday, Tuesday, Wednesday, Thursday and Friday.

Question 3:

If criminals, thieves and judges are represented below:

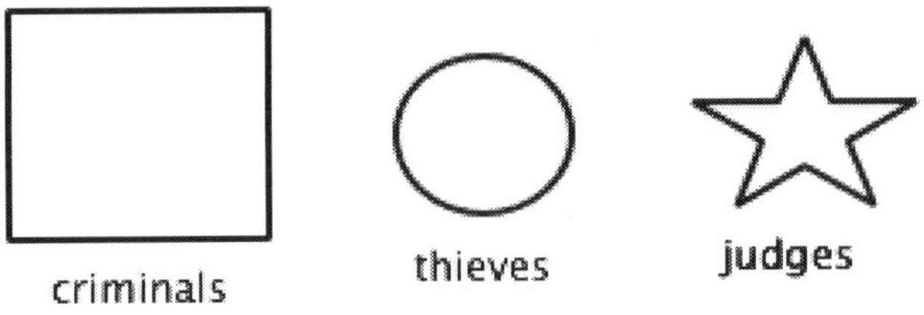

Assuming that judges must have clean record, all thieves are criminals and all those who are guilty are convicted of their crimes, which of one of the following best represents their interaction?

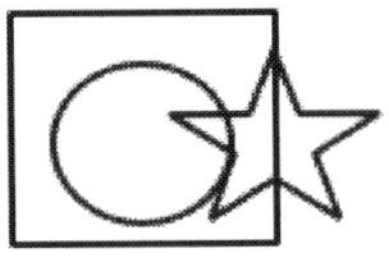
A.

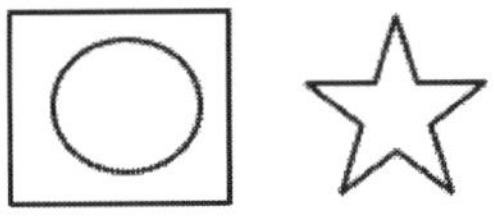
B.

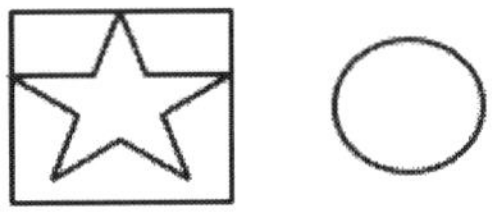
C.

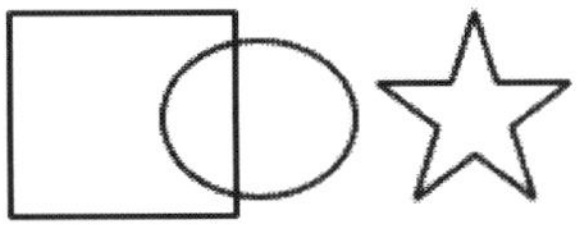
D.

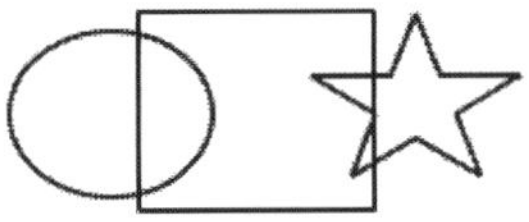
E.

Question 4:

Apples are more expensive than pears, which are more expensive than oranges. Peaches are more expensive than oranges. Apples are less expensive than grapes.

Which two of the following must be true?

A. Grapes are less expensive than oranges.
B. Peaches may be less expensive than pears.
C. Grapes are more expensive than pears.
D. Pears and peaches are the same price.
E. Apples and peaches are the same price.

Question 5:

A class of young students has a pet spider. Deciding to play a practical joke on their teacher, one day during morning break one of the students put the spider in their teachers' desk. When first questioned by the head teacher, Mr Jones, the five students who were in the classroom during morning break all lied about what they saw. Realising that the students were all lying, Mr Jones called all 5 students back individually and, threatened with suspension, all the students told the truth. Unfortunately Mr Jones only wrote down the student's statements not whether they had been told in the truthful or lying questioning.

The students' two statements appear below:

Archie: "It wasn't Edward. "
"It was Bella."

Darcy: "It was Charlotte"
"It was Bella"

Edward: "It was Darcy"
"It wasn't Archie"

Charlotte: "It was Edward."
"It wasn't Archie"

Bella: "It wasn't Charlotte."
"It wasn't Edward."

Who put the spider in the teacher's desk?

A. Edward
B. Bella
C. Darcy
D. Charlotte
E. More information needed.

Question 6:

On a specific day at a GP surgery 150 people visited the surgery and common complaints were recorded as a percentage of total patients. Each patient could use their appointment to discuss up to 2 complaints. 56% flu-like symptoms, 48% pain, 20% diabetes, 40% asthma or COPD, 30% high blood pressure.
Which statement must be true?

A. A minimum of 8 patients complained of pain and flu-like symptoms.
B. No more than 45 patients complained of high blood pressure and diabetes.
C. There were a maximum of 21 patients who did not complain about flu-like symptoms or high blood pressure.
D. There were actually 291 patients who visited the surgery.
E. None of the above.

Question 7:

During a GP consultation in 2015, Ms Smith tells the GP about her grandchildren. Ms Smith states that Charles is the middle grandchild and was born in 2002. In 2010, Bertie was twice the age of Adam and that in 2015 there are 5 years between Bertie and Adam. Charles and Adam are separated by 3 years.
How old are the 3 grandchildren in 2015?

A. Adam = 16, Bertie = 11, Charles = 13
B. Adam = 5, Bertie = 10, Charles = 8
C. Adam = 10, Bertie = 15, Charles = 13
D. Adam = 10, Bertie = 20, Charles = 13
E. Adam = 11, Bertie = 10, Charles = 8
F. More information needed.

Question 8:
A team of 4 builders take 12 days of 7 hours work to complete a house. The company decides to recruit 3 extra builders. How many 8 hour days will it take the new workforce to build a house?

A. 2 days
B. 6 days
C. 7 days
D. 10 days
E. 12 days
F. More information needed

Question 9:
Four young girls entered a local baking competition. Though a bit burnt, Ellen's carrot cake did not come last. The girl who baked a Madeira sponge had practiced a lot, and so came first, while Jaya came third with her entry. Aleena did better than the girl who made the Tiramisu, and the girl who made the Victoria sponge did better than Veronica.

Which **TWO** of the following were **NOT** results of the competition?

A. Veronica made a tiramisu
B. Ellen came second
C. Aleena made a Victoria sponge
D. The Victoria sponge came in 3rd place
E. The carrot cake came 3rd

Question 10:
John likes to shoot bottles off a shelf. In the first round he places 16 bottles on the shelf and knocks off 8 bottles. 3 of the knocked off bottles are damaged and can no longer be used, whilst 1 bottle is lost. He puts the undamaged bottles back on the shelf before continuing. In the second round he shoots six times and misses 50% of these shots. He damages two bottles with every shot which does not miss. 2 bottles also fall off the shelf at the end. He puts up 2 new bottles before continuing. In the final round, John misses all his shots and in frustration, knocks over gets angry and knocks over 50% of the remaining bottles.

How many bottles were left on the wall after the final round?

A. 2
B. 3
C. 4
D. 5
E. 6
F. More information needed

Question 11:
A bus takes 24 minutes to travel from White City to Hammersmith with no stops. Each time the bus stops to pick up and/or drop off passengers, it takes approximately 90 seconds. This morning, the bus picked up passengers from 5 stops, and dropped off passengers at 7 stops. What is the minimum journey time from White City to Hammersmith this morning?

A. 28 minutes
B. 34 minutes
C. 34.5 minutes
D. 36 minutes
E. 37.5 minutes
F. 42 minutes

Question 12:
I look at the clock on my bedside table, and I see the following digits:

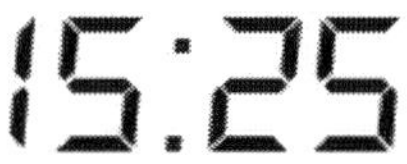

However, I also see that there is a glass of water between me and the clock, which is in front of 2 adjacent figures. I know that this means these 2 figures will appear reversed. For example, 10 would appear as 01, and 20 would appear as 05 (as 5 on a digital clock is a reversed image of a 2). Some numbers, such as 3, cannot appear reversed because there are no numbers which look like the reverse of 3.

Which of the following could be the actual time?

A. 15:52
B. 21:25
C. 12:55
D. 12:22
E. 21:52

Question 13:

Ryan is cooking breakfast for several guests at his hotel. He is frying most of the items using the same large frying pan, to get as much food prepared in as little time as possible. Ryan is cooking Bacon, Sausages, and eggs in this pan. He calculates how much room is taken up in the pan by each item. He calculates the following:

- Each rasher of bacon takes up 7% of the available space in the pan
- Each sausage takes up 3% of the available space in the pan.
- Each egg takes up 12% of the available space in the pan.

Ryan is cooking 2 rashers of bacon, 4 sausages and 1 egg for each guest. He decides to cook all the food for each guest at the same time, rather than cooking all of each item at once.

How many guests can he cook for at once?

A. 1
B. 2
C. 3
D. 4
E. 5

Question 14:

Northern Line trains arrive into Kings Cross station every 8 minutes, Piccadilly Line trains every 5 minutes and Victoria Line trains every 2 minutes. If trains from all 3 lines arrived into the station exactly 15 minutes ago, how long will it be before they do so again?

A. 24 minutes
B. 25 minutes
C. 40 minutes
D. 60 minutes
E. 65 minutes
F. 80 minutes

Question 15:

In how many different positions can you place an additional tile to make a straight line of 3 tiles?

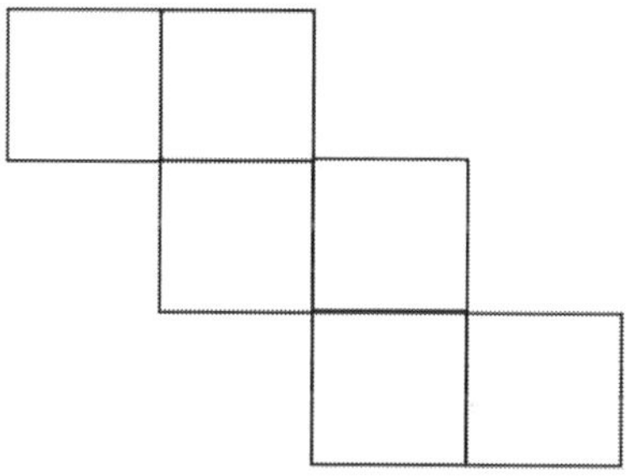

A. 6
B. 7
C. 8
D. 9
E. 10
F. 11

Question 16:

Ellie, her brother Tom, her sister Georgia, her mum and her dad line up in height order from shortest to tallest for a family photograph. Ellie is shorter than her dad but taller than her mum. Georgia is shorter than both her parents. Tom is taller than both his parents. If 1 is shortest and 5 is tallest, what position is Ellie in the line?

A. 1
B. 2
C. 3
D. 4
E. 5

Question 17:

Miss Briggs is trying to arrange the 5 students in her class into a seating plan. Ashley must sit on the front row because she has poor eyesight. Danielle disrupts anyone she sits next to apart from Caitlin, so she must sit next to Caitlin and no-one else. Bella needs to have a teaching assistant sat next to her. The teaching assistant must be sat on the left hand side of the row, near to the teacher. Emily does not get on with Bella, so they need to be sat apart from one another. The teacher has 2 tables which each sit 3 people, which are arranged 1 behind the other. Who is sitting in the front right seat?

A. Ashley
B. Bella
C. Caitlin
D. Danielle
E. Emily

Question 18:

Piyanga writes a coded message for Nishita. Each letter of the original message is coded as a letter a specific number of characters further on in the alphabet (the specific number is the same for all letters). Piyanga's coded message includes the word "PJVN". What could the original word say?

A. CAME
B. DAME
C. FAME
D. GAME
E. LAME

Question 19:

Lauren, Amy and Chloe live in different cities across England. They decide to meet up together in London and have a meal together. Lauren departs from Southampton at 2:30pm, and arrives in London at 4pm. Amy's journey lasts twice as long as Lauren's journey and she arrives in London at 4:15pm. Chloe departs from Sheffield at 1:30pm, and her journey lasts an hour longer than Lauren's journey.

Which of the following statements is definitely true?

A. Chloe's journey took the longest time.
B. Amy departed after Lauren.
C. Chloe arrived last.
D. Everybody travelled by train.
E. Amy departed before Chloe.

Question 20:

Jina is playing darts. A dartboard is composed of equal segments, numbered from 1 to 20. She takes three throws, and each of the darts lands in a numbered segment. None land in the centre or in double or triple sections. What is the probability that her total score with the three darts is odd?

A. $^1/_4$
B. $^1/_3$
C. $^1/_2$
D. $^3/_5$
E. $^2/_3$

Question 21

Should nurses be encouraged to make more significant decisions regarding treatment in the health care setting?

Select the strongest argument from the statements below.

A. No. Nurses are not able to make complex decisions that require a higher degree of training.
B. No. Nurses are not able to understand the complexity of medical care.
C. Yes. Nurses interact with the patients every day and therefore will be more qualified to make decisions than doctors.
D. Yes. Nurses provide valuable input to care delivery already as they deliver an important additional perspective.

Question 22

On a walk in the woods, James observes a variety of wildlife species. He finds that birds tend to fly off as soon as he approaches their position, whereas the many squirrels he sees tend to wait and observe his behaviour for some time. He also manages to see some deer in the distance and something he thinks was a fox.

Which of the following statements are true?

A. Squirrels are uncommon in the woods.
B. Birds are used to human presence.
C. He must be walking far away from any towns.
D. None of the above.

Question 23

"The physician must be able to tell the antecedents, know the present, and foretell the future – must mediate these things, and have two special objects in view with regard to disease, namely, to do good or to do no harm" – Hippocrates.
Which of the following statements is true with regards to the above statement?

A. A physician must be all-knowing and not make any mistakes.
B. It does not matter how well trained a physician is.
C. Avoidance of harm is one of the guiding principles of medicine.
D. Techniques of the past are still the best today.

Question 24

One of the biggest challenges facing the NHS is the discharge of patients from hospitals. This can generally have a variety of reasons, but most commonly it is due to the lack of adequate care being available for the patient outside of the hospital. The cuts to social care spending as well as a decreasing ability of families to care for their relatives compound this problem. Which of the following represent valid solutions to this problem?

A. Discharge patients irrespective of availability of social care.
B. Force families to care for their patients.
C. Charge wealthy patients for extended hospital stays.
D. None of the above.

Question 25

A farmer has a 200 head herd of animals consisting of cows, goats and pigs. The total value of the herd is £50,000. Every goat is worth £30 and every pig is worth £70. Due to local regulations, he must always have twice as many goats and twice as many pigs than he has cows. How many cows does the farmer have?

A. 100 B. 40 C. 60 D. 75

Question 26

In study of wild monkeys in the Amazon rainforest, a scientist finds that the monkeys mingle according to a complex set of rules based on their gender and age. He finds that young animals mingle with others irrespective of age and gender; adolescent males mingle only with young animals and adolescent females mingle exclusively with older females and the young monkeys. The majority of older males exhibit hostile behaviour to adolescent males. Older females treat adolescent males with suspicion but tolerate them in their proximity.

Which of the following statements are true with regards to the interactions of the group?

A. Young apes never mingle with older male apes.
B. Adolescent males have the widest range of social interactions in the herd.
C. This study is irrelevant as it is not complex enough.
D. There is a strict separation between adolescent males and females.

Question 27

Steve is going hiking with a friend. In the run up to the trip, they split up the equipment. Steve takes the tent and the provisions whilst his friend carries the sleeping bags, ground mats and cooking equipment.

Place yes or no depending on if the conclusion is correct.

A. Steve's friend is lazy as he lets you carry the majority of the equipment.
B. The two depend on each other for a comfortable trip.
C. The friend must be weaker as their load is lighter.
D. Steve and his friend are likely to spend several days on their hiking trip.

Question 28

Anna is visiting a concert with her four friends, Louise, Maria, Sophie and Jenny. The five manage to get a row of seats right in front of the stage.

Anna is the tallest and stands right in the middle next to Louise.
Sophie is left handed and prefers to sit on the far left.
Jenny met another friend and sits at the far end of the row next to Louise.

		Anna		

Please indicate which statements can be concluded to be true

A. Maria sits between Sophie and Anna.
B. Sophie sits at the edge of the concert hall.
C. Jenny left the group and sits with her other friend.
D. Louise sits on the second seat from the right.

Question 29

Sven is trying to set up a vegetable garden. He is allergic to tomatoes so will not be planting these. He decides to plant several rows of salad, carrots and courgettes. He also decides to plant raspberries and blackberries, even though they are not vegetables.

Which of the following conclusions are true?

A. Sven will grow more than 2 types of vegetables.
B. The garden will contain only green vegetables.
C. Allergies to tomatoes are very common.
D. None of the above.

Question 30

Louise is organizing a trip to Europe for her friends. They plan to leave London in June and visit 4 cities, starting the furthest north and move further south to then spend a week at the beach. They plan to visit Berlin, Amsterdam, Paris and Rome in that order.

Which of the following conclusions follow?

A. Paris is the most Southern city they visit.
B. Amsterdam is further north than Berlin.
C. They will be in at least 5 different countries in June.
D. None of the above

Question 31

James is planning to invest into a company by buying shares. He decides that he does not want to invest into any company that may take part in military supply. He finds that 40% of electronics firms contribute to military applications, but limited exclusively to computer technology firms. He also finds that all British steel companies are involved in producing specialty steel for the arms industry. The food industry, with exception to the beef industry does not seem to have any military contracts.

Decide if the statement is true or false?

A. James is free to invest in computer technology.
B. Investments into the chocolate industry are possible.
C. Most branches of industry are connected to military applications.
D. Investments in general are not a good idea due to the volatile political situation at the moment.

Question 32

A group of 5 friends live on the same road in a row of houses running parallel to the road.

Austin lives the furthest from Mark.
Steve lives two houses down from Austin.
David lives next to Mark.

Which of the following is true?

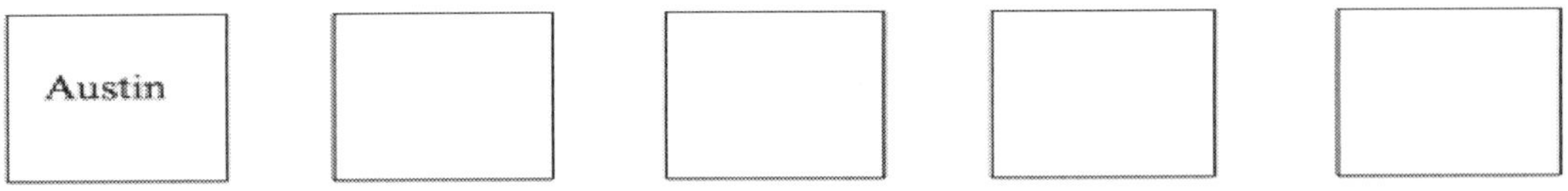

A. Steve lives equidistant from Austin and Mark.
B. The five live in a small town.
C. Peter lives next to Austin.
D. Peter and David are neighbours.

Question 33

A group of scientists investigate male pattern baldness for a popular shampoo producer that aims to release a product for that market. They find that male pattern baldness is becoming increasingly common in men aged between 30 – 60 and that it sometimes is associated with the use of anabolic steroids or type 2 diabetes. They also find that in the majority of cases there seems to be a genetic predisposition of unknown origin, but independent of external factors.

Which of the following is are reasonable conclusions from the above?

A. Baldness is not exclusive to men.
B. There is a connection between life-style choices and hair loss
C. A hair loss treatment in shampoo form promises to help for the majority of cases.
D. Anabolic steroids can cause hair loss.

Question 34

A farmer has a forest planted. It contains exclusively needle trees, except for some oaks and beeches. It also contains fruit trees.

Which of the following is true?

A. The forest will only deliver lumber.
B. There are only 2 types of trees in the forest.
C. One can harvest Christmas trees from the forest.
D. The forest covers a large area.

Question 35

Penguins live in large colonies in various climates of the Southern hemisphere. These colonies provide protection for the individual as well as offering companionship and breeding partners. Penguins are flightless but are excellent swimmers and spend about half of their life in the ocean. They live mostly of sea animals such as fish, krill and squid.

Which of the conclusions are false?

A. Penguins spend 50% of their life on land.
B. Penguins are herd animals.
C. Penguins live mostly off seafood.
D. Penguins live exclusively on ice.

Question 36

Should people stop burning fossil fuels immediately?

Select the strongest argument from the statements below.

A. Yes, because they represent old technology that has since been overcome.
B. Yes, there is little oil and coal in the UK and therefore fossil fuels are economically unsound.
C. No, fossil fuels represent a safe and plentiful source of energy.
D. No, we are too dependent on energy to be able to source adequate supply from non-fossil sources.

Question 37

In a national election 60% of the population go to vote. Some people did not like the candidates of any party.

Does this mean that 40% of people decided not to vote? Please choose the most appropriate answer

A. Yes, because the total would equate to 100%.
B. Yes, because there was discontent with the candidates up for election.
C. No, because not the entire population is allowed to vote.
D. No, because voting is more about intuition than actual decisions.

Question 38

With increasing parental age, the risk of congenital abnormalities in babies increases. This is thought to be due to a variety of factors including accumulation of genetic defects in egg cells as well as an increased degradation of sperm quality.

Which of the following consequences is true?

A. Older parents are less likely to have children with chromosomal abnormalities.
B. From a genetic perspective, it is safer to have children at a younger age.
C. Congenital abnormalities are due to poor sperm quality as sperm cells are present at birth and exposed to environmental mutagens.
D. None of the above

Question 39

5 drivers take part in a car race. The top three drivers are each separated by 1 second. The fastest driver, James, reached the finish line 10 seconds before the last, Lucas. Felix was 5 seconds faster than Lucas, but 3 seconds slower than Peter. Dorian finishes second.

Which of the following is true?

A. Peter finished 8 seconds before Lucas.
B. James finishes 2 seconds before Dorian.
C. Dorian finishes third.
D. None of the above.

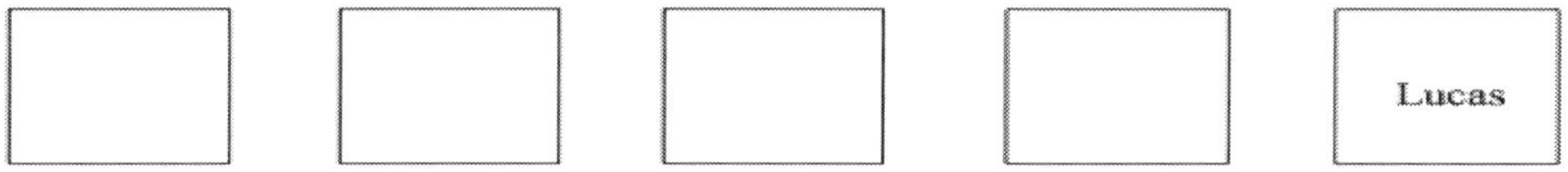

Question 40

A group of friends buys an assortment of junk food. They buy biscuits, chocolate and gummy bears. All but 2 of them like gummy bears. 6 like chocolate and 3 like biscuits. 1 doesn't like any sweets and therefore bought peanuts. Out of the 5 that like gummy bears, 2 like chocolate and 1 likes biscuits. 2 of the 3 that like biscuits also like chocolate.

Which of the following best represents the group's food preferences?

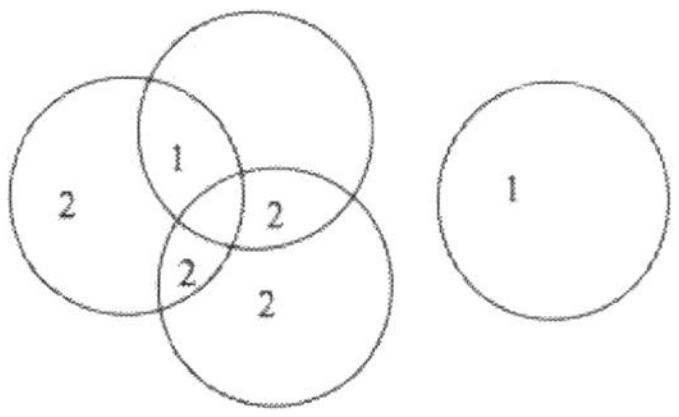

A.

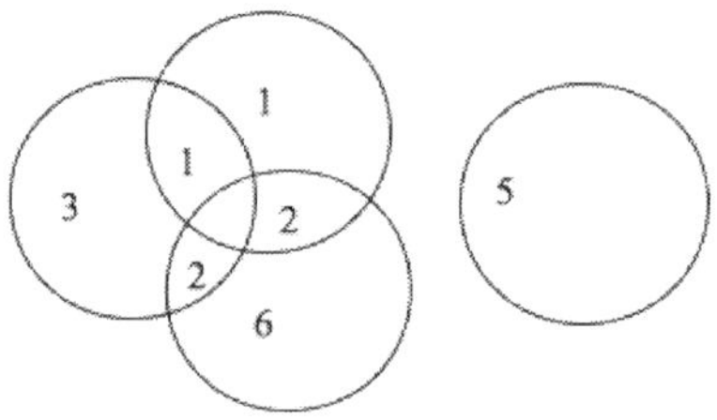

C.

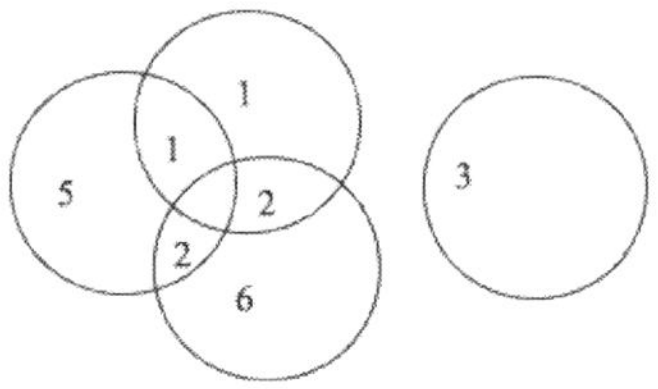

B.

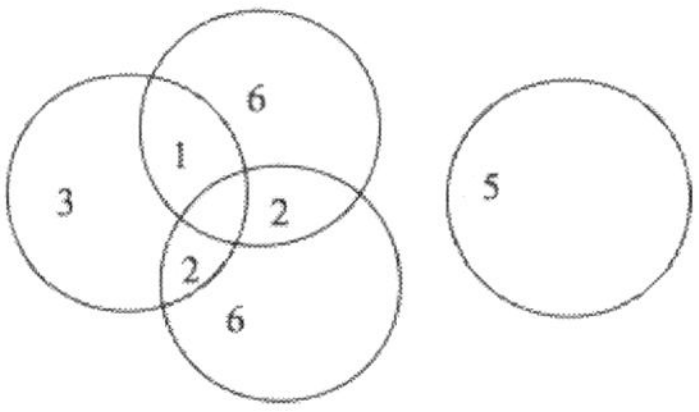

D.

Question 41

A popular confectionary manufacturer analyses their yearly sales. They have 5 main products. All numbers are given in 1 ton batches and each batch has the same value. Their first product has sold 10 000 batches. That is 10% more than the previous year. Product 2 has been sold in 500 batches, which represents a 95% drop in sales since the last year. Product 3 has been sold 12 000 times, representing an increase of 30% from last year. Products 4 and 5 have been sold 5000 times which is the same amount as the previous year in both cases.

Which of the following conclusions must be correct?

A. The company has made more money than the previous year.
B. The company has grown internationally.
C. The company has made less money than last year.
D. None of the above.

Question 42

A plastic surgeon claims that the majority of procedures he does fall into 4 main categories, listed according to prevalence: liposuction, nose reconstruction, facial lifting and eye surgery. They all have roughly equal durations, but the price of the surgeries varies. A nose reconstruction costs roughly £500, liposuction costs £300, facial lifting costs £700 and eye surgery costs £900. The prices are graded according to clinical difficulty.

Which of the following is not a valid conclusion?

A. The surgeon does only private work.
B. The surgeon does more liposuction that eye surgeries.
C. Eye surgery is the most challenging procedure.
D. Nose reconstruction is more difficult than liposuction but less difficult than facial lifting.

Question 43

In a group of 4 friends, each has a 50% chance that they are currently smoking. Given at least two of them are currently non-smokers.

Is the probability that there are 2 smokers 50%?

A. Yes, since there is a 50% chance of one of the friends smoking.
B. Yes, since two friends are non-smokers.
C. No, since any one of them might have smoked in the past.
D. No, since the chance of both of them being smokers is 25%.

Question 44

Studies show that children from families where both parents have university degrees are twice as likely to successfully complete a university degree themselves than children from families where only one of the two has a university degree. These families in turn are twice as likely to complete a university degree than children from families where neither parent has a university degree.

Which one of the following conclusions must be correct?

A. The education system must be reformed.
B. Families where only one of the parents have university degrees are more likely to be wealthy.
C. Universities are used to maintain old relationships of master and servant.
D. None of the above.

Question 45

On a particularly busy night in an accident and emergency department in a London hospital, the staff members conduct a study into the reason of visit. The study identifies 5 main reasons for patients to seek help.

A presentation due to respiratory causes was twice as likely as a presentation due to cardiovascular causes.
The chance of being admitted due to abdominal disease was 15%, making it proportionally 10% less common than cardiovascular causes. Traffic accidents and work accidents were equally as common.

Which of the following is true?

A. 5% of cases were due to traffic accidents.
B. 50% of cases were due to cardiovascular reasons.
C. The likelihood of a patient presenting with respiratory problems was 15%.
D. None of the above.

Question 46

A paediatric unit conducts a study into the prevalence of allergies in the children that are admitted to the unit. They find that 15% of children have allergies, with the majority of them, 65%, being food intolerances such as nut allergies. This was followed by contact allergies to latex, accounting for 10% of allergies. Other common allergies included dust and pollen.

Which of the following conclusions are correct?

A. Allergies are a problem affecting a large proportion of children.
B. Roughly 10% of all children have food allergies.
C. Nuts are the most common reason for allergies.
D. Dust and pollen allergies are much more common in adults.

Question 47

In the wild, chimpanzees have been observed to be using simple tools for food gathering as well as for hunting. It is not uncommon to see them fishing with sticks for algae or see them use rocks for opening nuts and seeds. In particular, over the last two decades, this has become an increasingly common observation.

Which of the following conclusions cannot be reasonably drawn?

A. Chimpanzees are becoming more intelligent.
B. Chimpanzees understand the effect of tools.
C. Chimpanzees are able to manipulate their environment.
D. None of the above.

Question 48

Carl and his friends want to build a treehouse. They know that they will need strong material as all 5 of them are supposed to be able to be on the treehouse at the same time. They calculate that the platform must be able to hold 225kg of weight for all of them as well as the structure of the house itself.

Carl is 10kg heavier than Alex.
Peter is the lightest of them, weighing 35kg.
Ben is the same weight as Alex
Luke weighs 5kg more than Alex and 10kg more than Peter.

Which of the following must be true?

A. Carl is neither the heaviest nor the lightest.
B. Ben weighs 10kg less than Carl.
C. The house can weigh up to 25kg.
D. Luke is the heaviest.

Question 49

A group of scientists study different subspecies of a spider family. They find that some of the subspecies share traits with one another, whilst others have nothing in common.

Group A shares some traits with group C.
Group C shares traits with group D but not with Group B.
Group C shares traits with A.
Group E shares traits with groups A.
Group E shares traits with group C but with neither Group A nor Group B.

Which of the following represents the interrelation between the groups the best?

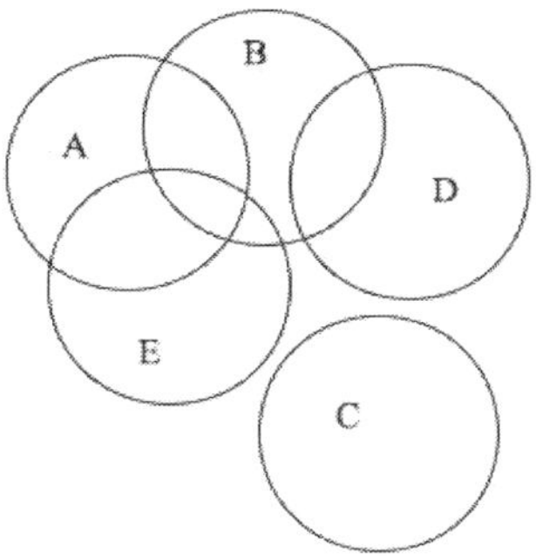

A.

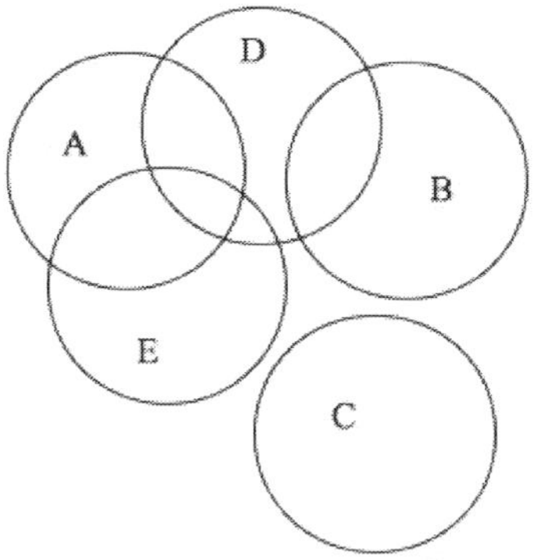

C.

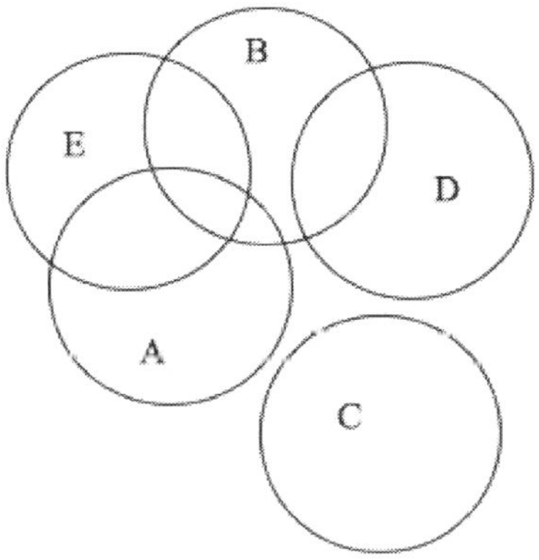

B.

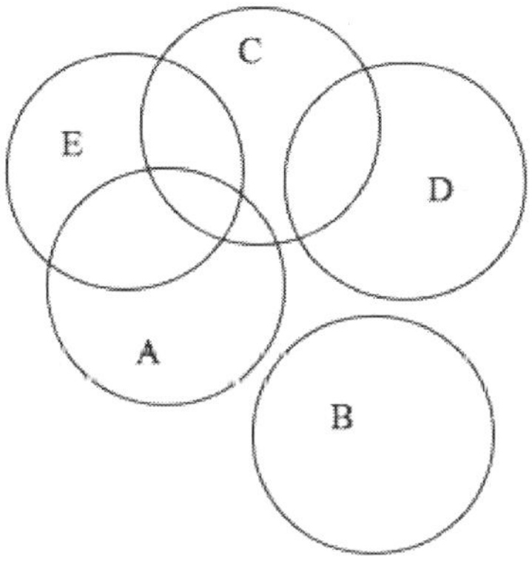

D.

Question 50

Ant colonies are organised as large units with clear distribution of responsibility amongst individual groups of individuals, coordinated by communication mechanisms. They are headed by a queen and thereby represent a female dominant society. Some species of ants feed of plant material, other species feed of animal material. Multiple colonies can exist in proximity leading to intraspecies competition but little interspecies competition.

Which of the following must be true?

A. Ants compete amongst individuals for food.
B. Ants of different colonies, but of the same species work together to displace ants from different species.
C. Ant colonies exist based on distribution of labour.
D. Ants are exclusively herbivores.

Question 51

Should the use of pesticides be outlawed by the government? Select the strongest argument from the list below.

A. Yes, pesticides should be outlawed as they are unnatural.
B. No, pesticides should not be outlawed as they allow the UK food industry to remain internationally competitive.
C. Yes, pesticides should be outlawed as they carry significant health risks for the consumer.
D. No, pesticides should not be outlawed as they represent an important branch of industry employing many workers

Question 52

Peter loves pink marbles. They represent the majority of marbles he owns. His sister likes marbles too. She has mainly blue ones but also some yellow and green ones. She trades him some of these for some of his pink ones. Now Peter also has a few yellow and green marbles, but he does not like them as much.

Select true or false for the conclusions below

A. Peter likes blue marbles.
B. Peter has less green marbles than pink ones.
C. Peter has no yellow marbles.
D. Peter should not play with marbles as they are a choking hazard.

Question 53

Ancient peoples in hunter gatherer societies lived a nomadic lifestyle, roaming freely through the forests of Europe. Before developing the technology needed for cultivation of grain, the majority of their food consisted of meat as this was available year around. After developing farming and setting up settlements, the proportion of non-meat food materials in their diet increased to include grain and other produce as well as by-products of animal farming.

Which of the following conclusions are false?

A. Hunting represented an important food source for our ancestors.
B. Farming formed the basis of settlement development.
C. Nomadic people tend to have a lower proportion of farm produced foods in their diet.
D. None of the above.

Question 54

Different studies have demonstrated that physical activity in children increases their cognitive performance.

Which one of the following conclusions can be drawn from this?

A. Exercise should play a bigger role in school life.
B. Leading a sedentary life style can have detrimental effects on intellectual development of children.
C. Children that are members in sports clubs are likely to perform better at school.
D. All of the above.

Question 55

Recently NASA discovered several planets that stand in a similar constellation to their sun as our planet does with our sun. This led to general conclusion that there are further inhabitable planets in the universe.

Which of the following assumptions must be met in order for this conclusion to be true?

A. The new planets must meet other pre-requisites for life such as air and water.
B. The planets are already inhabited.
C. The sun the new planets are related to must be stronger than ours.
D. None of the above.

Question 56

Different birds have different food preferences. Species A mainly eats sunflower seeds, but if that is not available may fall back to pumpkin seeds. Species B has grown particularly strong jaws allowing them to break open the hard shells of hazelnuts which represent their favoured food source. Species C mainly lives off berries, but will also eat the smaller seeds or insects if berries are not available. Species D lives off smaller insects.

Which of the following is true?

A. Species B lives off berries.
B. Species D has a strong beak to kill its insect pray.
C. Species A exclusively eats pumpkin seeds.
D. Species C is adapted to all seasons.

Question 57

NHS employees should be encouraged not to smoke, drink or be overweight as they represent important role-models to society.

Which represents the biggest problem with this statement?

A. Healthcare professionals are not role-models for society.
B. Politicians are more important in guiding public opinion.
C. This statement limits freedom of choice.
D. Drinking, smoking and obesity represent important health risks.

Question 58

A group of scientists conducted a study into the purchasing behavior of young men. The find that having positive experiences such as holidays has the greatest effect in encouraging purchase, whereas advertising depicting products themselves without a theme has the least effect on encouraging purchase. Other effective techniques to encourage purchase seem to be financial success or social interaction such as with friends.

Which of the following statements are correct?

A. Financial gain is powerful advertising tool.
B. Advertising is most effective if exclusively focused on the product itself.
C. Young women are most encouraged to make purchases by positive experiences.
D. None of the above.

Question 59

A company groups applicants into different populations depending on the type of experiences they bring to the table.

Most applicants posses good excel skills, but only few have good photoshop skills.
Some of those that have good photoshop skills, speak more than one language.
A proportion of those that speak more than one language also have excellent communication skills.
Very few applicants speak only English, but have great experience from previous jobs.

Which of the following represents the distribution of applicants the most accurately?

A.

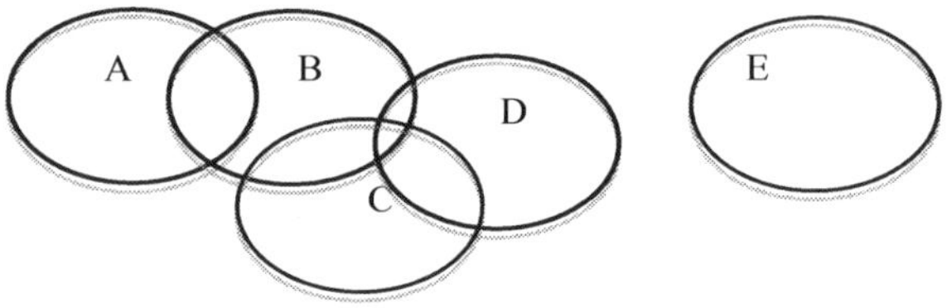

B.

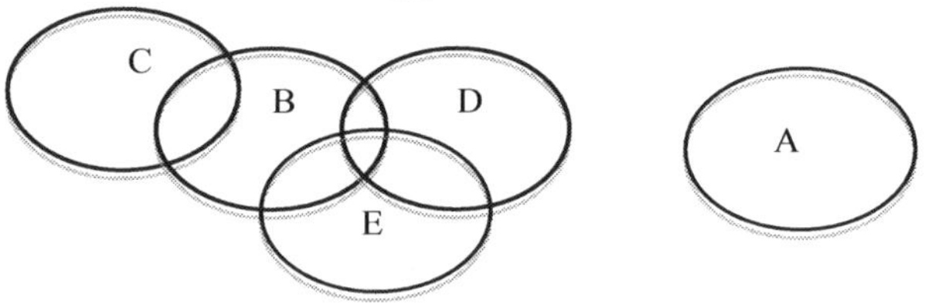

C.

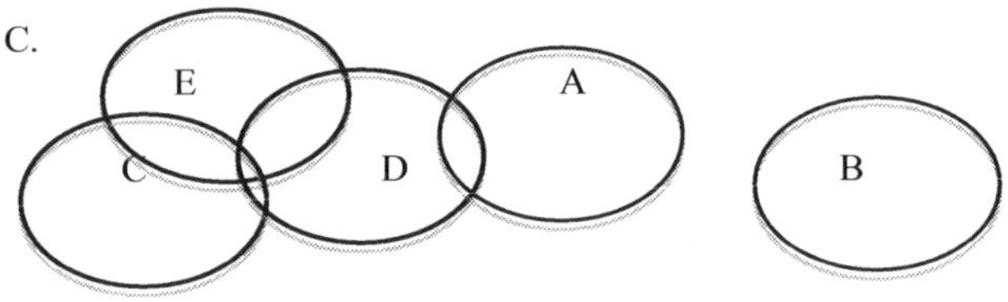

D.

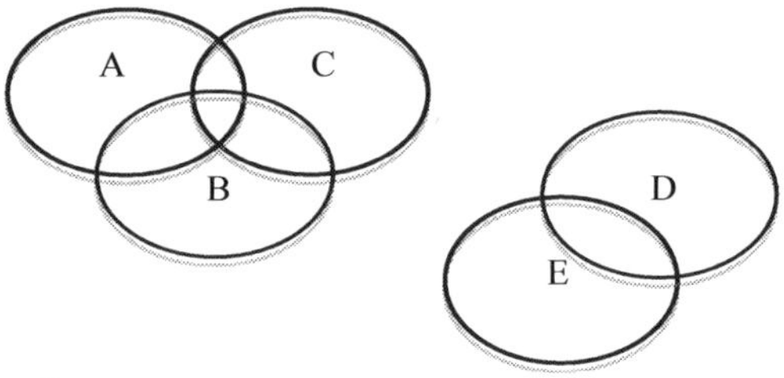

Question 60

A group of five friends compare the results of a recent maths test. Tom finds he achieved the highest score in all three sections. Richard has the second best score in sections A and B but the worst score in section C. Tony has the same result as Richard in section C, and worse results than Anthony in sections A and B. Anthony is in the middle field achieving 50% of all possible points in all three sections. Steve finished better than Richard in section C, but worse than Anthony in sections A and B.

Which of the following is false?

A. Tom has the best results.
B. Steve has a higher score than Tony.
C. Anthony has worse results for section A and B than Richard.
D. Richard finishes well in section C.

Question 61

A tobacco company orders research into the effects of a new cigarette that is supposed to be less toxic than the current most common cigarettes on the market. The results show that the new cigarette has a lower tar content than competitor brands, but the amount of nicotine is twice as high and so is the amount of carbon monoxide that's inhaled. They also find that there is significantly more nitrous oxide released from the new cigarette than from competition blends.

Which of the following is correct?

A. The new cigarette leads to less carbon monoxide being inhaled.
B. The new cigarette contains more tar being inhaled.
C. The competitors blend had to be smoked in twice the amount to reach the same nicotine level.
D. Overall the new cigarette blend is associated with less toxicity.

Question 62

A train travels from Elmsworth to Southwarf. The trip takes a total of 120mins. After 30mins of travel the train reaches the Eastwich where it stops for 5mins. After that it travels for another 45mins to reach Northtown. From Northtown the trip to Southwarf takes another 30mins, but the train waits for 5mins at the station before setting off on the journey.

Which of the following is correct?

A. The trip from Elmsworth to Northtown takes 70mins.
B. Eastwich lies 60mins away from Southwarf.
C. The train waited for 5mins at Northtown.
D. All of the above.

Question 63

A sports club publishes the results of a local football tournament. There are a total of 5 teams taking part but only the first 2 teams will receive a prize. In the scoring system, a victory will deliver 3 points, a loss will deliver 0 and a draw will deliver 1 point to each team. In the tournament each team plays each other team once.

Team A wins against team E and C, but draws against team B and loses to team D.
Team B never wins but finishes with 3 points.
Team C wins against Team E and draws with Team B.
Team D does not lose or draw any games.

Which of the following are correct?

A. Team D will finish with the second most points.
B. Team E draws with team B.
C. Team C will finish first.
D. It is customary for the best 3 teams to receive a prize.

Question 64

Every year there is a discussion surrounding the discontinuation of daylight saving time.

Which of the following represents the strongest argument in support of this?

A. Daylight saving is not necessary as it was introduced during the resource shortage of World War 1 and now this war is long over.
B. It is confusing to citizens who forget to change their watches.
C. It causes Jetlag.
D. Especially in the early months of spring it places the end of school in a dangerous twilight time causing increased casualties to road traffic accidents.

Question 65

Tim plans to run a marathon. For that he asks his friends to place themselves at different intervals from the start line to hand him snacks and sports drinks. He places his friend Chris at 15km after the start line. Anne stands 31km after the start line followed by Tara 5km after her. His friend Peter is placed 2km before the finish. Philip stands 10km up race from Chris.

Which of the following is true?

A. Chris stands 10km from Anne.
B. Philip is the first friend Tim will pass.
C. The distance between snack stops decreases towards the end of the race .
D. All of the above.

Question 66

"When conducting research, all funding with corporate interest should be refused."

Select the strongest argument supporting this statement.

A. The government should fund all research.
B. Corporations never deliver enough funding.
C. Research should not be about the money.
D. Corporate funding can restrict impartial research.

Question 67
Lisa likes to put her 5 dolls in a specific order when she puts them away on her shelf at the end of the day.

Tina always sits next to Annette.
Annette sits the furthest from Stephanie.
Patricia sits next to Tina.

Stephanie				

Which of the following is correct?

A. Patricia sits next to Annette.
B. Tina must sit at the edge.
C. Sophie must sit next to Stephanie.
D. Patricia does not sit in the middle.

Question 68
When it comes to the actions of the individual, there are several priorities influencing behaviour. Factors like socialization and inter-personal relationships can influence this decision making as well as some degree of individual variability. It is for this reason that we can find all kinds of behavioral patterns in people from all different walks of life, independent of the cultural background, but they all follow similar patterns.

Which of the following conclusions can be drawn from the above?

A. People make choices based on fixed patterns that show little variability.
B. Certain behavioral traits are associated with specific social classes.
C. Poor people will always act differently than rich people.
D. None of the above.

Question 69
Steve ranks his 5 university applications.

He really wants to go to Cambridge.
He ranks Sheffield in third place, behind Imperial.
He places Southampton between Cardiff and Sheffield.

Cambridge				

Which of the following is correct?

A. Cardiff must be his last choice.
B. Sheffield is higher up in his ranking than Imperial.
C. His first choice is Oxford.
D. All his universities are private schools.

Question 70
If we don't change our wasteful, consumerist behavior, we as a species will fail.

Which of the following represents the strongest argument in support of this question?

A. Consumerism is bad.
B. Due to the increasing shortage of resources, we must start to conserve resources more.
C. Capitalism is based on consumerism.
D. Our current behavior is damaging to the Earth upon which we rely for sustenance.

Question 71
Tim is going to the dentist. He hates going to the dentist. In order to make the visit easier for him, he tries to distract himself with little games that keep his mind occupied and prevent him from focusing on what is going on around him. His favorite coping mechanism is reciting poetry in his head. He also likes to tell himself stories that distract him.

Which of the following is true?

A. Tom hates dentists.
B. Tim likes poetry.
C. Coping mechanisms are the best way to deal with stressful situations.
D. All of the above.

Question 72
A group of scientists research swarm patterns of small fish. They find that there is a great degree of coordination between the individual fishes in the swarm in order to maintain a tight group. They also find that swarm patterns seem to be particularly successful in more murky water in comparison to very clear water. There is also a difference in success rate depending on the eyesight of the number one predator in the area, worse eye sight seems to increase protection to the individual.

Which of the following conclusions can be drawn?

A. Large fish never swim in swarm patterns.
B. The water temperature is a central factor in swarm formation.
C. The better the eyesight of the predator, the more success swarm patterns show in protecting the individual.
D. There seems to be a visual component to the success of swarm formations in protecting the individual.

Question 73
A political party is trying to determine the most popular topics in order to prepare their manifesto for the next general election. They produce a survey asking people to select the topic they find most pressing. 50% of people consider health care to be essential. Defense spending is considered the most essential by only 10% of people filling in the survey. Education comes in as the second highest priority, accounting for 25%. The remaining people consider infrastructure to be the most relevant.

Which of the following is correct?

A. Healthcare is not an issue in this population.
B. The population must feel very secure.
C. The study is flawed as it has too few choices.
D. Infrastructure is an important issue for 15% of people.

Question 74
A local political leader conducts a survey into the key interests of his constituents. He finds that the issues can be reduced to five main issues: Education, housing, health care, smoking policy and public cleanliness. Education is the most important point accounting for 28% of votes, followed by housing which is most important to 5% less of the voters. The least important issue is smoking policy, a priority for only 11% of people, which places it behind public cleanliness policy which represents 16% of all votes.

				Smoking

Which of the following conclusions is incorrect?

A. Health care is more important than public cleanliness policy.
B. Housing is more important than public health.
C. Smoking is the least important issue.
D. Housing policy accounts for 22% of votes.

Question 75
The mating behavior of birds heavily relies on the use of loud calls that are designed to attract the attention of a female to the male where the loud call originates. They are species specific, though there can also be a certain degree of mimicry when it comes to breeding calls. The amount of different calls varies depending on the season and increases with the amount of birds that are actively looking for a sexual partner.

Which of the following conclusions can be drawn from the above text?

A. It never happens that one bird uses another species' mating call.
B. Birds are the most active in the summer.
C. Females sing to attract males.
D. None of the above.

Question 76
Elephants are highly social animals. They live in groups that are led by a single older female elephant, and the main aim of the group is to protect the young whilst providing the most stable social environment for the young to grow up. For this reason, young males are often excluded from the groups in order to prevent conflict for hierarchical reasons and to encourage the young males to find their own herd, thereby also contributing to genetic variability by preventing inbreeding.

Which of the following statements about elephant behavior is correct?

A. Elephants live in group led by males.
B. Elephant groups include young animals that are protected by the group.
C. Female elephants share the responsibility of leading the group.
D. All of the above.

Question 77
A group of monkeys is found to prefer yellow fruit to all other types of fruit. They will also eat red fruit. They never eat green fruit.

Which of the following statements is true?

A. The monkeys prefer red fruit to green fruit.
B. The monkeys eat four different colored fruits.
C. As the monkeys don't eat the green fruits, they must be poisonous.
D. The statement is flawed as the data is too limited.

Question 78
A group is only as strong as its weakest member.

Which of the following statements most supports this theory?

A. Groups consist of individuals, so without them, there is no group.
B. A large group is better than a smaller one.
C. Groups are based on division of labour, therefore struggling members will limit efficiency.
D. All of the above.

Question 79
A mobile phone company takes stock of the sales of their 5 different handsets. In total they sold 10,000 handsets in the last year.

Set A sold the most, accounting for 4,000 units sold.
Set B and C sold to equal shares.
Set D sold 1,500 units.
Set E sold worst, with only 500 units sold.

		Set C		

Which of the following statements is true?

A. Set C sold 2,000 units.
B. Set B sold 2,500 units.
C. Set E must be the most expensive.
D. Set D is the second most sold handset.

Question 80

Different types of trees prefer different conditions. A study delivers the following results:

Walnut trees like moist ground but secrete a poison that prevents any other trees from growing around them.
Willow trees like darker and moist areas.
Beeches grow high and grow in pretty much all areas.
Oaks dislike moist areas.

Which of the following best represents the individual relationships?

A.

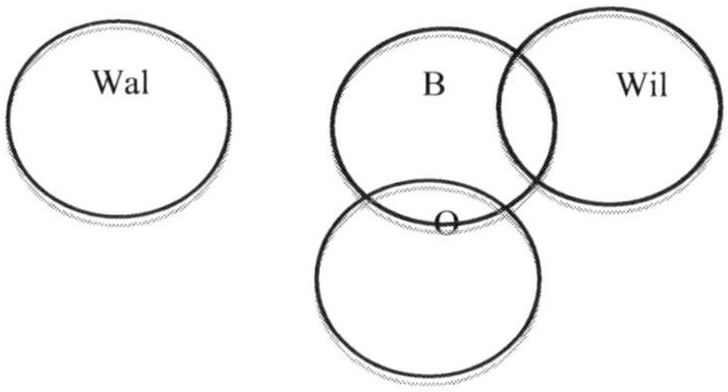

B.

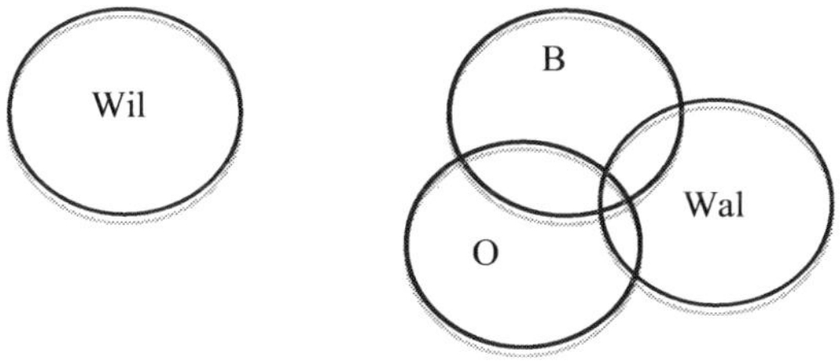

C.

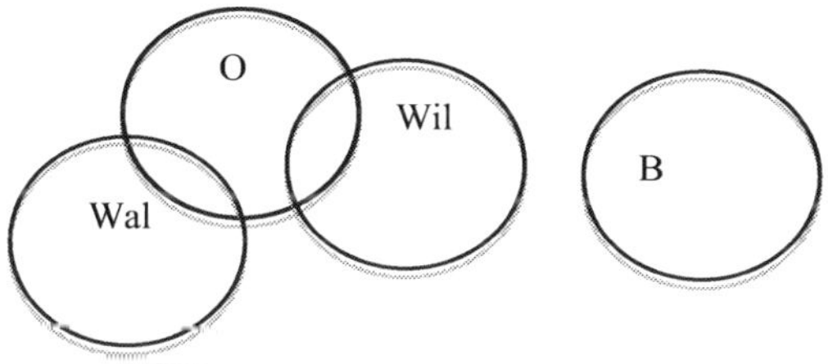

D.

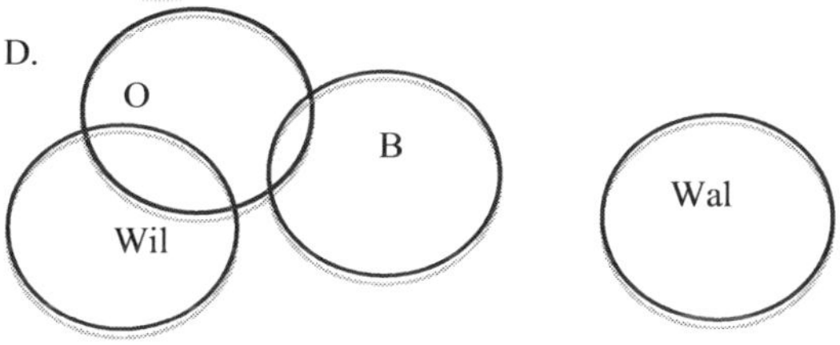

Question 81

Five friends decide to order take-away. They decide to order Chinese food, as 80% of the group are happy with Chinese. They order three portions of egg fried rice, two portions of beef spring rolls, 2 portions of sweet and sour chicken and one portion of sweet and sour duck. They also order two fish dishes.

Which of the following conclusions can be reasonably drawn?

A. 4 of the friends wanted Chinese food.
B. There are vegans in the group.
C. One friend wanted Pizza instead of Chinese.
D. One of the friends must have an allergy to eggs as they only order three portion of egg fried rice.

Question 82
After a local sports tournament, the leader table of countries is published, based on gold medals achieved. All different groups have the same number of athletes and there is a total of 5 groups.

Group A achieves 5 gold medals, 7 silver medals and no bronze medals.
Group B achieves 6 gold medals, 2 silver medals and 1 bronze medal.
Group C Ranks highest.
Group D achieves 1 gold medal and 10 silver medals as well 3 bronze medals.
Group E achieves 3 bronze medals.

				Group E

Which of the following is correct?

A. Group A ranks higher than group B.
B. Group C has achieved at least 7 gold medals.
C. Group D finishes last.
D. Group C has more Bronze medals than group D.

Question 83
Scientists have found that due to the change in temperatures during the winter, the behavior of birds that normally fly South for warmer climates is changing. They now are more likely to stay in their normal habitat without migrating. This results in a constant presence of the birds which influences predator as well as prey populations. Feeding habits of humans in developed countries have however helped to counterbalance the increased pressure on prey populations.

Which of the following conclusions cannot be drawn from the text?

A. Migratory birds provide important prey to predators.
B. Climate change has reduced bird migration
C. It must be getting colder in the South which prevents bird migration.
D. Predatory animals provide a degree of population control on migratory birds.

Question 84
Tim only owns black clothes – except for sports clothes, where he also owns some green ones. His parents then gave him a pair of blue trousers for his birthday.

Select true or false for each of the following statements

A. Tim has no coloured clothes.
B. Tim owns red clothes.
C. Tim only owns suits.
D. Most of Tim's sports clothes are green.

Question 85
A rowing club celebrates their 100th birthday by holding a 2000m race. Anthony, Peter, Eugene, David and John compete against each other.

Anthony finishes the race after David.
Peter is 3 seconds faster than Eugene.
John is one second slower than Eugene, but faster than David.

		John		

Select true or false for each of the following statements

A. David is last to finish.
B. Peter has the fastest time.
C. John is between Eugene and David.
D. Anthony is slower than Peter.

Question 86

In order to ensure a fair distribution of health care funds, healthy behavior must be enforced through the penalizing of unhealthy actions such as smoking or eating unhealthy foods.

Select the strongest argument against the statement above.

A. Penalties rarely work to change behaviour.
B. Health care funds cannot be allocated fairly.
C. Penalizing unhealthy actions restricts freedom of choice.
D. In order to distribute heath care funds fairly, the richest in society must pay more.

Question 87

Scientists investigate the feeding behavior of bears. Bears are omnivores that feed on meat as well as plants. They find that bears will always prefer berries over any other type of food. Scientists believe that this is due to their sweet taste. They also find that bears do not tend to hunt, but rather tend to eat the meat of freshly deceased animals. They have been seen chasing away other predators in order to steal their catch. This suggests that bears actually are more gatherers than hunters and will only actively attack if cornered or if considering their offspring to be in danger.

Which of the following conclusions can be drawn from the above text?

A. Bears frequently hunt small animals like rabbits and squirrels.
B. Bears prefer seeds over berries.
C. Bears tend to abandon their young if threatened.
D. None of the above.

Question 88

Ants are investigated for their social behaviour. Scientists come to the following conclusions:

Some ants are exclusively responsible for construction work.
Some ants take part in hunting and a proportion of those also play a role in protection of the nest.
Male ants exclusively exist for reproduction.

Which of the following most accurately depicts the relationship between the different roles of ants?

A.

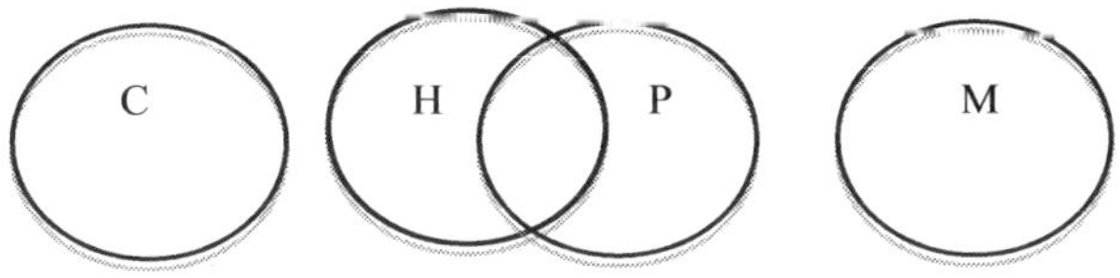

B.

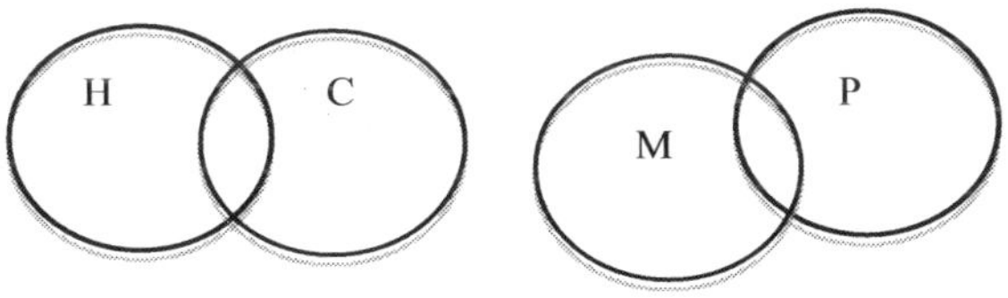

C.

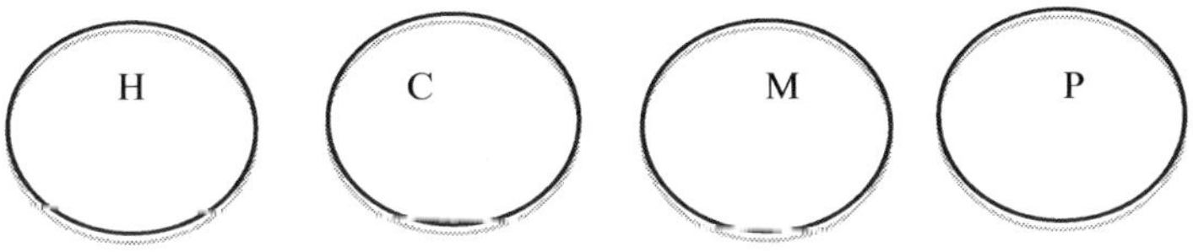

D.

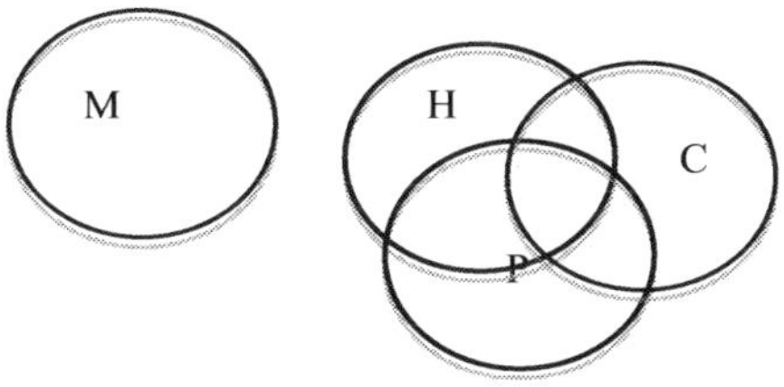

Question 89

Annette is planting a garden. She really likes raspberry jam, so exclusively plants raspberry bushes. There are also some blackberry bushes there. Her husband then decides to plant some cherry trees as well.

Select whether the statements below are true or false.

A. There are no trees in the garden.
B. There is only fruit in the garden.
C. Annette does plant cherry trees.
D. Annette did not plant anything but raspberry bushes.

Question 90

In order to improve our health, we must make an effort to avoid unhealthy foods.

Which of the following arguments most strongly opposes this statement?

A. Health is always dependent on the individual.
B. The definition of unhealthy foods is too imprecise to be of any use
C. This statement encourages fat shaming.
D. All of the above.

Question 91

Stanley decides to build a wardrobe for his new bedroom. He measures the room and finds that he will need to make his wardrobe 75cm wide in order to have space for all his clothes and he decides to make it 2 meters high in order to take full advantage of the ceiling space available. He decides to use the more expensive Walnut wood because he prefers the darker color in comparison to pine. He also decides to use nails instead of screws because he does not have a drill and does not want to buy one. This increases the risk of the wardrobe collapsing.

Which of the following statements is correct?

A. The wardrobe will be large.
B. Nails hold less securely than screws.
C. Pine is darker than Walnut.
D. Peter will need to help him.

Question 92

In order to deliver the highest quality product at the most affordable price possible, a company conducts research into different materials to use for their product. They know that their product needs to be deliver a good compromise of cost, tensile strength, weather resistance and head resistance.

Material A delivers good cost effectiveness and weather resistance, but poor tensile strength and little heat resistance.
Material B delivers good tensile strength, weather resistance and hear resistance, but is very expensive.
Material C is a 50/50 mix of Materials A and B resulting in good tensile strength and excellent weather resistance and heat resistance.

Which of the following conclusions is true?

A. Material A is ideal for a good product.
B. Material B must be steel.
C. Material C must be expensive.
D. Materials A and B do not interact to achieve new properties.

Question 93

A magazine ranks 5 different companies according to annual income.

Company A makes $100,000, which is twice as much as company B.
Company C makes 10% less than company A.
Company D is the smallest company and only makes $75,000.
Company E makes the least.

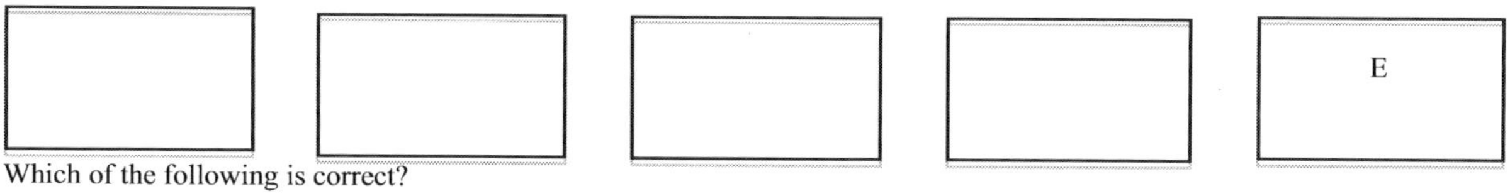

Which of the following is correct?

A. Company A makes the most.
B. Company B makes more than company C.
C. Company D is amongst the larger companies.
D. Company E must be going bankrupt.

Question 94

Cheryl analyzes the relationships of her friends for a school project. She finds that Sarah gets along well with Tina and Marylin, but not at all with Peter and Astrid. Peter gets along with everybody but Sarah. Tina gets along well with Peter and Sarah, but not with Astrid. Astrid gets along well with Peter.

Which of the following best represents the interaction of Cheryl's friends?

A.

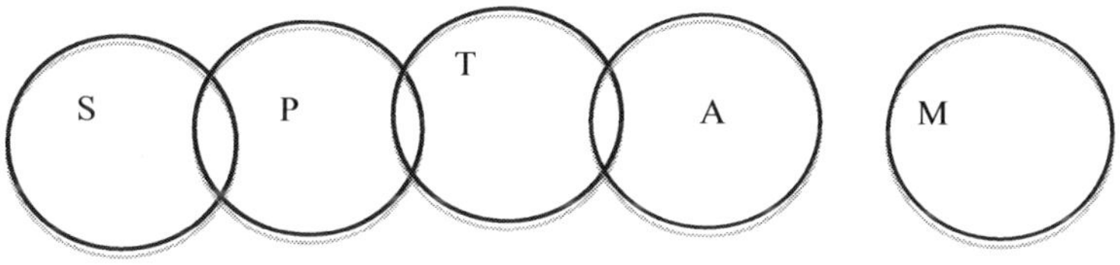

B.

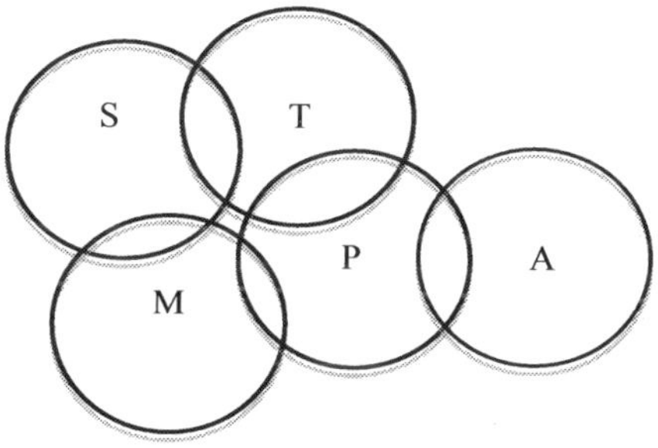

C.

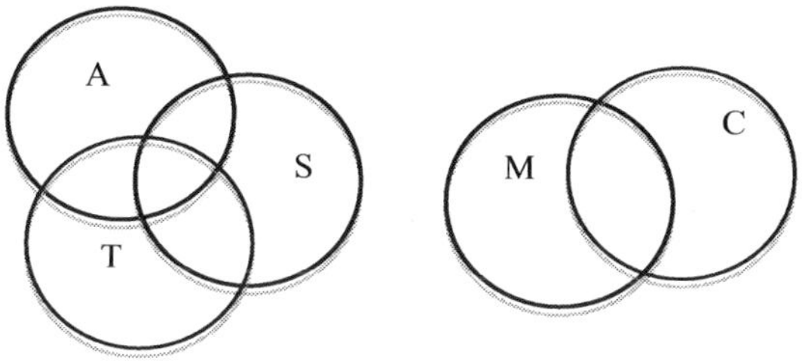

D.

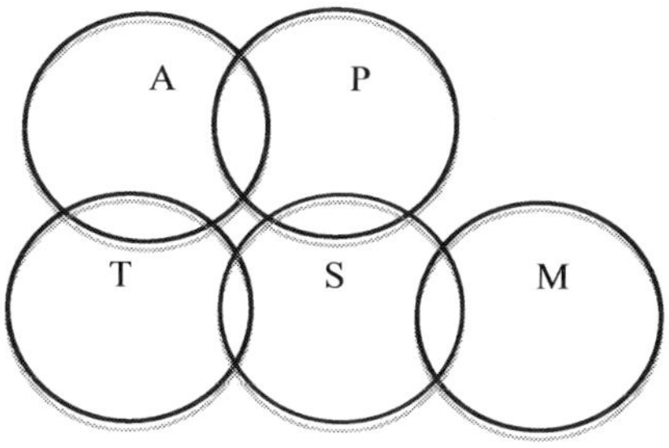

Question 95

A group of scientist investigates the link between population density and the density of newspapers. They find that as populations grow, the amount of newspapers increases until it reaches a ceiling from where it declines as population growth continues. In addition to that they find that the remaining newspapers can increasingly easily be classed into two opposing camps that tend to approach issues from polar opposites.

Which of the following statements is true with regards to the text above?

A. The media is a tool to make us believe in the theories of the politicians.
B. At a certain point population growth is inversely proportional to newspaper density.
C. There are always only two sides to a story.
D. None of the above.

Question 96

A school conducts a survey of their 200 students to find out about their individual job aspirations. They find that they are essentially limited to 5 categories.

10% of children want to be politicians.
40% of children have not chosen a profession yet.
50 children want to be doctors.
20 children want to be actors.
More children want to be teachers than actors.

Which of the following statements is correct?

A. More children want to be politicians than actors.
B. The majority of children want to be doctors.
C. 80 children don't know what they want to be yet.
D. More children want to be politicians than teachers.

Question 97

Philipp and Tom play for Port Town United FC. Philipp scores in every game of the football season. Tom only scores in half the games. In the last game, neither Tom nor Philipp score. In every game Tom scores, Philipp scores at least the same number of goals as Tom. In every game that Tom scores, Port Town never lose. Neither Philipp nor Tom have been sent off in the season.

Which of the following statements is supported by the text?

A. Philipp scores more goals than Tom.
B. Tom scores in the last game of the season.
C. The last game of the season must have been a loss.
D. Tom is better than Philipp.

Quantitative Reasoning

The Basics

The Quantitative Reasoning subtest tests your ability to quickly interpret data and perform relevant calculations upon them. Section 3 contains 36 questions and you have 24 minutes to answer them, giving a total of 40 seconds per question – slightly more generous than the verbal reasoning section. As with all UCAT sections, you have one additional minute to read the instructions at the start.

There are different types of question you can be asked in Section 3, but all involve interpreting a numerical data source and performing calculations. This is all about testing your natural ability with numbers, how easily you understand numbers and how well you can make calculations based upon new data. You won't find advanced mathematics, so you are at absolutely no disadvantage by not taking A-level maths. Common sources include food menus, timetables, sales figures, surveys, conversion tables and more. All questions have 5 options of which only one is correct.

In this section, the whiteboard you are provided can be useful – use it to scribble down working and intermediate numbers as required.

There is an on screen calculator – a basic calculator for performing arithmetic. You should ideally **practice with a non-scientific calculator** when working through this book, as that will give the closest simulation to what you will get on the day. When you move on to trying the online UCAT practice papers, the calculator is available on screen as you will see it in the test. In addition to using it to solve questions, practice different calculations to build your speed using it – though this sounds boring, it will save you valuable time on the day. Something many candidates do not realise is that the calculator can be operated using the keyboard controls. Try this out for yourself in practice, and if it works for you it is yet another way to boost your speed when you come to the UCAT for real. If not then it's fine, it can be used with the mouse too and you will at least be properly prepared, knowing the best approach for you.

Preparation

Be comfortable using the on-screen calculator

As discussed, it's important to know exactly how the calculator works so that you use it quickly and most effectively during the test. Also make sure you know which functions the calculator has, and does not have. Practice using the calculator until you're really familiar with it to ensure you waste no time on the day. Use the automated practice section of the UCAT website for this – that way, you practice using the same software you will use on the day.

Practice common question styles

Be especially comfortable with things like bus and rail timetables, sales figures, surveys, converting units and working with percentage changes in both directions. These are commonplace in the UCAT –, but could prove awkward if you're rusty. Likewise be sharp on your simple arithmetic – it might seem basic, but a good knowledge of times tables will save you a lot of time. Even if you're not answering questions, you can hone your skills by practicing reading charts, graphs and tables quickly.

Familiarise yourself with the format of diagrams

Working through plenty of practice questions will help here, as you'll see similar questions coming up again and again. Commonly you will need to use timetables, data tables and different types of graphs to answer Section 3 questions. Make sure you are comfortable with all of these styles of questions.

When looking at an unfamiliar diagram, a clear approach will help you quickly grasp what it shows. Candidates who let the time pressure stop them from properly interpreting the data are much more likely to lose marks. Avoid this common pitfall by following our approach below to quickly read complex data.

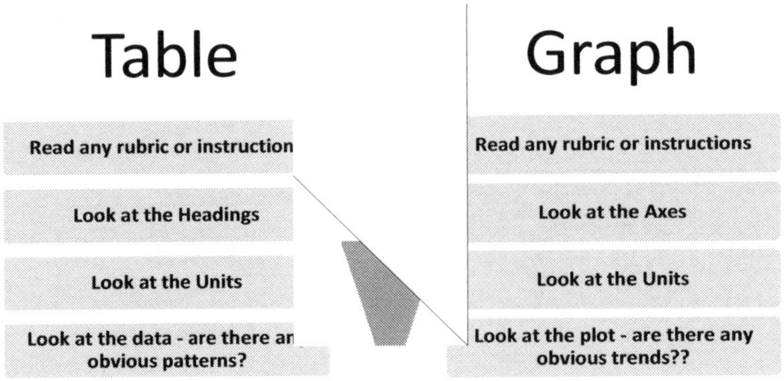

Mental Speed

The main challenge in most questions is finding the right data and selecting the appropriate calculation to perform, rather than the actual calculation itself. However, time is tight so you should be confident with addition, subtraction, multiplication, division, as well as working out percentages, fractions and ratios. Although there is an on-screen calculator in the test, you can save time by doing the basic sums in your head – being confident in your mental arithmetic ability will help you use the time most effectively. There are some good websites and apps to practice quick-fire mental arithmetic – using these you can quickly refresh these essential skills.

Answering Questions

Estimation

Estimation can be very helpful, particularly when the answers are significantly different. If, for instance, answers are an order of magnitude or more away from each other, you can ignore the fine print of the numbers and still get the right answer. If it's a particularly complicated calculation, quickly ask yourself roughly what answer you are expecting. With the simple UCAT calculator it can be easy to slip up – but if you've already made a quick estimation then you may be alerted to your mistake before you put the wrong answer down. Another important use of estimation is to generate educated guesses if you're short on time. In Section 3 there are five answers per question, so your odds of blindly guessing correctly are low. But here a simple estimation can help. A quick glance or simplified sum might help you eliminate a few answers in only seconds, boosting the chance your guess is correct.

Flagging for review

Flagging for review is so quick and easy, it can always be a useful tool. If you're finding a question difficult, or you've decided it is likely to take too long to solve, put a guess (or quick estimation if possible), flag for review and move on. This allows you to revisit the question at the end if there's time whilst using your time more efficiently elsewhere. When doing this you should make an initial guess, as this ensures you have at least a chance of being correct if you don't have enough time to come back again.

Pace yourself

In this section you have an average of 40 seconds per question, and this is a very useful guide to have. Of course some questions will take more or less time, but you should aim to work steadily forwards at roughly that pace. So after 6 minutes you should be about 9 questions in, and after 12 minutes should have completed about 18 questions and so on. By keeping a regular rhythm to your work, you ensure you don't leave lots of potentially easy questions at the end untouched. It's far better to skip a few tricky questions with a guess to make sure you make a decent effort at all questions, rather than wasting time with the hardest questions and missing out on easier marks.

Read the question first

If the data looks complex, it makes sense to look at the question first before beginning to interpret the data. Just like data-heavy questions in section 1, it can take a few moments to interpret the data provided. By reading the question first, you focus your mind, giving you a better focus to approach the data with and ensuring you only spend time analysing data you actually need to work from.

Top tip! Don't spend too long on any one question. In the time it takes to answer one hard question, you could gain three times the marks by answering three easier questions. *Make the most of every second!*

Example Questions

Example 1

An online company provides personalised sports kit with discounts for bulk purchases. Shipping rates are £4.99. All prices are quoted in pounds and are per item.

Having read the instru[redacted] you know what the tabl[redacted] show. Now look straight [redacted] question below so you [redacted] what to do with the data.

[redacted]			
1-10	4.99	5.59	5.99

No of I	Monotone Print	ulti-tone Prin	Embroidered Logo
	0.99	1.99	3.99
26-	0.29	0.89	2.99

A local hockey team requires 26 polo shirts with embroidere the back.
How much will this cost?

A. £194.01
B. £217.62
C. £222.61
D. £225.21
E. £240.81

This is a typical question. Find the right data in the table and start adding it up

Answer: C

This question highlights the need to read the question carefully as to use the correct data from the tables and is a relatively common type of question. If you look closely at the tables, you will realise that the number of items bracketed together changes between the tables. Watch out for this, or similar changes in unit, in the test. If you only skim over the tables you are in danger of missing this and will therefore get the question wrong. However, the calculation required is simple as is often the case, the question is more looking at your ability to pick out relevant data.

Price per polo shirt = 5.09 (base price) + 2.99 (embroidered logo) + 0.29 (monotone print) = £8.37
Price for 26 polo shirts as specified = 8.37 x 26 (number of items required) – £217.62
Total Price = 217.62 + 4.99 (shipping) = £222.61

Example 2

Sarah's route to work consists of an 8 minute walk followed by the 200 bus from Styal centre to Wilmslow station, the train from Wilmslow to Manchester Piccadilly and finally a 6 minute walk to her offices.

Styal centre	07.14	07.30	07.57
Wilmslow Centre	07.36	07.52	08.22

Alderley Edge	07.32	07.48	08.20
Manchester Oxford Road	08.23	08.39	09.11

If Sarah needs to arrive at her offices by 9.00, what time must she leave her house?

A. 07.08
B. 07.24
C. 07.30
D. 07.37
E. 07.49

Answer: D

Bus and train timetables are common questions and it is worth being comfortable working through them logically. On first glance of the question, there appears to be a lot of information. However, if you read the question carefully, you can simply work through the timetables from the end of the question. Split Sally's journey down into stages and consider each in turn – this splits the question so it is easily manageable and makes it less likely to make mistakes.

Sally must be at the offices for 09.00, therefore she must get into Manchester Piccadilly by 08.54 (6 minute walk). The latest train that gets into Manchester Piccadilly by 08.54 arrives in at 08.46. This train leaves Wilmslow Station at 08.12. The latest 200 bus that gets to Wilmslow Station by 08.12 arrives at 08.02. The 08.02 bus to Wilmslow Station leaves Styal Centre at 07.45. It takes Sally 8 minutes to walk to the bus stop therefore she must leave her house at 07.37.

Quantitative Reasoning Questions

SET 1

The country of Ecunemia has a somewhat complicated tax code. There are four states that make up Ecunemia: Asteria, Bolovia, Casova and Derivia. Each state has its own tax code, including different tax rates on different items. The table below represents the tax a **customer** has to pay when they purchase an item from a store.
E.g. a £100 coat in Asteria would cost £110.

	Asteria	Bolovia	Casova	Derivia
Clothes	10%	15%	10%	10%
Food	5%	0%	10%	0%
Imports from other states	20%	5%	10%	15%

The customer must add the tax onto the advertised purchase price. In the case of an item falling into multiple categories (for example, in the case of Imported Food) the higher tax rate is paid and the lower rate is ignored.

Question 1:
A shopper visits a certain supermarket. Without tax, the shopper spends \$50 on food, \$30 on clothes and nothing on imported items. She spends \$88 in total. Which state is this supermarket in?

A. Asteria
B. Bolovia
C. Casova
D. Derivia

Question 2:
Someone runs a supplier in Bolovia, supplying supermarkets in each state in Ecumenia. Each year they supply each state with 250 items of clothing, which the supermarket sells for \$40 (including tax), and the supplier gets all of this revenue, minus the tax paid. A competitor in Asteria goes out of business, and this supplier has the opportunity to buy the manufacturing plant for \$20,000, and transfer to this state.

If the supplier purchases the site, and moves to Asteria, how many years will it take to make back the cost of purchasing the site?

A. 5 years
B. 12 years
C. 23 years
D. 26 years

Question 3:
John goes into a store and spends \$100. Of this, \$12 is tax. Which of the following is possible?

A. He shopped in Asteria and bought no imported goods.
B. He shopped in Casova.
C. He shopped in Derivia and bought at least \$50 of food (excluding tax).
D. He shopped in Bolovia and spent \$10 on imported goods (excluding tax).

Question 4:
Sibella is on a road trip through Ecunemia, driving through different states. On the journey she buys \$100 of the finest Asterian ham, \$30 of the finest Bolovian caviar, a \$10 case of Casovan orange juice and spends \$100 on a Derivian dress (all of these prices without tax). Which of the following cannot have been the total amount Sibella spent, including tax?

A. \$256
B. \$264
C. \$273
D. \$288

SET 2

As a probe drops through the ocean, the pressure it experiences increases. For every 10 metres the probe drops down, the pressure it experiences increases by 10,000 Pascals (Pa).

Question 5:
A particular probe can survive 200 pounds per square inch without incurring damage. Given that the conversion factor between these units is 7000 Pa = 1 pound per square inch and assuming that pressure at sea level is 0 Pascals, how deep can the probe drop into the ocean without incurring damage?

A. 14 m
B. 140 m
C. 1.4 km
D. 14 km

Question 6:
A different probe is dropped into the ocean and falls downward. This probe can withstand 300,000 Pa of pressure without breaking. A model of the effect of the fluid states that the object's depth in the fluid is $d = \frac{1}{2}\sqrt{(t^3)}$, where d is depth in metres and t is time in seconds. How long will it take for this probe to break?

A. 65 seconds
B. 71 seconds
C. 75 seconds
D. 78 seconds.

SET 3

The fictional drug Cordrazine is used to treat four separate conditions. The following table gives the amount of drug used in each case to treat each condition, written in the form *x* mg/kg: i.e. for every kilogram you weigh, you take *x* mg of the drug. The recommended course for the drug is also listed, in the form of number of times a day and how many weeks you need to take the drug.

Condition	Dosage	Course
Black Trump Virus	4 mg/kg	3 times daily for 4 weeks
Swamp Fever	3 mg/kg	Once daily, 1 week
Yellow Tick	1 mg/kg	2 times daily for 12 weeks
Red Rage	5 mg/kg	2 times daily, 3 weeks

Question 7:
Over the course of treatment, John, an 80 kg male, takes 26.88 grams of the drug. Which disease was he prescribed the drug for?

A. Black Trump Virus
B. Swamp Fever
C. Yellow Tick
D. Red Rage

Question 8:
Carol is a 60 kg female who is prescribed the drug (precisely and at different times) three times in one year. Two of the cases are for Yellow Tick. In total she takes 40.32 grams of the drug. Which was the third disease she was prescribed the drug for?

A. Black Trump Virus
B. Swamp Fever
C. Yellow Tick
D. Red Rage

Question 9:
Clarence takes the drug twice in his life. Once he takes it for Swamp Fever at age 18, when he weighs 80 kg, and he takes it later in life at age 40 for Black Trump Virus, when he weighs 110 kg. What is the ratio of the amount he takes each time?

A. 1:23
B. 1:22
C. 1:21
D. 1:20

Question 10:
Danny has liver disease. His system cannot cope with more than 15.5 grams of Cordrazine every 4 weeks. Danny has a medical condition usually treated with Cordrazine, but doctors have advised him to not complete a course of the treatment, as he would exceed the dose that his system is able to cope with. Which of the following statements is possible?

A. Danny suffers from Red Rage and weighs 75 kg.
B. Danny suffers from Swamp Fever and weighs 100 kg.
C. Danny suffers from Black Trump and weighs 45 kg.
D. Danny suffers from Yellow Tick and weighs 75 kg.

Question 11:
Eileen has kidney failure. Her system cannot cope with more than 10 grams of Cordrazine every 4 weeks. She suffers from Red Rage, but doctors have recommended she does not use Cordrazine to treat it, as this would exceed the 10 g dosage her system can cope with. Which of the following weights is the minimum that would support this recommendation?

A. 40.34 kg
B. 42.53 kg
C. 45.81 kg
D. 47.62 kg

SET 4

A bakery sells four varieties of cakes. The cakes contain the following ingredients:

	Sponge (520g)	Madeira (825g)	Pound (710g)	Chocolate (885g)
Flour (g)	125	250	150	200
Butter (g)	125	175	185	175
Egg (g)	120	180	180	120
Milk (g)	25	45	45	150
Sugar (g)	125	175	150	200
Cocoa (g)	-	-	-	40

Question 12:
Which cake contains the highest proportion of flour?

A. Sponge
B. Madeira
C. Pound
D. Chocolate.

Question 13:
The cake recipes are scaled up for a large order. One cake weighs 2.6 kg and contains 625 g of flour. What variety of cake is it?

A. Sponge
B. Madeira
C. Pound
D. Chocolate

Question 14:
Eliza is having a wedding and wants to produce a 4-tiered wedding cake. She wishes each tier to be of different size, and scaled such that that the bottom cake is 50% heavier than normal (e.g. the cake contains 50% more ingredients), the second cake is 25% heavier than normal, the third cake is 10% heavier than normal and the top cake is normal-sized, where each cake is of the same type.

Which of the following is a possible weight of sugar for the cake (rounded to 2 s.f.)?

A. 940 g
B. 970 g
C. 1,000 g
D. 1,030 g

Question 15:
It is known that flour costs £0.55 per 1.5 kg and sugar costs £0.70 per 1 kg. Which of the following is the closest to the cost ratio of flour to sugar in a Madeira cake?

A. 1:2
B. 3:4
C. 4:5
D. 5:6

Question 16:
Milk costs £0.44 per kilogram and flour costs £0.55 per 1.5 kg. What is the cost ratio of flour to milk in a chocolate cake?

A. 1:1
B. 2:3
C. 8:7
D. 10:9

SET 5

The Kryptos Virus is particularly virulent. The infection rate is dependent upon the gender of the recipient. A random sample of 100 men and 100 women are taken from a population and tested for the Kryptos virus using Test A. The results of Test A are displayed below:

	Men	Women
Have virus	45	63
Do not have virus	55	37

Question 17:
What percentage of people tested have the virus?
A. 45%
B. 54%
C. 55%
D. 63%

Question 18:
A population of 231,768 is divided: 53% women, 47% men. Use the data in the table to estimate the number of people in the population that have the Kryptos virus. Assume that the infection rates in each gender will be the same as for the sample population in Test A. Which of the following is the number of people expected to be infected with Kryptos virus in this population?
A. 123,587
B. 123,589
C. 125,541
D. 126,406

Question: 19
3/9 of the men and 5/7 of the women testing positive for Kryptos in Test A have visited the city of Atlantis. Which of the following is the correct percentage of people in the test group testing positive for Kryptos who have **NOT** visited Atlantis?
A. 40%
B. 44%
C. 50%
D. 55%

Question 20:
It is known that Test A is not always correct. Test B is a more accurate test. The 45 men who tested positive for the Kryptos virus using Test A were then re-tested with Test B - only 20 tested positive. Assuming the same proportion of men and women experienced false positive results with Test A, how many women in the test group do we expect to actually have the Kryptos virus?
A. 20
B. 28
C. 35
D. 42

Question 21:
It is decided the women who tested positive under test A should be retested using test B. This time 29 women test positive for the Kryptos Virus. Considering both the men and women tested, what percentage of people who tested positive in Test A also tested positive in Test B (to the nearest whole number)?
A. 40%
B. 45%
C. 50%
D. 55%

SET 6

A business has 3 manufacturing plants and 3 stores. Each plant can ship to each store, and the following table shows the flat rate cost, in pounds sterling (£), of the business sending a truck from the plant to the store.

	Store 1	Store 2	Store 3
Plant A	100	190	530
Plant B	120	180	600
Plant C	140	200	450

Question 22:
Currently the businesses strategy is to send material from Plant A to store 2, from Plant B to store 3 and from Plant C to store 1. One truck is sufficient for a day's delivery. What is the daily cost of this plan?

A. £850
B. £930
C. £970
D. £1,030

Question 23:
The store wishes to optimize their shipping costs by sending material from Plant C to store 3, noticing that the delivery cost is lower. They then choose the two other options that save the most money. What percentage saving is achieved by this strategy relative to the strategy in the previous question (to the nearest whole number)?

A. 18%
B. 20%
C. 22%
D. 24%

SET 7

The table below shows the number of books sold by a bookshop in one day:

	Below 18	Above 18
Non-Fiction	12	30
Horror	50	45
Sci-Fi/Fantasy	23	90
Other Fiction	103	159

Question 24:
The shop also ran an author's visit event in the evening in which 106 people purchased the author's book. These books are **NOT** counted in the above table. What proportion of the books sold on this particular day were sold at the author's visit event (to the nearest whole number)?

A. 13%
B. 17%
C. 21%
D. 25%

Question 25:
Non-fiction books cost, on average, £10, and fiction books cost, on average, £6. What percentage of the shop's revenue (excluding the author's visit event) came from non-fiction books?

A. 10%
B. 13%
C. 19%
D. 23%

Question 26:
Assume that the shop makes this number of sales of each type of book every day. One week, the shop adopts a new marketing strategy and markets non-fiction books more heavily. The result is that the number of non-fiction sales double during this week, but all of the other book sales stay in line with previous sales. How much does the shop earn this week?

A. £24,250
B. £25,620
C. £26,950
D. £27,890

Question 27:
The following week, the shop decides to market the horror books more heavily, resulting in the sales of horror books doubling, and the sales of non-fiction books returning to the normal level. How much does the shop's income increase this week compared to the non-fiction marketing week? Sales of all other books can be assumed to be the same as un-marketed weeks.
A. 1%
B. 2%
C. 3%
D. 4%

SET 8

The following table shows the taxing structure for Italian city hotels:

City	Tax
Venice	1 euro per star per room per night. Rooms with children under 16 are tax exempt.
Rome	Per person, per night: 5 euros for 3 star, 6 euros for 4 star, 7 euros for 5 star, up to a maximum of ten nights worth, after which no tax is charged. Rooms with children under age 10 are tax exempt.
Padua	Per person, per night: 2 euros for 3 star or below, 3 euros for 4 star or above. Rooms with children under 16 are tax exempt.
Siena	2 euros per person per night in high season, 1 euro per person per night in low season. Rooms with children under 12 are tax exempt.

Unless specifically mentioned, assume that all of the people below are aged 18 or over.

Question 28:
A family goes on a tour of Italy in the High season. They are 2 adults and 2 children, aged 9 and 13. They spend two nights in each of Venice, Rome, Padua and Siena. They stay in 3 star hotels for the entire trip, and have two rooms (an adult room and a child room). How much tax do they pay for their trip?
A. EUR 35
B. EUR 56
C. EUR 60
D. EUR 65

Question 29:
Claude is comparing cities. He can either spend 7 nights in Rome in a 4 star hotel, or 8 nights in Padua in a 5 star hotel. Which of the following is the ratio between the tax he pays in Rome and the tax he pays in Padua?

A. 8:3
B. 7:4
C. 6:2
D. 1:4

Question 30:
Alice goes on a trip for 2 days to Venice in a 3 star hotel and for 3 days to Padua in a 4 star hotel. What is the percentage more tax she pays in Padua relative to Venice?

A. 25%
B. 50%
C. 75%
D. 100%

Question: 31
How long does Reuben have to stay in a 4 star hotel in Rome so that the tax would be less than or equal to the tax he incurs if staying the same length of time in a 4 star hotel in Padua?

A. 10 days
B. 15 days
C. 20 days
D. 25 days

SET 9

Peter is building a house that contains rooms of different sizes. The sitting room is 10m x 20m, the hallway is 3m x 10m, and the master bedroom is 15m x 15m. In addition, the house has another square-shaped bedroom, a kitchen and a bathroom.

Question 32:
Assuming that the second bedroom walls are 60% of the length of the master bedroom, what is the area of the second bedroom?

A. 64 m^2
B. 81 m^2
C. 100 m^2
D. 121 m^2

Question 33:
Suppose the kitchen has a floor area of 100 m^2 and the bathroom has a floor area of 4 m^2, and the second bedroom has the floor area calculated in the previous question. What percentage of the area of the house is taken up by the master bedroom?

A. 30%
B. 35%
C. 40%
D. 45%

Question 34:
After building the house, Peter decides to add an extension to the sitting room, turning it into a combined lounge and dining room. He extends the room by increasing the length of the longer wall by 5 metres. The lounge is 3 metres high. How much extra wall (in m^2) does Peter have to build, assuming that he is extending directly outwards and cannot move or re-use any wall?

A. 15m^2
B. 30m^2
C. 45m^2
D. 60m^2

Question 35:
A larger extension is considered, and two builders offer Peter separate quotes. The first builder offers to build wall at a cost of £15 per m^2, but there is also a flat fee of £200 just for starting the job. The second builder offers to build wall at a cost of £16 per m^2 but with no flat fee at the start. If Peter builds 300 m^2 of wall, what is the ratio of builder 1 cost to builder 2 cost (to 3 s.f.)

A. 1.00:1.00
B. 1.00:1.02
C. 1.02:1.00
D. 2.00:3.00

SET 10

The table below shows the service prices for competing mobile phone plans A-D. Any SMSs or call minutes beyond those free with the plan are charged individually at listed price.

	A	B	C	D
Monthly fee	£0	£5	£10	£15
# Free SMSs	0	200	1000	Unlimited
# Free call minutes	0	0	100	Unlimited
Price/SMS	10p	20p	20p	-
Price/call minute	10p	20p	20p	-

Question 36:
John buys Plan B for one month and calls for 15 minutes and sends 207 SMSs. How much does he pay this month?
A. £5.00
B. £6.60
C. £7.80
D. £9.40
E. £11.20

Question 37:
Robin buys Plan A, and makes no calls. How many SMSs can Robin send before Plan B would have been cheaper?
A. 6
B. 21
C. 51
D. 101
E. 121

Question 38:
Mary wants to call for 5 minutes and send 5 SMSs every day in September. Which plan should she choose for the lowest cost?
A. A
B. B
C. C
D. D
E. A and B are both the lowest

Question 39:
Evan buys Plan B but Chris buys Plan C. Which of these options is cheaper for Evan than Chris per month?
A. They each call for 29 minutes and send no SMSs.
B. They each call for 26 minutes and send 174 SMSs
C. They each send 351 SMSs and call for 8 minutes.
D. They each call for 4 minutes every day of the month.
E. They each send 223 SMSs and make no calls.

Question 40:
Rachel doesn't send any SMSs and buys Plan C. What is the maximum percentage by which she can exceed her free call minutes allowance without Plan D being cheaper?

A. 5 %
B. 10 %
C. 25 %
D. 50 %
E. 75 %

SET 11

A muffin recipe calls for ingredients in the amounts listed in the table below:

Ingredient	Density	Amount
Flour	600 gram/dm^3	2 cups
Sugar	850 gram/dm^3	1 cup
Milk	1050 gram/dm^3	½ cup
Butter	950 gram/dm^3	4 tablespoons

1 cup = 2.5 decilitres (dl); 1 tablespoon = 15 millilitres (ml); 1 cubic decimetre (dm^3) = 1 litre

Question 41:
How many cups of ingredients are called for overall by the recipe (to 2 decimal places)?

A. 3.54
B. 3.66
C. 3.74
D. 3.82
E. 3.86

Question 42:
What weight ratio of milk to butter does the recipe call for (to 1 decimal place)?

A. 2.3:1
B. 2.7:1
C. 3.1:1
D. 3.4:1
E. 3.9:1

Question 43:
Jane wants to use only a ½ cup measure for baking. What is the smallest number of cups of flour she would need for it to be possible to measure all required ingredients in ½ cups?

A. 2
B. 10
C. 25
D. 30
E. 50

Question 44:
To make pancakes, the amount of flour and milk are reversed. What is the average density of pancake batter, assuming that there are no interactions that change the densities of the individual ingredients when they are mixed?

A. 930 grams/dm^3
B. 970 grams/dm^3
C. 1,050 grams/dm^3
D. 1,070 grams/dm^3
E. 1,100 grams/dm^3

Question 45:
If Peter wanted to make 10 muffins weighing 100 grams each, how much butter would he need to 1 decimal place? Assume that the finished product weighs the same as the initial dough.

A. 55.1 grams
B. 62.3 grams
C. 70.7 grams
D. 76.4 grams
E. 81.3 grams

Question 46:
When Peter's ten 100 gram muffins are done, assuming no losses to cooking, what percentage of the weight will be made up by flour, to the nearest whole number?

A. 35 %
B. 39 %
C. 43 %
D. 46 %
E. 52 %

SET 12

New ocean crust is formed at spreading ridges. The area of the crust formed is dependent on temperature. The volume of crust formed in a given time interval depends on the **crust cross sectional area** and on the spreading rate (the rate at which newly formed crust moves away from the spreading ridge, an independent variable).

The relationship between **crust volume** formed in a time interval, **cross sectional area** and **spreading rate** is:

Crust volume per time = cross sectional area x spreading rate

The table below gives the crustal cross sectional area, spreading rate and temperature at Locations A-D:

	A	B	C	D
Cross Sectional Area (km^2)	10	20	30	40
Spreading rate (mm/year)	150	20	100	50
Temperature (°C)	1300	1400	1500	1600

Question 47:
Assuming that the trends in this table can be reliably extrapolated, at which temperature would the crust volume formed in a year be expected to be 0 km^3?

A. 1,200 °C
B. 1,400 °C
C. 1,600 °C
D. 1.800 °C
E. 2,000 °C

Question 48:
If the temperature at Location A increased by 50%, what would be the spreading rate?

A. 25 mm/year
B. 50 mm/year
C. 100 mm/year
D. 150 mm/year
E. 225 mm/year

Question 49:
What volume of crust is formed in a year at Location B?

A. 400 m^3
B. 400 °C km^3
C. 40,000 km^3
D. 400,000 m^3
E. 560,000 °C km^3

Question 50:
If the spreading rates of Locations A and C were exchanged, what would be the ratio of crust volume formed at the two locations each year (to 1 decimal place)?

A. 1:1.0
B. 1:3.3
C. 1:4.5
D. 1:5.6
E. 1:6.0

Question 51:
If the same crustal volume was produced in the same amount of time at 2 locations, E with temperature 1300 °C and F with temperature 1450 °C, how many percent faster/slower was the spreading rate at location E than F?

A. 250 % faster
B. 25 % slower
C. 400 % faster
D. 40 % slower
E. 500 % faster

Question 52:
If the temperature at Location D was decreased by 10%, what would be the crustal volume formed in 3 years?

A. 2,000 m^3
B. 2,000 °C km^3
C. 3,200 km^3
D. 3, 200,000 m^3
E. 3, 600,000,000,000,000 mm^3

SET 13

A new drug to treat vision problems in diabetics is tested on volunteers. It is also tested on control groups of diabetics without vision problems and healthy volunteers with or without vision problems. Some volunteers are given one inactive placebo pill which they are told is the drug. There are the same number of people in each group testing either the drug or placebo, as indicated below.

The table below shows the number of volunteers in Groups A-D who self-reported improved vision and their measured average accuracy reading letters before and after taking the drug or a placebo.

	Group A		Group B		Group C		Group D	
	Drug	Placebo	Drug	Placebo	Drug	Placebo	Drug	Placebo
Number Improved	15	9	8	6	9	7	7	8
Accuracy Before (%)	27	27	60	60	29	29	68	68
Accuracy After (%)	36	31	66	61	31	32	70	70

Group A: 50 diabetics with vision problems (25 in each group)
Group B: 46 diabetics without vision problems (23 in each group)
Group C: 44 healthy volunteers with vision problems (22 in each group)
Group D: 48 healthy volunteers without vision problems (24 in each group)

Question 53:
What is the average percentage of participants who self-report vision improvements after receiving an inactive pill to the nearest percent?

A. 26 % B. 31 % C. 32 % D. 33 % E. 36 %

Question 54:
By what ratio is visual accuracy in reading letters increased by the drug in diabetics with poor sight relative to healthy volunteers with poor sight (to 2 decimal places)?

A. 1:0.78 B. 3.50:1 C. 4.21:1 D. 4.50.1 E. 4.83:1

Question 55:
If there are 10 women in Group A and their average accuracy was 45 % after receiving the drug, what was the average accuracy of the men in the group after receiving the drug?

A. 16 % B. 27 % C. 30 % D. 36 % E. 41 %

Question 56:
If the general population has 100 000 diabetics with vision problems, how many of these people would be expected to self-report improvements in their vision because of the effects of the drug?

A. 24,000 people
B. 32,000 people
C. 36,000 people
D. 60,000 people
E. 96,000 people

Question 57:
When the drug dose was doubled, the placebo groups showed no change in numbers or accuracy, but the number of Group A volunteers who reported improved vision jumped to 18. Assuming that drug effectiveness is dose dependent, what percent of volunteers in Group A taking the drug would be expected to self-report improved vision if the dose was tripled?

A. 54.0 % B. 72.0 % C. 84.0 % D. 90.0 % E. 100.0 %

Question 58:
Which of the following statements is supported by the data in the table?

A. The placebo is more effective than the drug.
B. The drug acts to improve vision in diabetics and healthy volunteers.
C. Volunteers who see well are more motivated to improve vision than those with vision problems.
D. Thinking you have taken a drug to improve vision improves your vision.
E. The data are inconclusive.

SET 14

Dave weighs 200 pounds and has a Basal Metabolic Rate (BMR) of 2000 calories. Elizabeth weighs 140 pounds and has a BMR of 1500 calories. The table below shows the calorific value of the foods they eat:

	Cereal	Sandwich	Apple	Chocolate	Lasagna	Chicken	Vegetables
Calories	400	500	100	350	700	250	200

To lose one pound of fat requires a 3500 calorie deficit, obtained by eating fewer calories than the BMR or burning calories by exercising. Running burns 5 calories per hour per pound you weigh at any running speed.
Cycling burns calories according to the following relationship, where M is mph cycling speed:

Calories burned per mile = 50 calories + (5 calories x (M-10))

Question 59:
Dave wants his workout to take one hour on a 5 mile track. What is the maximum number of calories he can burn by running or cycling?
A. Burn 125 calories running
B. Burn 125 calories cycling
C. Burn 1,000 calories running
D. Burn 1,000 calories cycling
E. Burn 1,250 calories running

Question 60:
Dave doesn't want to eat less than his BMR and can only run for 30 minutes a day, but cycles 20 miles every day in an hour. How long will it take him to lose 10 pounds?
A. 5 days
B. 7 days
C. 10 days
D. 14 days
E. 30 days

Question 61:
Elizabeth and Dave both want to lose 10% of their body weight without dieting or cycling. What is the ratio of minutes a day Elizabeth would have to run to those Dave would have to run to achieve their goal at the same time to 1 decimal place?
A. 1:0.5
B. 1:0.7
C. 1:1.0
D. 1:1.4
E. 1:2.0

Question 62:
If Elizabeth eats cereal for breakfast, a sandwich for lunch, chicken and vegetables for dinner and does no exercise, in how many full days will she have reached her goal of 10% weight-loss?
A. 327 days
B. 354 days
C. 372 days
D. 416 days
E. 435 days

Question 63:
If Elizabeth also began cycling 10 miles in 1 hour every day, how much faster would she reach her goal than in question 62?
A. 1.00
B. 2.50
C. 3.00
D. 3.33
E. 4.33

Question 64:
Elizabeth eats one chocolate everyday; 3 times as much chicken as chocolate and twice as much cereal as chicken. If she exchanged these foods with 3 different foods in the table in the same proportions, what is the ratio of her rate of weight change before and after the switch, assuming she is trying to obtain the lowest weight she can?
A. 1:1
B. 1:2
C. 1:5
D. 2:1
E. 5:1

SET 15

Visitors to an amusement park pay for food, rides and games with coupons. Coupons can be bought individually for £1 each or in multipacks at a discounted price. A £70 wristband can gives free entry and access to all rides (but not games or food) without using coupons. The table below shows the cost in coupons for each activity:

	Entrance	Rollercoaster	Fun House	Swings	Carnival Games	Candy Floss
All Day	10	4	2	3	1	2
Night	5	3	2	2	1	2

Question 65:
Susan buys a 20 coupon multi-pack at 10 % off single coupon price. She rides the rollercoaster five times at night. What percent off did she get on the first rollercoaster ride compared to buying single day tickets (to 1 decimal place)?

A. 10.0 %
B. 22.5 %
C. 25.0 %
D. 32.5 %
E. 33.3 %

Question 66:
One weekend the single coupon prices are raised 20 %. Greg wants to ride the rollercoaster 10 times, buy 3 candy floss, play a carnival game, go through the fun house 2 times and ride the swings during the day. What is the ratio of the cost with a wristband to the cost without a wristband to 2 decimal places?

A. 1:0.93
B. 1:0.98
C. 1:1.02
D. 1:1.10
E. 1:1.12

Question 67:
Andy went to the amusement park one night. He rode the rollercoaster 50 % more times than he rode the swings, and rode the swings 20 % more times than he played carnival games. He used a whole number of coupons that were cheaper than getting a wristband. How much did Andy pay?

A. £31
B. £44
C. £49
D. £56
E. £70

Question 68:
Anna and James each spent one pound less than the cost of a wristband on single coupons one day at the amusement park. Anna went on the rollercoaster for half of her rides and the fun house for the rest. James went on the swings every odd ride and in the fun house every even ride. Neither of them went on any other rides or bought any food. What is the ratio of the number of rides Anna went on to the number James went on?

A. 1:0.78
B. 1:0.81
C. 1:1.23
D. 1:1.28
E. 1:2.56

Question 69:
A 10-weekend season pass covers all costs in the park and is available for £1,000. Erik goes to the park one day every weekend and buys a wristband each time. On the first weekend he buys one candyfloss, and the next four weekends increases the number of candyfloss he buys by 100%, relative to the previous weekend. The four weekends after that he increases the number of candyfloss he buys by 50% each weekend, relative to the previous weekend. On the 10th weekend he is sick of candyfloss and buys none.
What is the ratio of the cost without and with a season pass (to 2 decimal places)?

A. 0. 7 : 1
B. 0.92 : 1
C. 1 : 0.92
D. 1 : 1.15
E. 1.15 : 1

SET 16

The table shows the prices a pizzeria charges for their pizza:

	Italian		Pan Pizza		
Type	Cheese	Toppings	Cheese	Topping	Stuffed Crust
Price Small	£6.00	+50p/topping	£10.00	+50p/topping	+£1.00
Price Medium	£8.00	+£1.00/topping	£12.00	+£1.00/topping	+£1.50
Price Large	£10.00	+£1.50/topping	£14.00	+£2.00/topping	+£2.00

The pizzeria also offers three discount deals: 20% off orders from £20 - £29.99, 30% off orders from £30 - £49.99, and 50% off orders over £50. Small pizzas have 6 slices, medium pizzas have 8 slices, and large pizzas have 10 slices

Question 70:
Josh gets 2 large stuffed-crust 2 topping pan pizzas, 1 medium 3 topping Italian pizza and 3 small cheese pan pizzas. How much does he pay?

A. £31.00
B. £40.50
C. £52.50
D. £81.00
E. £96.00

Question 71:
Janet bought cheese pan pizzas for the cheapest cost per slice and got £35 off as a discount deal. How many slices did she buy?

A. 35
B. 48
C. 50
D. 64
E. 70

Question 72:
Joey bought some plain cheese pizzas for a total price of £60 post-discount. All the plain cheese pizzas were the same. What is the price of the one type of pizza he could **NOT** have bought?

A. £6.00
B. £8.00
C. £10.00
D. £12.00
E. £14.00

Question 73:
Lea always buys 30 slices of cheese pan pizza with 2 toppings and stuffed crust. What is the ratio of the cost of buying all large to all small pizzas (to 2 decimal places)?

A. 1:0.50
B. 1:0.75
C. 1:0.80
D. 1:1.00
E. 1:1.25

Question 74:
Kate and two friends each order cheese pan pizzas (with no toppings) and get 30% off their order. They ordered the pizzas to pay the smallest price which gets this discount, but ended up with 25% more slices than they could eat. How many slices did they manage to eat?

A. 16
B. 18
C. 20
D. 25
E. 32

SET 17

Sarah has three journalist jobs she splits her time across. The table shows a breakdown of what she earns at each job. Her salary is composed of a fixed starter wage she earns for showing up and an hourly wage on top of that. Her hourly wage increases in each job the more hours she works at that job. She must pay for her own travel expenses. Each travel cost occurs once per job she completes, and is not affected by the length of the job in hours.

	Travel Cost	Fixed Starter Wage	Hourly Wage	Average Job Length	Hourly Wage Growth
Job A	£5	£10	£10 per hour	2 hours	£5 per 50 worked
Job B	-	£5	£15 per hour	1 hours	£10 per 100 worked
Job C	£10	£5	£20 per hour	4 hours	£5 per 100 worked

Question 75:
If Sarah works for 1 hour at each job, what will be the ratio of the earnings expressed as [Job A Earnings:Job B Earnings:Job C Earnings] (to 2 decimal places)?

A. 1.00:0.75:1.00
B. 1.00:1.00:0.75
C. 1.00:1.25:1.00
D. 1.00:1.33:0.75
E. 1.00:1.33:1.00

Question 76:
Sarah worked 25 2-hour jobs, 4 1-hour jobs and 1 4-hour job for Job A in her first month. How much did she earn?

A. £625.00
B. £730.00
C. £770.00
D. £980.00
E. £1,020.00

Question 77:
Sarah can work 50 2-hour jobs per month. For which single job should she work these hours to earn the most from 2 hour jobs at the end of the month?

A. A
B. B
C. C
D. A and B are the same
E. B and C are the same

Question 78:
Sarah pays 10% income tax if her monthly salary exceeds £1275. How many hours should she work in her first month for Job C, if all jobs are the average job length, to earn the highest amount possible whilst not paying tax, to the nearest half-hour?

A. 60.0 hours
B. 62.5 hours
C. 65.0 hours
D. 68.0 hours
E. 75.0 hours

Question 79:
At the start of her third month, Sarah has worked 200 hours at Job C. She works 100 hours at average job length this month. How much of her month's earnings go to 10% income tax?

A. £150.00
B. £187.50
C. £200.00
D. £287.50
E. £300.00

Question 80:
Job B wants her to work a minimum of 50 hours a month for them, and Job A and Job C require that she works at least the same hours for them as she does at any other jobs she has, or no hours at all. Assuming all jobs are the average job length, which arrangement would give her maximum earnings in her first 100-hour work month?

A. 50 hours for A and 50 hours for B
B. 50 hours for A and 50 hours for B
C. 50 hours for B and 50 hours for C
D. 100 hours for B
E. None of the above.

SET 18

The table below shows the number of cars passing a toll booth going into the town centre and how many passengers the cars carried, including the drivers. It also shows the number of passengers who got off at the town's central underground station each day.

	Mon	Tue	Wed	Thu	Fri	Sat
Number of cars	1,517	1,632	987	1,465	2,024	478
Total car passengers (incl. Drivers)	1,873	2,421	1,116	2,101	2,822	1,339
Underground passengers	2,346	1,798	3,103	2,118	1,397	576

Question 81:
Taking the underground costs £5. On Wednesdays this fare is reduced 15% and it is cheaper for some drivers to leave the car at home. How much more revenue is generated on Wednesday than the next highest grossing day?
A. £1,457.75
B. £3,537.25
C. £5,275.75
D. £1,1730.00
E. £1,3187.75

Question 82:
On weekdays, what is the ratio of the average number of people being driven (not driving) in cars to the average number of people riding on the underground (to 2 decimal places)?
A. 1:0.25
B. 1:0.78
C. 1:3.97
D. 1:7.60
E. 1:9.60

Question 83:
What is the ratio of the average number of people per car on Tuesday compared to the average number of people per car on Saturday?
A. 1:0.67
B. 1:0.85
C. 1:1.27
D. 1:1.33
E. 1:1.89

Question 84:
What is the ratio of the number of Underground passengers on Monday compared to that on Saturday?
A. 1:0.13
B. 1:0.25
C. 1:0.40
D. 1:1.50
E. 1:4.08

Question 85:
The tollbooths charge £4 per car and an additional £1 per passenger (including the driver). 80% of this payment is tax. How much tax is paid at the tollbooths next week from Monday-Friday if there are 4,219 commuters everyday split in the ratio of 2:1.7:1 - underground passenger : car passenger (including driver) : car ratio?
A. £1,938.45
B. £4,219.00
C. £4,560.50
D. £5,198.40
E. £6,498.96

SET 19

Music practice rooms are available seven days a week, with each day being split into three sessions: morning (8am-2pm), day (2pm-8pm) and night (8pm-2am). The table below gives the prices for the hourly rental of the music practice rooms. Some information is missing. The "two sessions" column indicates the hourly charge if two sessions are booked on the same day.

Type of room	Deposit	Cost per Hour			
		1-2 hours (night session)	3-6 hours (night session)	Two sessions	All day
Basic (no piano)	£10.00	-	-	£11.00	£8.00
Standard (upright piano)	£25.00	£20.00	£18.00	£16.00	£12.00
Superior (baby grand piano)	£50.00	£30.00	£26.00	£22.00	£16.50
Deluxe (grand piano)	-	£45.00	£38.00	£30.00	£20.00

NB: All prices above include VAT (25%)

Question 86:
The hourly rate for a day session is 10% more expensive than a night session. What is the total cost, excluding the deposit, for 3 hours in the Superior room during a day session?

A. £59.40
B. £70.20
C. £78.00
D. £84.18
E. £85.80

Question 87:
The total cost for two 6 hour sessions in the Deluxe room is £460. How much is the deposit?

A. £64
B. £75
C. £82
D. £100
E. £136

Question 88:
Mike books a Basic room and a Standard room for a full night session. The total cost is £221 including deposit. What is the hourly rate for a full night session in a Basic room?

A. £12.50
B. £13.00
C. £15.00
D. £16.83
E. £18.83

Question 89:
The hourly rate for a morning session up to 6hrs is 5% cheaper than a night session. The deposit remains the same. A Superior room is booked for 90 minutes one morning, all costs paid up front. How much is paid at the start of the session? (Assume half hours can be booked at half the hourly rate.)

A. £97.25
B. £92.75
C. £95.00
D. £90.50
E. £90.25

Question 90:
A Basic room is booked for 18 hours each day for three full weeks. What is the total cost of this booking excluding VAT and deposit?

A. £1,935.36
B. £2,419.20
C. £2,459.52
D. £3,024.00
E. £3,074.40

SET 20

A group of 180 people took part in a perception study and were asked to count how many differences they could spot between two similar pieces of short video footage. The results are given below

		Age (years)					
		10 to 16	16 to 22	22 to 34	34 to 48	48 to 65	65+
Differences correctly spotted	<5	9	10	10	16	15	19
	5 to 10	7	12	9	8	8	5
	11 to 15	11	8	6	2	8	9
	15+	3	2	0	1	2	0

Question 91:
What percentage of people under the age of 22 spotted more than 10 differences?
A. 31.3% B. 33.3% C. 38.7% D. 46.7% E. 63.2%

Question 92:
75% of the results for the people who spotted 5 to 10 differences correctly were removed from the study. What percentage of the remaining people aged 16-22 spotted more than 15 differences?
A. 6.3% B. 6.9% C. 8.5% D. 8.7% E. 9.4%

Question 93:
25% of people who correctly spotted over 10 differences, also *incorrectly* spotted over 10 differences. How many people was this?
A. 11
B. 12
C. 13
D. 14
E. 15

Question 94:
10,000 people aged 48 or older take this test. Using the data, estimate how many spotted fewer than five differences to the nearest 50.
A. 2,300
B. 2,900
C. 4,500
D. 5,100
E. 5,150
F. 5,200

Question 95:
The test is repeated with the same population. The number of 16-34 year olds who spot 11-15 differences increases by 50%. All other age groups experience no change. What is the new ratio between 16-34 year olds and the total number of people in the other age groups who spot 11-15 differences?

A. 1:3
B. 4:17
C. 14:44
D. 14:51
E. 21:51

SET 21

The pie chart below shows the favourite sports of some high school students. Every student plays only their favourite sport in games lessons. The school has 1300 students, with an exact 50:50 split between boys and girls.

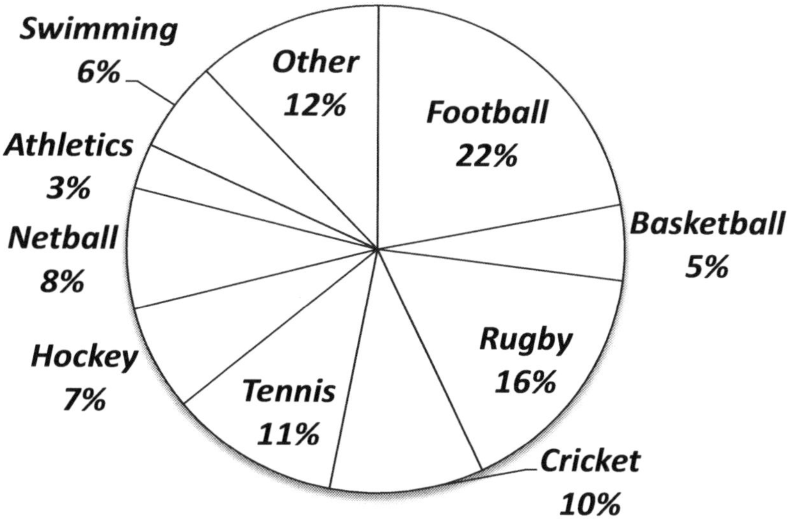

Question 96:
What is the difference between the number of boys that play football and the number that play netball in games lessons?
A. 90
B. 91
C. 104
D. 180
E. 182
F. 286

Question 97:
The senior football teams are picked from the two most senior years – a total of 350 students. Only those whose favourite sport is football play. At least 11 people are needed per team. What is the maximum number of teams that could be made? Assume that the values given in the chart are representative of these years.
A. 4
B. 5
C. 6
D. 7
E. 8

Question 98:
All those whose favourite sport is basketball are boys and all those whose favourite sport is netball are girls. 80% of the basketball boys are invited to play netball. What proportion of the netball-playing population do they then make?
A. 17%
B. 25%
C. 33%
D. 42%
E. 50%

Question 99:
One quarter of students in the *Other* category have a favourite sport which is a ball sport. In the whole school, how many students have a favourite sport which is a ball sport?
A. 39
B. 117
C. 572
D. 1,066
E. 1,183

Question 100:
Only boys play cricket. Only girls play hockey. The gender split for tennis follows that of the school as a whole. How many more boys play cricket or tennis than girls play hockey or tennis?
A. 39
B. 58
C. 59
D. 111
E. 112

SET 22

The number of apples picked by a company per year is given below, along with the quality of the apples. 30% of edible apples are sold as they come. Passable apples and the remaining edible apples are processed into cider.

Apples which are No Good are not used for human consumption, and are instead discarded for animal food.

	1998	1999	2000	2001	2002	2003
Edible	1,100,547	1,398,663	1,563,327	1,443,599	1,763,870	1,931,784
Passable	2,983,411	2,691,553	3,008,941	2,790,456	2,651,399	2,439,012

No Good	400,001	391,747	398,014	568,440	494,309	571,221

Question 101:
What is the percentage increase in the number of apples used for human consumption from 1998 to 2003?
A. 7%
B. 10%
C. 22%
D. 76%
E. 93%

Question 102:
What percentage of all No Good apples was produced in the year most apples could not be used for humans?
A. 11.6%
B. 11.8%
C. 13.9%
D. 19.9%
E. 20.2%

Question 103:
2004 saw a three-fold increase on 2003 in the number of No Good apples. The total number of apples fit for consumption remained the same. What was the difference in number between processed and No Good apples in 2004 to the nearest apple?
A. 2,077,598
B. 2,224,675
C. 2,478,954
D. 2,675,133
E. 2,765,131

Question 104:
The next six-year period saw an overall 20% increase on the period 1998-2003 in the total number of edible apples picked. How many were sold as they came between 2004 and 2009?
A. 3,588,698
B. 3,321,646
C. 3,312,644
D. 2,392,465
E. 2,208,430

Question 105:
Generally, 20 apples give 1 litre of cider. Given that 2004 saw the same number of apples fit for human consumption as 2003, roughly how many litres of cider were produced in 2004?
A. 122,000 l
B. 189,600 l
C. 215,400 l
D. 247,100 l
E. 988,400 l

SET 23

Jen tracks her daily jogs using an app which gives her data on her performance. Her app tells her that her average speed is 5 mph.
Conversion factor: 1 mile = 1.6 km

Question 106:
On wet days, Jen's average speed decreases by 8%. How many kilometres does she cover in 40 minutes?

A. 3.1 km
B. 3.3 km
C. 4.9 km
D. 5.3 km
E. 7.4 km

Question 107:
Jen begins training for a marathon (26 miles). She starts off by trying to complete a marathon over the space of four equally long jogs. Estimate how long each jog is. Assume dry conditions.

A. 42 minutes
B. 46 minutes
C. 1 hour 18 minutes
D. 1 hour 25 minutes
E. 1 hour 30 minutes

Question 108:
After starting marathon training, her average speed decreases to her old wet speed; her average wet speed remaining 8% slower than this. Estimate, therefore, how long it would take her to cover 12km in the rain.

A. 1 hour 38 minutes
B. 1 hour 46 minutes
C. 2 hours 17 minutes
D. 2 hours 37 minutes
E. 2 hours 50 minutes

Question 109:
After bringing her average speeds back to their original values, Jen starts a new regime. She goes on four jogs, each being 50% further than the last. Her first jog is 4km long. How long does the final jog take in dry conditions?
A. 1 hour 8 minutes
B. 1 hour 41 minutes
C. 1 hour 50 minutes
D. 2 hours 9 minutes
E. 2 hours 42 minutes

Question 110:
Lots of training later, Jen completes the marathon in a time of 3hrs 42mins on a dry day. What is the percentage increase in Jen's dry average speed compared to her original one?
A. 7%
B. 12%
C. 41%
D. 52%
E. 53%

SET 24

The table below gives the prices per person per week for different luxury holiday accommodations with different swimming facilities. Some types of accommodation offer a choice between swimming facilities. Some information is missing. Additional days are charged at 1/7 of the weekly cost.

	Studio	Apartment	Villa	Palazzo
No pool	£50.00	£70.00	£95.00	£155.00
Shared pool	£60.00	£80.00	-	-
Private pool	-	£100.00	-	£325.00
Beachfront	-	-	£220.00	£480.00

Question 111:
Villas are available with a private pool, and currently they are on sale: 20% off the standard price, where the standard price sits halfway between that of an apartment with a private pool and a palazzo with a private pool. How much would this cost for two people for one week?

A. £323 B. £332 C. £340 D. £415 E. £664

Question 112:
A group of twelve rents out a beachfront palazzo for four weeks. A booking fee is required from each member of the group, in this case charged at 10% of the weekly cost per person. What is the total cost of the booking?

A. £23,040 B. £23,161 C. £23,616 D. £25,344 E. £25,614

Question 113:
A couple rents an apartment with a shared pool for 20 days. The total cost is £492.89. How much is the booking fee?

A. £35.55 B. £35.57 C. £35.75 D. £37.55 E. £37.75

Question 114:
A family of four stays at a beachfront villa for two weeks, with no booking fee. Due to a complaint, they are refunded 20% of the standard charge. How much does the family pay?

A. £1,408 B. £1,760 C. £1,920 D. £2,340 E. £2,620

Question 115:
A company hires three palazzi with private pools for a week for the grand total of £19,500. The booking fee is 10% of the total cost. Assuming each palazzo has the same number of people staying in it, how many people are there in each palazzo?

A. 18 B. 20 C. 22 D. 54 E. 60

SET 25

FastFoodCo is a fast food take-away that delivers directly to customers' homes. Delivery rates are £3.00 for orders less than £10, £1.50 for orders from £10 - £15 and free for orders over £15. Below is a selection from their menu (delivery and food prices exclude 20% VAT, which is payable on all orders). VAT is added after delivery and any discounts have been taken into account.

Item	Cost
Green Curry	£3.95
Chicken Curry	£2.95
Noodles	£2.95
Chicken Tikka	£4.95
Vegetarian Curry	£3.95

Question 116:
John orders a green curry, noodles and a vegetarian curry. What is the total price?
A. £16.62
B. £14.82
C. £14.52
D. £12.35

Question 117:
Katy orders 3 noodles, 2 chicken tikkas and a green curry. Her total is:
A. £22.44
B. £25.67
C. £27.24
D. £29.04

Question 118:
John orders 2 noodles and a vegetarian curry. What is his total price?
A. £15.42
B. £14.24
C. £13.62
D. £12.14

Question 119:
Katy orders a green curry, 3 noodles and a vegetarian curry. What is her total?
A. £21.89
B. £20.10
C. £18.52
D. £18.09

Question 120:
A final 'two for the price of one' offer is applied for noodles. John orders 4 noodles, 2 chicken tikkas and a green curry. What is his total?

A. £18.20
B. £21.33
C. £22.51
D. £23.70
E. £24.31

SET 26

The graph below shows the first quarter profits (in GBP) of four suppliers of prescription medicine.

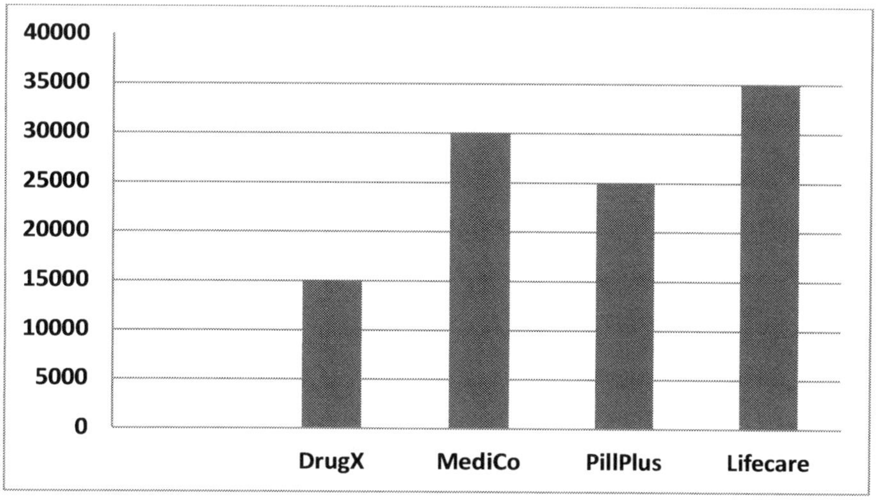

Question 121:
What percentage of total first quarter profits were earned by MediCo?
A. 26.6%
B. 28.6%
C. 30.4%
D. 33.3%

Question 122:
What percentage of the total first quarter profit is from MediCo and Lifecare combined?
A. 56.8%
B. 59.5%
C. 61.9%
D. 62.3%

Question 123:
PillPlus offers a 10% discount on all products in the second quarter. As a result, their sales increase and profit increases by 15%.

Assuming that the profits of all other suppliers remain constant into the second quarter, what percentage of the total second quarter profits did PillPlus make?
A. 16.4%
B. 23.8%
C. 26.4%
D. 27.3%

Question 124:
During the third quarter, all profits fall by 10% from second quarter values. Lifecare then buys DrugX. What percentage of the third quarter profits was made by Lifecare?
A. 46.0%
B. 46.6%
C. 47.9%
D. 48.2%

Question 125:
Production costs are increased in the fourth quarter, resulting in all profits falling by a further 5%, despite an increase in sales. The information given in question 124 still applies. How much money does Lifecare make in this quarter?
A. £41,800
B. £42,750
C. £43,490
D. £47,002

SET 27

The chart below shows the cost of a variety of cars and optional extras. All prices are excluding 20% VAT, which must be paid by all customers.

Model	Price	Leather Seats	Sound System	Easy-Park Technology
Racer	£15,000	£395	£195	£395
Stuntman	£12,500	£345	£145	£295
Saloon	£21,500	£495	£245	£445
Pod	£18,000	£445	£395	£495

Question 126:
What is the total cost of the Stuntman, with all optional extras?
A. £15,942
B. £15,904
C. £15,894
D. £15,616

Question 127:
What is the price difference between the Saloon and the Pod (with all optional extras)?
A. £3,900
B. £4,020
C. £4,040
D. £4,100

Question 128:
What is the difference in price between the Racer (with no optional extras) and the Stuntman with all optional extras?
A. £2,040
B. £2,048
C. £2,058
D. £2,142

Question 129:
There is a 10% discount on the Racer and all its optional extras. What is the difference in price between the Pod with no optional extras and the Racer with all optional extras?
A. £4,236.20
B. £4,285.50
C. £4,336.20
D. £4,438.40

Question 130:
A final offer on the Saloon is 20% off, including all options. What is the difference in final price between the Saloon with Leather seats and Easy-Park technology and the Pod with only basic features?
A. £18.60
B. £37.20
C. £48.30
D. £57.60

SET 28

The graph below shows the total amount of CO_2 (in Tonnes) emitted by the country Aissur in each year from 2000 onwards.

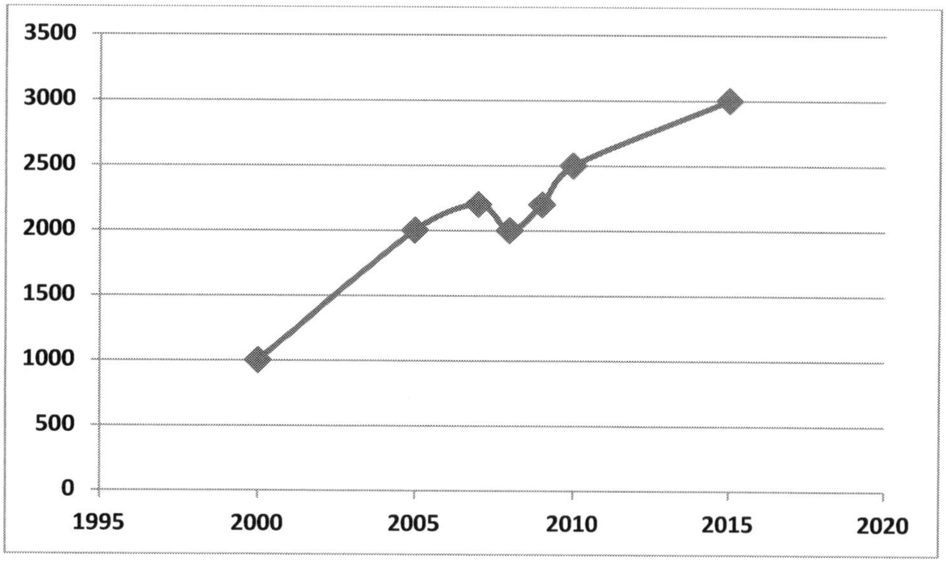

Question 131:
What was the rate of increase of CO_2 emissions between 2000 and 2005?
A. 250 Tonnes/year B. 225 Tonnes/year C. 200 Tonnes/year D. 100 Tonnes/year

Question 132:
The economic crash of 2008 caused global CO_2 emissions to decrease due to a decrease in industrial output. How much less CO_2 was emitted in the year 2010 compared to if emissions had continued to rise at the same rate seen from 2000 to 2005.
A. 500 Tonnes B. 750 Tonnes C. 1,000 Tonnes D. 2,500 Tonnes

Question 133:
What is the percentage increase in CO_2 emissions from 2005 to 2015?
A. 25% B. 33% C. 50% D. 150%

Questions 134 – 135 require the following information:
In 2015, the government of Aissur voted on a new energy bill. The bill seeks to reduce the rate of CO_2 increase over the past 5 years by 50% over the next 5 years, and keep the increase at this level thereafter.

Question 134:
If the new energy bill is successful in meeting its aims, how much CO_2 will be saved by the end of 2020 relative to the 2010 – 2015 trend continuing?
A. 200 Tonnes B. 250 Tonnes C. 500 Tonnes D. 750 Tonnes

Question 135:
What will the total CO_2 be in 2020 according to this new act?
A. 2,750 Tonnes B. 3,000 Tonnes C. 3,250 Tonnes D. 3,500 Tonne

SET 29

The chart below shows the price per item for different styles of printing. The price is lower when larger orders are made, as shown in the table.

Type	1	10+	100+
Single sided black & white	£0.10	£0.07	£0.05
Single sided colour	£0.25	£0.20	£0.15
Double sided black & white	£0.15	£0.12	£0.10
Double sided colour	£0.45	£0.30	£0.25

Question 136:
What is the price per job of 74 single sided black & white sheets?
A. £3.70
B. £5.18
C. £5.24
D. £7.40

Question 137:
How many double-sided colour sheets can you buy for £100?
A. 222
B. 333
C. 400
D. 425

A 10% discount is offered for orders above 50 units, applying to the whole order. All other offers still apply.

Question 138:
What is the price of 150 units of double sided black & white?
A. £13.50
B. £15.50
C. £16.20
D. £20.25

Question 139:
Compared to buying 150 double sided black & white sheets individually, how many sheets worth (at the standard price for 1 sheet) is saved by buying in one transaction at the discounted price?
A. 65 sheets
B. 60 sheets
C. 53 sheets
D. 50 Sheets

Question 140:
What is the total cost of an order of double sided pages, with 227 requiring black and white printing and 34 requiring colour printing?
A. £22.38
B. £29.61
C. £32.90
D. £34.32

SET 30

4 sets of 300 volunteers take part in a clinical trial for a new drug, which is aimed at reducing the effects of asthma. The responses received are recorded below.

Group	Positive	Negative	No Effect
1	75%	20%	5%
2	65%	30%	5%
3	70%	15%	15%
4	55%	25%	20%

Question 141:
How many people reacted positively overall?

A. 135
B. 265
C. 523
D. 795

Question 142:
How many more people reacted negatively from set 2 compared to set 3?

A. 15
B. 33
C. 45
D. 56

Question 143:
What proportion of those tested overall reacted negatively?

A. 21%
B. 23%
C. 26%
D. 28%

After modifications to the drug, a new survey of 300 volunteers was taken. The results of this are shown below:

Group	Positive	Negative	No Effect
5	82%	15%	3%

Question 144:
What was the percentage increase in the success rate (i.e. the percentage of people reacting positively) in the 5th group compared to the first 4 groups?

A. 7.81%
B. 15.75%
C. 17.93%
D. 23.77%

Question 145:
Across all groups, including group 5, how many people reacted negatively to the drug?

A. 275 B. 315 C. 355 D. 380

SET 31

The graph below shows the total number of views for two rival local television dramas, The Last Chase and The Final Frontier, across the 4 yearly quarters in 2014.

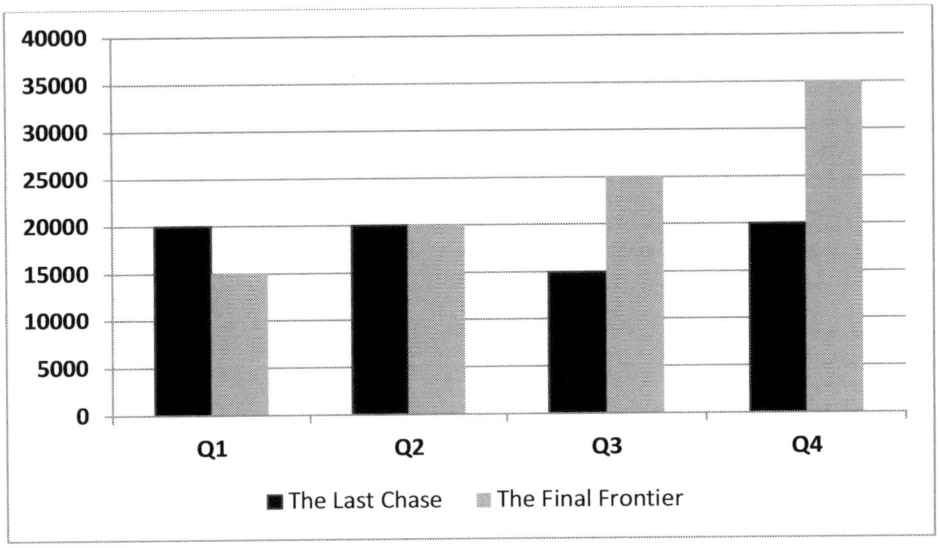

Question 146:
What is the difference between the total number of views of the Final Frontier and The Last Chase during 2014?
A. 10,000 B. 15,000 C. 20,000 D. 25,000

Question 147:
Broadcasters earn £2,500 from advertisements per 1,000 views. What is the difference in money earned through advertising between the two shows in 2014?
A. £45,000 B. £50,000 C. £55,000 D. £60,000

Question 148:
If the number of views of The Final Frontier continues to increase at same rate it did from Q1 – Q3 of 2014, how many views will it have during the final quarter of year 2015?
A. 50,000 B. 55,000 C. 60,000 D. 65,000

Question 149:
If the number of views of The Final Frontier continues to increase at same rate it did from Q1 – Q3 of 2014, how many views will it have in 2015 in total?
A. 180,000 B. 190,000 C. 200,000 D. 250,000

Question 150:
Under different circumstances, at the end of the third quarter of 2014, the broadcasters decide to terminate The Last Chase. As a result, half of The Last Chase's views instead transfer to The Final Frontier. How many views will The Final Frontier have at the end of the final quarter of 2014 under these circumstances?
A. 25,000 B. 35,000 C. 37,500 D. 45,000

SET 32

The table below shows the average time, in minutes, spent waiting for GP appointments by patients, according to a series of surveys from 2014. On average, 20% of patients who wait between 11 and 30 minutes and 40% of those who wait for more than 30 minutes register a complaint during a customer satisfaction survey. No patients who waited for 10 minutes or less registered complaints.

	0-10	11-30	30+	Survey size
England	60%	30%	10%	100,000
Scotland	55%	25%	20%	50,000
Wales	50%	25%	25%	25,000
Northern Ireland	60%	25%	15%	25,000

Question 151:
How many patients waited for less than half an hour for an appointment in Scotland?
A. 12,500
B. 27,500
C. 40,000
D. 45,000

Question 152:
What percentage of patients across the UK waited for more than half an hour for an appointment?
A. 10%
B. 15%
C. 20%
D. 25%

Question 153:
How many complaints are received from this survey at the end of the year?
A. 20,250
B. 21,500
C. 23,000
D. 24,250

Question 154:
What proportion of patients complained about waiting times by the end of the 2014 survey?
A. 12.1%
B. 11.5%
C. 11.0%
D. 10.7%

Question 155:
In January 2015, the government announced a target to reduce the number of patients waiting for longer than 30 minutes for an appointment by 50%, and by 25% for those waiting between 11-30 minutes. Proportionally, what will be the decrease in the number of complaints recorded by an identical survey at the end of 2015, if all targets are met?
A. 40%
B. 38%
C. 36%
D. 34%

SET 33

The graph below shows the price of crude oil in US Dollars during 2014:

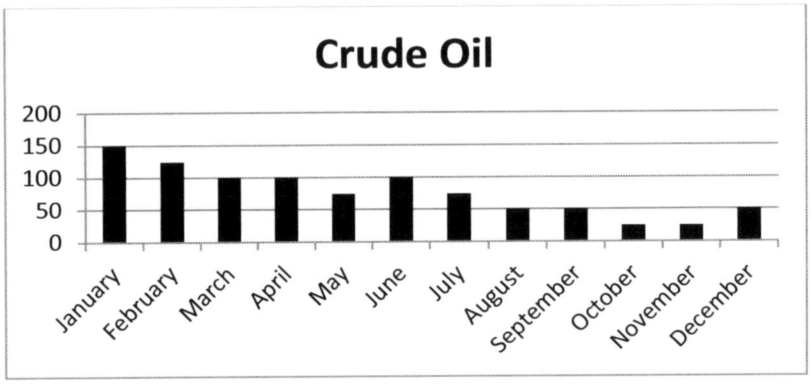

The total oil production, in millions of barrels per day, is shown on the graph below:

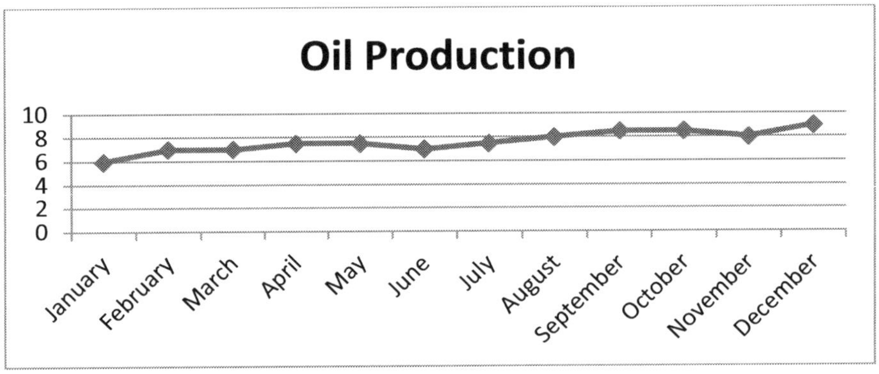

Question 156:
At what rate did the price of oil fall between January and March of 2014?

A. $16.70 per month
B. $20.00 per month
C. $22.70 per month
D. $25.00 per month

Question 157:
What was approximate total oil production in 2014?

A. 1,750 million barrels
B. 2,146 million barrels
C. 2,300 million barrels
D. 2,700 million barrels

Question 158:
How much did oil sales total in July 2014?

A. $0.56 Billion
B. $16.9 Billion
C. $17.4 Billion
D. $21.1 Billion

Question 159:
Oil prices have been falling due to a high supply. On average, the price of extraction & production of oil makes up 40% of the total price. The rest of the price is profit. How much profit was made from oil sales during June 2014?

A. $8.4 Billion
B. $12.6 Billion
C. $13.0 Billion
D. $21.0 Billion

Question 160:
Profit from oil extraction is 60% of the total sale price. This profit is split between the oil companies and the nation producing the oil in a ratio of 5:2. Of the oil company profits, 30% are used for corporation tax in the companies' home countries. Given that the overall sales value was $204 billion over the year, how much corporation tax was paid in 2014 (to 2 decimal places).

A. $26.23 Billion
B. $36.74 Billion
C. $43.71 Billion
D. $67.57 Billion

SET 34

The chart below shows the severity of asthma amongst a sample of 5 groups of 50 people of different ages. The average cost of asthma inhalers per patient is £50 per year. The population of the United Kingdom averaged 50 million during the period of interest. Children aged 0-5 years made up 7% of the population and children aged 5-10 years made up 10% of the population.

Children below the age of 10 who suffer from mild asthma have a half chance of developing respiratory problems in adult life. This figure is 90% for children below the age of 10 who suffer severe asthma. Children without asthma will not develop respiratory problems.

A review into doctors' practices concluded that between 1990 and 1995, 35% of mild asthma diagnoses of children between 0-10 were incorrect.

Age	No Asthma	Mild	Severe
0-5	80%	15%	5%
5-10	75%	20%	5%
10-21	85%	12%	3%
21-30	95%	3%	2%
30+	95%	4%	1%

Question 161:
How many people surveyed suffer from asthma?

A. 25 B. 35 C. 45 D. 55

Question 162:
What is the proportion of children surveyed who are likely to develop respiratory problems?

A. 13.00% B. 13.25% C. 13.50% D. 14.25%

Question 163:
How many 0-10 year olds from the survey have been incorrectly diagnosed with asthma?

A. 6.1% B. 6.9% C. 7.4% D. 8.0%

Question 164:
What proportion of children below the age of 10 who were correctly diagnosed with asthma will develop respiratory problems?

A. 9% B. 10% C. 11% D. 12%

Question 165:
How much money was wasted on mistakenly prescribing medication to children who were wrongly diagnosed with asthma from 1990 to 1995?

A. £133 million B. £157 million C. £187 million D. £255 million

SET 35

The following table shows data related to equity shares issued by five public sector companies on 1 March 2015.

Company	Number of equity shares (million)	Current market price Per share (£)	Percentage of equity share held by UK government
A	10	60	75%
B	20	50	50%
C	30	40	33.33%
D	40	30	25%
E	50	20	12.5%

Question 166:
If the government disinvested 50% of its stake in A at current market price, what (in £) is the amount of revenue generated by the government through the disinvestment?
A. 375 Million B. 325 Million C. 275 Million D. 225 Million

Question 167:
If the government disinvested 25% of its stake in B at current market price, the amount of revenue generated by the government through the disinvestment would be (in £):
A. 125 Million B. 150 Million C. 175 Million D. 200 Million

Question 168:
The government disinvested its entire stake in C at a price of £35 per share. What would have been the additional revenue generated by the government had it done the given disinvestment at the given market price?
A. £25 Million B. £50 Million C. £75 Million D. £100 Million

Question 169:
If the share price of D fell to £25 on 2 March 2015, then what was the decline in the total value of D's shares held by the government from that of the previous day?
A. £25 Million
B. £50 Million
C. £75 Million
D. £100 Million

Question 170:
If the share price of E rose to £25 on 2 March 2015, then what was the increase in the total value of E's shares held by the government over that of the previous day (in £)?
A. £30.25 Million
B. £30.75 Million
C. £31.25 Million
D. £31.75 Million

Question 171:
Which of the following will fetch higher revenue for government?
A. Redeeming all its stock from company A.
B. Redeeming all its stock from company B.
C. Both of the above will fetch the same value.
D. None of the above.

SET 36

The table below shows the production of some agricultural crops in Harvestland in the years 2011-12 and the targets that were earlier set for that growing season.

Crop	Targeted production For 2011-12 (tonnes)	Actual production for 2011-12 (tonnes)	% Increase in production from 2010-11
Food grains	120	100	25
Oil seeds	60	50	25
Sugarcane	50	40	10
Cotton	40	30	20
Jute	25	20	25

Question 172:
The production of food grain (in tonnes) in 2010-11 was:
A. 40
B. 60
C. 80
D. 100

Question 173:
What was the difference in targeted production in 2011-12 and actual production in 2010-11 for oil seeds (in tonnes)?
A. 10
B. 20
C. 30
D. 40

Question 174:
How much more sugarcane should have been produced in order to meet the target in 2011-12 (in tonnes)?
A. 5
B. 10
C. 15
D. 20

Question 175:
What was the combined production of Cotton and Jute in year 2010-11 (in tonnes)?
A. 11
B. 21
C. 31
D. 41

Question 176:
How much more food grain was produced than oil seeds in 2010-11 (in TONNES)?
A. 10 B. 20 C. 30 D. 40

Question 177:
Cotton constituted what percentage of total crops in year 2011-12?
A. 10 B. 12.5 C. 15 D. 17.5 E. 30

SET 37

The table given below shows the sales volume of four products A, B, C and D manufactured by a company from January to April in the year 2014.

	January	February	March	April
Product A	9,500	10,250	10,500	11,000
Product B	6,500	7,000	7,250	7,500
Product C	3,500	3,750	4,000	4,250
Product D	2,500	3,100	3,500	4,000

Question 178:
In February, sale of product B constituted what percentage of total sales of all 4 products put together?
A. 26%
B. 27%
C. 28%
D. 29%

Question 179:
Which of the following products recorded maximum percentage increase from March to April?
A. Product A
B. Product B
C. Product C
D. Product D

Question 180:
In May 2014, the sales of product C witnessed an increase of 20% over the previous month. The sales of D were the same as those of C. What was the percentage increase in the sales of D in May relative to April?
A. 22.5 %
B. 25.0 %
C. 27.5 %
D. 30.0 %

Question 181:
By what percentage did the combined sales of product A and product C increase from January to April?
A. 17.0 % B. 17.1 % C. 17.2 % D. 17.3 %

Question 182:
Assume a different scenario, that May 2015 witnessed a 20% growth in sales for products A and B, and a 30% growth in sales for products C and D over April values. What was the total sales value in May for all the products combined?
A. 32,925 B. 33,925 C. 34,925 D. 35,925

Question 183:
Assume a different scenario, that May 2015 witnessed 20% growth in sales of product A and 10% growth in sales for the other 3 products (B, C and D). Sales of A constituted what percentage of total sales in May 2015?

A. 40.25 % B. 41.25 % C. 42.25 % D. 43.24 %

SET 38

A courier company uses three modes of transportation for delivering consignments – Road, Rail and Air. The following table shows the percentage distribution of the total number of consignments delivered, the revenue generated and the cost incurred, across the three modes of transportation in 2014.

Mode of transportation	Number of consignments (%)	Revenue (%)	Cost (%)
Rail	30	35	25
Road	45	20	25
Air	25	45	50

Question: 184
In 2012, the profit made by Courier Company was 30% of the total revenue. The company made a profit of £2.5 million. What was the total revenue?

A. £3.6 Million
B. £7.2 Million
C. £8.3 Million
D. £25 Million

Question 185:
In 2014, the cost per consignment was the lowest through which method?

A. Rail
B. Road
C. Air
D. Equal between road and rail

Question 186:
In 2014, the cost per consignment through rail was £5 and the revenue per consignment through rail was £20. What was the ratio of the total revenue through rail to the total cost through rail? Assume the number of consignments is equal to that given in the table.

A. 4:1 B. 5:1 C. 6:1 D. 7:1 E. 8:1

Question 187:
In 2013, the total costs of the company are £54,000. What is the total cost of air transportation in the year 2013?

A. £13,500
B. £17,000
C. £27,000
D. £32,000
E. More information needed

Question 188:
In 2014, if the total number of consignments delivered was 17,145, then what was total number of consignments delivered using rail and road?

A. 11,670 B. 11,974 C. 12,463 D. 12,859

SET 39

The following table provides partial information about the composition of three different alloys, A, B and C. Each of these alloys contains five different elements: Zinc, Tin, Lead, Copper and Nickel, and no other substances. An alloy, Alloy G, the composition of which is not given in the table, contains alloys A, B, C in the ratio 2:1:3. It is also known that in Alloy G, Tin, Lead and Copper are present in equal quantities.

Alloy	Zinc	Tin	Lead	Copper	Nickel
A	10%	40%			10%
B	25%	15%	50%	5%	5%
C	15%		20%		35%

Question 189:
Find the percentage of Lead in alloy A.
A. 8.33 %
B. 4.16 %
C. 2.70 %
D. 2.08 %

Question 190:
Find the percentage of Tin in alloy C.
A. 31.3 %
B. 15.8 %
C. 10.6 %
D. 7.9 %

Question 191:
An alloy X contains A, B and C in equal proportion. What is the percentage of Zinc in this alloy?
A. 12.50 %
B. 16.67 %
C. 25.00 %
D. 33.33 %

Question 192:
Find the percentage of Tin and Copper combined in alloy C.
A. 15 %
B. 20 %
C. 25 %
D. 30 %

Question 193:
Find the percentage of Tin in alloy G.
A. 11.11 %
B. 21.11 %
C. 31.11 %
D. 41.11 %

Question 194:
How many elements have exactly the same concentration in Alloy G?
A. One B. Two C. Three D. Four

SET 40

The following table chart represents the number of people in the USA surveyed by CNN-Time in an opinion poll for "***The most influential person of the year 2001***". The number of people surveyed is 11,500.

Response	Percentage
Voted in favour of George Bush	39
Voted in favour of Donald Rumsfield	5
Voted in favour of Robert Guiliani	4
Voted in favour of Bill Clinton	2
Voted in favour of Lady Politicians	17
Non-respondents	33
Total	**100**

Question 195:
How many people voted in favour of Hillary Clinton, who received 60% of total votes polled for lady politicians?
A. 1,173 B. 1,223 C. 1,253 D. 1,273

Question 196:
If everyone who voted in favour of Robert Guiliani is a citizen of New York, then out of all the people surveyed, the number of citizens from New York is:
A. 460
B. 960
C. 1,040
D. Cannot be determined.

Question 197:
Out of the respondents, 20% are not US citizens. Given that only US citizens voted for George Bush, determine the percentage of US citizens who voted in favour of Bush.
A. 42.8% B. 45.3% C. 46.6% D. 48.8%

Question 198:
Out of the total people surveyed, 40% are employees of the Federal Government and out of these 10% are in favour of Rumsfield. Find the number of people who are in favour of Rumsfield but are NOT employees of the Federal Government.
A. 105 B. 110 C. 115 D. 120

Question 199:
A mid-year survey has also been done on the same group of people. In that survey 16% of the people were in favour of Bill Clinton. Find the decrease in the number of people who voted in favour of Bill Clinton from mid-year survey to the actual survey.
A. 1,210 B. 1,410 C. 1,610 D. 1,810

Question 200:
A mid-year survey has also been done on the same group of people. In that survey 40% of the people were in favour of Bush. Find the decrease in the number of people who voted in favour of Bush from mid-year survey to the actual survey.
A. 115 B. 230 C. 460 D. 920

SET 41

Shop A sells merchandised mugs and also offers to print flyers at the prices shown below:

Number of flyers	Colour printing	Black and white printing
0-9	20p	5p
10-99	10p	4p
100+	5p	2p

Number of mugs	Basic mug cost per mug	Medium mug cost per mug	Premium mug cost per mug	Cost for logo/picture per mug
0-49	20p	30p	50p	5p
50-99	15p	26p	45p	4p
100-499	10p	20p	34p	3p
500+	7p	10p	20p	2p

Question 201:
Before Christmas, the shop offers an extra 15% discount. Customer A decides to buy 5 premium mugs and 4 basic mugs with a unique picture printed on the basic mugs. How much will this cost?

A. £2.50
B. £2.59
C. £2.76
D. £2.81
E. £2.98

Question 202:
Customer B needs 750 premium mugs, 130 basic mugs and 80 flyers, after Christmas. She wants a logo printed on the basic mugs. She wants black and white flyers. To the nearest pound, how much will she have to pay?

A. £160
B. £170
C. £172
D. £388
E. £395

Question 203:
Customer C wants to spend £250. How many medium mugs with a logo can she buy with this money if she also wants to buy 50 colour flyers?

A. 1200
B. 1225
C. 2041
D. 2452
E. 2500

Question 204:
The price of extra logo printed on the mug decreased by 1p, the price of premium mug decreased by 2p and the price of colour flyer decreased by 1p across all quantities in 2015. In percentage terms, how much cheaper would have been to order 70 medium mugs with logo and 150 colour flyers in 2015 instead of 2014?

A. 4%
B. 5%
C. 7%
D. 8%
E. 11%

Question 205:
The shop made a profit of £325,750 in 2015. This was a compound average growth rate of 1.2% between 2012 and 2015. What was the profit in 2012?

A. £188,513
B. £231,862
C. £314,299
D. £318,071
E. £362,059

SET 42

In St. Mary College, all students must have at least one device to interact with digital, interactive study materials. There are thirty students who have all three gadgets: Smartphone, tablet and laptop.

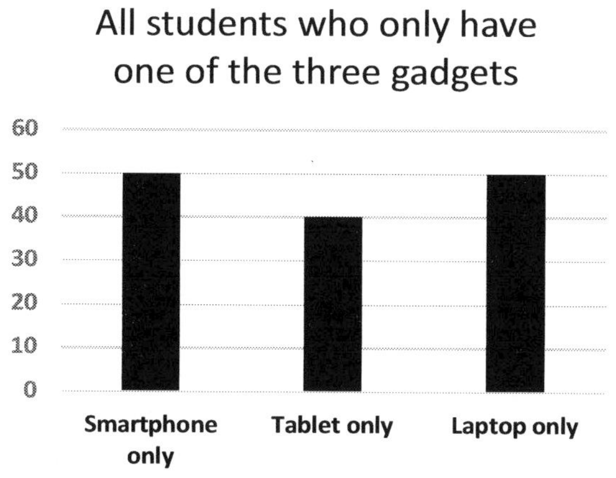

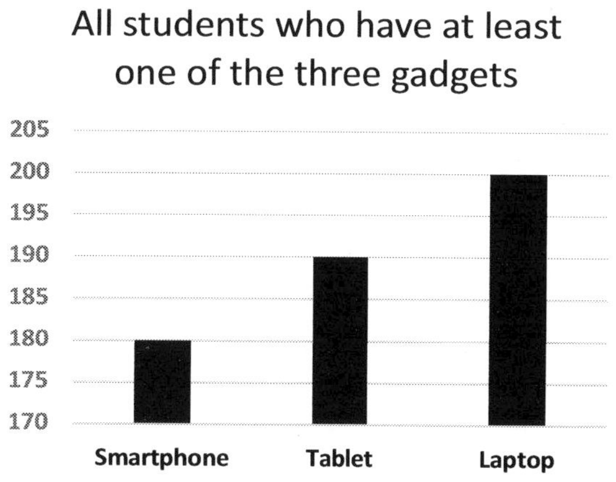

Question 206:
How many students are studying at St. Mary College in total?
A. 325
B. 340
C. 345
D. 350
E. 360

Question 207:
How many students have both a tablet and smartphone but no laptop?
A. 40
B. 45
C. 50
D. 55
E. 65

Question 208:
How many more students have a smartphone than both a tablet and laptop?
A. 80
B. 85
C. 95
D. 100
E. 80

Question 209:
What percentage of all students have both a smartphone and a laptop?
A. 20.5%
B. 23.1%
C. 23.5%
D. 25.4%
E. 25.9%

Question 210:
Five more students come to St. Mary College. Three of the students have both a smartphone and a tablet. Two of the students have a smartphone only. What percentage of all students in the college have a smartphone now?
A. 34%
B. 45%
C. 54%
D. 55%
E. 60%

SET 43

Train Timetable [Cambridge to London Liverpool Street]

Cambridge	**6.45**	**7.00**	**7.10**	**Then every 20 minutes**	**23.10**
Whittlesford Parkway	7.25	7.40	7.50	Then every 20 minutes	23.50
Audley End	7.35	7.50	8.00	Then every 20 minutes	00.00
Bishops Stortford	7.42	7.57	8.07	Then every 20 minutes	00.07
Sawbridgeworth	7.53	8.08	8.18	Then every 20 minutes	00.18
Tottenham Hale	8.03	8.18	8.28	Then every 20 minutes	00.28
Liverpool Street	8.14	8.29	8.39	Then every 20 minutes	00.39

Question 211:
How many trains leave from Cambridge Station going to Liverpool Street between 2pm and 6.00pm?

A. 10
B. 12
C. 15
D. 18
E. 20

Question 212:
At 2.45pm, Antonia is at Sawbridgeworth station waiting for the next train to London Liverpool Street. What is the earliest time can she expect to arrive at Liverpool Street?

A. 3.01pm
B. 3.09pm
C. 3.19pm
D. 3.31pm
E. 3.51pm

Question 213:
How many trains run from Cambridge Station to Liverpool Street all day?

A. 46
B. 47
C. 50
D. 51
E. 56

Question 214:
It is 3pm and Mark wants to take the next train from Cambridge Station to Tottenham Hale for a 1 hour meeting straight at the station. What is the earliest time that Mark could schedule the meeting?

A. 4.25pm
B. 4.28pm
C. 4.45pm
D. 4.55pm
E. 5.02pm

Question 215:
If the distance between Audley End and Bishops Stortford is 10.5 miles. What is the speed of the train?

A. 60 miles/hour
B. 70 miles/hour
C. 80 miles/hour
D. 90 miles/hour
E. 100 miles/hour

SET 44

The list of the longest rivers in the UK by length in 2014.

River	Length (miles)	Drainage Area (square mile)	Average Discharge (m^3/s)
River Severn	220	4,409	61.17
River Thames	215	4,994	65.8
River Trent	185	4,029	84
River Great Ouse	143	3,236	15.7
River Wye	134	1,597	3.4
River Ure	129	560	2.4
River Tay	117	431	2.3

Question 216:
What is the total length of the five longest rivers in the UK?
A. 897
B. 905
C. 1026
D. 1143
E. 1234

Question 217:
In 2015, the drainage area of the River Thames increased by 1345.5 square miles. In percentage terms, how much did the drainage area of the seven longest rivers in England increase in 2015 if the other rivers the same?
A. 2%
B. 7%
C. 17%
D. 93%
E. 97%

Question 218:
In percentage terms, how much bigger was the drainage area of the River Thames than the River Wye in 2014?
A. 213%
B. 276%
C. 313%
D. 345%
E. 425%

Question 219:
What was the difference in length between the two rivers with the highest and lowest average discharge?
A. 68 miles
B. 91 miles
C. 117 miles
D. 185 miles
E. 213 miles

Question 220:
What was the average drainage area of the six longest rivers in England in 2014?
A. 2750
B. 3138
C. 3210
D. 3455
E. 4235

SET 45

Scottish GDP breakdown by Sector

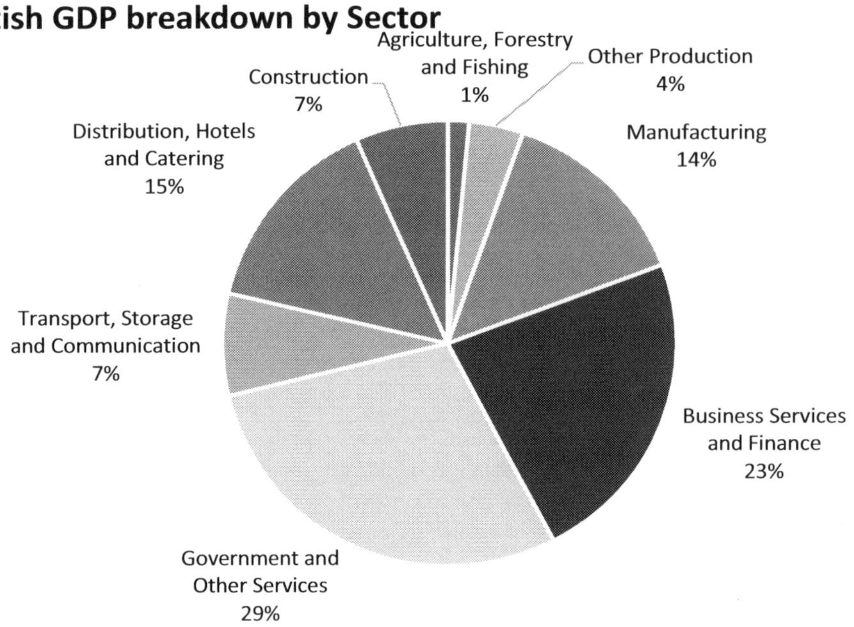

UK GDP breakdown by Sector

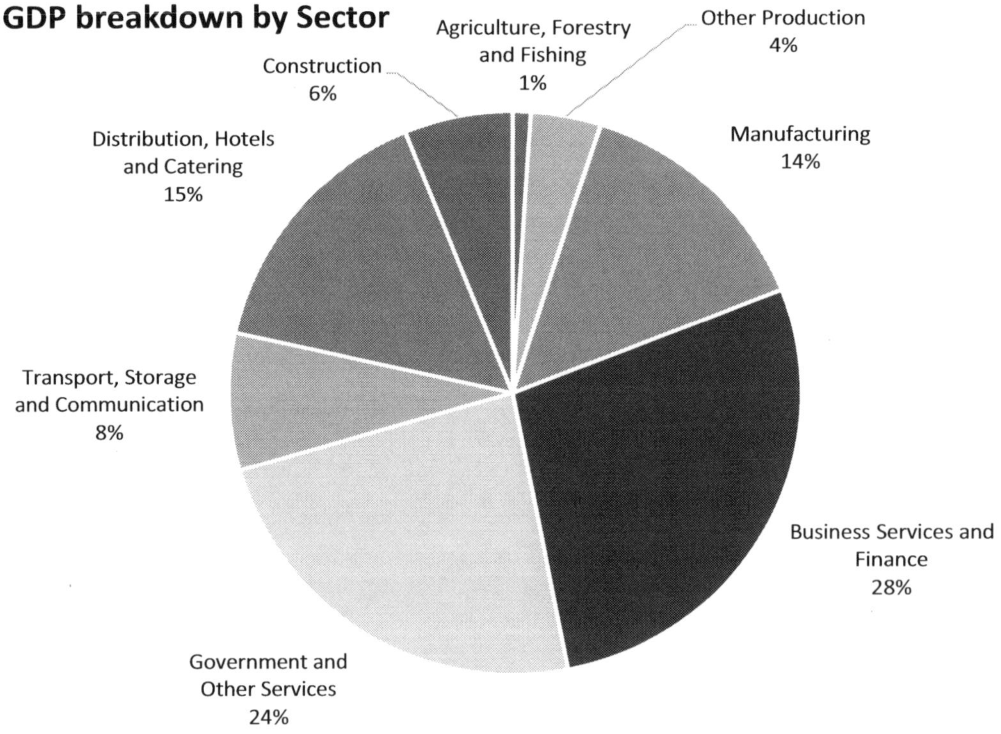

Question 221:

Which industry has the largest contribution to Scottish GDP?

A. Agriculture, Forestry and Fishing
B. Construction
C. Government and Other Services
D. Manufacturing
E. Other Production

Question 222:

In 2015, UK GDP increased by 5% overall to 4.2tn pounds. How much was the UK GDP in 2014?

A. 3.9tn
B. 4tn
C. 4.1tn
D. 4.2tn
E. 4.41tn

Question 223:

How much bigger is the contribution of Business Services and Finance to total UK GDP than the contribution of Manufacturing to Scottish GDP?

A. 3%
B. 4%
C. 5%
D. 7%
E. 14%

Question 224:

Scottish GDP was £1.2tn in 2014. What is the share of Agriculture, Forestry and Fishing in Scottish GDP in 2015 if there was an overall increase in GDP by 3%? Assume the percentage share of GDP for Agriculture, Forestry and Fishing does not change from 2014 to 2015.

A. £0.007tn
B. £0.012tn
C. £0.015tn
D. £0.022tn
E. £1.11tn

Question 225:

What are the top three contributing sectors to UK GDP?

A. Agriculture, Forestry and Fishing; Manufacturing; Construction
B. Government and Other Services; Manufacturing; Construction
C. Business Services and Finance; Government and Other Services; Manufacturing
D. Distribution, Hotels and Catering; Business Services and Finance; Government and Other Services
E. Distribution, Hotels and Catering; Business Services and Finance; Manufacturing

SET 46

Top-5 TV Shows	Viewers (millions)		% people watching show in Year 2	
	Year 1	Year 2	Females	Males
The Voice	3.4	4.1	5%	2%
Britain's Got Talent	5.2	5.6	4.5%	4%
Big Brother	1.3	1.4	9%	15%
Geordie shore	9.2	12.5	21%	19%
Fresh Meat	5	3	19%	5%

Question 226:
In percentage terms, how much did the most-watched TV show increase in the number of viewers between year 1 and year 2?
A. 29%
B. 33%
C. 36%
D. 41%
E. 42%

Question 227:
How many more viewers did The Voice and Britain's Got Talent have together in year 2 than in year 1?
A. 0.1 million
B. 0.2 million
C. 0.5 million
D. 0.7 million
E. 1.1 million

Question 228
Which is the least-watched TV show by males in year 2?
A. Big Brother
B. Fresh Meat
C. The Voice
D. Britain's Got Talent
E. Can't tell

Question 229:
In percentage terms, what was the total increase in the number of viewers across all TV shows from year 1 to year 2?
A. 5%
B. 10%
C. 15%
D. 20%
E. 25%

Question 230:
If the total population of females in year 2 was 30 million, how many males watched Geordie Shore in year 2?
A. 1.75 million
B. 2.38 million
C. 2.9 million
D. 6.2 million
E. 6.3 million

SET 47

Mobile Phone Plans

	Basic Plan Charges		**Premium Plan Charges**	
	Included minutes	**Cost per additional minute**	**Included minutes**	**Cost per additional minute**
Text Messages	250 free texts	15p per text	500 free texts	22p per text
Standard Calls	50	4p	75	6p
Mobiles (same network)	150	9p	500	15p
Mobiles (other networks)	100	15p	250	25p

Monthly fee for basic and premium plan fees: £45.29 and £47.89 respectively.

Question 231:
Each month, Claire sends 300 text messages and makes 75 mobile calls in the same network, each one minute on average. Which plan would be cheaper for Claire and by how much per month?

A. Basic plan by £4.90
B. Basic plan by £5.90
C. Premium plan by £3.90
D. Premium plan by £4.90
E. Premium plan by £5.90

Question 232:
Adam wants to spend maximum £60 per month on a mobile plan. Excluding any included minutes, what is the maximum number of additional minutes he can use if he has the premium plan?

A. 105 minutes
B. 145 minutes
C. 201 minutes
D. 245 minutes
E. 283 minutes

Question 233:
All basic plan charges increase by 1p; the basic plan fee remains unchanged. Andrew sends 45 texts, and uses 125 minutes in the same network and 325 minutes in other networks on average. How much is he worse off?

A. 0p
B. 75p
C. £1.55
D. £2.05
E. £2.25

Question 234:
Daisy does not send any text messages ever. She makes 800 minutes of calls in the same network. Which plan would be cheaper for Daisy and by how much?

A. Basic plan by £2.10
B. Premium plan by £5.75
C. Premium plan by £9.33
D. Premium plan by £10.90
E. Premium plan by £11.89

Question 235:
Kevin sends only text messages, 450 per month on average. If there were a 15% price increase in the monthly fee for both basic and premium plans, how much would Kevin save by changing to premium plan now?

A. £23.43
B. £25.01
C. £27.01
D. £27.10
E. £28.91

SET 48

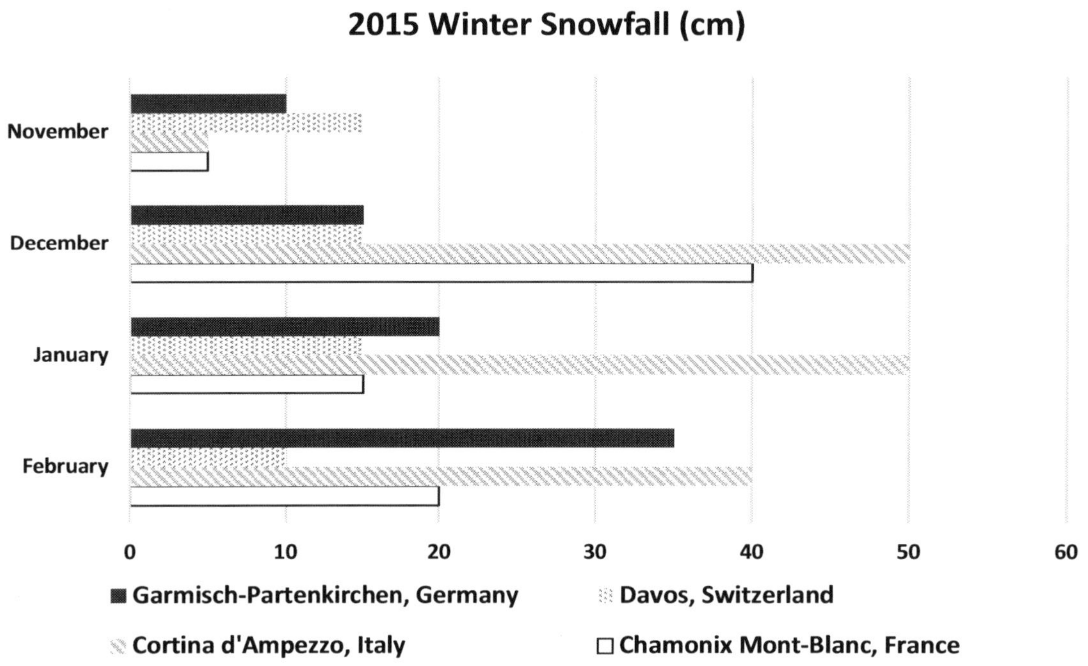

Question 236:
What was the mean monthly snowfall in cm across Davos and Chamonix Mont-Blanc during winter in 2015?
A. 12.325 cm
B. 16.875 cm
C. 19.738 cm
D. 26.842 cm
E. 43.123 cm

Question 237:
During Winter 2015, where was the average monthly snowfall the highest?
A. Davos
B. Chamonix Mont-Blanc
C. Cortina d'Ampezzo
D. Garmisch Partenkirchen
E. Can't tell

Question 238:
In percentage terms, how much more snow fell in December than in February overall?
A. 8%
B. 12%
C. 14%
D. 20%
E. 22%

Question 239:
In November 2014, 30cm snow fell in the four areas together. In percentage terms, how much more snow fell in November 2015 in the four areas together?
A. 5%
B. 17%
C. 19%
D. 24%
E. 29%

Question 240:
How much snow fell in Cortina d' Ampezzo and Garmisch Partenkirchen in November and February together?
A. 20 cm
B. 30 cm
C. 60 cm
D. 90 cm
E. 145 cm

SET 49

Please find below Kevin's expenses for December 2015.

Date	Client	Detail of expense	Cost
01.12.15	HSBC	Mileage to and from presentation in Cambridge	£16.80
01.12.15	Soros Fund Management	Single ticket - Train journey to meeting in London	£15.40
13.12.15	HSBC	Breakfast with client	£35.90
16.12.15	Black Rock	Return ticket – Train journey to meeting in London	£20.00
20.12.15	MKB	Lunch with client	£49.50

Mileage paid at £0.25 per mile for the first 100 miles each month and £0.10 thereafter

Question 241:
The greatest proportion of December expenses related to which client?
A. HSBC
B. Soros Fund Management
C. Black Rock
D. MKB
E. Can't Tell

Question 242:
What is the total expense in December?
A. £121.50
B. £137.60
C. £142.45
D. £146.50
E. £210.40

Question 243:
In percentage terms, how much more did Kevin spend on meals than on train tickets?
A. 35%
B. 41%
C. 59%
D. 149%
E. 141%

Question 244:
How many miles did Kevin travel by his car in December?
A. 50.5 miles
B. 67.2 miles
C. 67.9 miles
D. 78.4 miles
E. 112.6 miles

Question 245:
The company decides to change its policy from 2016 and only 75% of travel expenses and 90% of accommodation and meal expenses will be reimbursed. How much money would Kevin have lost in December if the new policy had been implemented already in 2015?
A. £8.54
B. £14.22
C. £13.05
D. £21.59
E. £39.15

SET 50

The table below shows the cost of jet ski renting. There are four different jet skies: Alpha, Beta, Gamma and Delta. The deposit is non-refundable.

Type	Deposit	Cost per hour	Total cost for first hour
Alpha	---	£30	£50
Beta	£20	£90	£110
Gamma	£25	£115	£140
Delta	£100	£150	£250

Question 246:
How much is the deposit for Alpha jet ski?
A. £20
B. £30
C. £40
D. £50
E. £60

Question 247:
What is the difference between the total cost of renting a Beta and a Gamma jet ski for 6 hours each?
A. £150
B. £155
C. £200
D. £205
E. £215

Question 248:
Aron has £500 for jet ski renting. Which jet skis can he afford to rent for an hour?
A. Alpha only
B. Alpha and Beta and Gamma
C. Alpha and Beta and Gamma and Delta
D. Beta only
E. Gamma only

Question 249:
Andrew and Thomas want to rent Alpha and Gamma jet ski for three hours. How much will they pay in total?
A. £360
B. £480
C. £660
D. £690
E. £960

Question 250:
If the deposit for Delta jet ski is increased by 5% on Sundays, what will be the total cost of renting a Delta jet ski for 8 hours on a Sunday?
A. £990
B. £1200
C. £1305
D. £1605
E. £1900

SET 51

Flight tickets to various regions from the UK

	In The Air	Good Fly	Take Me There	Around the World
North America	250£	290£	560$	360 €
South America	190£	275£	370$	300 €
Europe	80£	100£	210$	110 €
East Asia	290£	280£	570$	400 €
Australia	290£	300£	610$	450 €

Assumed exchange rate is 1£ = 2$ = 1.5€

Question 251:
What is the price of the cheapest offer to East Asia in pounds (£)?
A. £238
B. £252
C. £267
D. £276
E. £280

Question 252:
On average how much more expensive is it to choose a non-European destination with Good Fly than to choose a European one? (rounded up to one digit)
A. £185.2
B. £186.3
C. £186.9
D. £189.8
E. £191.0

Question 253:
Take Me There decides to offer a 50$ discount on every travel to the Americas. In percentages, how much more expensive is the discounted ticket to North America than the original price offered by In The Air?
A. 2%
B. 4%
C. 5%
D. 7%
E. 11%

Question 254:
Around The World only sells 10 tickets to Australia and 5 tickets to South America.
Good Fly only sells 25 tickets to Europe and 12 tickets to Australia. Rounded to two decimals, what is the difference between the total revenues of these two companies, in percentage of the higher revenue?
A. 33.33%
B. 34.86%
C. 34.43%
D. 35.35%
E. 36.36%

Question 255:
The £ to $ exchange rate changes in a way that £1 = 2.5$. In pounds, what is the difference between the original and the new ticket price of Take Me There to Australia?
A. £55 B. £58 C. £61 D. £64 E. £75

SET 52

Indian GDP

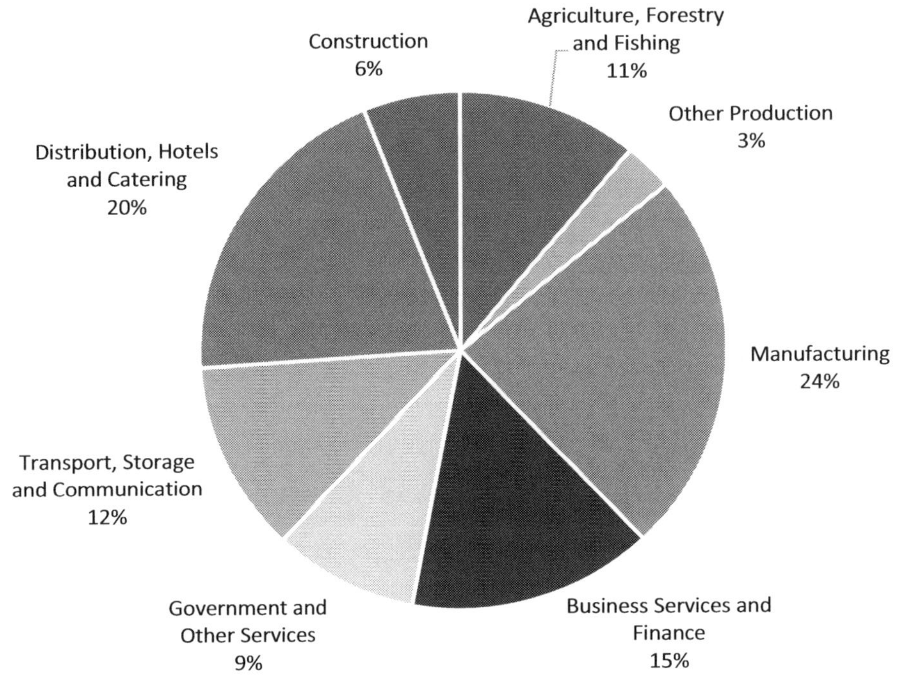

UK GDP

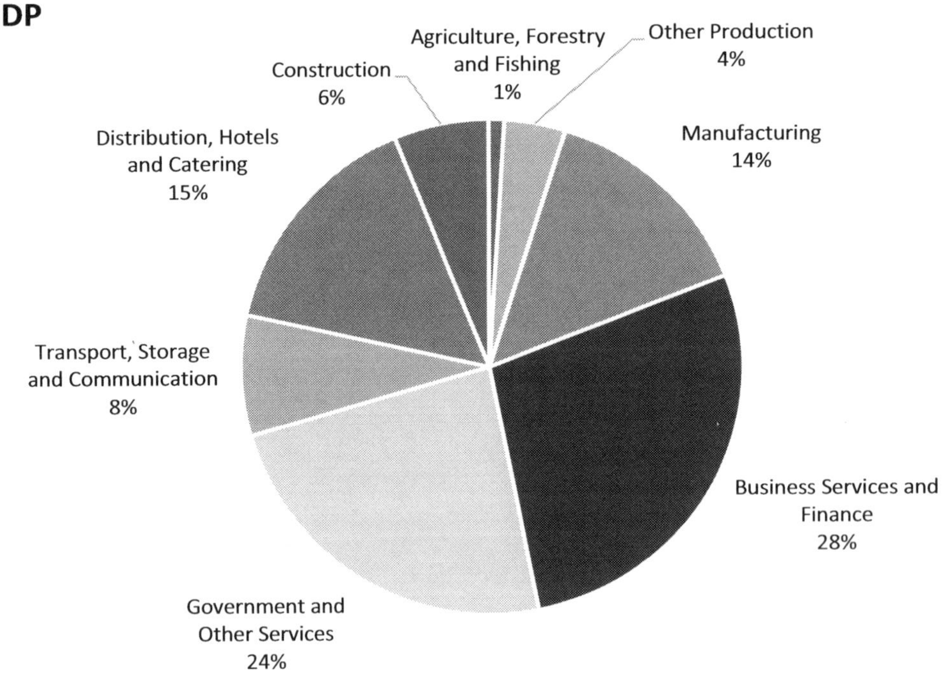

Question 256:
Which industry has the largest contribution to Indian GDP?
A. Agriculture, Forestry and Fishing
B. Construction
C. Government and Other Services
D. Manufacturing
E. Other Production

Question 257:
Expressing 'Government and Other Services' as a percentage of 'Business Services and Finance', what is the difference between these ratios in India and the UK?
A. 10%
B. 12%
C. 26%
D. 34%
E. 67%

Question 258:
What are the top **three** contributing sectors to Indian GDP?
A. Business Services Finance; Distribution, Hotels and Catering; Manufacturing
B. Agriculture, Forestry and Fishing; Business Services Finance; Manufacturing
C. Distribution, Hotels and Catering; Government and Other Services; Business Services and Finance
D. Construction; Manufacturing; Transportation, Storage and Communication
E. Distribution, Hotels and Catering

Question 259:
If the Indian GDP was £2 trillion and the UK GDP was £4.2 trillion in 2014. How much more did the bottom two performing sectors contribute to the UK GDP than to the Indian GDP?
A. £10 Billion
B. £15 Billion
C. £21 Billion
D. £30 Billion
E. £40 Billion

Question 260:
If the Indian GDP was £2 trillion and the UK GDP was £4.2 trillion in 2014. In monetary terms which sector was the largest?
A. Business Services and Finance in the India with £400 Billion
B. Business Services and Finance in the UK with £400 Billion
C. Manufacturing in India with £1.176 trillion
D. Business Services and Finance in the UK with £1.176 trillion
E. Business Services and Finance in the UK with £2 trillion

SET 53

The table below shows the average value of 1 Japanese Yen (JPY).

	2010	2011	2012	2013
GBP	0.021	0.020	0.019	0.022
USD	0.010	0.013	0.013	0.015
EUR	0.015	0.016	0.015	0.015
CAD	0.123	0.115	0.119	0.125

Question 261:
How much USD could you get for 1500 Yen in 2011?
A. USD 19.50
B. USD 21.00
C. USD 21.90
D. USD 25.50
E. USD 100.50

Question 262:
What was the GBP/USD average exchange rate in 2013 based on the information available?
A. 0.85
B. 0.92
C. 1.26
D. 1.47
E. 1.54

Question 263:
In percentage terms, what was the increase in JPY/CAD exchange rate between 2011 and 2012?
A. 3.5%
B. 3.9%
C. 4.5%
D. 5.1%
E. 11.5%

Question 264:
How much more JPY would I have received for USD 1300 in 2010 than in 2013?
A. JPY 43,333
B. JPY 45,000
C. JPY 45,225
D. JPY 46,310
E. JPY 47,450

Question 265:
Which exchange rate has been the least volatile between 2010 and 2013?
A. CAD
B. USD
C. EUR
D. JPY
E. GBP

SET 54

The table below shows changes in car use and population in four American cities between 2009 and 2014.

		Boston	Chicago	Denver	El Monte
2009	Population	4 million	3.5 million	2 million	0.8 million
	Number of cars	235,675	345,526	231,456	54,000
2014	Population	4.4 million	3.3 million	2.1 million	1.5 million
	Number of cars	542,000	350,685	249,990	62,044

Question 266:
In which city was the population growth the largest between 2009 and 2014?
A. Boston
B. Chicago
C. Denver
D. El Monte
E. Can't Tell

Question 267:
In which city was the growth in the number of cars used the largest between 2009 and 2014?
A. Boston
B. Chicago
C. Denver
D. El Monte
E. Can't Tell

Question 268:
In which city was the number of cars per person the lowest in 2014?
A. Boston
B. Chicago
C. Denver
D. El Monte
E. Can't Tell

Question 269:
In which city was the change in the number of cars per person the largest between 2009 and 2014?
A. Boston
B. Chicago
C. Denver
D. El Monte
E. Can't Tell

Question 270:
What is the difference between the number of cars per person in 2009 and 2014 in Boston?
A. 0.0064
B. 0.035
C. 0.054
D. 0.064
E. 0.065

SET 55

The table shows the change in tax rates and bands from tax year 2014-15 to 2015-16.
Family: Adam, Lewis, Courtney and Bruno

Income Tax Bands	2014-15 Rate	2015-16 Rate	2014-15 (GBP)	2015-16 (GBP)
Starting rate	15%	10%	≤ 2,450	≤ 2,730
Basic rate	25%	25%	2,450 < to ≥33,500	2,731 < to ≥ 37,000
Higher rate	40%	40%	33,500 <	37,000 <

Question 271:
Adam earned £37,000 in 2014-15. How much income was deducted from his salary during that year?
A. £4560
B. £6730
C. £8129.50
D. £9110.75
E. £9530

Question 272:
Bruno and Lewis each have a part-time job at a local pub and each earned £7,000 per year in 2014-15. What is the difference between their annual incomes after income tax has been deducted?
A. £0
B. £50
C. £176
D. £450
E. £745

Question 273:
Courtney received £42,000 in the tax year 2014-15. What was her average monthly income tax deduction?
A. £878.98
B. £898.98
C. £910.15
D. £960.83
E. £1024.58

Question 274:
Adam earned a performance bonus of £4,000 in 2014-15, increasing his salary from £37,000 to £41.000. By how much did his income tax change from what it would have been for this year without the performance bonus?
A. £1200
B. £1600
C. £1800
D. £2100
E. £3400

Question 275:
How much did the starting rate upper bound change from 2014-15 to 2015-16?
A. £80 decrease
B. £150 decrease
C. £280 decrease
D. £150 increase
E. £280 increase

SET 56

The table below shows the annual summary for performance evaluation of four partners at a management consulting firm. The bonus earned is calculated by multiplying the total sales by the bonus rate.

Partner	Projects Acquired (No.)	Total Sales	Bonus	Customer Satisfaction Rate
Adam	5	£45,000,000	**1%**	**97%**
John	2	£150,453,000	**5%**	**90%**
Richard	3	£180,000,000	**4%**	**75%**
Daniel	7	£654,150,000	**10%**	**25%**

Question 276:
Who received the highest bonus?
A. Adam
B. John
C. Richard
D. Daniel
E. Can't Tell

Question 277:
What is the average sales per project generated by Daniel?
A. £83,755,000
B. £93,450,000
C. £96,345,000
D. £99,950,000
E. £100,145,000

Question 278:
How much bonus did Richard and Adam receive together?
A. £5,500,000
B. £6,000,000
C. £6,350,000
D. £7,250,000
E. £7,650,000

Question 279:
Whose customer satisfaction rate was the highest?
A. Adam
B. John
C. Richard
D. Daniel
E. Can't Tell

Question 280:
How much was the total sales generated by the four partners together?
A. £1,029,603,000
B. £1,135,150,000
C. £1,529,540,000
D. £1,529,110,000
E. £2,130,042,000

SET 57

The table below shows the daily share price movements of four UK companies:

Name	Current Share Price (in pence)	Percentage Change from Previous Day	High	Low	Volume
HSBC	25.432	-0.03%	27.000	25.123	7,345,321
BP	286.123	+4.5%	286.456	284.567	4,431,748
GSK	134.432	+0.13%	142.511	131.678	1,125,469
British Land	54.923	+1.11%	54.934	54.914	4,999,432

Market Capitalisation is calculated as: number of shares outstanding (volume) multiplied by share price

Question 281:
What was the share price of GSK yesterday?
A. £132.873
B. £134.157
C. £134.257
D. £134.345
E. £135.012

Question 282:
What was difference between the daily highest and lowest price of British Land?
A. £0
B. £0.01
C. £0.02
D. £0.025
E. £0.3

Question 283:
What was the market capitalisation of HSBC yesterday assuming that the volume is unchanged?
A. £186,250,178.618
B. £186,350,178.618
C. £186,450,178.618
D. £186,650,178.618
E. £186,862,262.351

Question 284:
Which company's actual share price changed the most from yesterday?
A. HSBC
B. British Land
C. BP
D. GSK
E. Can't Tell

Question 285:
What is the difference between the latest market capitalisation of BP and British Land?
A. 993,441,229.268
B. 993,941,234.268
C. 994,114,112.268
D. 994,241,299.268
E. 1,113,345,891.268

SET 58

The table below is a summary of students who signed up for the following courses at St. Mary Grammar School:

Courses	Women	Men
Psychology	10	6
Maths	8	7
Physics	10	15
Programming	4	5
Literature	12	8
History	7	7

Students can take more than one course.

Question 286:
For which course is the ratio of women and men most similar to that of Psychology?
A. Mathematics
B. Physics
C. Programming
D. Literature
E. History

Question 287:
For which course is the ratio of women and men most similar to that of Physics?
A. Mathematics
B. Psychology
C. Programming
D. Literature
E. History

Question 288:
What is the total number of women in St. Mary Grammar School?
A. 34
B. 51
C. 64
D. 145
E. Can't Tell

Question 289:
What is the total proportion of women to men?
A. 0.25
B. 0.5
C. 0.96
D. 1
E. Cannot Say

Question 290:
If three new students arrive at St. Mary Grammar School and they are all women studying Psychology. What is the change in the ratio of women to men studying Psychology?
A) 0.1
B) 0.3
C) 0.5
D) 0.7
E) 1.2

SET 59

This graph below shows the employment statistics (in percentages) of the men and women living in the UK in September 2015. A person is considered being in employment if they are shown as employed, self-employed, or "employed other".

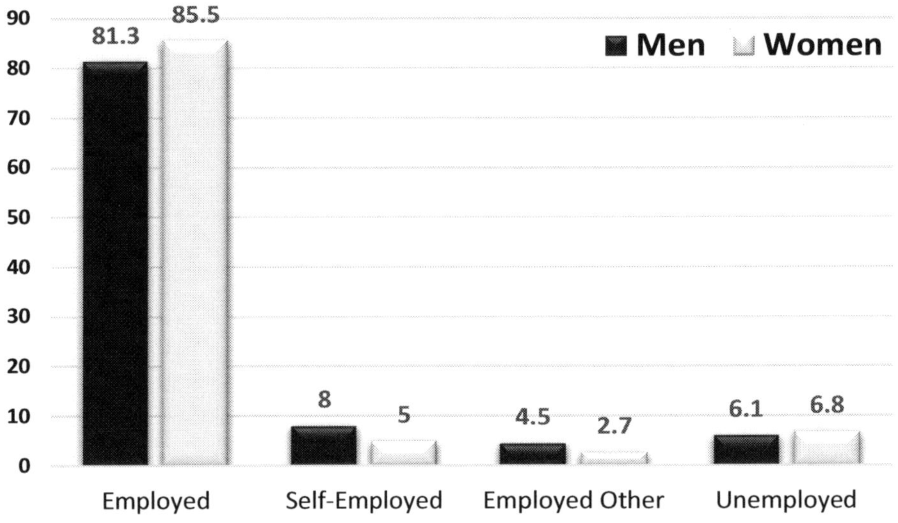

Question 291:
The difference between the percentage of women and men in employment is:
A. 0.6 B. 0.7 C. 1.2 D. 3.2 E. 4.2

Question 292:
The proportion of men to women self-employed or unemployed is:
A. 0.1
B. 0.5
C. 0.9
D. 1.2
E. 1.7

Question 293:
If there are overall 21 million women in employment in the UK how many women are self-employed?
A. 0.59 million
B. 0.86 million
C. 0.93 million
D. 1.07 million
E. 1.13 million

Question 294:
If there are 31 million men and 32 million women living in the UK, how many more women are unemployed than men?
A. 285,000
B. 423,000
C. 659,500
D. 735,000
E. 810,000

Question 295:
What is the proportion of employed to unemployed women in the UK?
A. 2.87
B. 5.43
C. 8.51
D. 13.7
E. 15.91

SET 60

This chart shows the expenses of the Jones household for this month. Overall they spent 360 pounds.

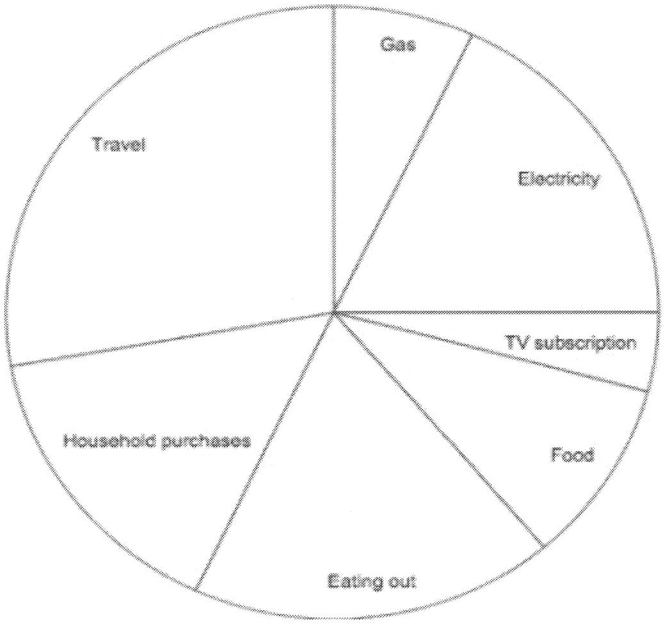

Question 296:
How much was their energy cost (electricity and gas) this month?
A. 65 pounds
B. 85 pounds
C. 90 pounds
D. 155 pounds
E. 200 pounds

Question 297:
What is the ratio of household purchases, travel and gas costs to energy costs (electricity and gas)?
A. 0.5:1
B. 1:1
C. 1.5:1
D. 2:1
E. 3:1

Question 298:
Which cost item was the greatest this month?
A. Gas
B. Travel
C. Electricity
D. Household purchases
E. Energy

Question 299:
If the total cost of household purchases, travel and gas costs was 180 pounds. How much were the energy costs in total this month?
A. 80 pounds
B. 87.5 pounds
C. 89.5 pounds
D. 90 pounds
E. 95 pounds

Question 300:
Which was the smallest cost item this month?
A. Gas
B. Travel
C. Electricity
D. Household purchases
E. TV subscription

Abstract Reasoning

The Basics

The abstract reasoning section of the UCAT will test your ability to think beyond the information that is readily available to you in form of the information provided by the question. The idea behind this section of the paper is to test how well the candidate is able to respond to questions that may go beyond the scope of their knowledge or require them to apply their existing knowledge in an unusual way. This is thought to be helpful in determining how well a student will be able to interpret information such as scans, X-rays or other test results as a clinician.

This section of the test examines pattern recognition and the logical approach to a series of symbols in order to match symbols to one group or another. There are a number of different question types, but all require one key skill – the ability to recognise patterns in a set of shapes

In this section of the UCAT, you have to answer 55 questions in only 13 minutes (with one additional minute to read instructions). Thus, it is mathematically the most time pressured section of the UCAT. But in terms of timing, think of it in terms of the image sets. There are multiple questions per image set. Since the main investment in time is in figuring out the pattern, you have a greater proportion of the time to spend on the first question in each set. Then all subsequent questions in that set will be easy and quick to answer. By far the hardest task is deducing the rules – once you have them, matching the options to the correct set is straightforward. Therefore as a rule of thumb, if the image set has 5 questions on it you have about 60 seconds to work out the pattern. Then, match the options to the set they each belong in using the remaining time allocation.

Timings

As with the rest of the test, you have to keep an eye on the time to keep track of how you're doing. Make sure that you stay within your time limit of 78 seconds for each block of 5 questions, and quicker for data sets with fewer questions. When divided up to 15 seconds per question it might not seem like a lot, but actually given the format of the questions you will begin to realise that it is enough. As mentioned above, for the 5-question sets keep ticking on at a steady rate of about 55–60 seconds to find the rule then about 18–23 seconds to decide which set the 5 different options fit into. Your **practice will increase both your speed and overall likelihood of finding the rule**, but despite thorough preparation you still may fail to spot the pattern. If you can't see it, don't despair – simply make reasonable guesses (you have a 33% success rate by chance alone), flag for review (in case you have spare time at the end to check back and have another go) and move swiftly on.

Top tip! Give yourself plenty of time to systematically work out the rules. Once you have found them, answering the questions will be quick.

Pattern Recognition

By far the most important ability in this section is to correctly identify patterns, as regardless of question style the matching process is straightforward once you have identified the rules. Some people are naturally better at this than others. You might be the sort of person who sees these patterns easily and can quickly put a name to the rule, or you might be the sort of person who finds it takes them more time and effort to work out what's going on. In reality, everyone lies at a different position on this scale, but one thing is certain. **You can improve your speed and accuracy on this section by having a methodical system** that can be repeated and applied to all shape-sets. One such system is the **NSPCC** system. This provides a logical structure for working through each set of images and looking for different components of a possible pattern.

In this system, the letters stand for:

Number ➔ Size ➔ Position ➔ Colour ➔ Conformation

Using this system, you consider each of the following aspects of the images in sequence, looking each time for commonly used patterns. We recommend this because it begins by looking for the simplest and most common potential patterns – if they are present, you are sure to get the pattern quickly and easily. If the first few patterns you look for are not present, then you look further on in the sequence to check for harder and less commonly tested patterns until you arrive at the answer.

Practice

It's very important to practice for this section as the style of questions are unlikely to be familiar. **Practicing well gives you three key advantages.** Firstly, you get used to the types of patterns which are likely to be asked in the real exam. This makes it more likely you will spot the patterns quickly as you will have seen them before, and it also trains up your implicit recognition system, meaning that if you take an "educated guess" you are more likely to be right. Secondly, it gives you practice implementing a pattern recognition system, like **NSPCC**. With practice you will become better at using the system, and therefore quicker and more accurate overall. Thirdly, you will gain a feeling for the time it takes to answer different types of question. This will allow you to better plan your time on the day, making the most out of every second you have.

Guessing

If you practice well you shouldn't have to guess very many questions, but it might be necessary if you just can't figure out a pattern. Guessing in this section of the test has a reasonable probability of success. Since there are only three or four options per question there is a 25-33% chance of guessing any one question correctly, and if all 5 questions in a data set are guessed then there is and 87% chance of gaining at least one mark from the set – better than in any other section of the UCAT. However there is more to it than that.

Whilst the best way to answer these questions correctly is to formally deduce the rule and apply it (using a pattern recognition system like **NSPCC** helps here), humans *do* have an innate instinct for pattern recognition. This innate instinct is not necessarily right and can lead you astray, but in a quick guessing situation, it can be applied cleverly to boost your chances of guessing correctly. That is to say, in some questions the overall look of the image will feel as though it should be placed in a particular set – you wouldn't be able to say exactly why, but to you it would look much more like one group than the other. Learning to harness this power can help give you a much better guessing accuracy. Below is a simple example to demonstrate:

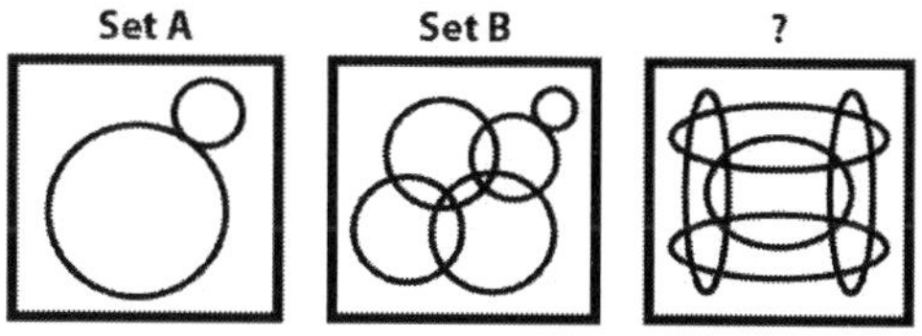

By quickly looking at the images provided for Set A and B, you get a general feel for what the contents are like. If asked which set the question image belongs to, you might be tempted to say Set B – it kind of looks more complicated and cluttered then Set A. It just looks more like the image. Now whilst this reasoning does not provide a comprehensive rule, in instances like this it can lead you to the correct answer quickly – even if you don't properly identify the underlying pattern.

Using the NSPCC system

The **NSPCC** system is a good way of working through possible patterns in a structured way. Whilst no structured response can be perfect, this system will solve over 90% of patterns quicker and more reliably than by trusting intuition alone.

Using the system, it is important that you are thorough. Sometimes the pattern can be subtle and you could easily miss out on it if not taking care. You have to examine the details closely: count corners, sides of shapes, check where they are etc. **You shouldn't be looking AT the shapes; you should be looking FOR patterns.** You should be working quickly, checking one thing, and if it's not that checking the next item in your list until you find the rule. Now to look at the system step by step.....

Number

Looking at "number" is about *counting* as many things as possible. How many dots? How many squares? How many sides? How many corners? How many right angles? Also have a look at how many different types of shapes you can find in the frames. Sometimes you might find one type of shape only in Set A and not in Set B for example. A good rule of thumb: block arrows have 7 sides, so don't count all the sides individually every time you see one!

Size

It is quite common to find patterns in the size of the shapes. Is one shape always bigger than the others? Is there always a big shape in the centre, or in the corner? Are there smaller shapes inside larger ones?

Position

Look for patterns in where shapes are positioned. You might, for instance, always find a square in the top right corner in one set and a circle in the top right corner of the other set. Look for Look also for touching and overlap of shapes – when you see this, make careful note of the type of contact. Is it tangential? Does it cut the shape in equal pieces, or is it off centre? Is there a certain shape that always makes this contact?

Colour

The shading of different shapes can constitute a pattern. Whilst this is often the easiest pattern to spot, it takes its place lower down in the system as it can often be a distracter. Most diagrams contain some amount of shading, but only occasionally is the primary pattern centred upon this. Look for shapes that are always shaded. Are all triangles black in one set and all circles black in the other, for example? On the other hand, are some shapes never shaded?

Conformation

These are the hardest patterns to spot, as they are the more complex patterns that can't be found by looking at the more geometric aspects. Conformation describes the pattern by which the shapes are arranged within the box – so you have to take a step back and look at the box as a whole in order to spot them. Look for patterns to the arrangement, like shapes arranged in a horizontal, vertical or diagonal line. Look also for the influence of one shape on another. For example, the presence of a white circle might signal a 90 degrees clockwise rotation of one shape and the presence of a black circle might signal a 90 degrees anticlockwise rotation, for example. When there are arrows, look at where they are pointing: are they all pointing in the same direction or at the same thing? You're looking for second order patterns, how things change with other aspects of the image.

Question Answering Strategy

There are four styles of question in this section, but all of these require the same pattern-recognition skills.

The **first style** of questions is the original style of question that used to be the only style in this section of the UCAT. It also tends to be the style that accounts for the majority of the questions in this section, however this is not an official rule and it will not necessarily be the same this year. In this type of question, you are provided with two sets of six shapes, Set A and Set B. All of the images within each set are linked to each other by a common rule, but the rule must be different for Set A and Set B. The task is to identify the rules for each set, then for the 5 options you need to decide where they belong. If an option follows the same rule as the shapes in Set A, then it belongs in Set A, and likewise for Set B. If the image obeys neither the rule for Set A nor the rule for Set B, then it is correct to say it belongs in neither set and you choose the "neither" option. Approach this style of question by spending the majority of the time deducing the rule by using a system like **NSPCC**. Then when you have decided on the rule for each set, work through the options, selecting which set each fits best. If you don't figure out the rule in time – don't worry. It is expected that you won't work out them all in the time pressure of the exam. In that case, simply use an educated guessing strategy to give yourself a good chance of picking up some marks and then move on.

normally quicker to answer as it is more intuitive. In addition, you have three different transition points that you can compare to each other to help deduce whether you have correctly identified the rule. To answer this style of question well, start by scanning quickly across all four shapes – this gives you a general understanding of what is happening in the sequence. Then, focus on the element that is changing and apply your system to find out exactly *how* it is changing. Once again, if you're struggling, you can probably use your intuition to make a decent educated guess and move on. Consider flagging for review so you know where to focus your efforts if you have any additional time at the end.

The **third style** of question is also a sequence style of question. You are provided with two shapes with a rule linking them. The rubric states shape one **is to** shape two by this rule. Then you are provided with shape three, and you have to apply this rule to find out how the rule transforms shape three into shape four (you are given four options). Once again, the key to accuracy is in deducing the rule that links the shapes. Focus on the same elements in shape one and shape two and notice any changes that have taken place. This style of question has a more straightforward strategy as there are many fewer options to examine; as you can directly compare the two boxes you can usually deduce the rule without needing to use a system, but remember it is always there if needed. Be certain to check the rule applies to *all* elements in the boxes, otherwise you will need to revise the rule to account for the box as a whole rather than just one or two of the elements. Once you are satisfied with the change, apply the rule to the next shape and select the answer. Ideally you should imagine what the answer is *before* focusing on the options, otherwise you could be biased by a similar but incorrect option, but if you are struggling to do this then use your intuition to select the option that feels as though it is the best fit.

The **fourth style** of question is very similar to the first and original style. You are provided with two sets of six shapes, Set A and Set B, each linked by a common rule. Once again apply the same system to deduce the rule for each set. The only difference comes when it is time to select your answer. Instead of being asked which set a shape fits into, you are provided with four options and asked to select the one that fits into one set or the other. So once you know the rule, test the options to see which one fits the set you are asked for.

Example 1

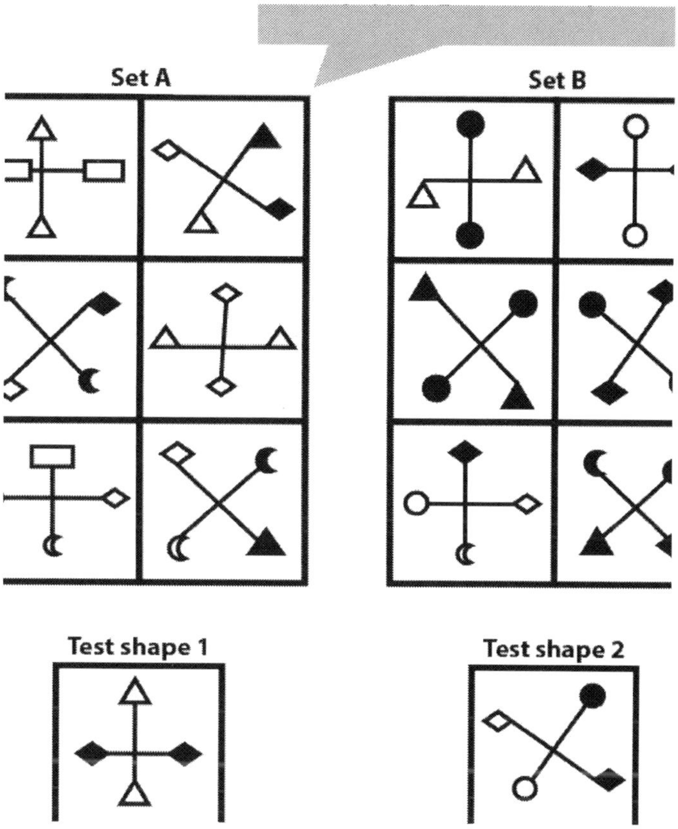

Start by applying the NSPCC system. Number: count the number of shapes, sides, angles and so on looking for a pattern (I can't see one). Size: are all shapes the same size (yes they are). Position: is there a pattern to where certain shapes are (not obviously). Colour: Is there a pattern to the shading (yes, the shading is dependent upon the shape of the cross). If you didn't get that, look back now to identify what the pattern is before reading on.

We can use our observations to devise the following rules:
Set A: (+)-shaped crosses have four white shapes and (X)-shaped crosses have two white and two black shapes. **Set B**: (+)-shaped crosses have two white and two black shapes and (X)-shaped crosses have four black shapes.

Applying these rules tells us Test Shape 1 belongs to Set B and Test Shape 2 belongs to Set A.

A Final Word

This section is all about pattern recognition. The more you see the better you will become. Once you're familiar with the main types of patterns which come up, you'll be able to solve the majority of questions without difficulty. Remember that **you're looking to identify a rule** for each set of boxes, something which links them all together. Then, you can decide which set each question item fits into (or indeed neither). Start using the **NSPCC** system, then practice makes perfect!

Abstract Reasoning Questions

SET 1

Set A Set B

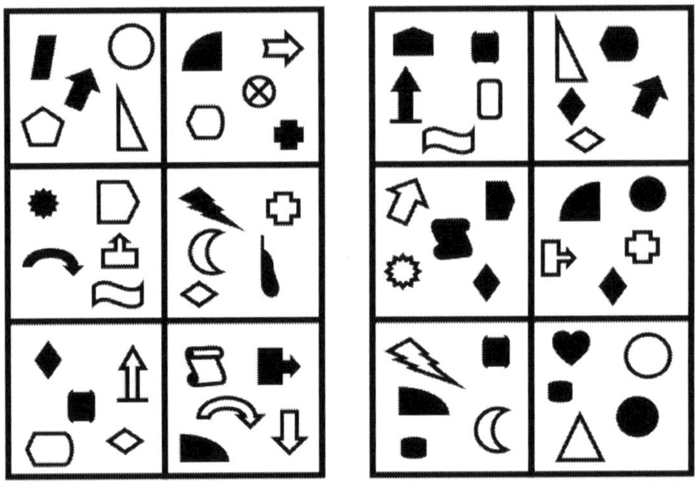

Questions 1-5

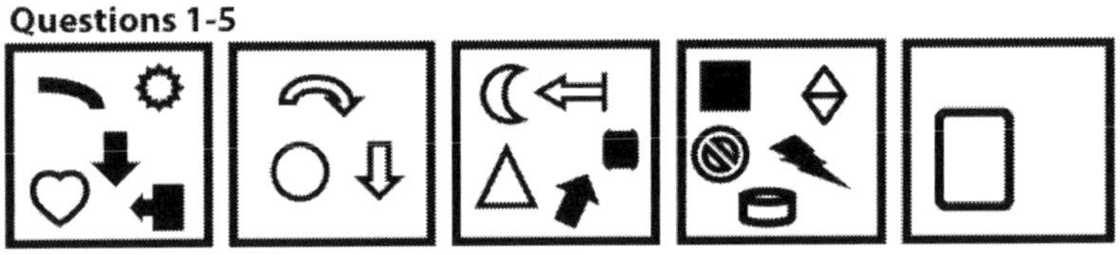

SET 2

Set A Set B

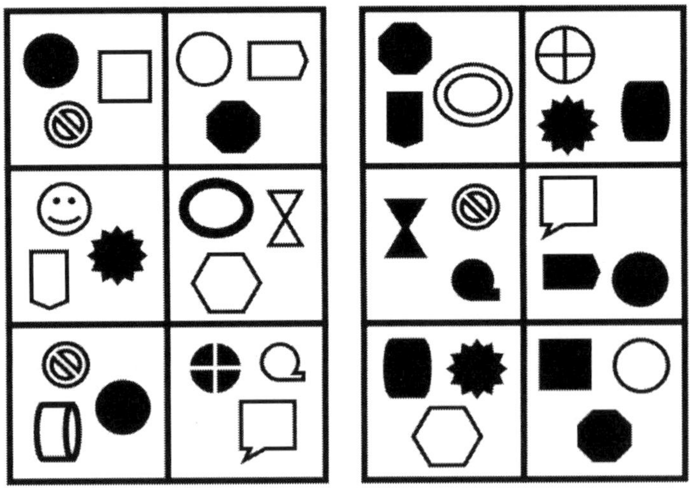

Questions 6-10

SET 3

Set A Set B

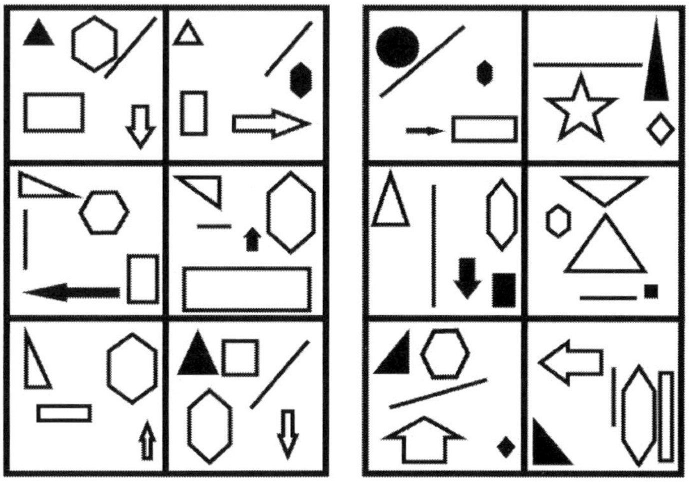

Questions 11-15

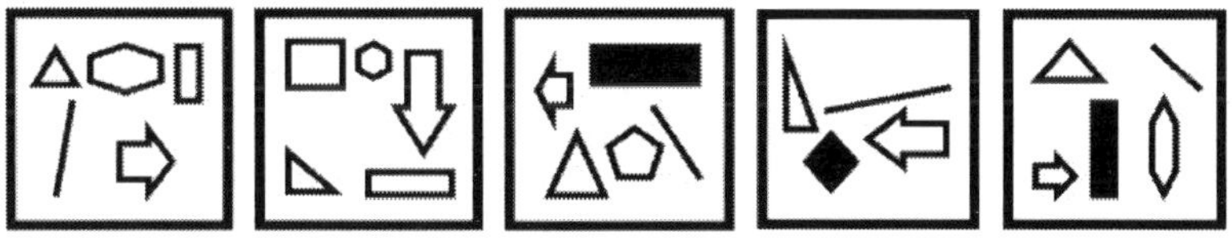

SET 4

Set A Set B

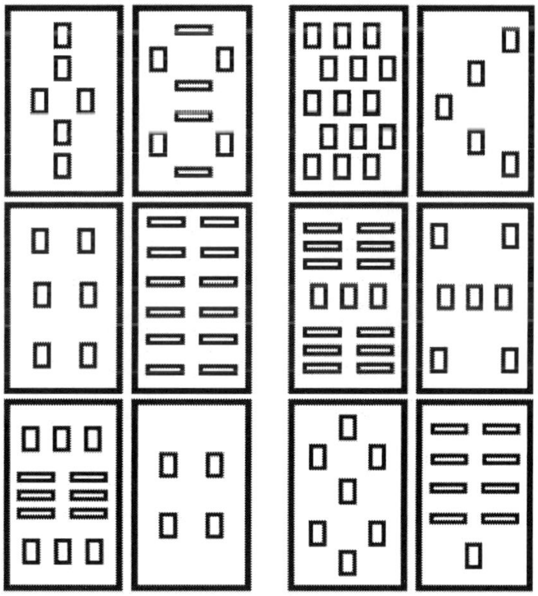

Questions 16-20

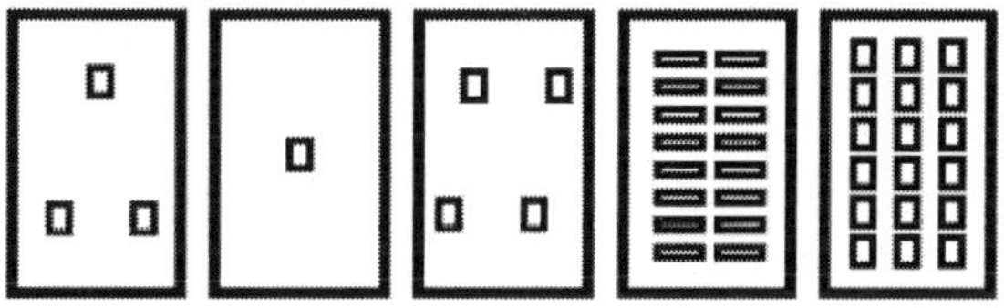

SET 5

Set A

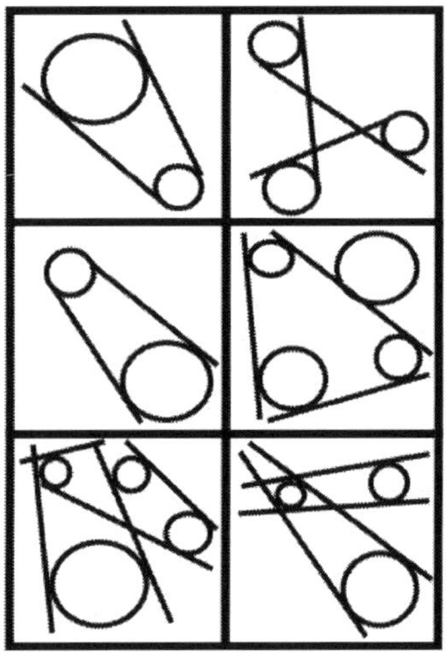

Set B

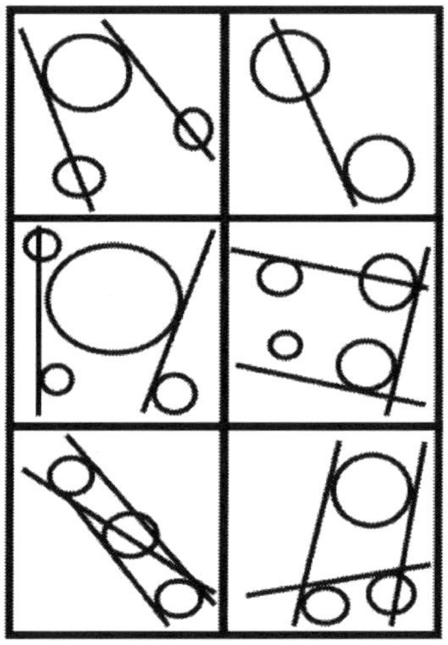

Questions 21-25

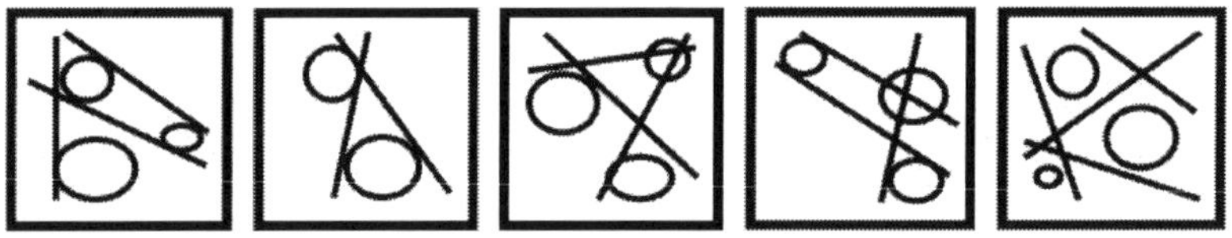

SET 6

Set A

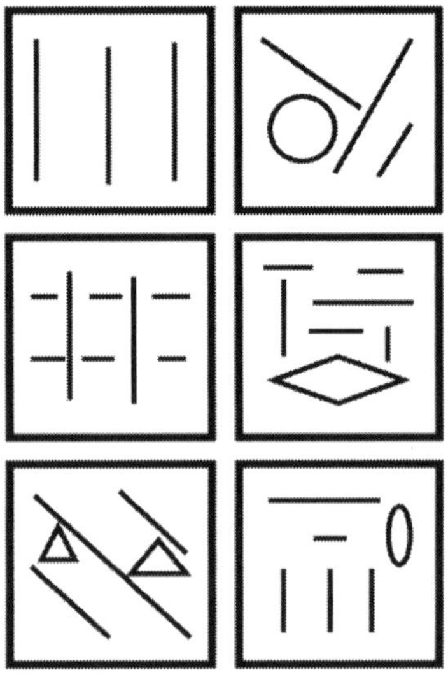

Set B

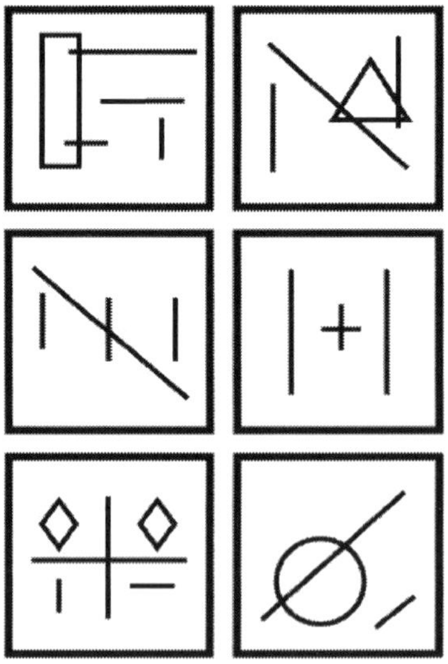

Questions 26-30

SET 7

Set A Set B

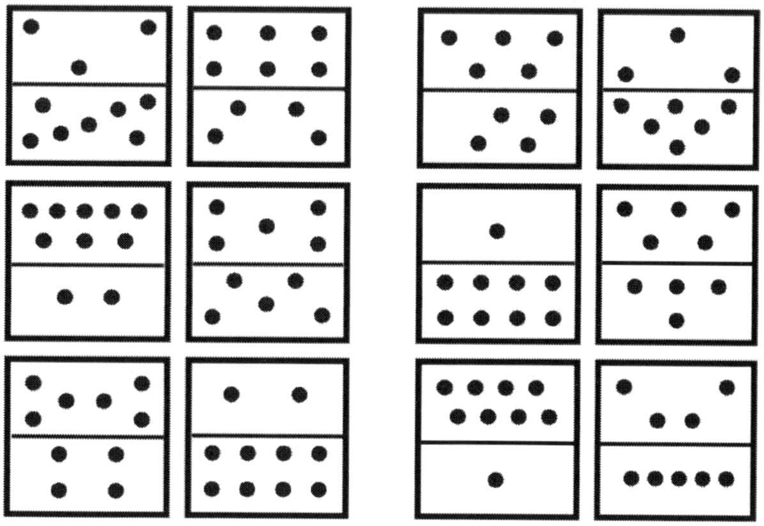

Questions 31-35

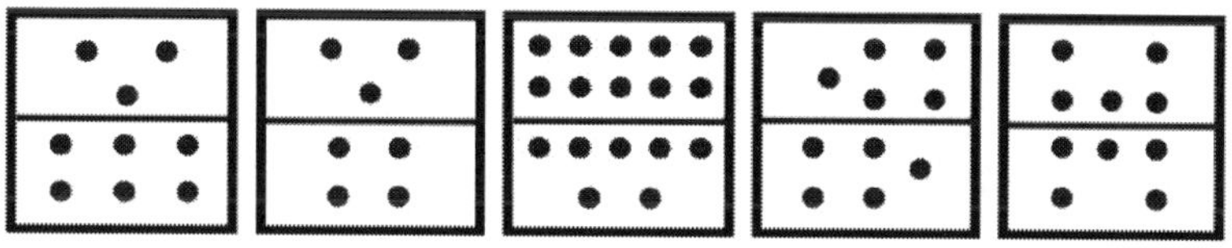

SET 8

Set A Set B

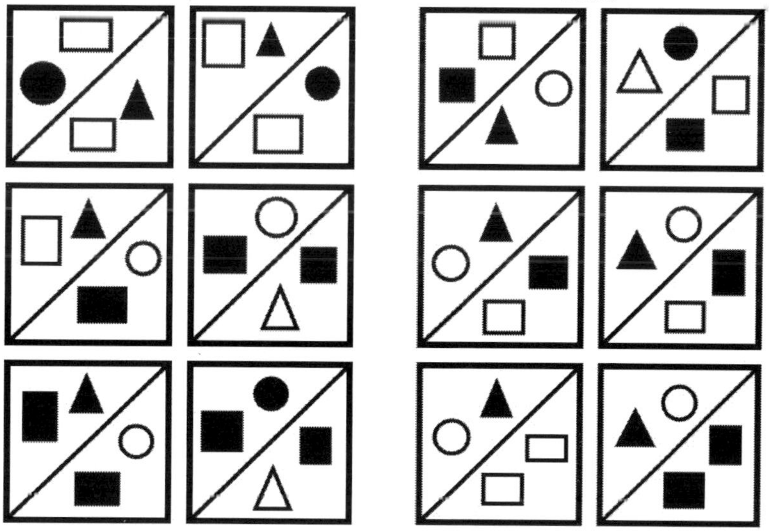

Questions 36-40

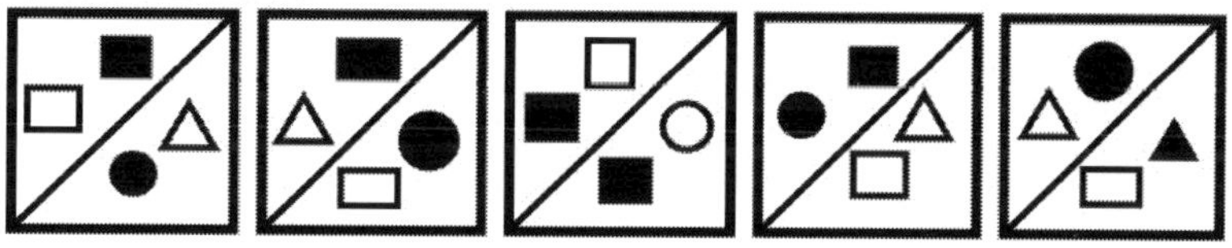

SET 9

Set A Set B

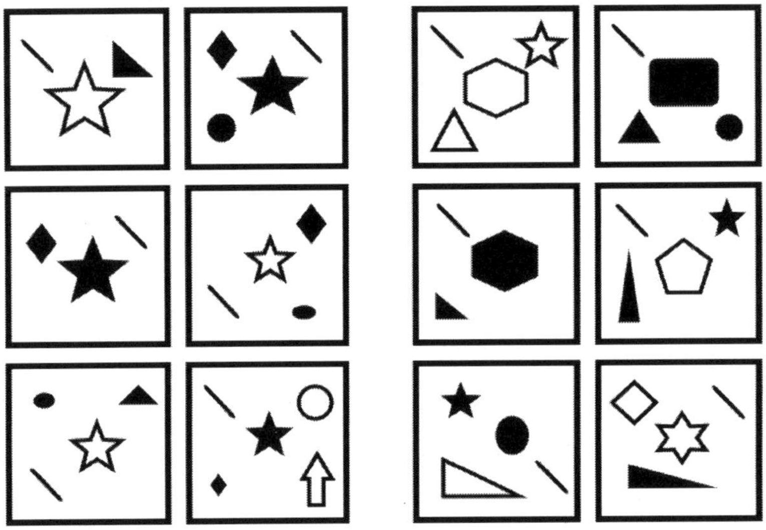

Questions 41-45

SET 10

Set A Set B

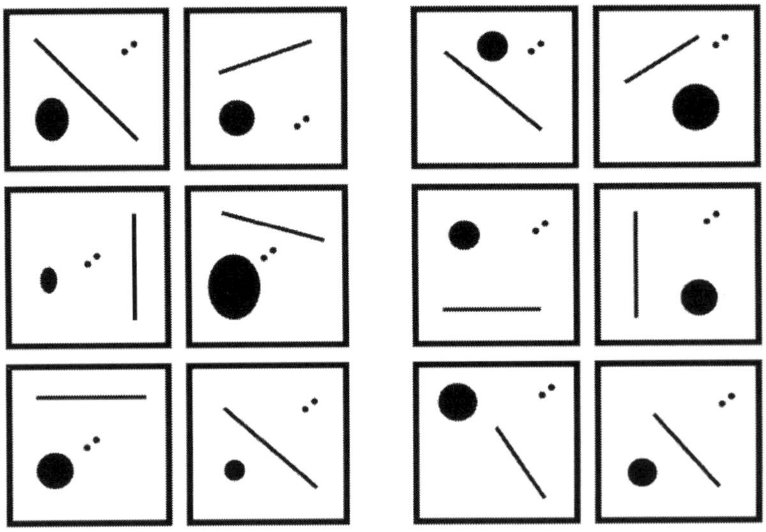

Questions 46-50

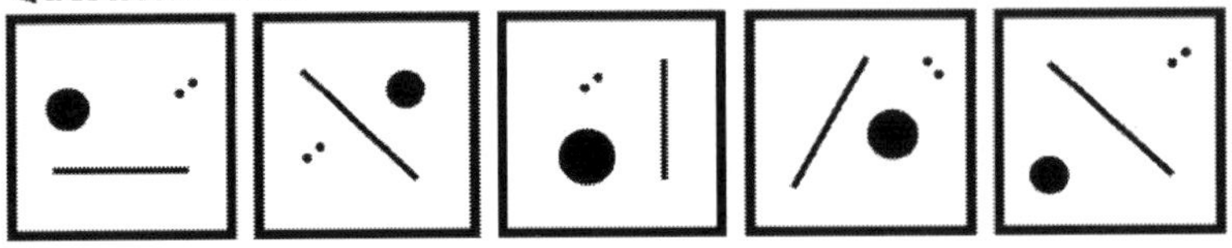

SET 11

Set A Set B

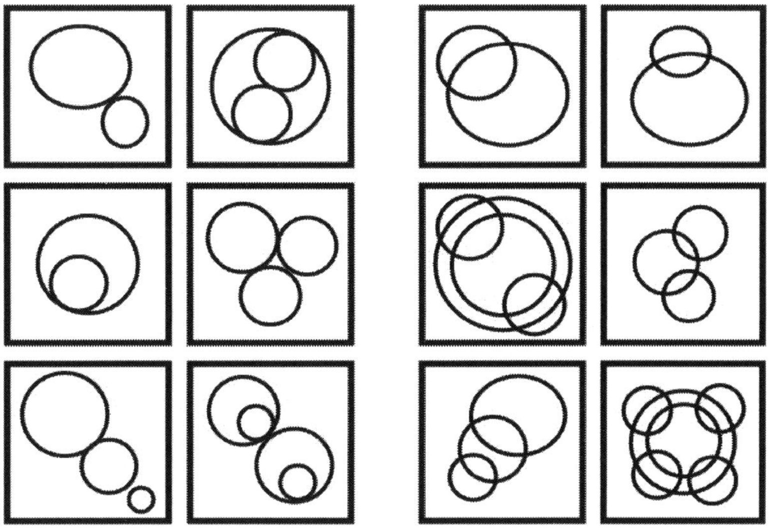

Questions 51-55

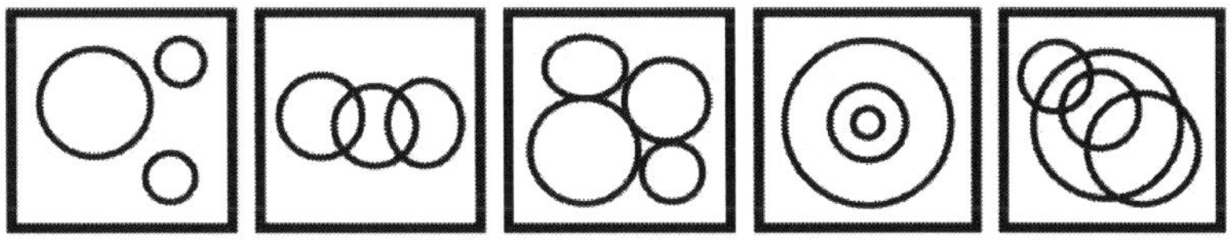

SET 12

Set A Set B

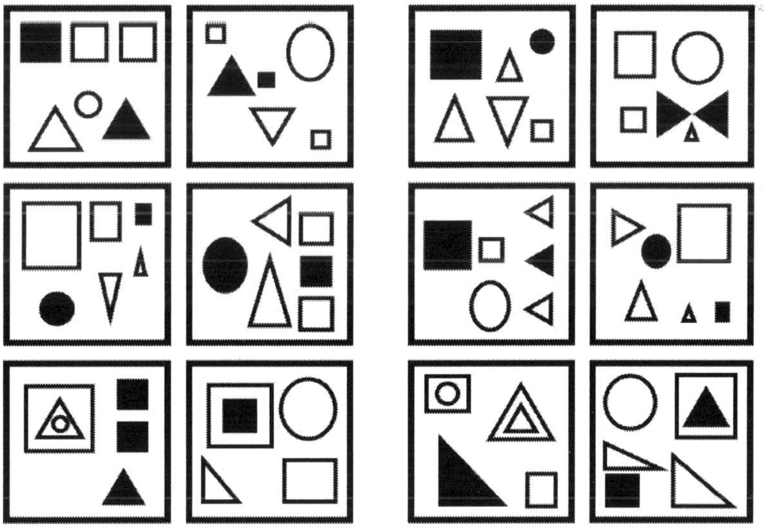

Questions 56-60

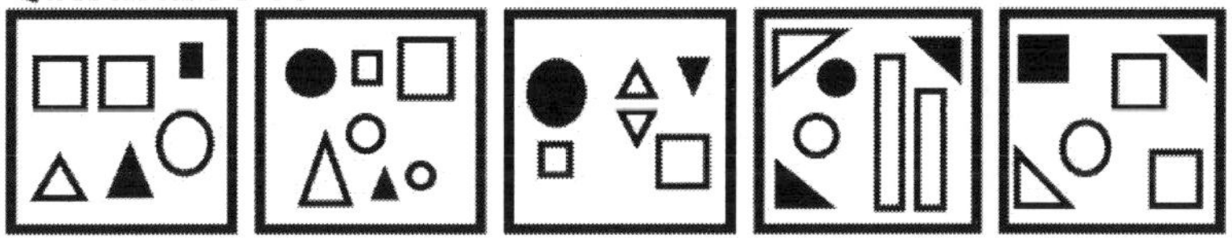

SET 13

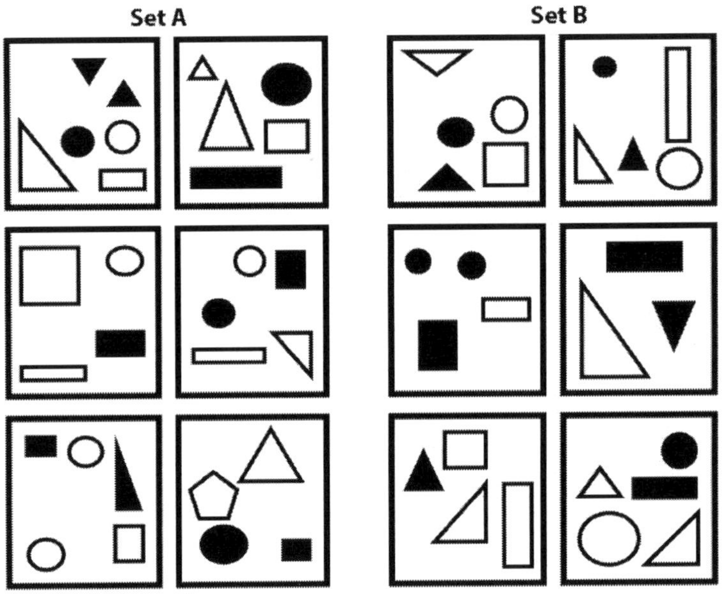

Questions 61-55

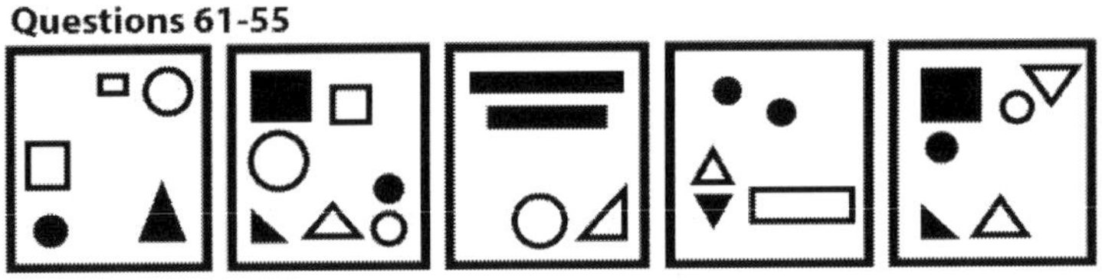

SET 14

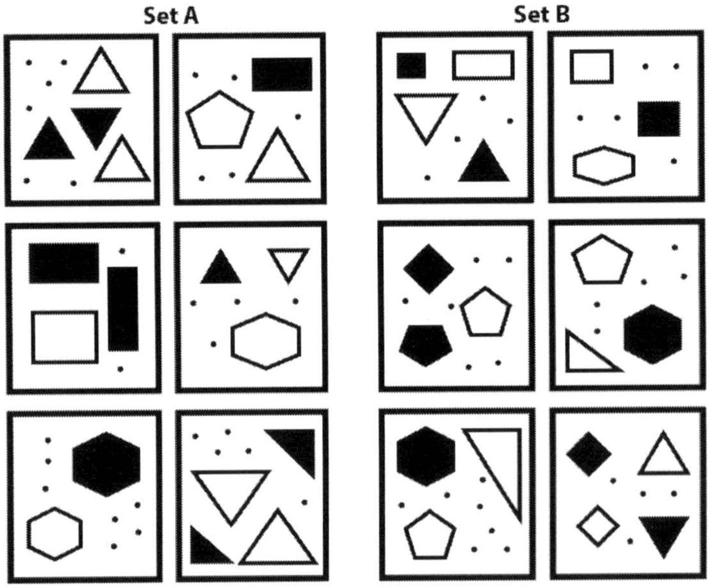

Questions 66-70

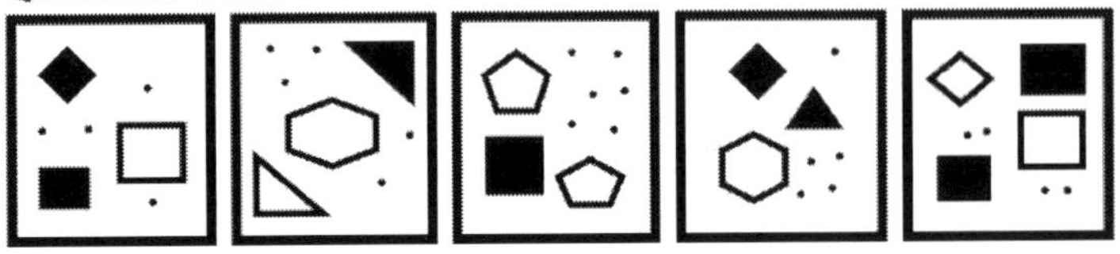

SET 15

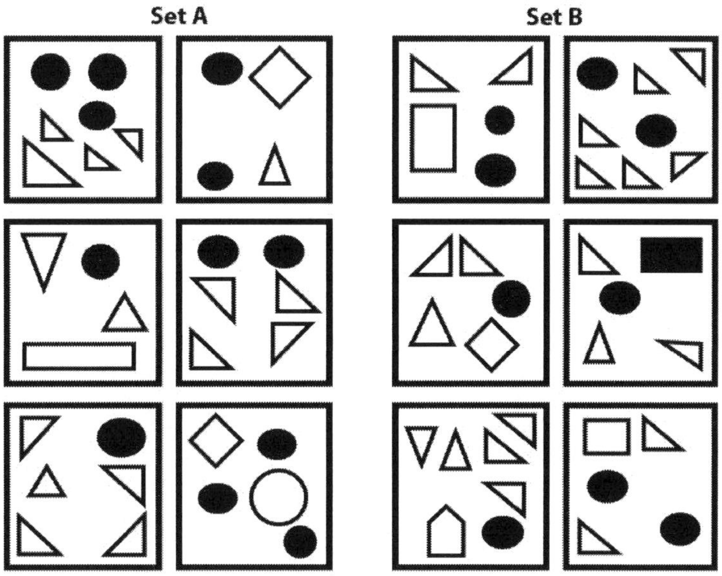

Questions 71-75

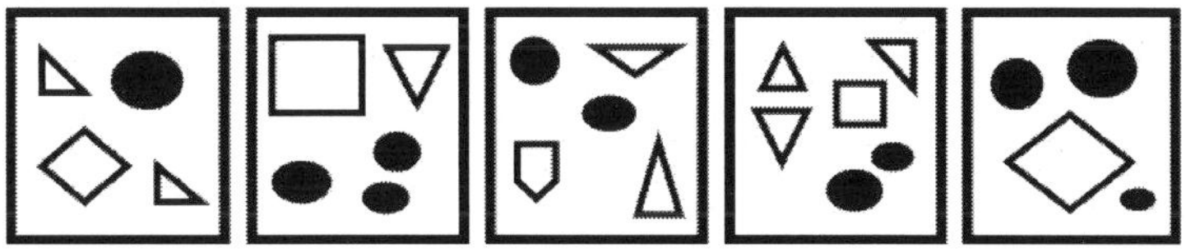

SET 16

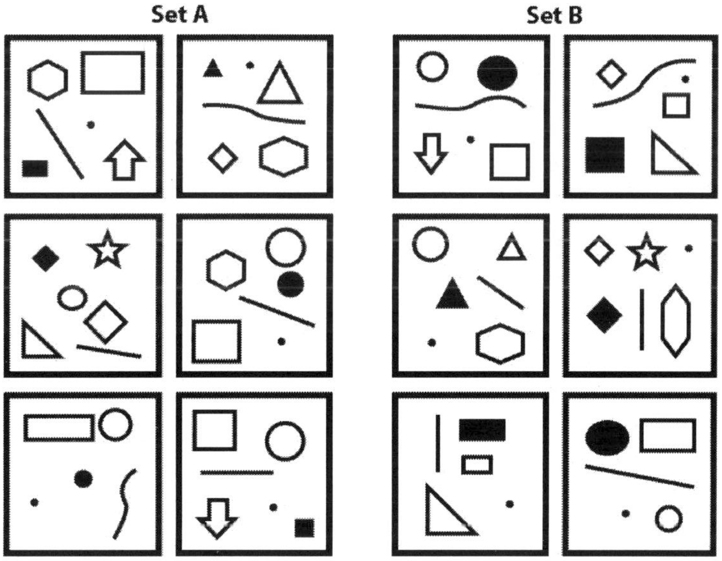

Questions 76-80

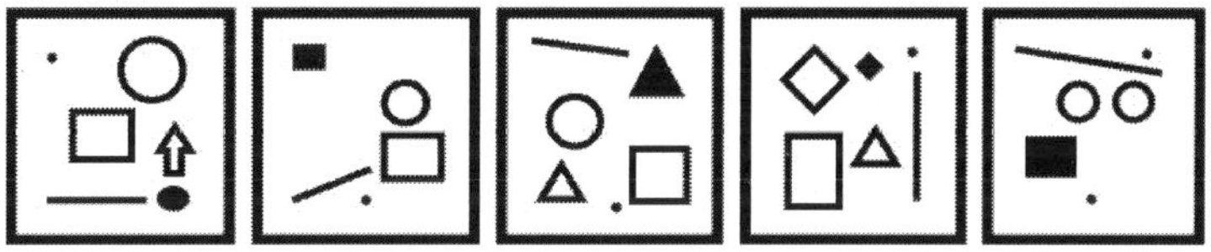

SET 17

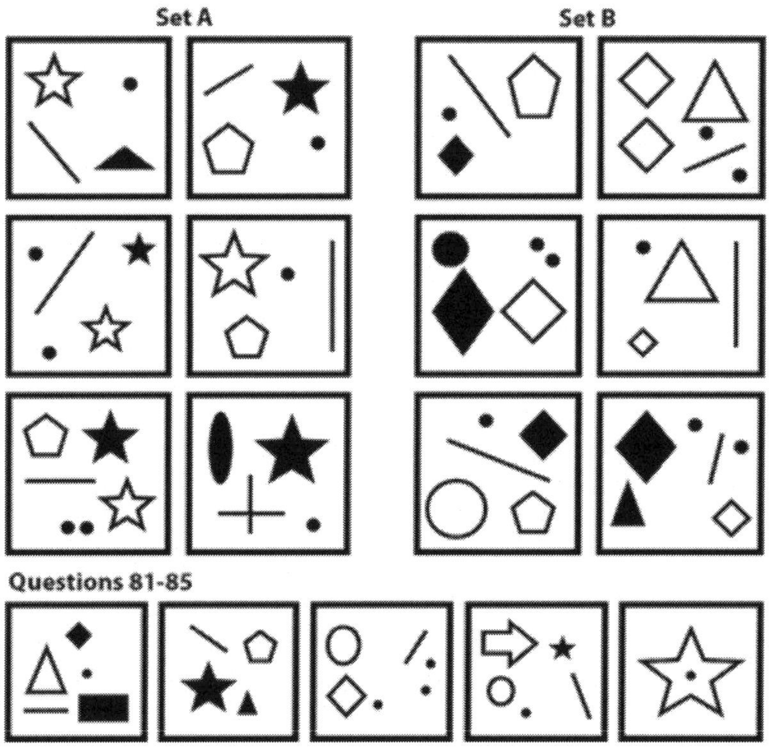

SET 18

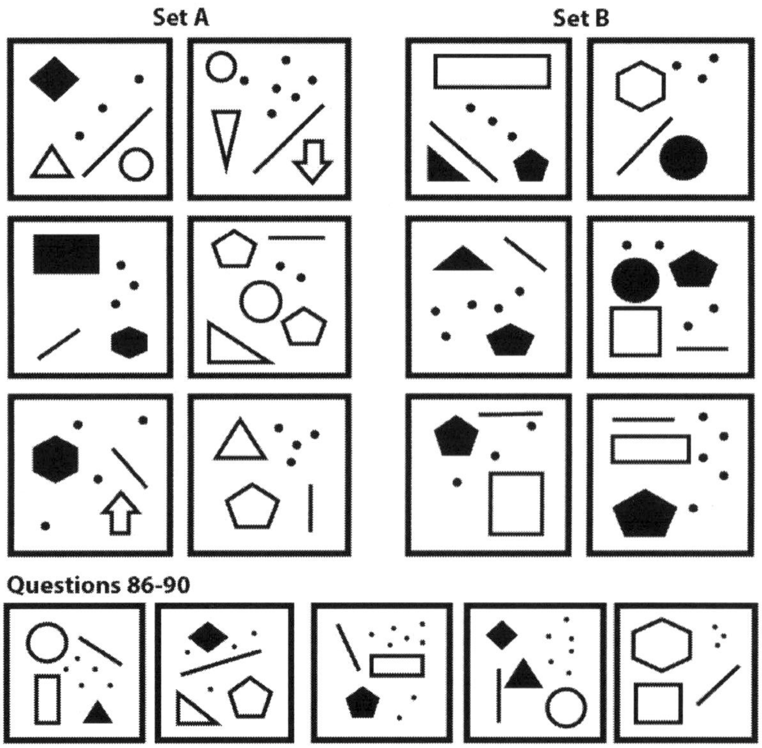

SET 19

Set A Set B

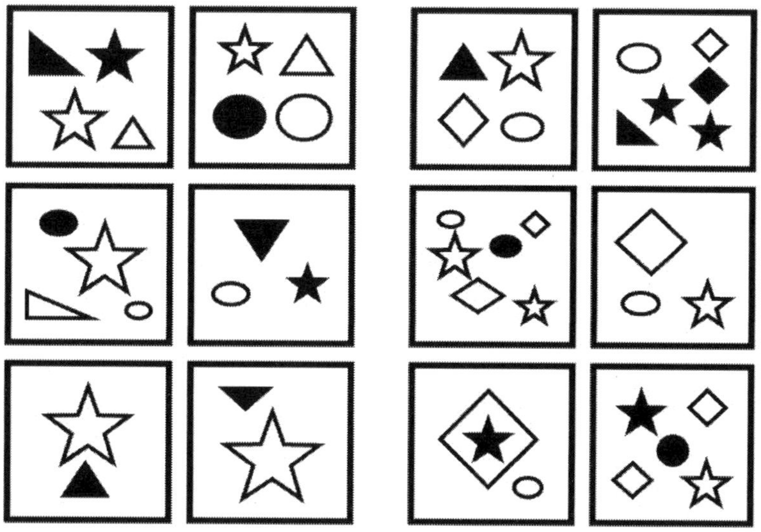

Questions 91-95

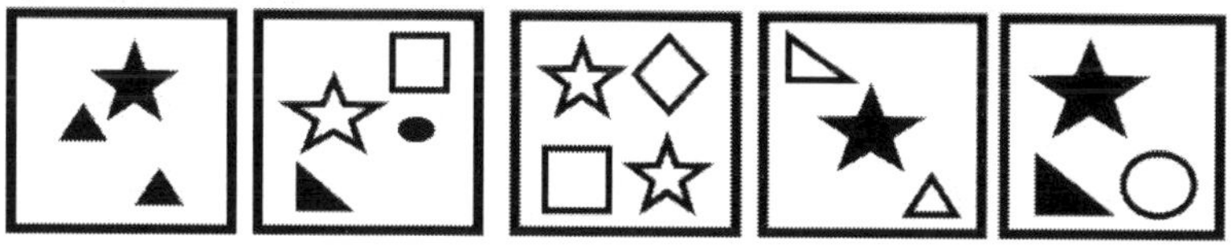

SET 20

Set A Set B

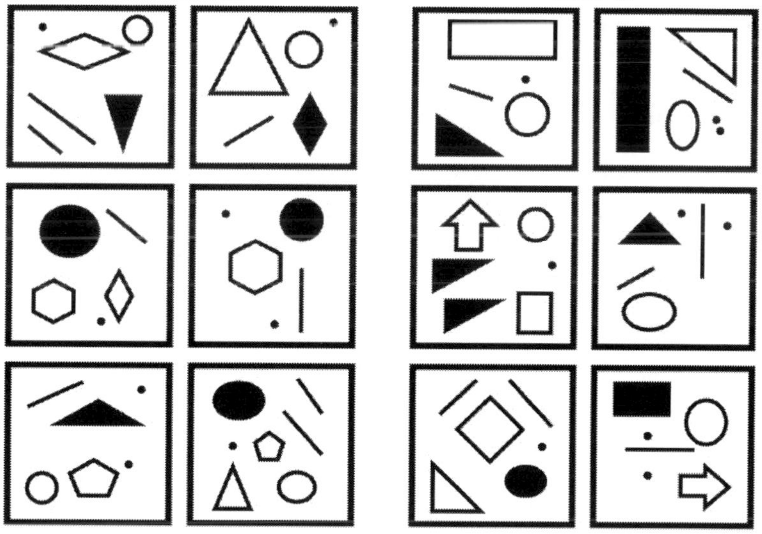

Questions 96-100

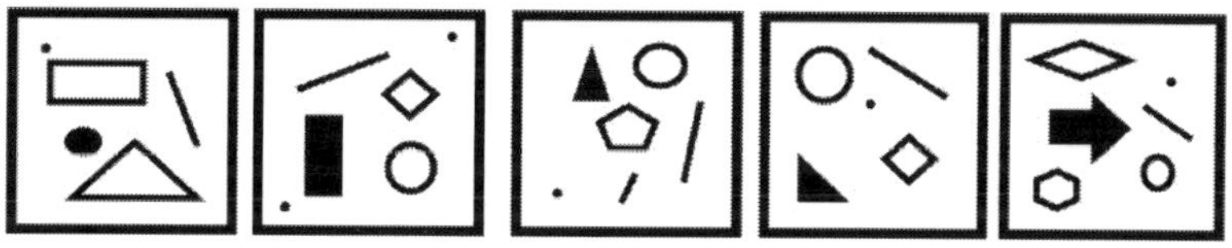

SET 21

Set A Set B

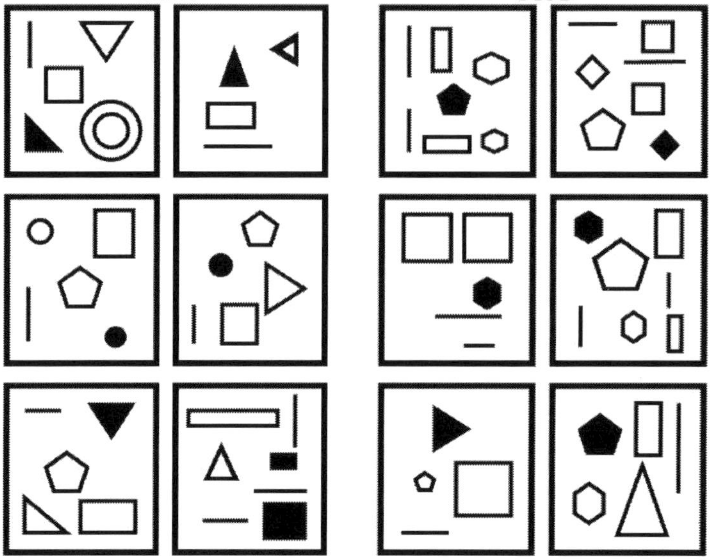

Questions 101-105

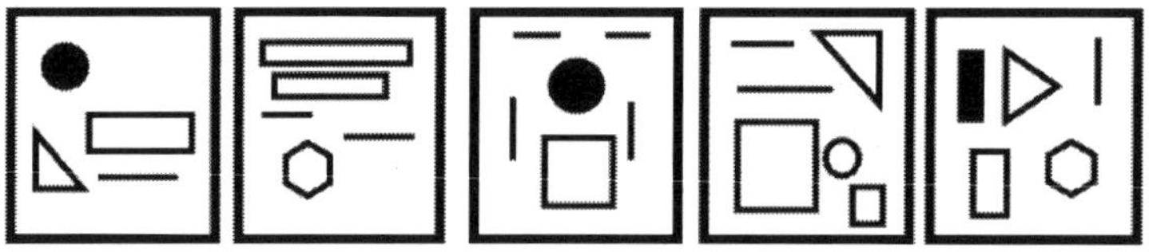

SET 22

Set A Set B

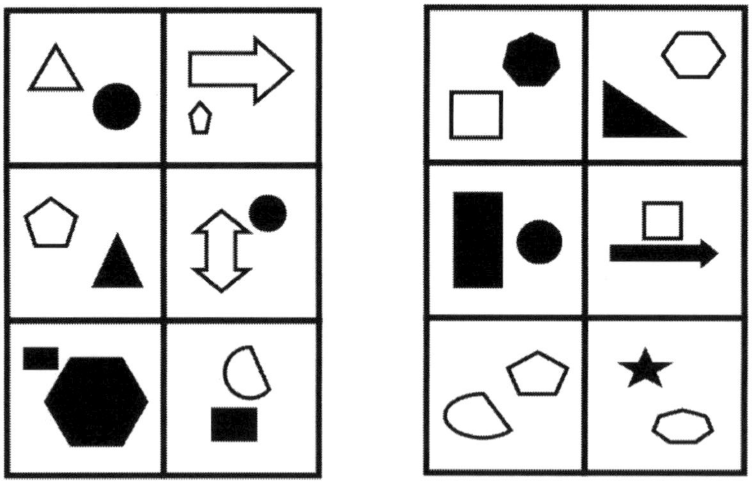

Questions 106-110

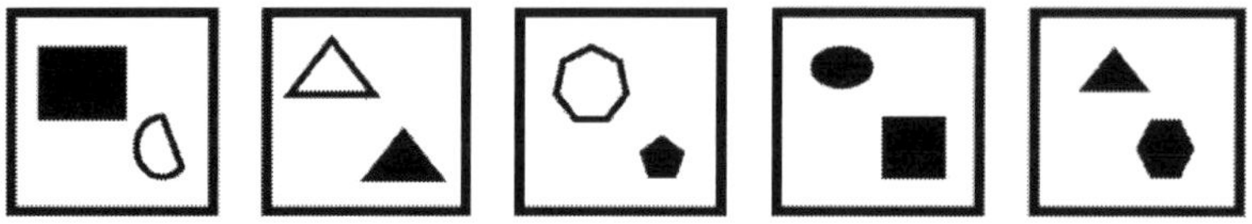

SET 23

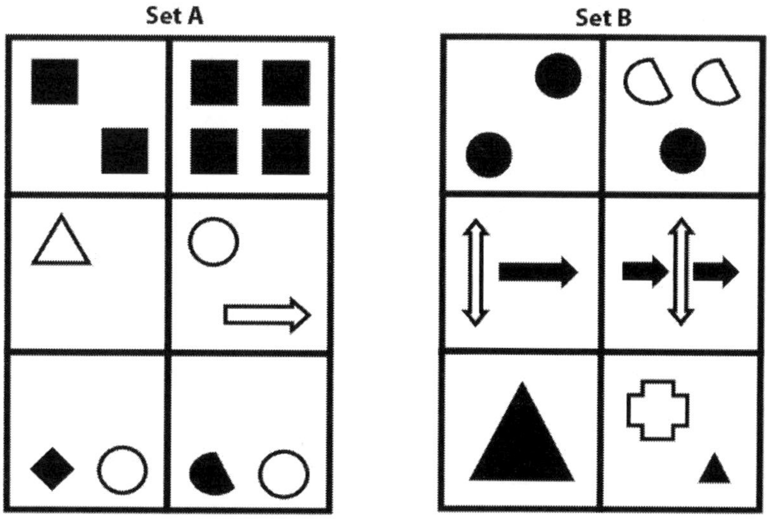

Questions 111-115

SET 24

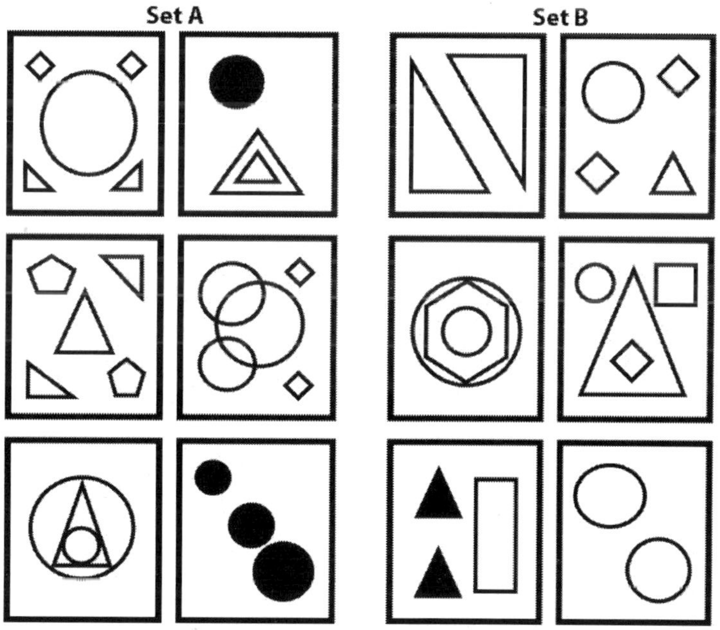

Questions 115-120

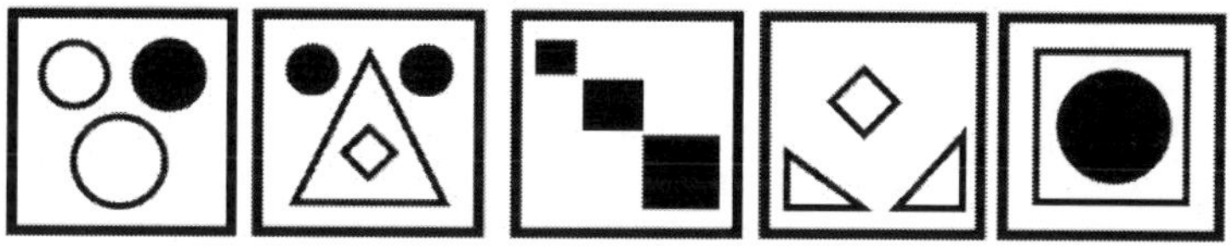

SET 25

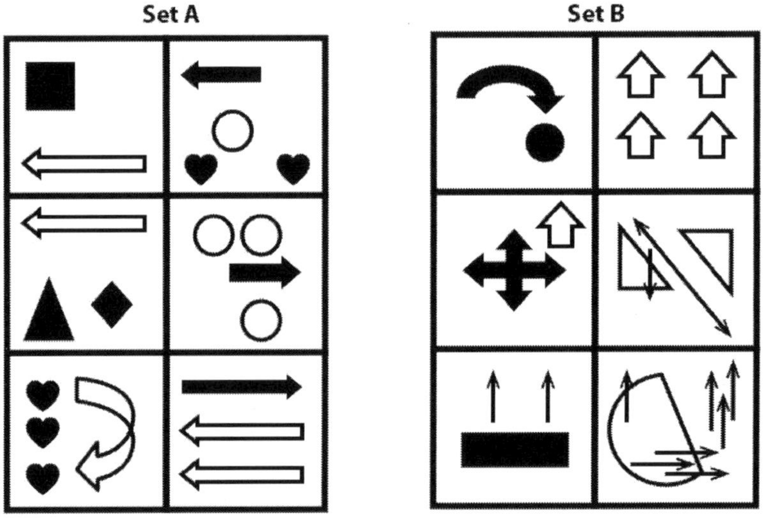

Questions 121-125

SET 26

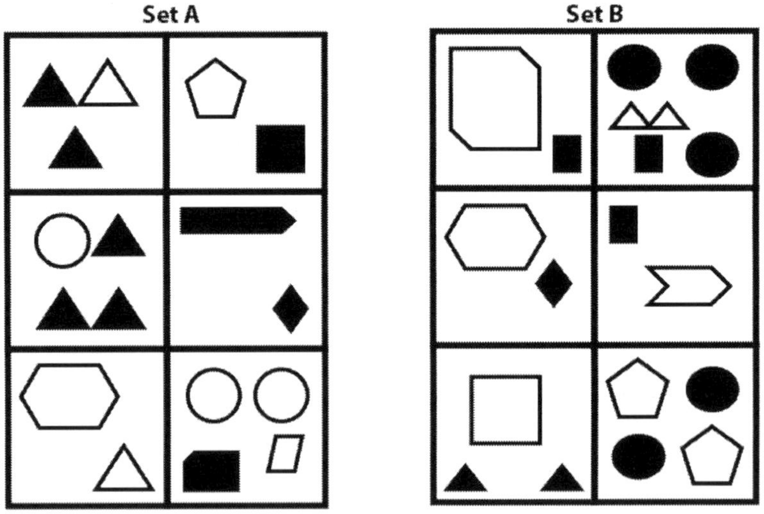

Questions 126-130

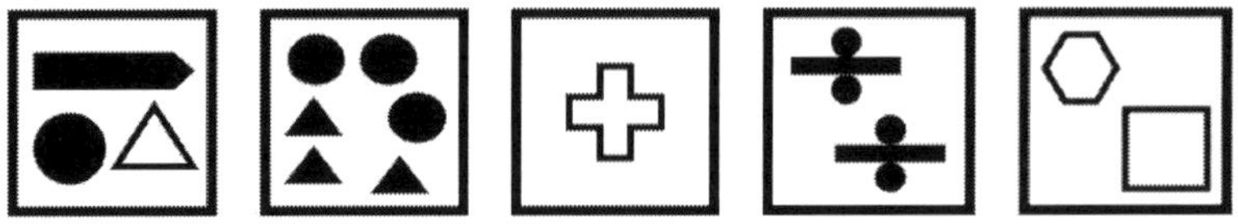

SET 27

Set A

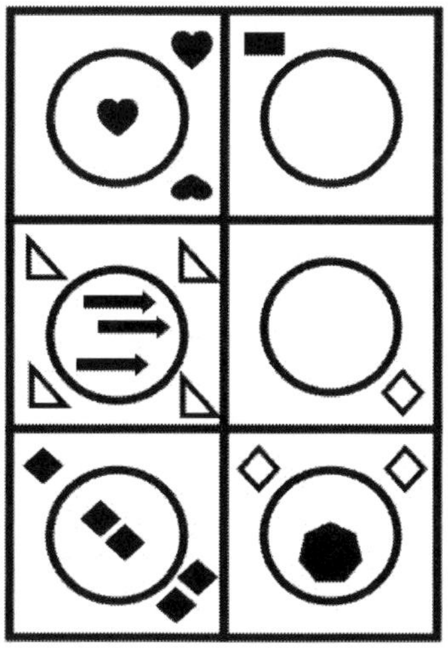

Set B

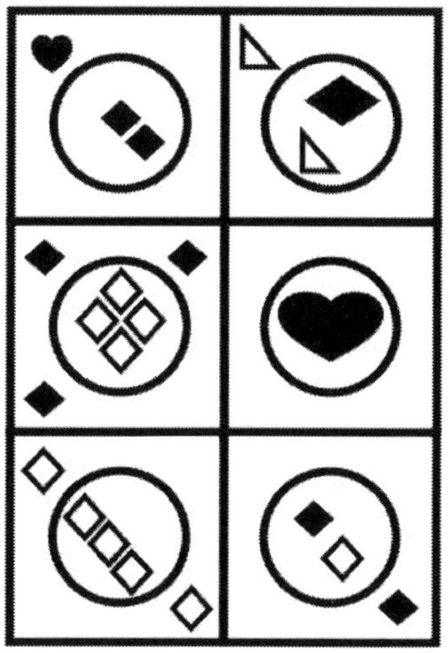

Questions 131-135

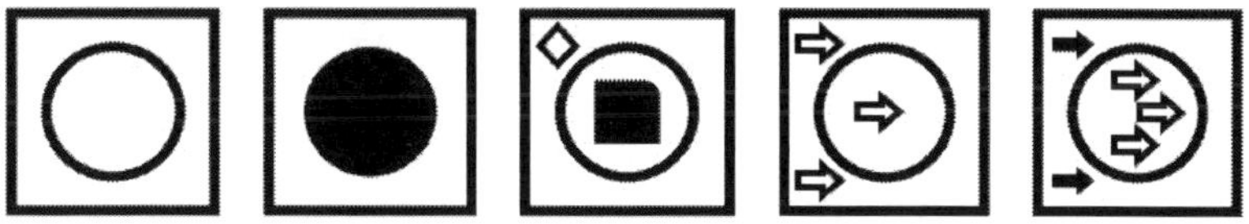

SET 28

Set A

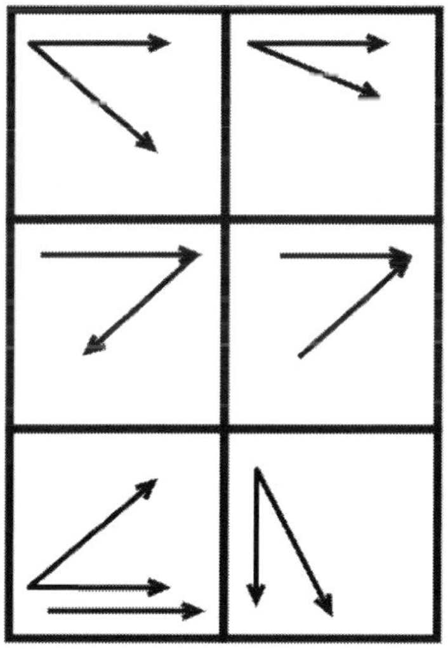

Set B

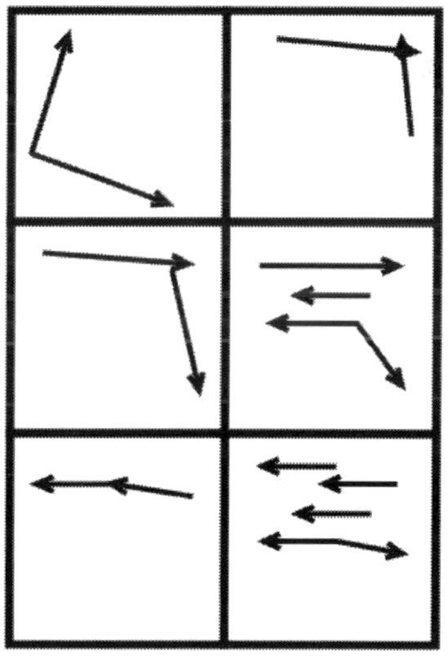

Questions 136-140

SET 29

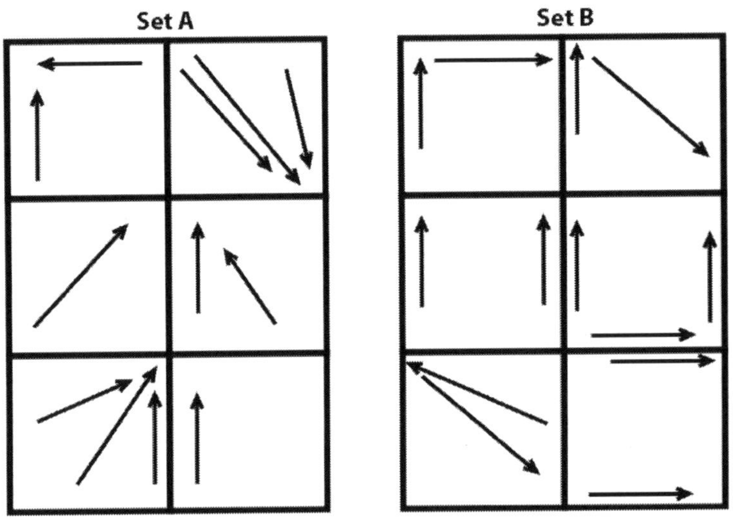

Questions 141-145

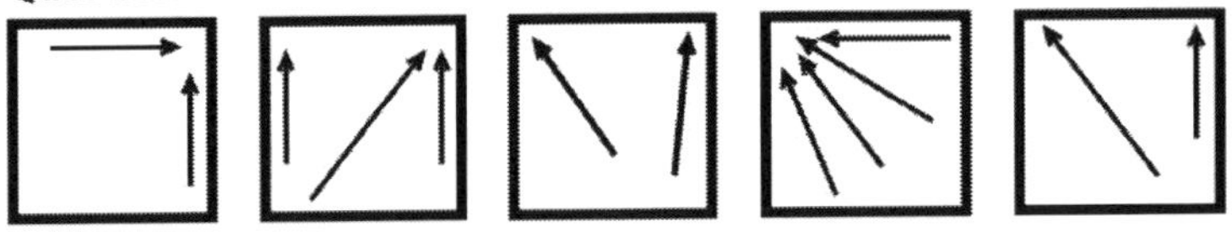

SET 30

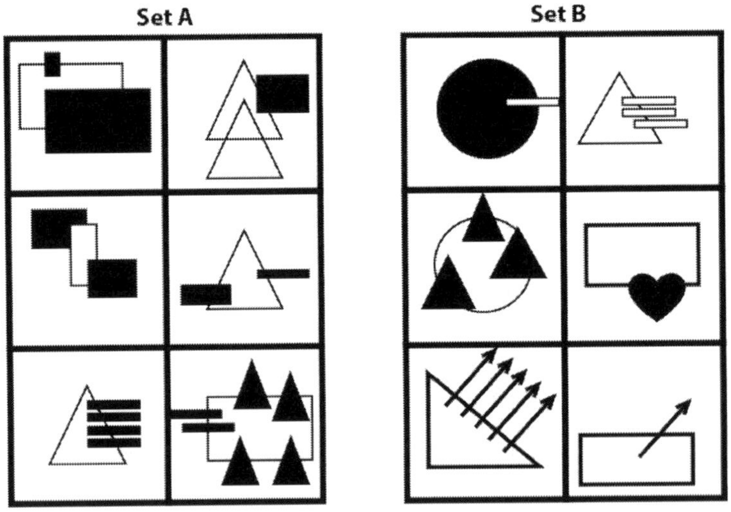

Questions 146-150

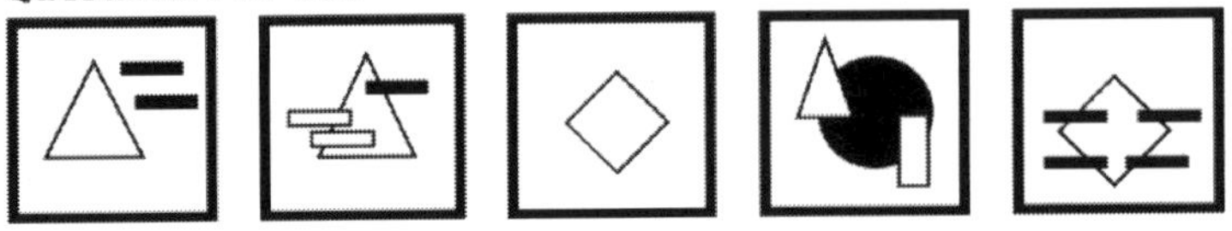

SET 31

Set A

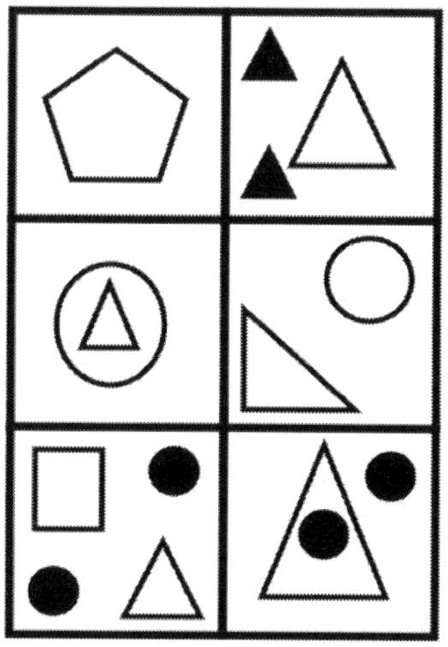

Set B

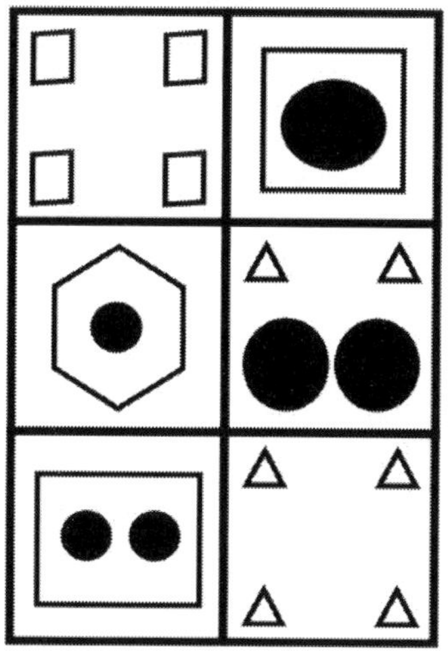

Questions 151-155

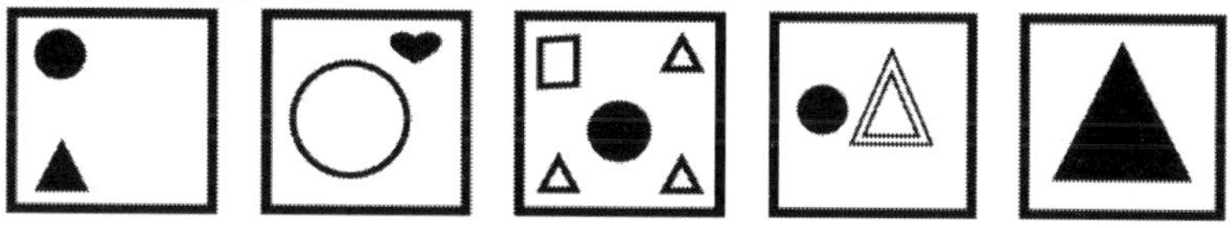

SET 32

Set A

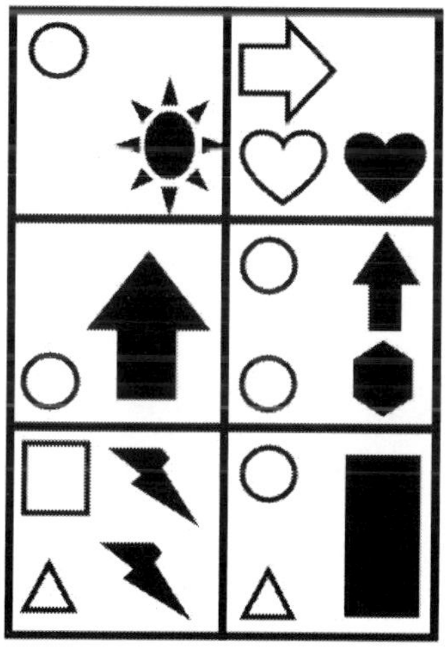

Set B

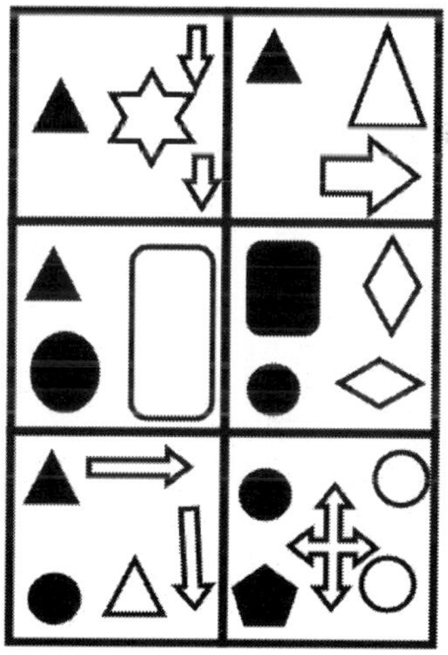

Questions 156-160

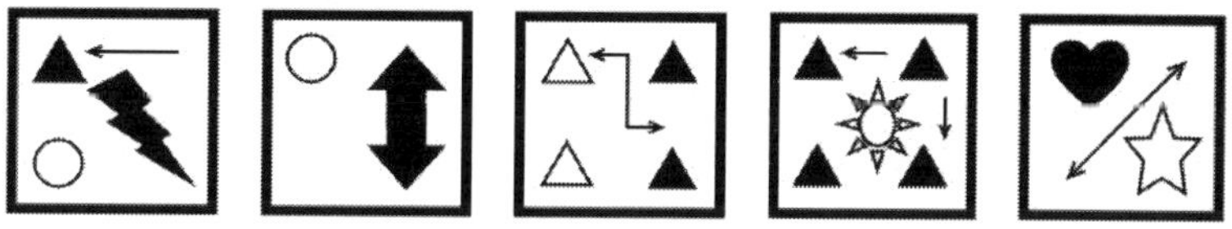

SET 33

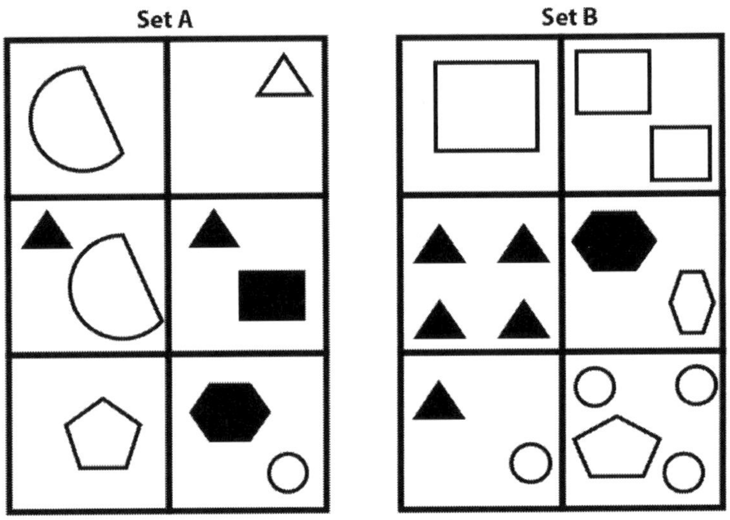

Questions 161-165

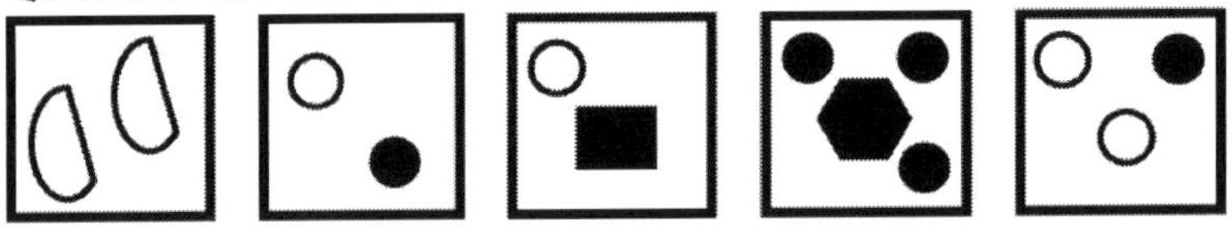

SET 34

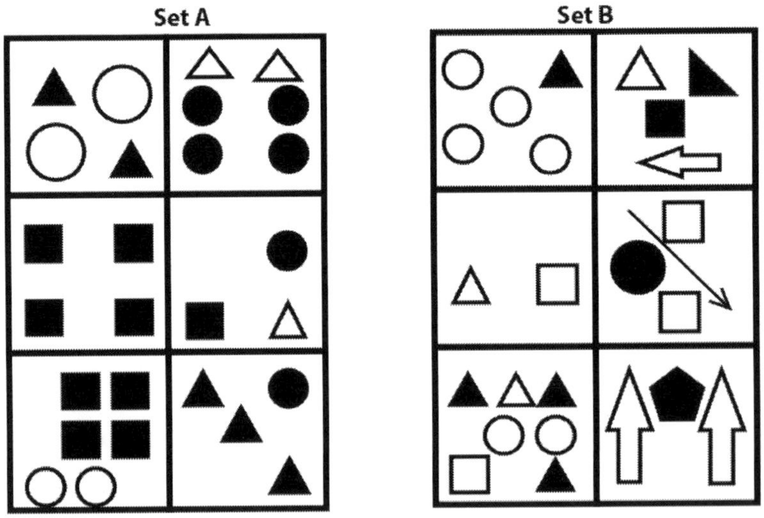

Questions 166-170

SET 35

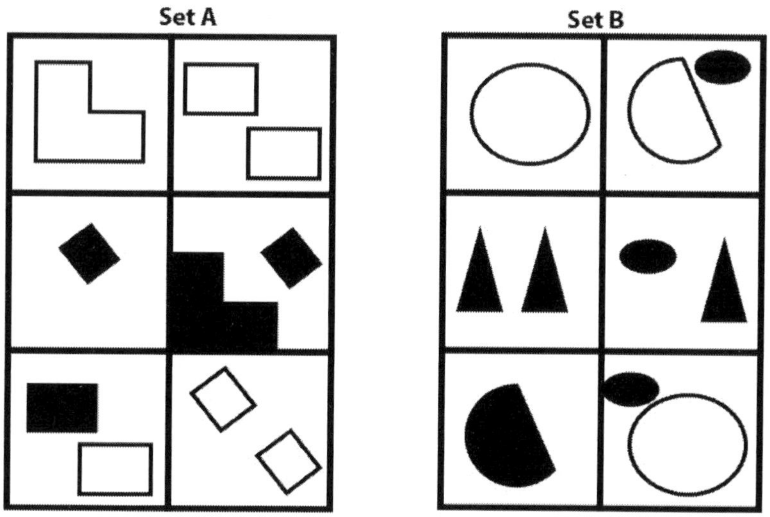

Questions 171-175

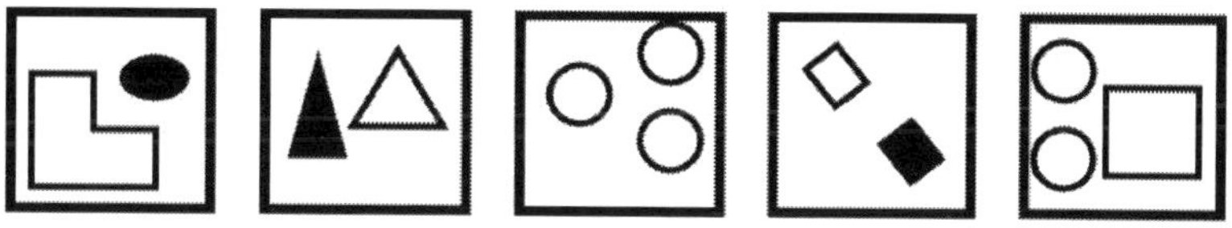

SET 36

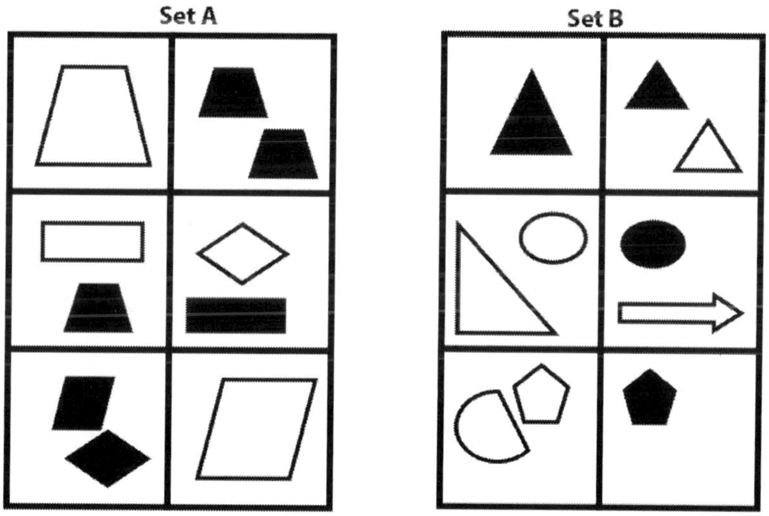

Questions 176-180

SET 37

Set A

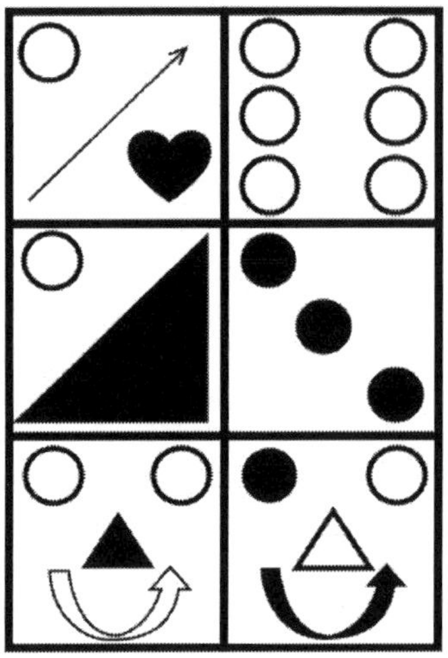

Set B

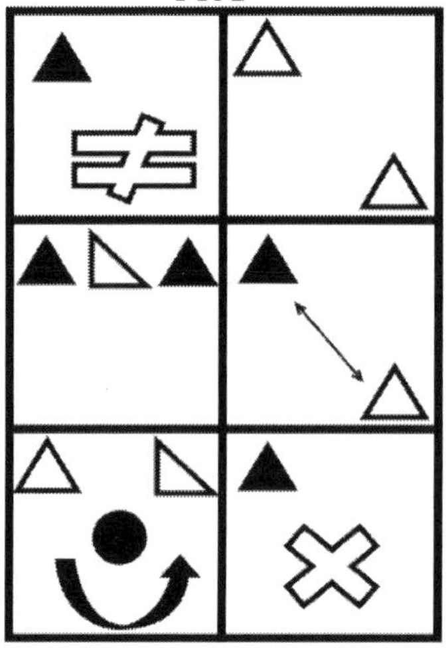

Questions 181-185

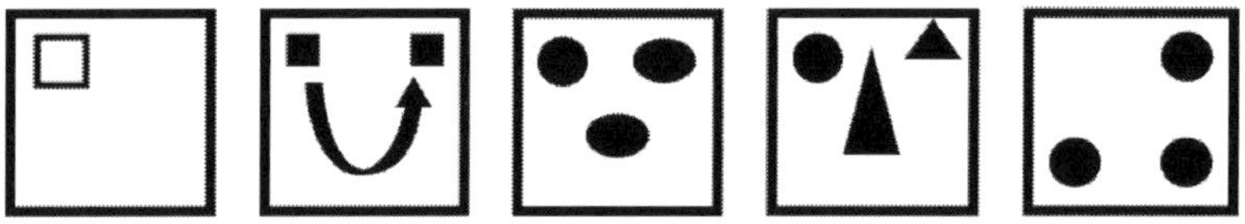

SET 38

Set A

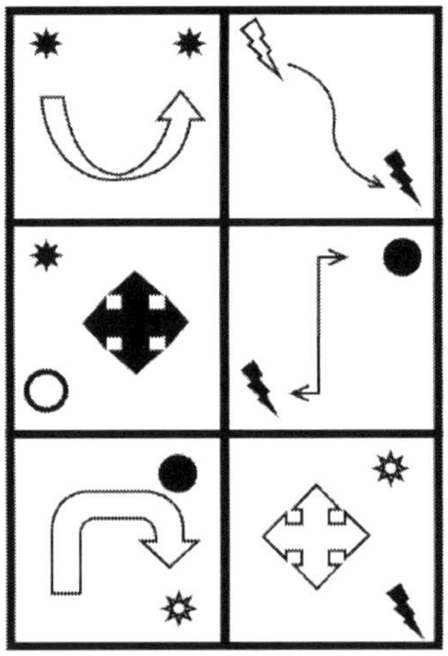

Set B

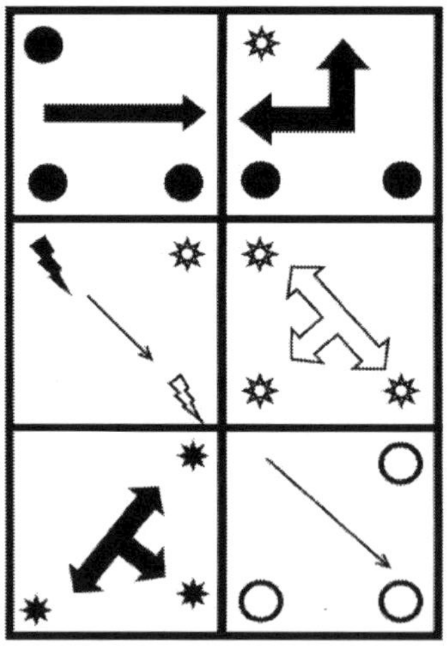

Questions 186-190

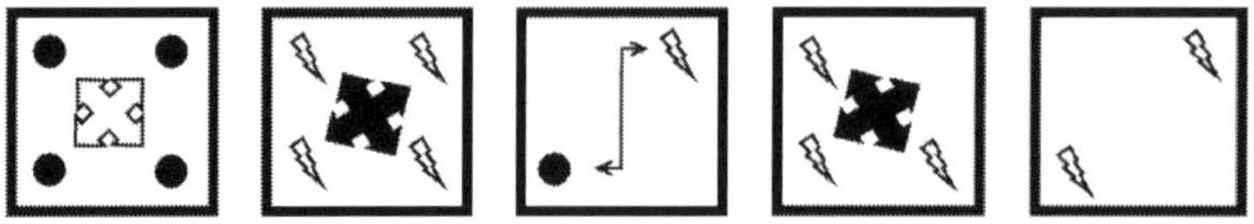

SET 39

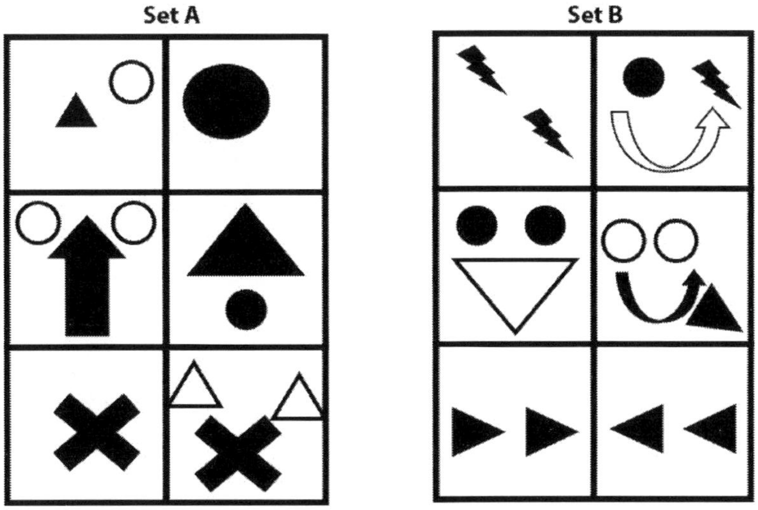

Questions 191-195

SET 40

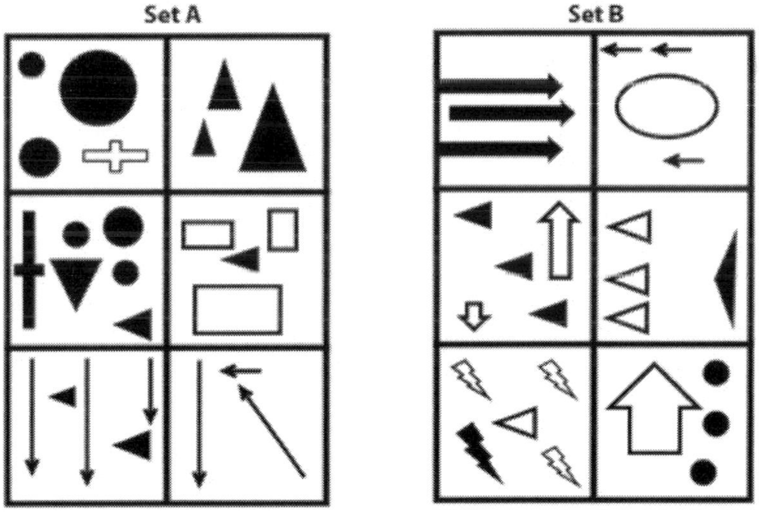

Questions 196-200

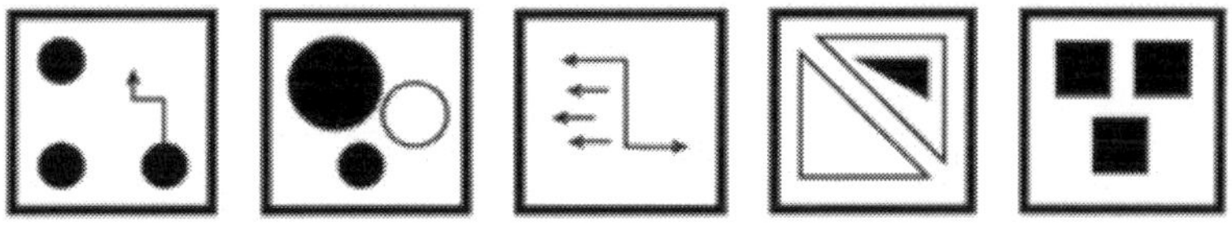

For Questions 201 – 250: which answer option completes the series?

Q201

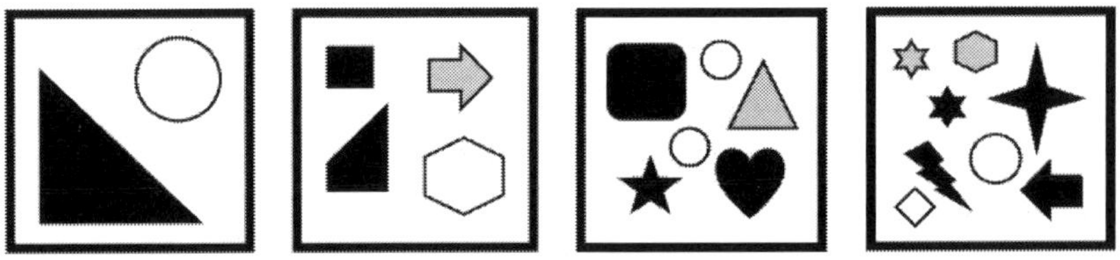

A) 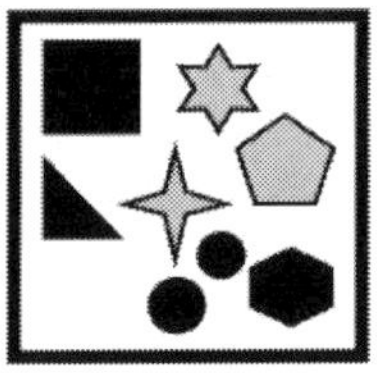 B)  C)  D) 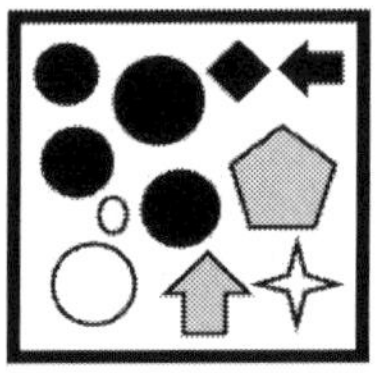

Q202

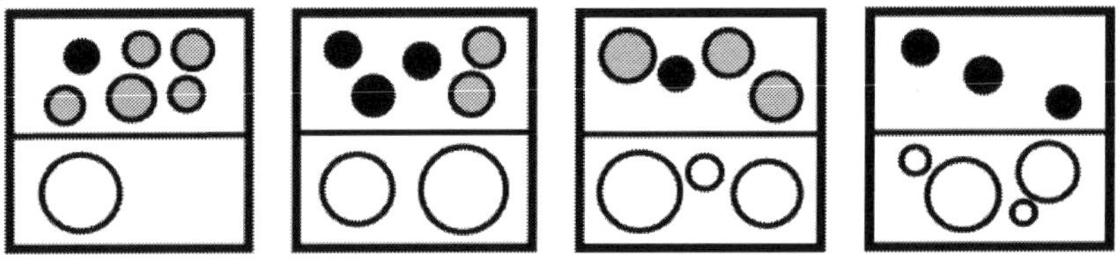

A) 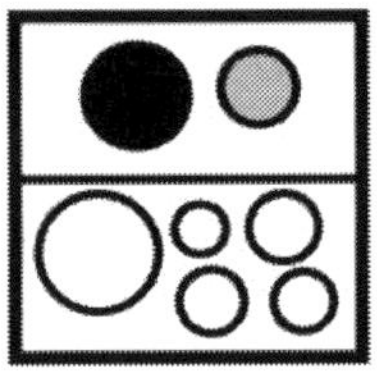 B) 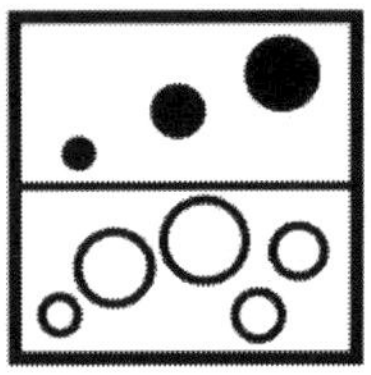 C) 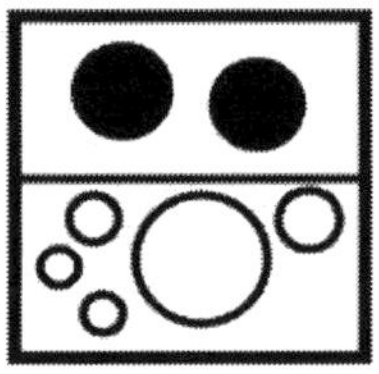 D) 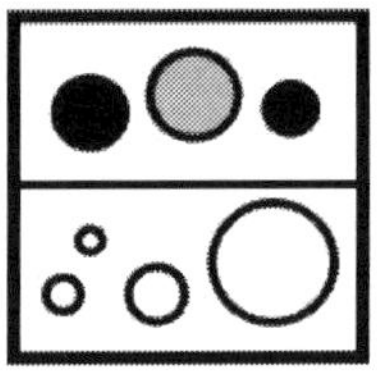

Q203

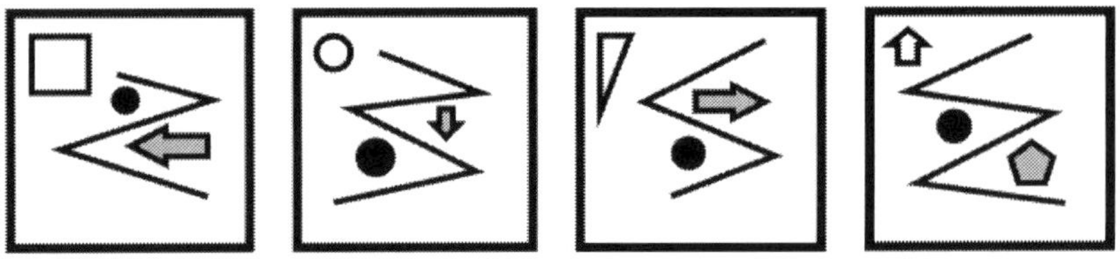

A) 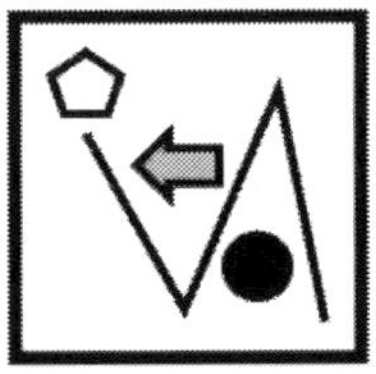 B) 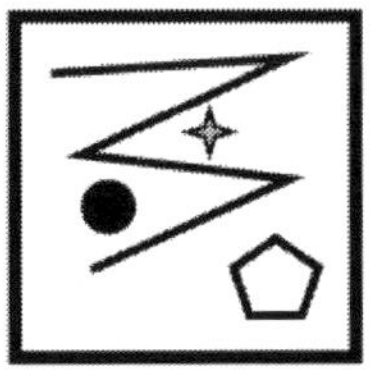 C) 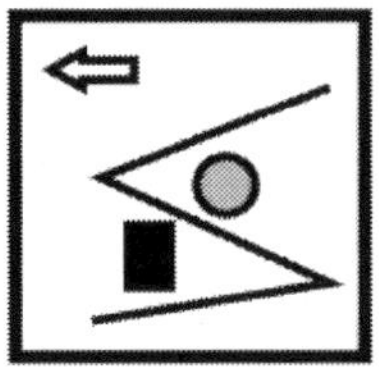 D) 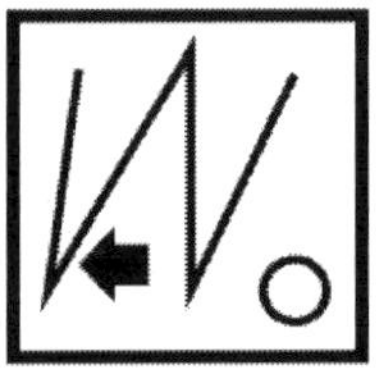

Q204

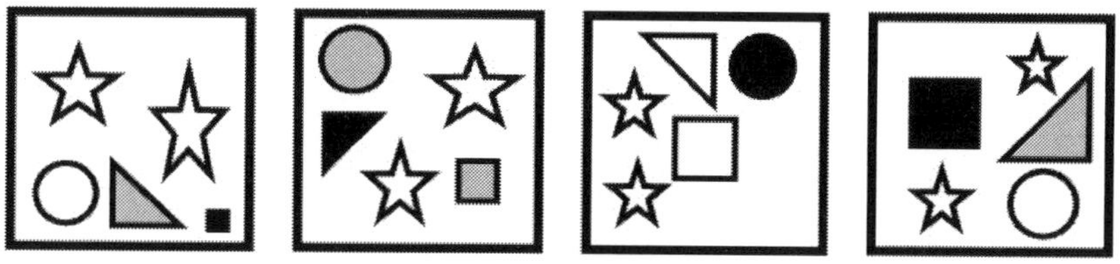

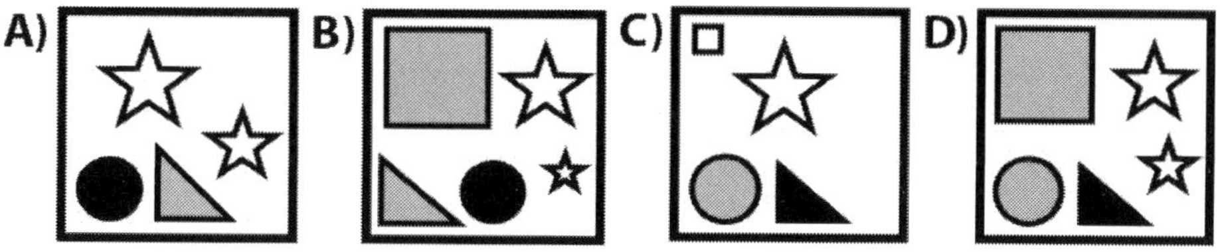

Q205

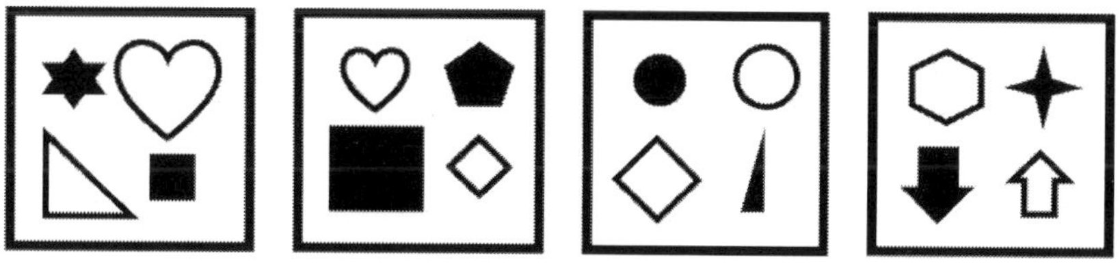

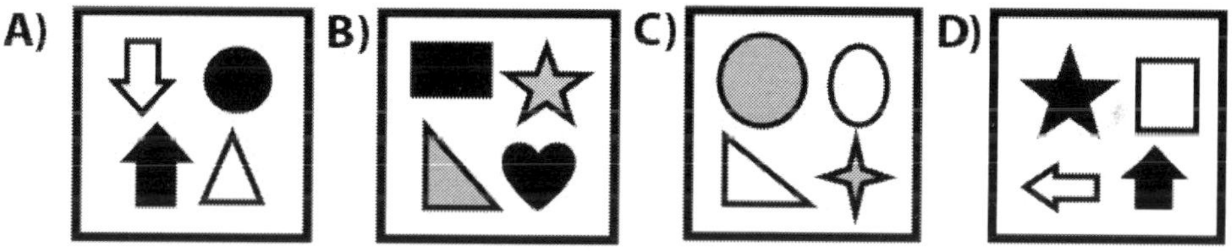

Q206

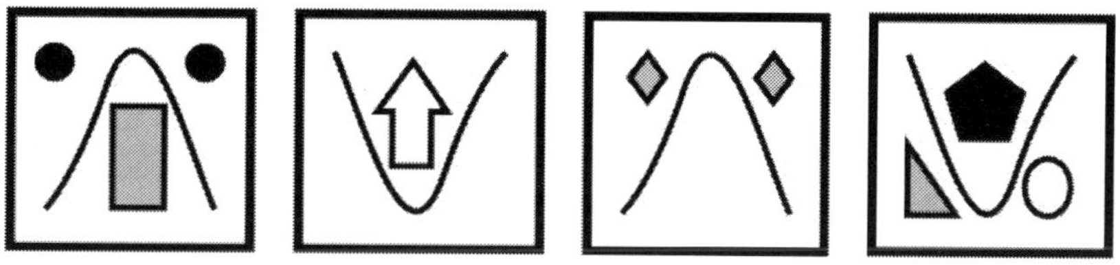

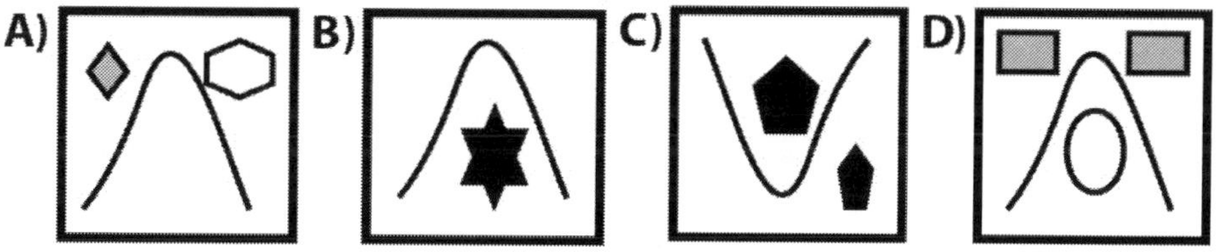

Q207

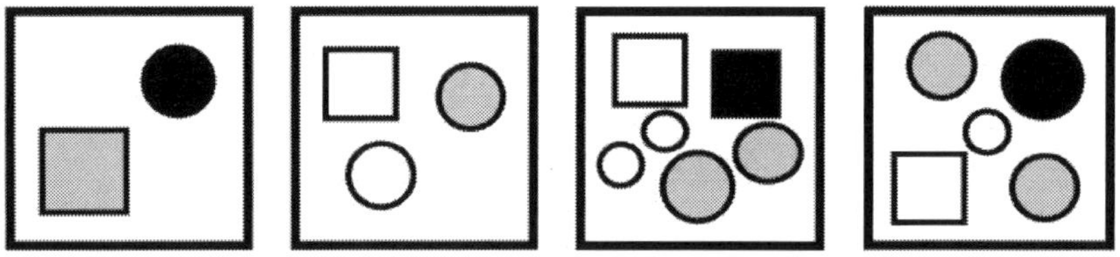

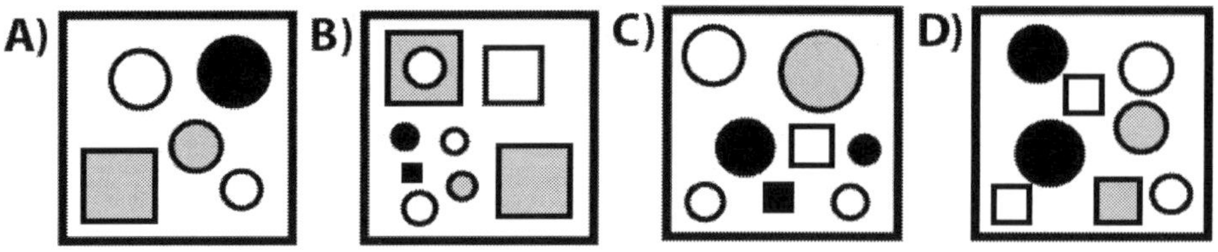

Q208

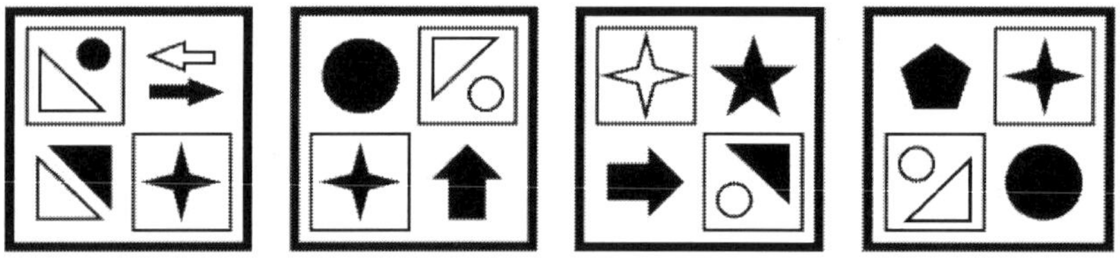

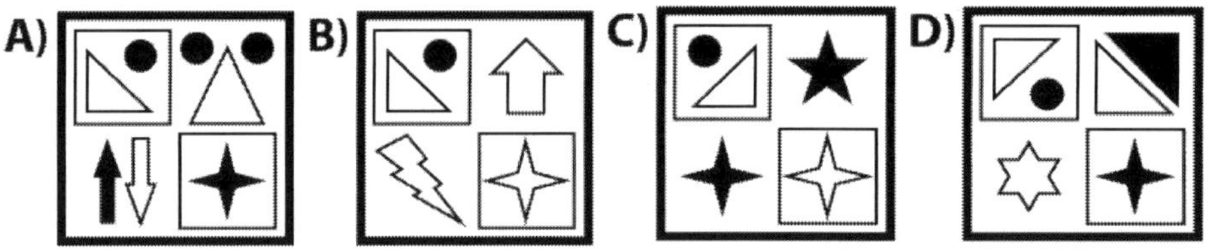

Q209

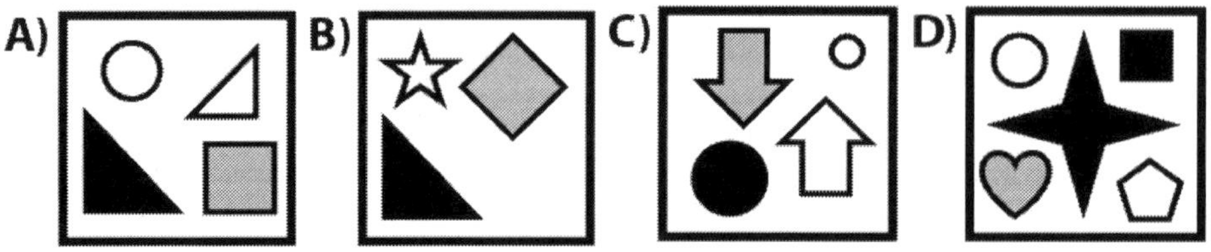

Q210

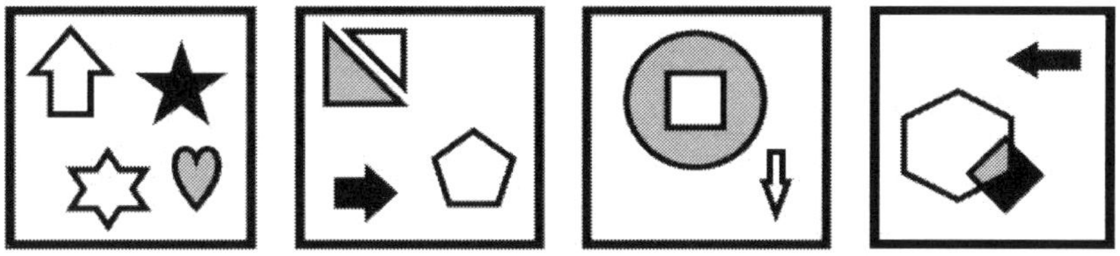

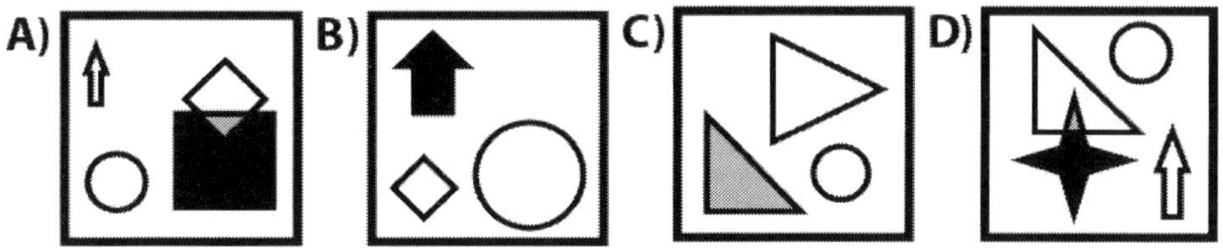

Q211

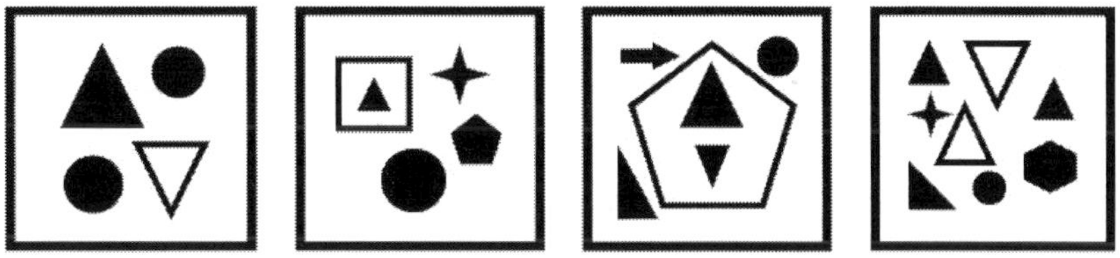

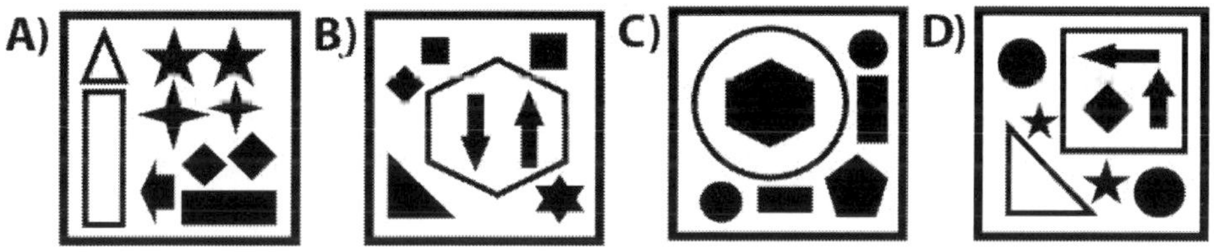

Q212

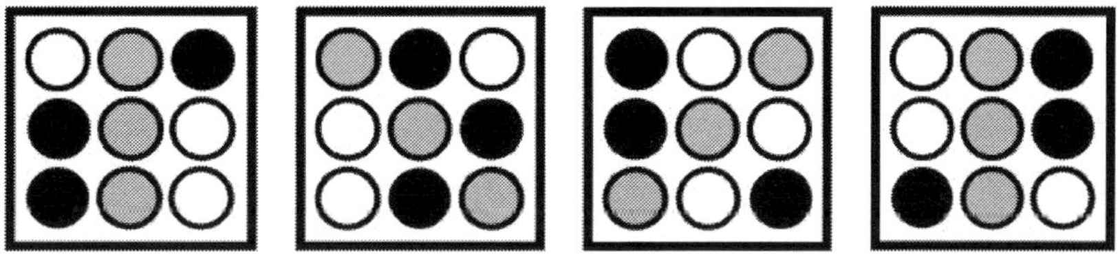

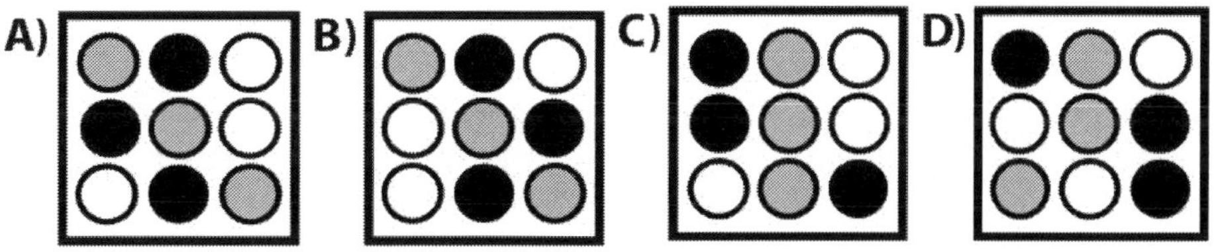

Q213

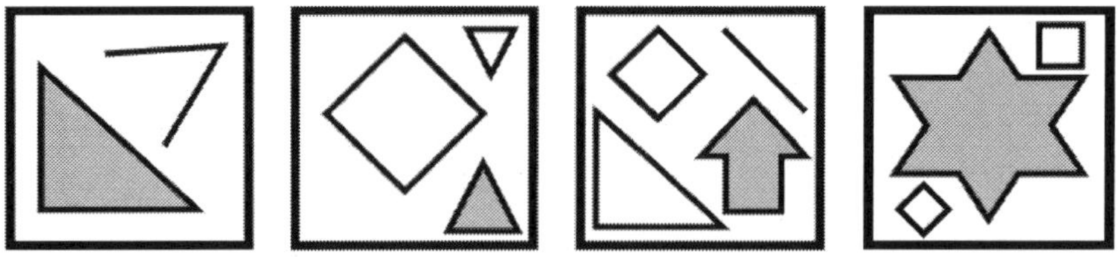

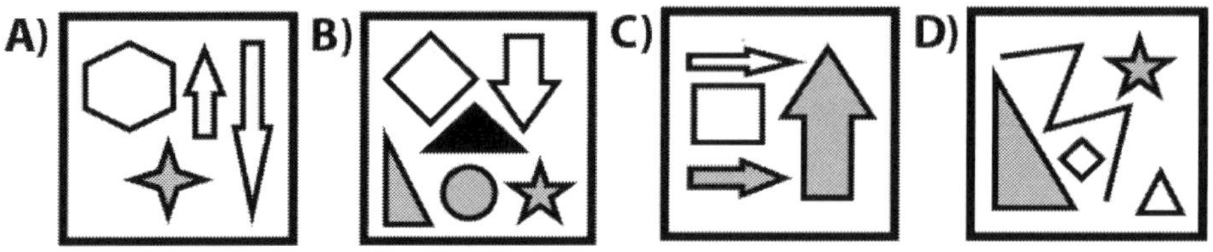

Q214

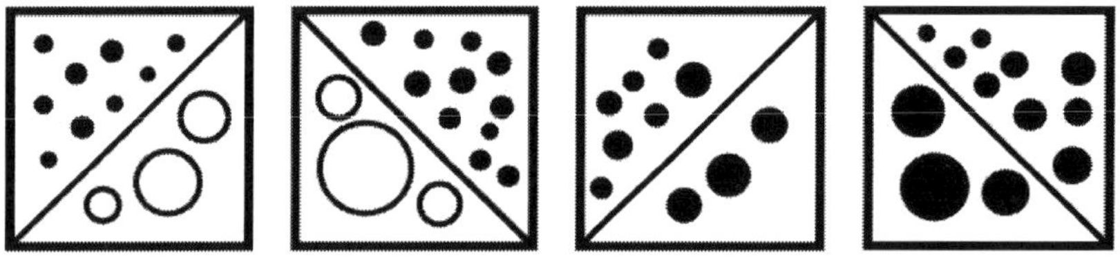

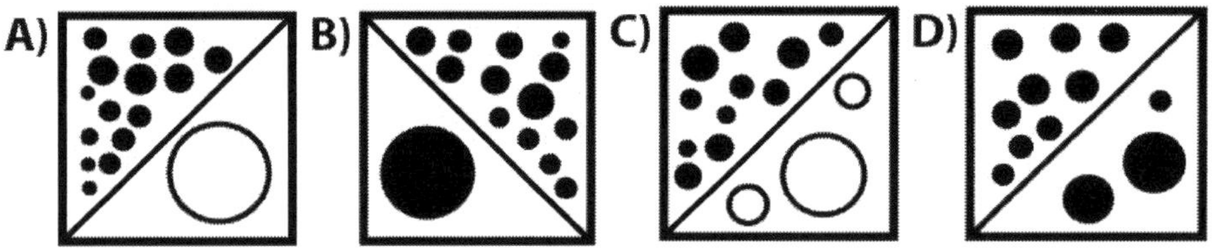

Q215

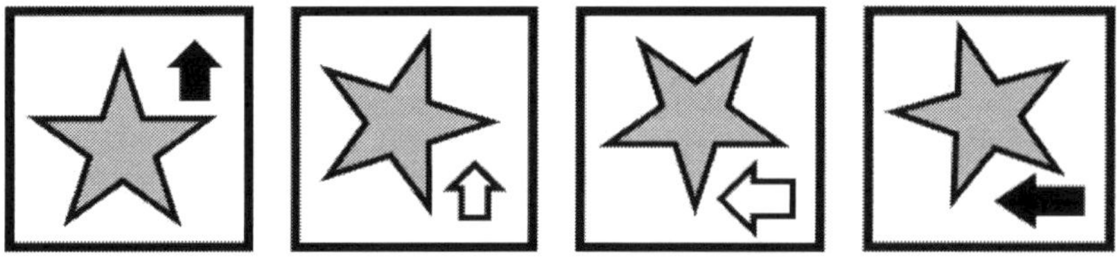

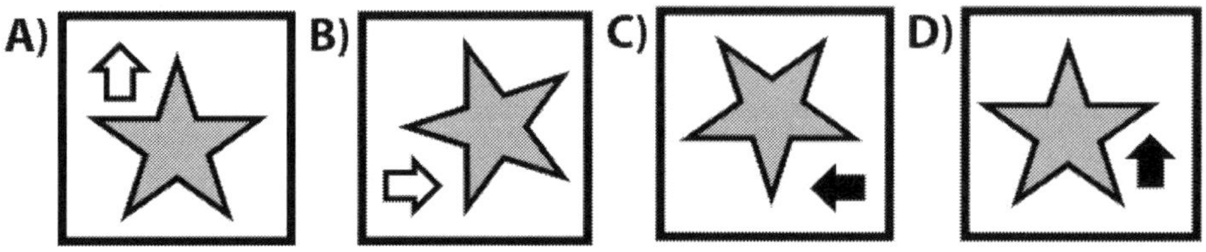

Q216

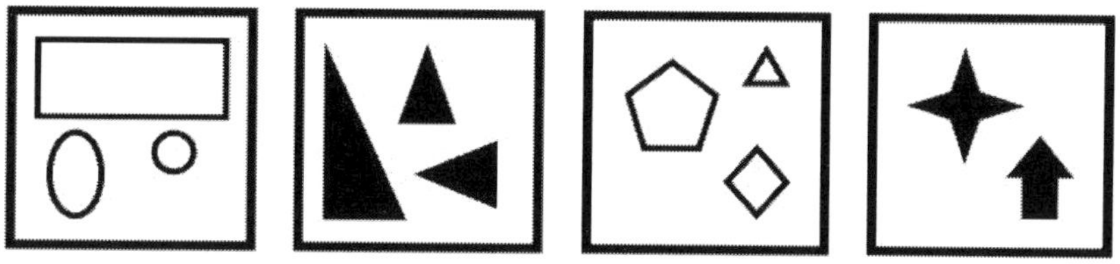

A) 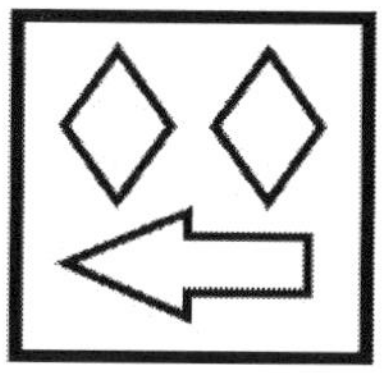
B) 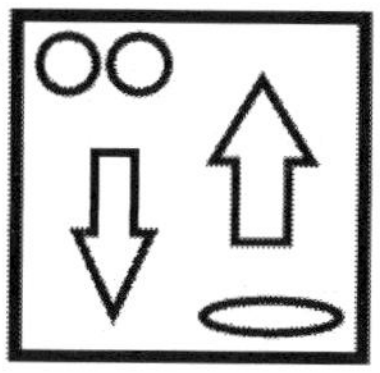
C) 
D) 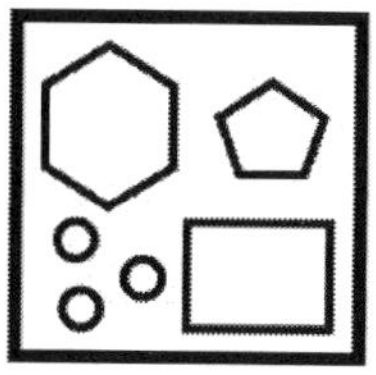

Q217

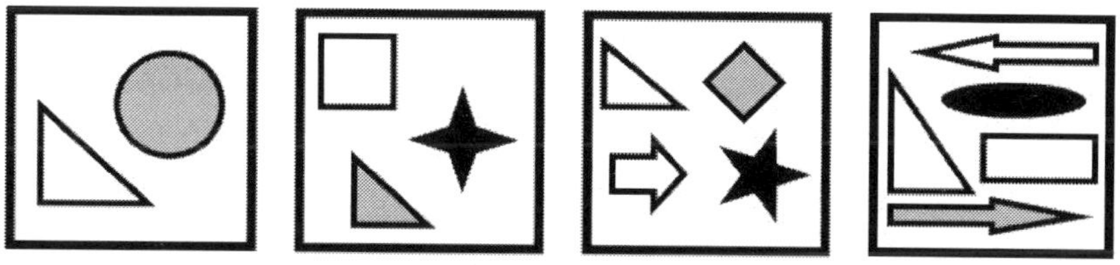

A) 
B) 
C) 
D) 

Q218

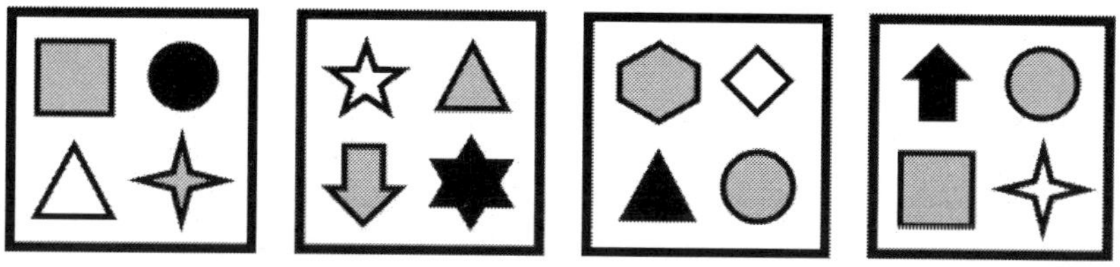

A) 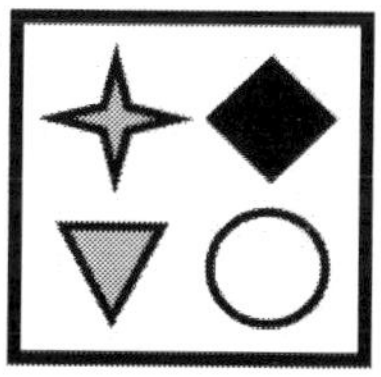
B) 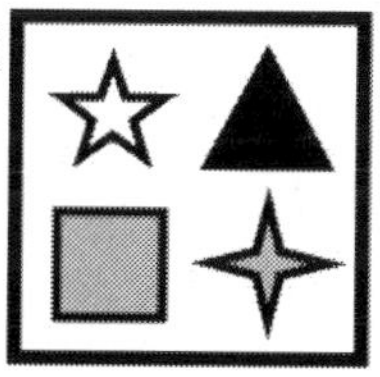
C) 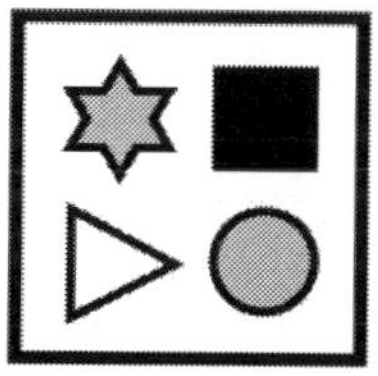
D) 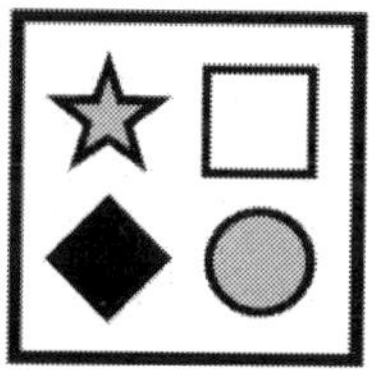

Q219

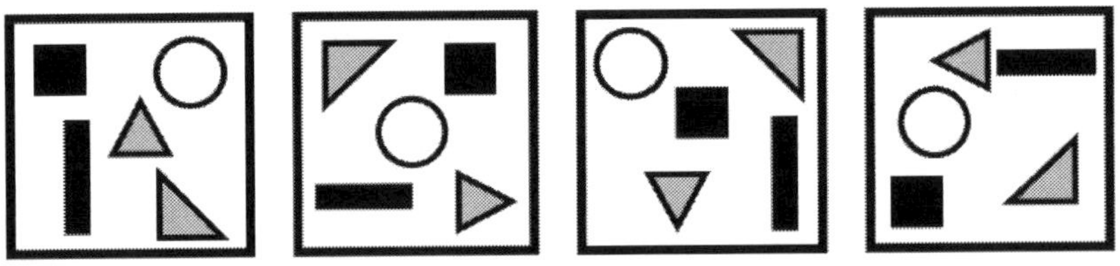

A) 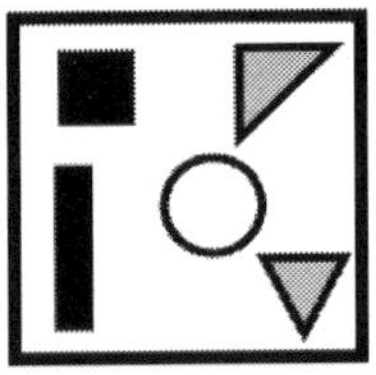
B) 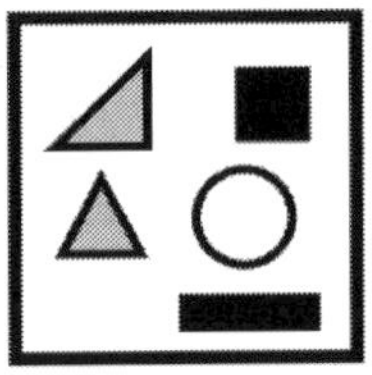
C) 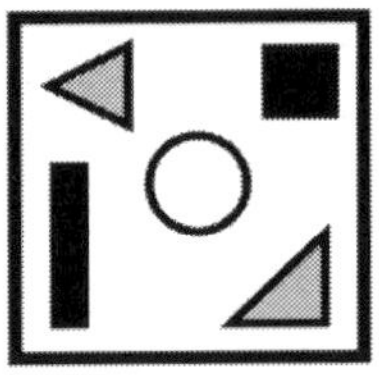
D) 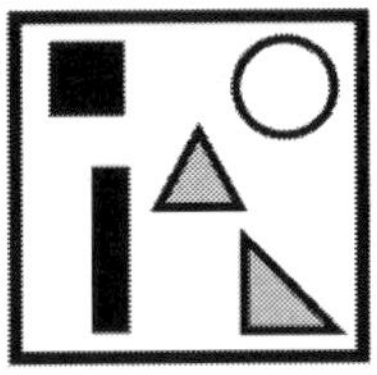

Q220

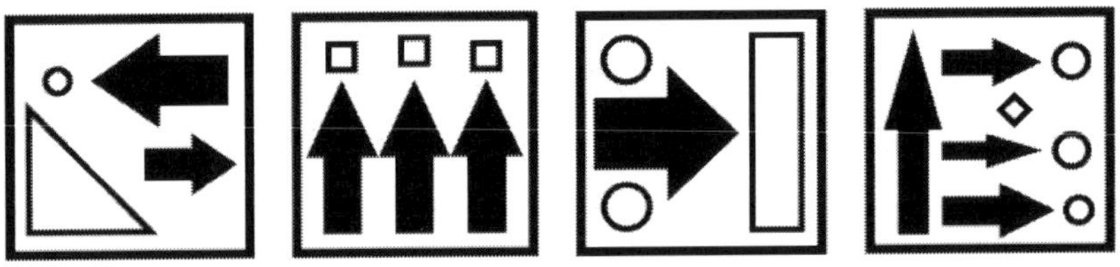

A) 
B) 
C) 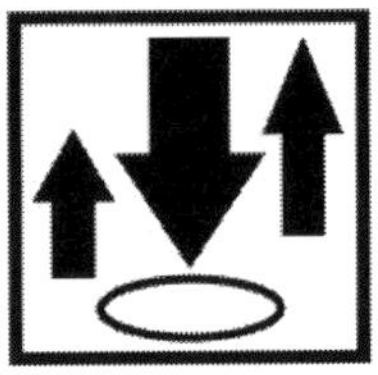
D) 

Q221

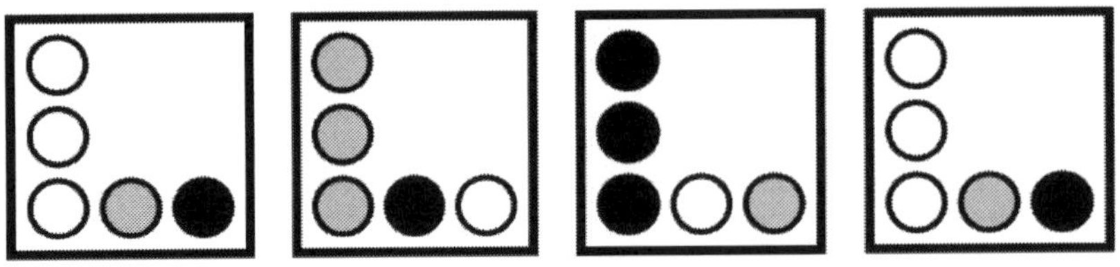

A) 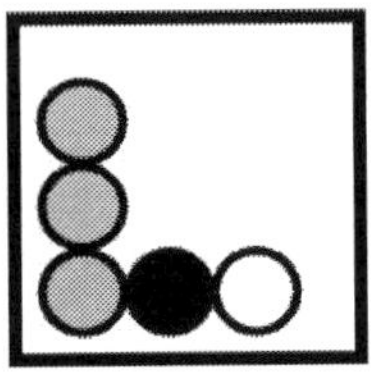
B) 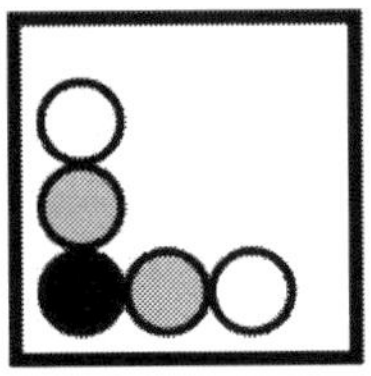
C) 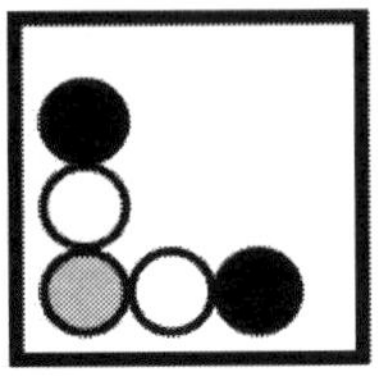
D) 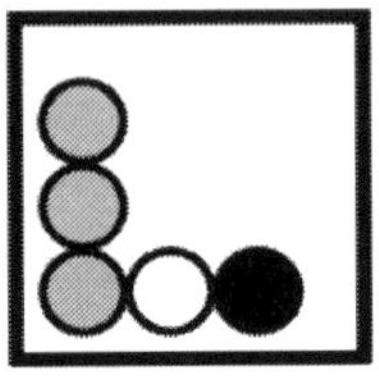

Q222

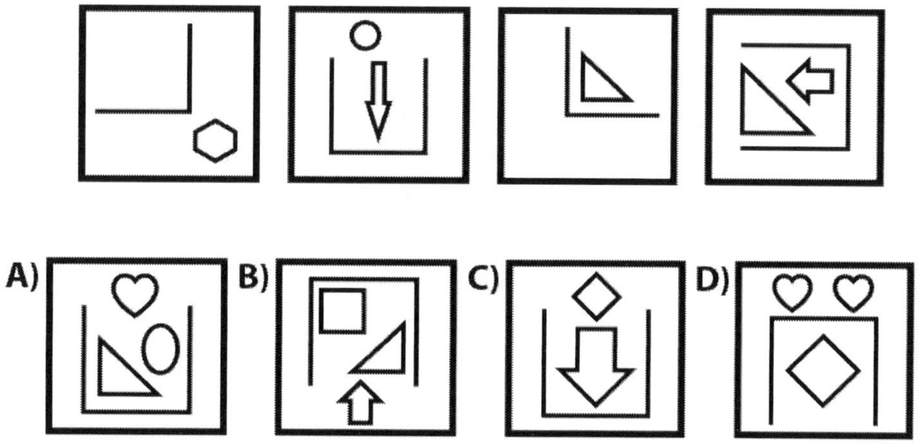

Q223

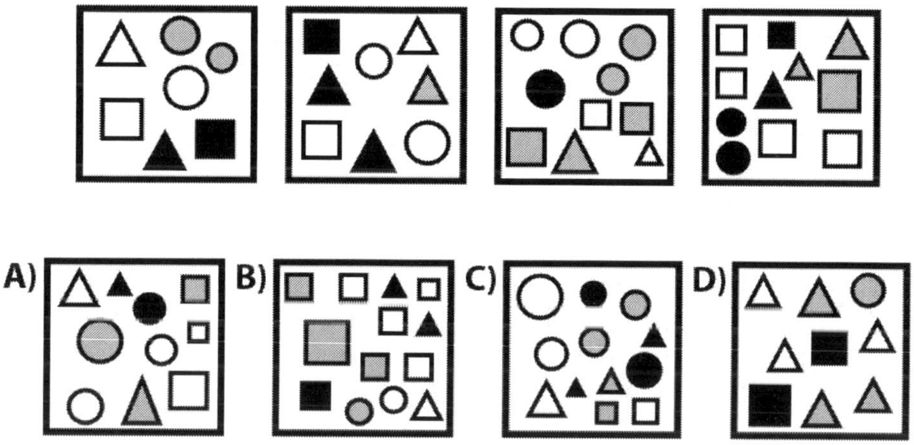

Q224

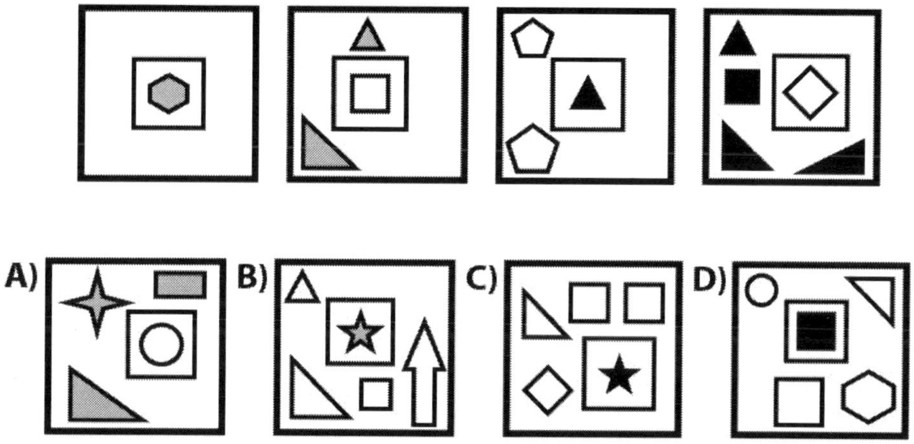

Q225

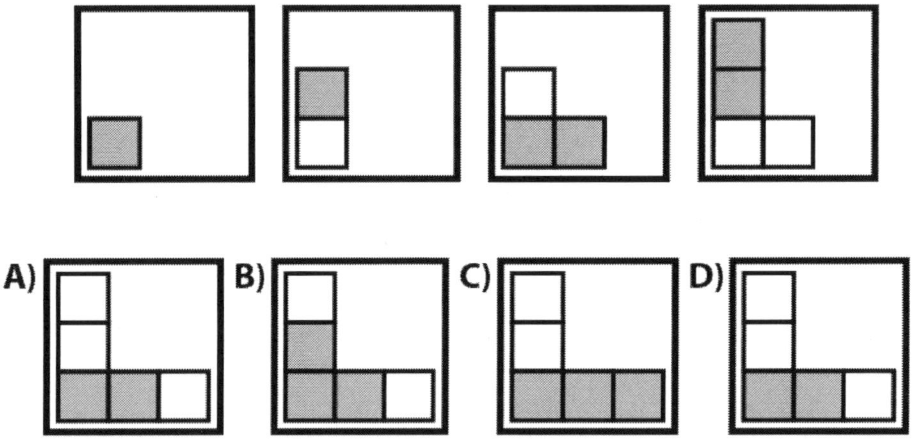

Q226

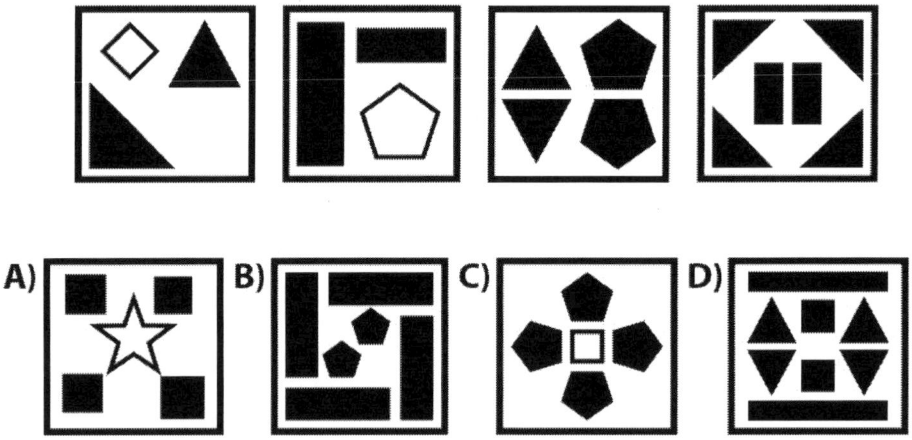

Q227

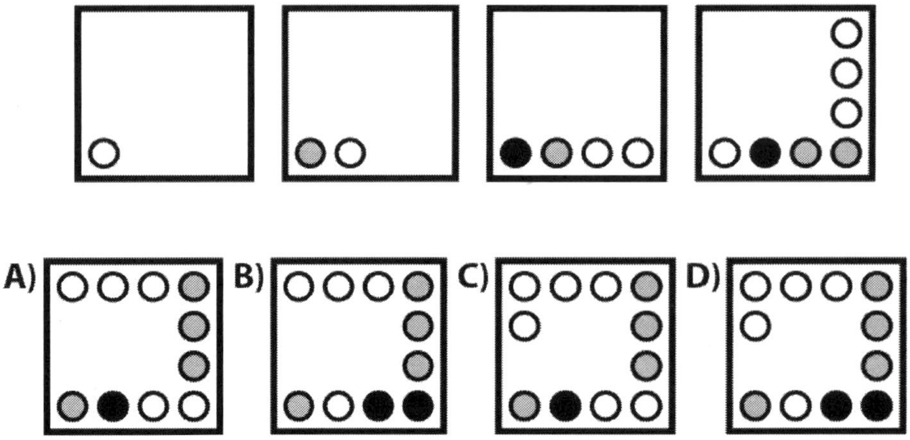

Q228

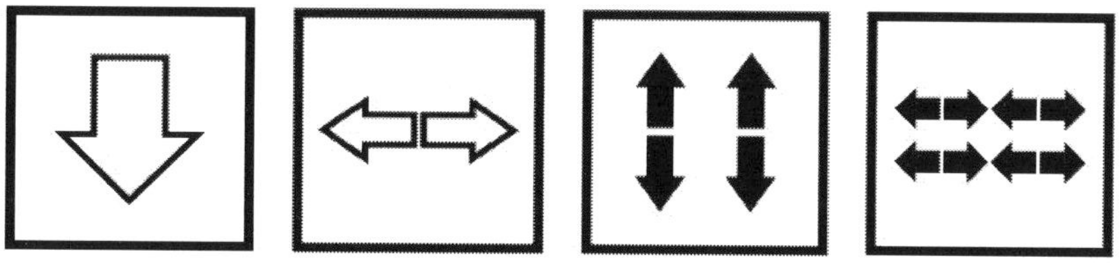

A) 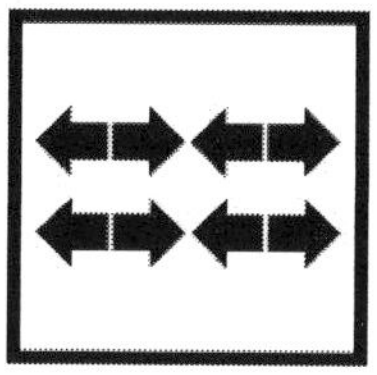 B) 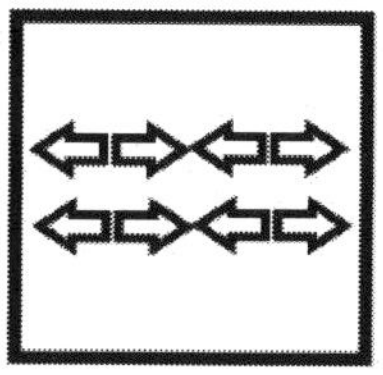 C) 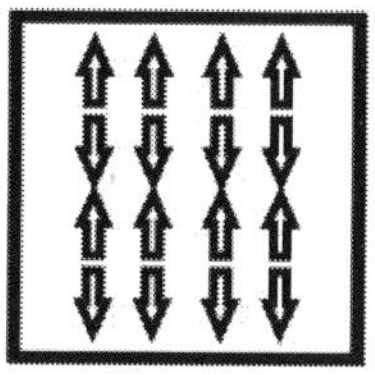 D) 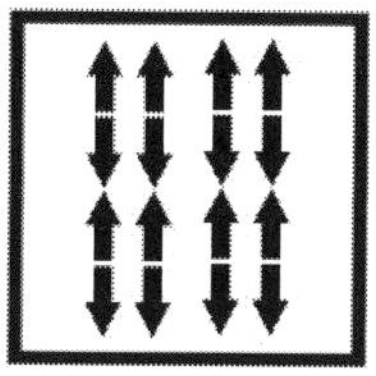

Q229

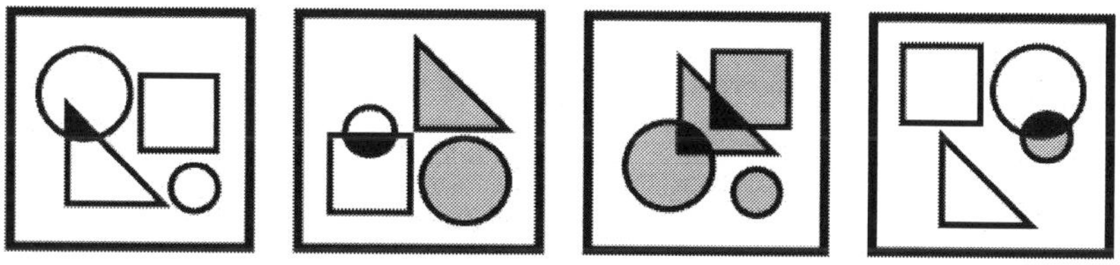

A) 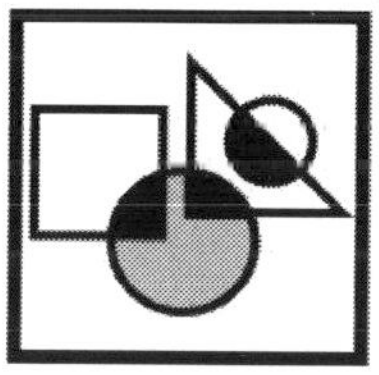 B) 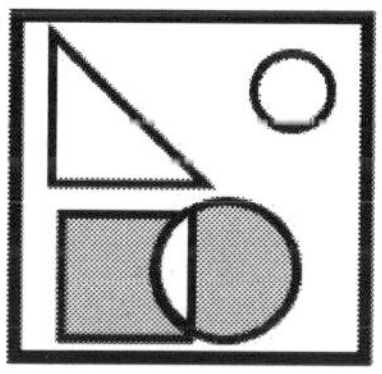 C) 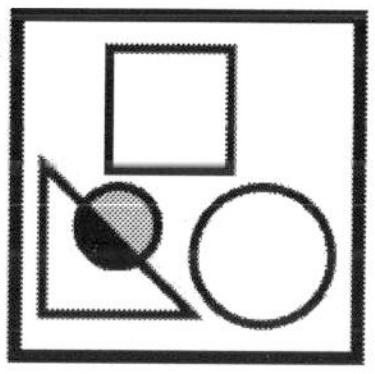 D) 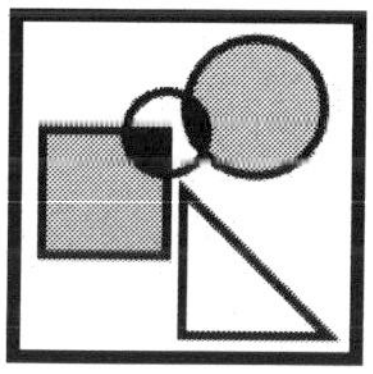

Q230

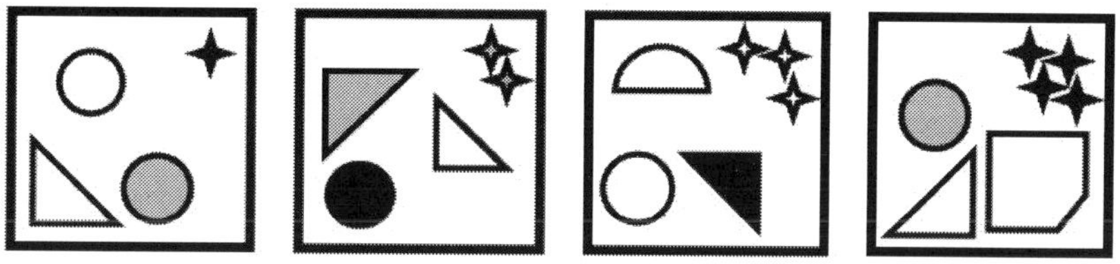

A) 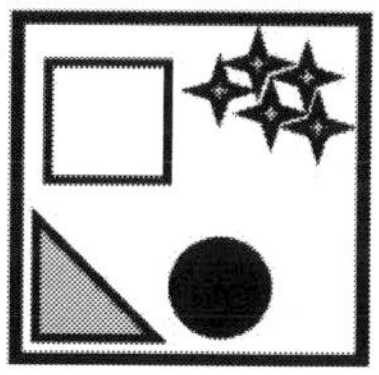 B)  C) 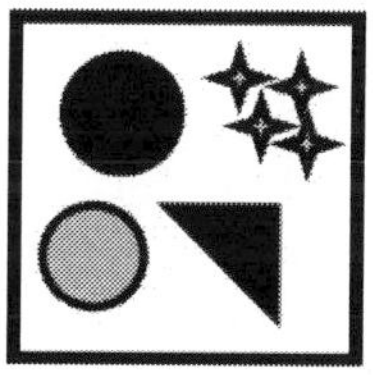 D) 

Q231

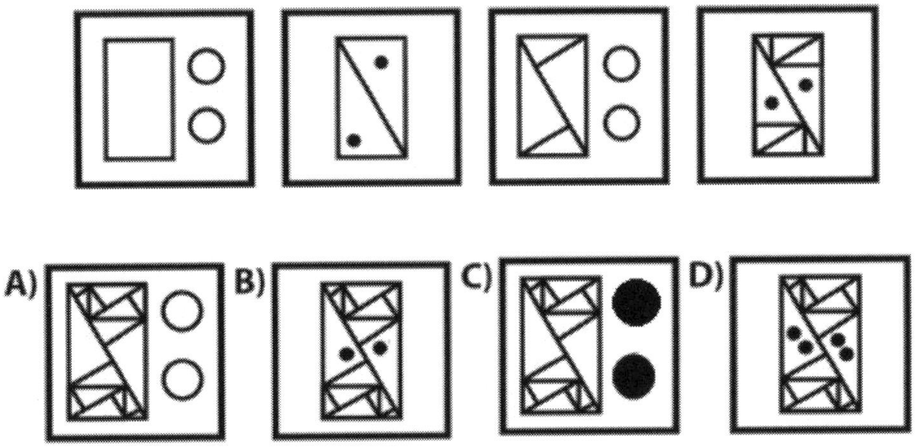

Q232

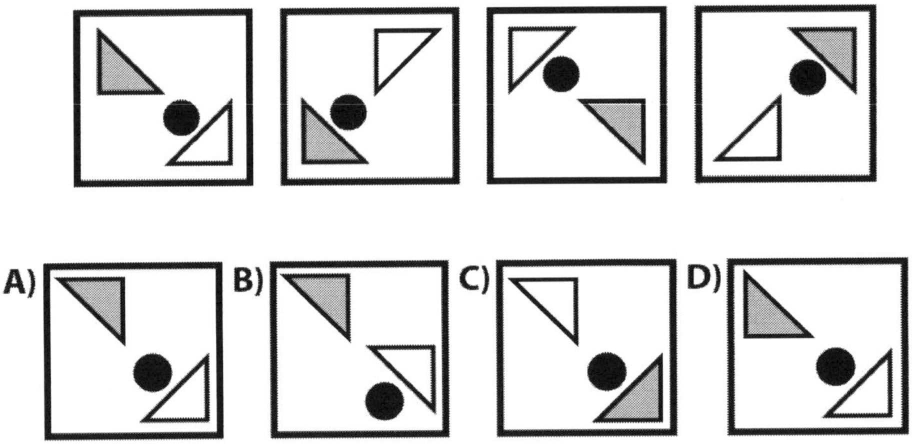

Q233

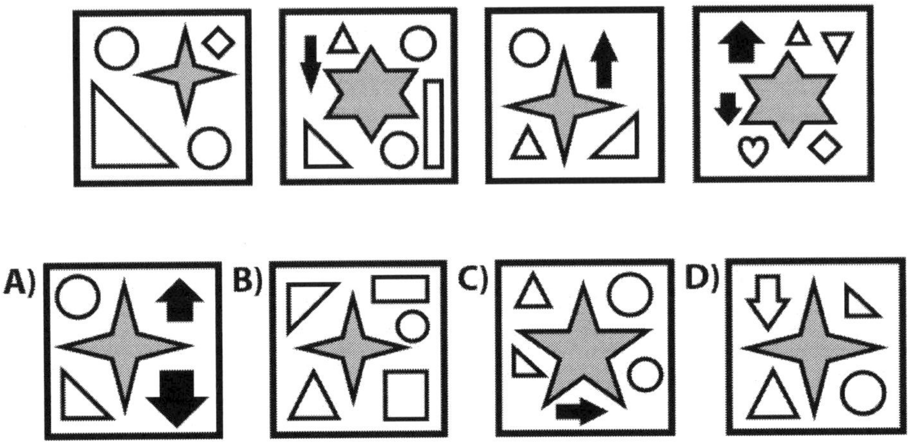

Q234

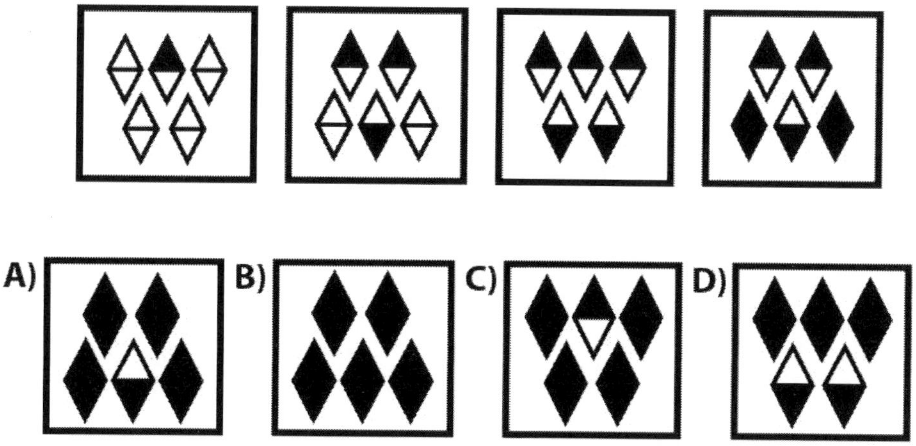

Q235

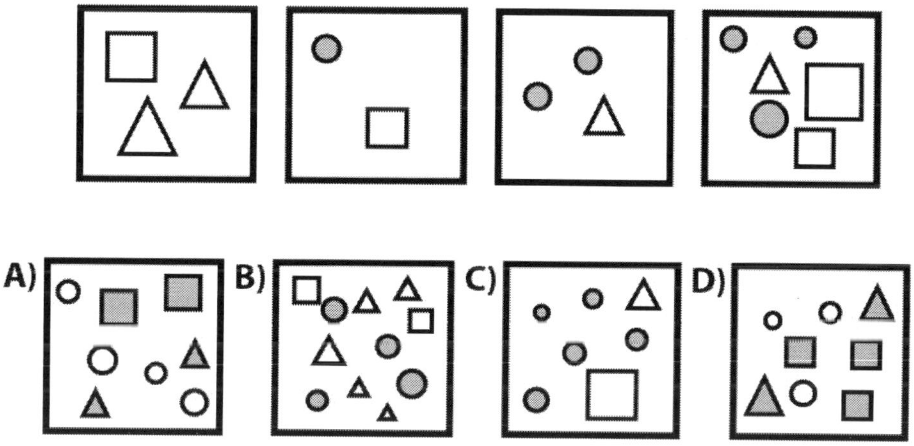

Q236

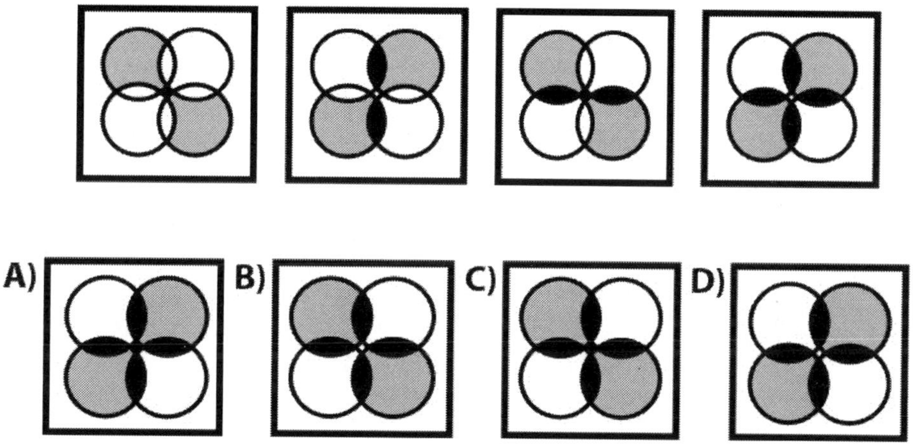

Q237

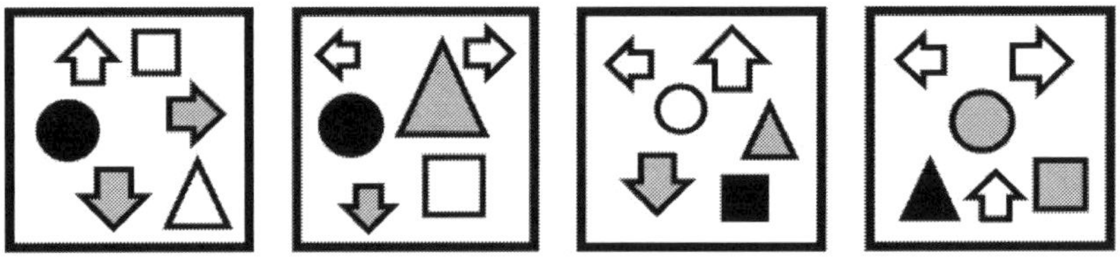

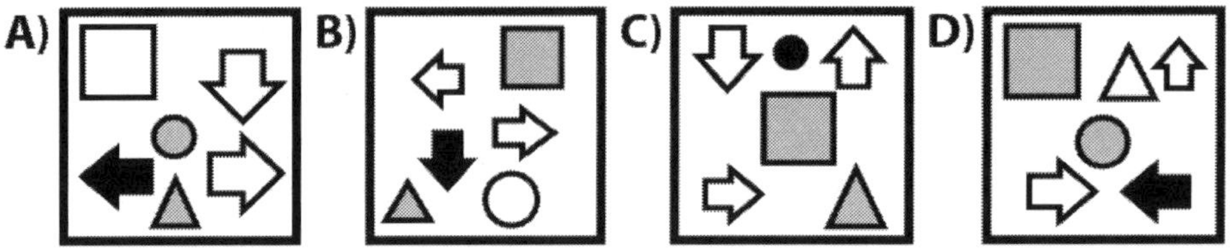

Q238

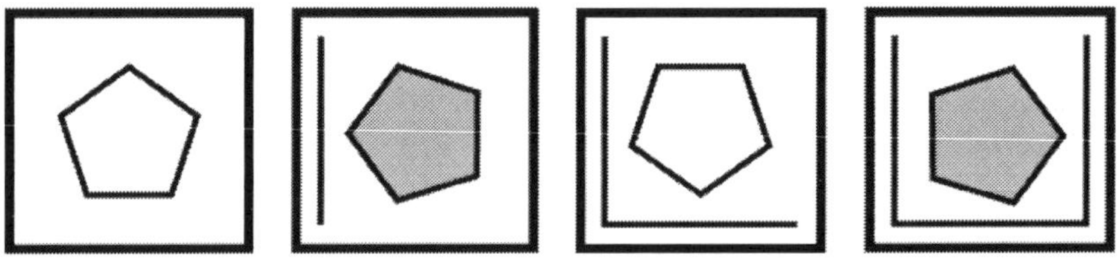

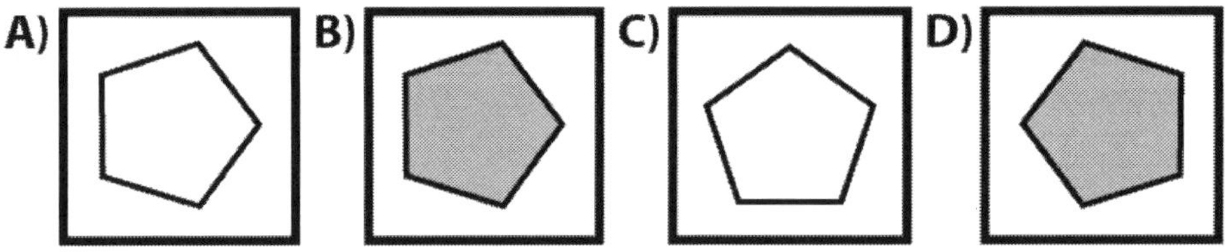

Q239

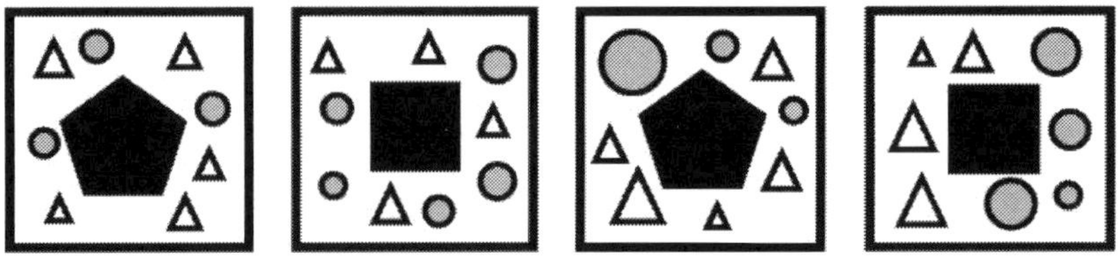

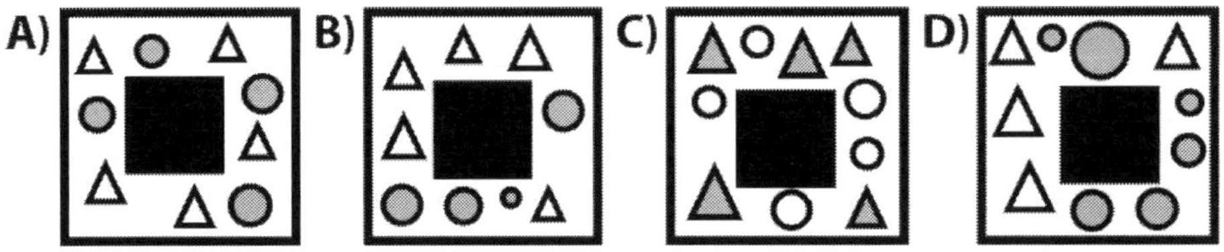

Q240

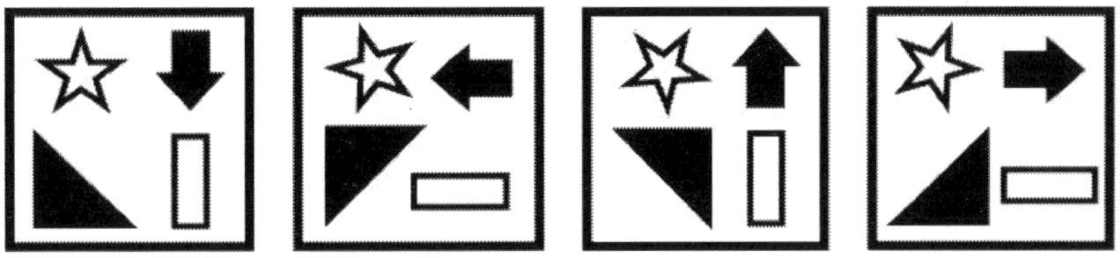

A)  B)  C)  D) 

Q241

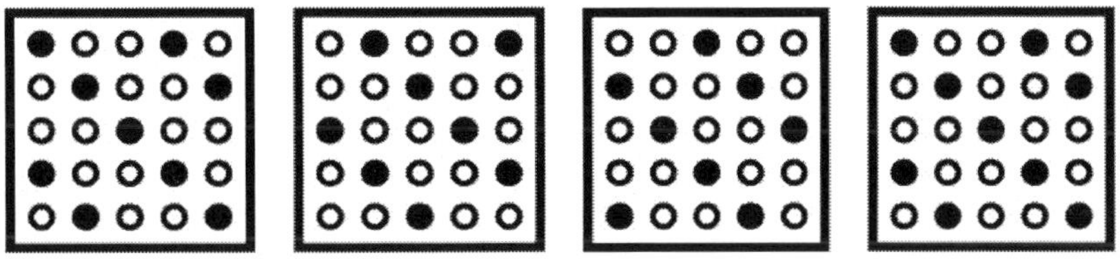

A) 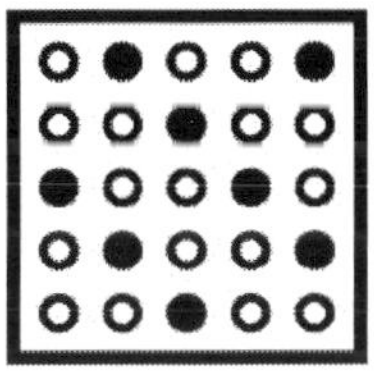 B) 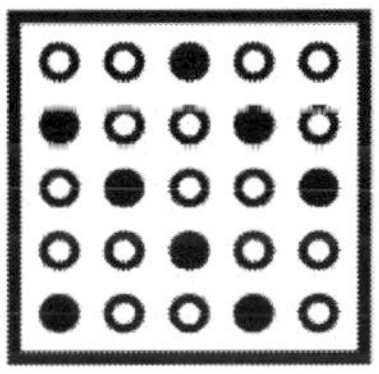 C) 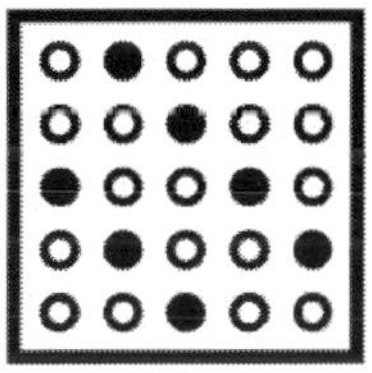 D) 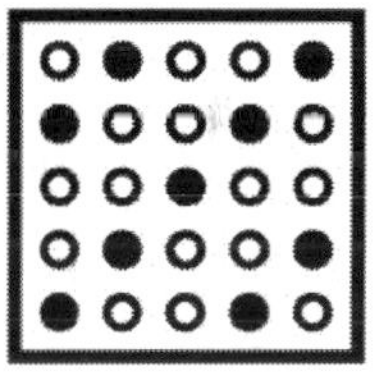

Q242

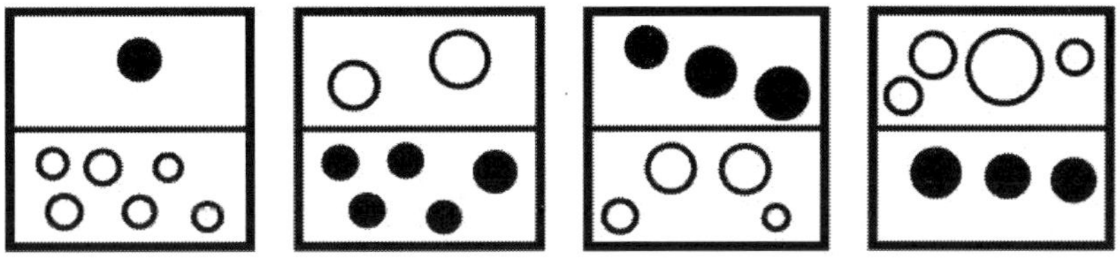

A) 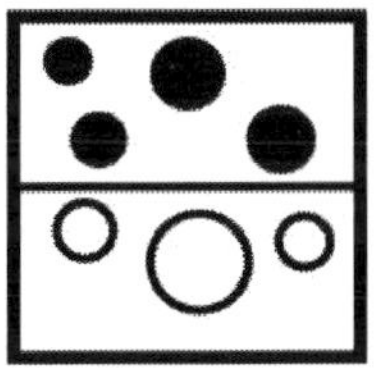 B) 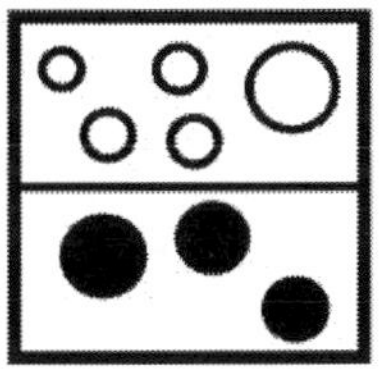 C) 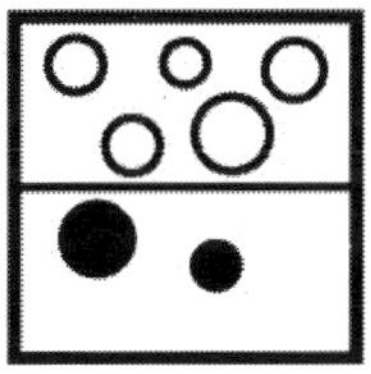 D) 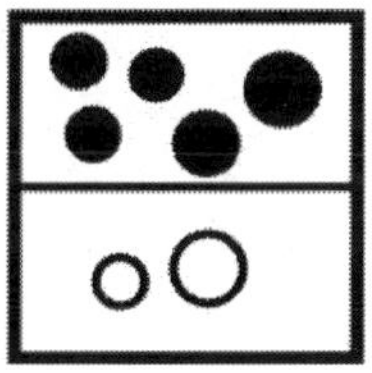

Q243

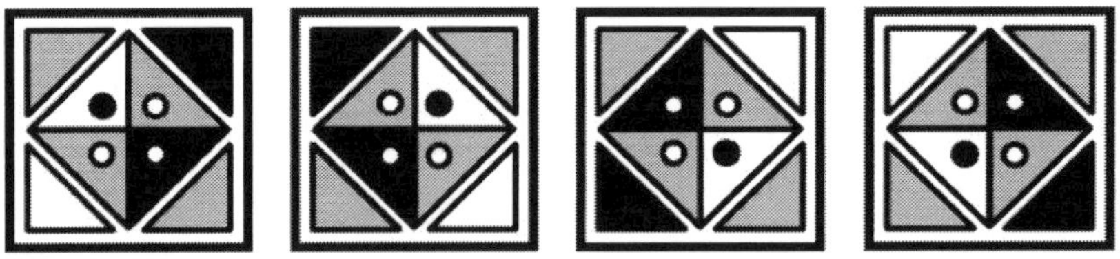

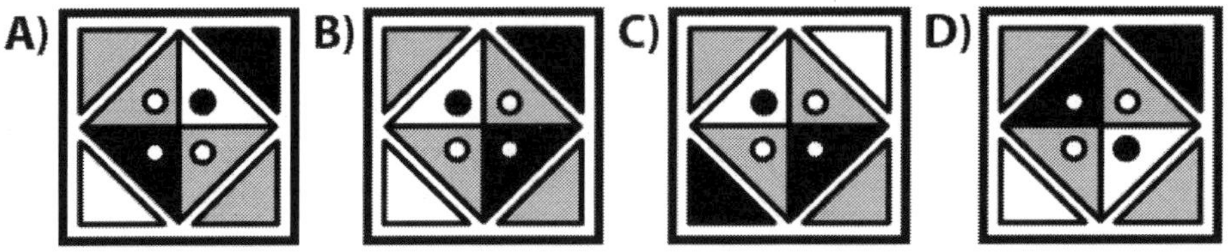

Q244

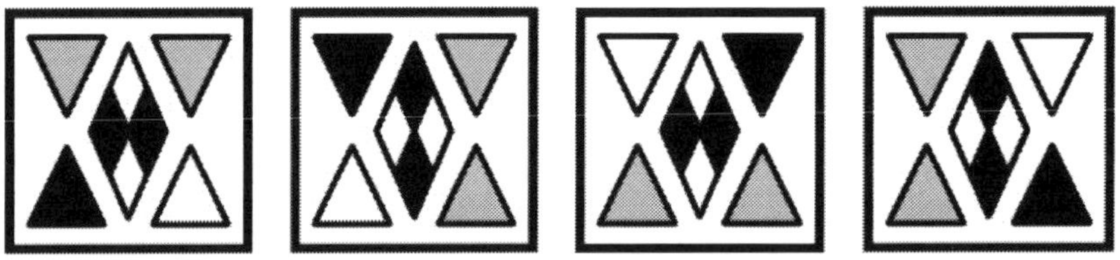

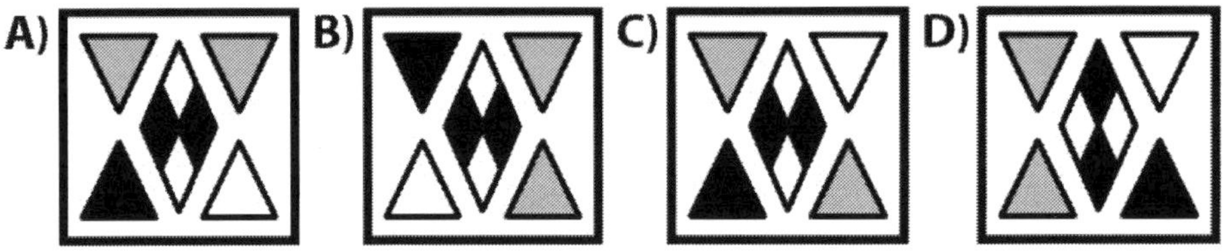

Q245

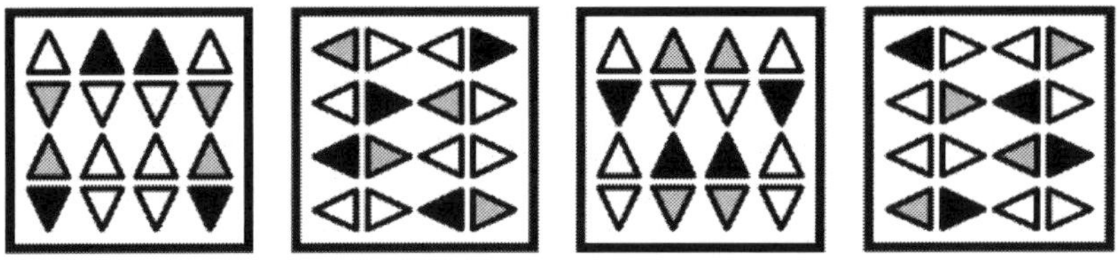

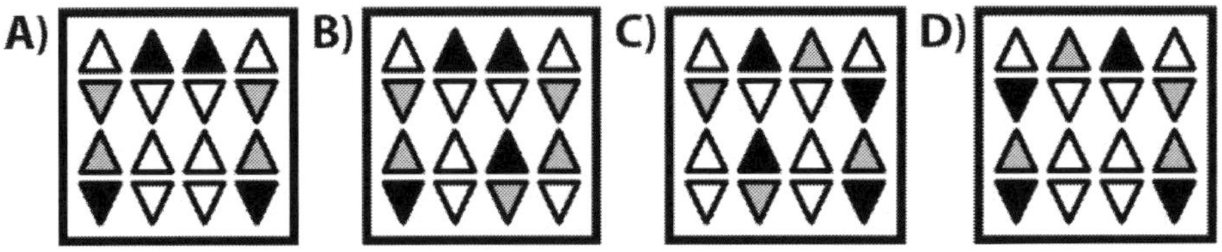

Q246

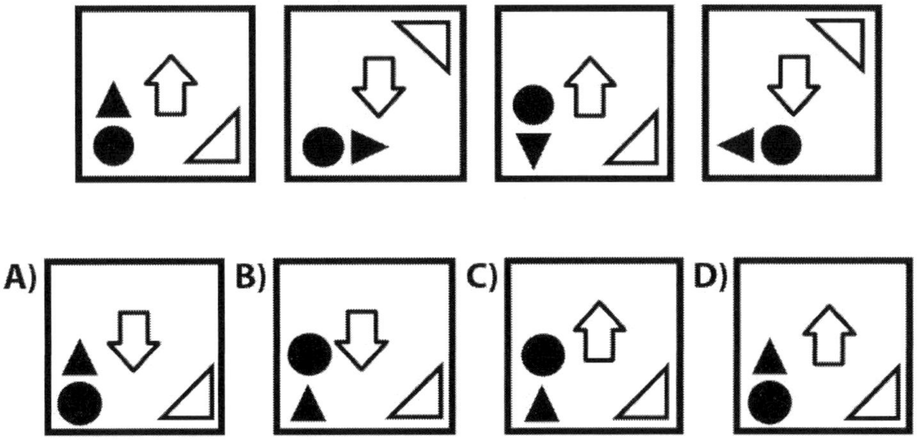

Q247

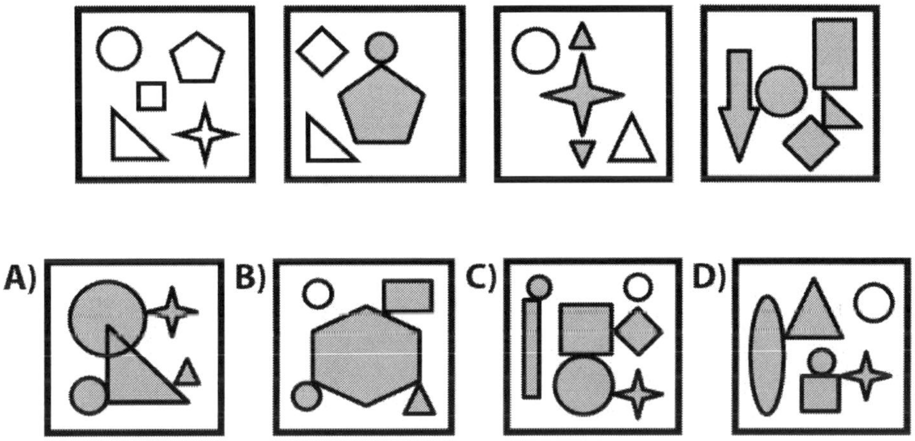

Q248

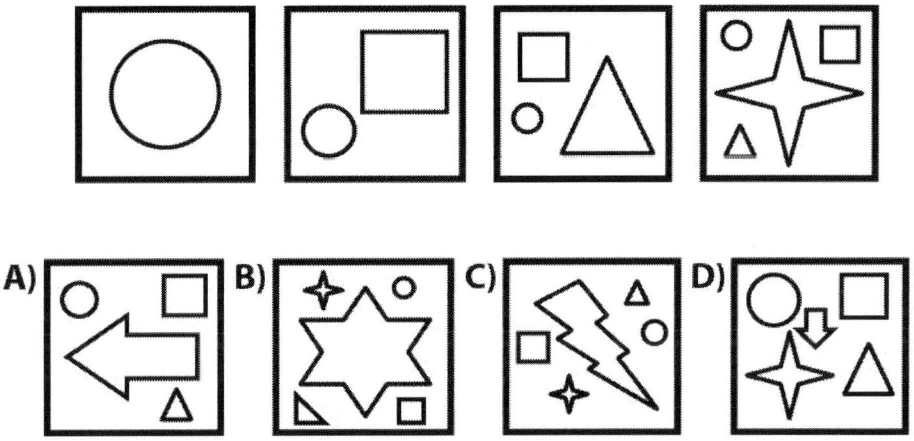

Q249

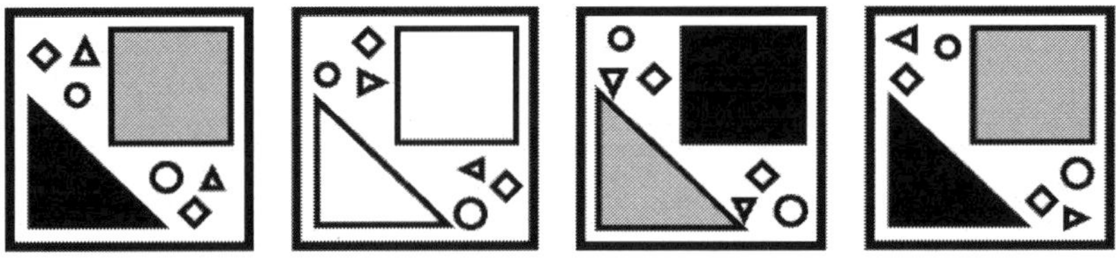

A) 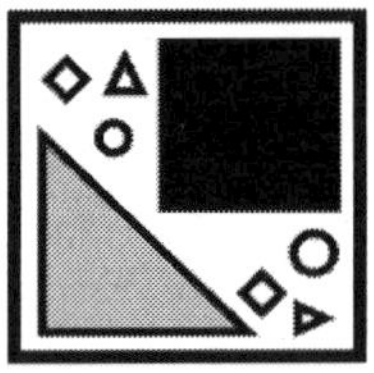 B) 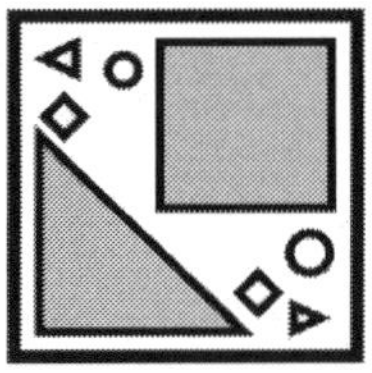 C) 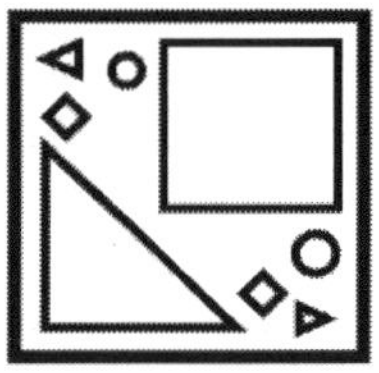 D) 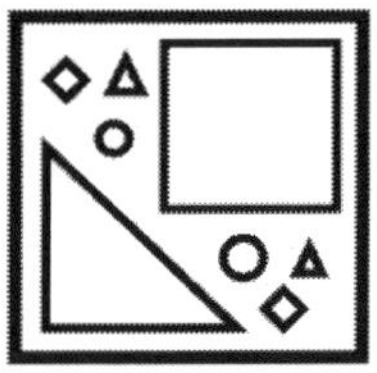

Q250

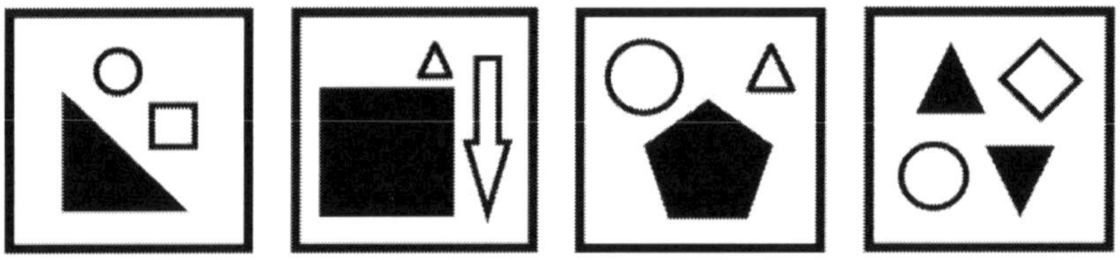

A) 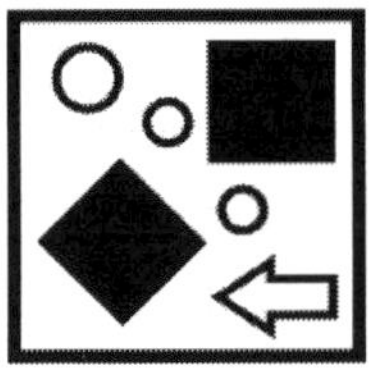 B)  C)  D) 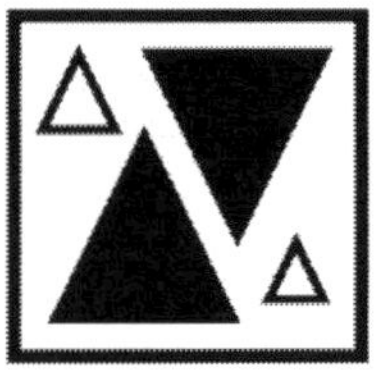

For Questions 251 – 300, which answer option completes the statement?

Q251

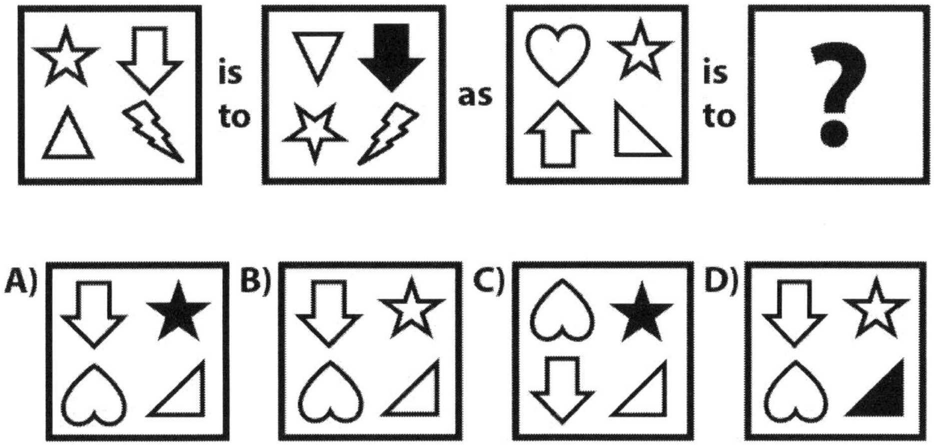

Q252

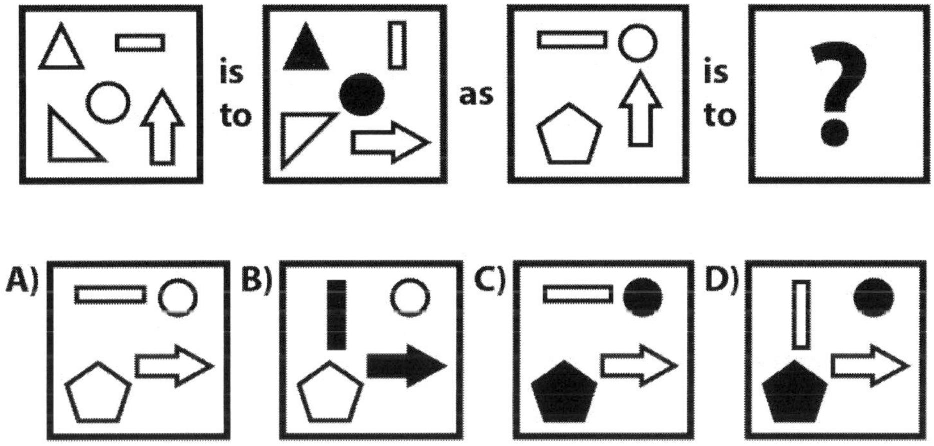

Q253

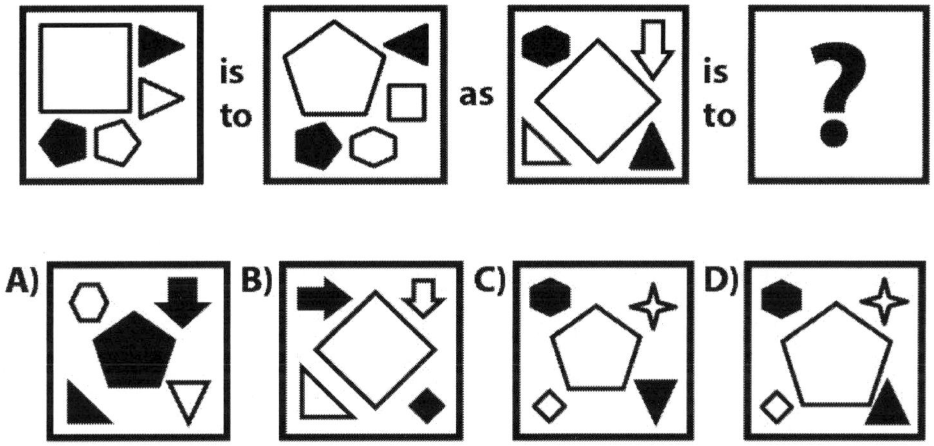

Q254

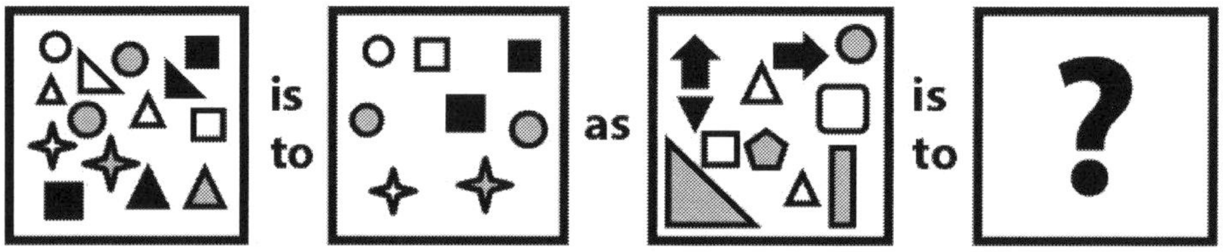

A) 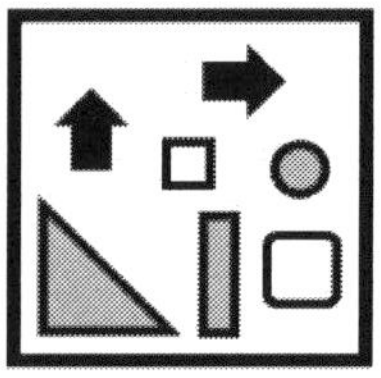

B) 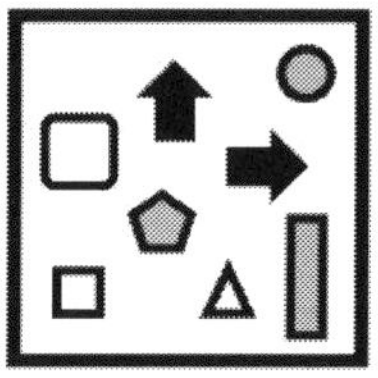

C) 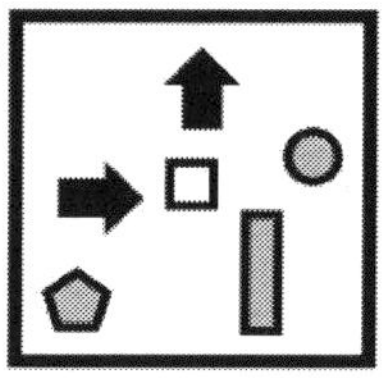

D) 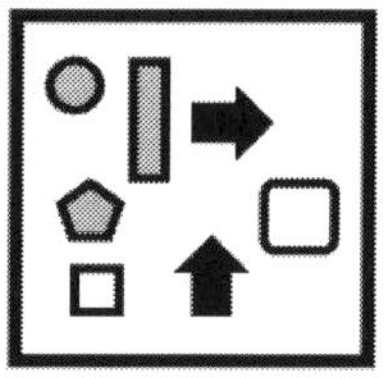

Q255

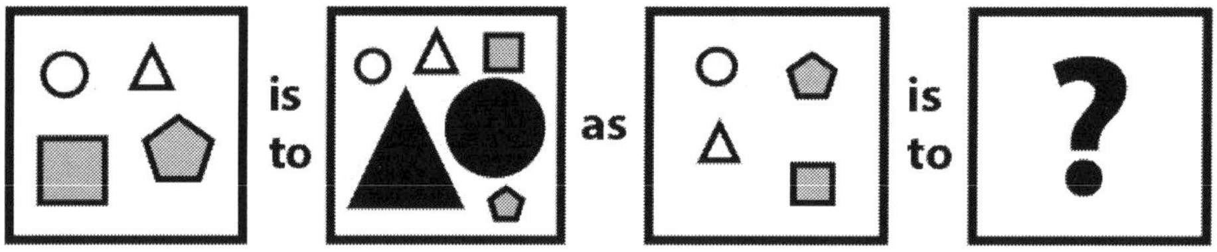

A) 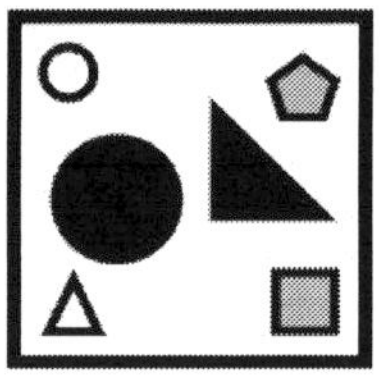

B) 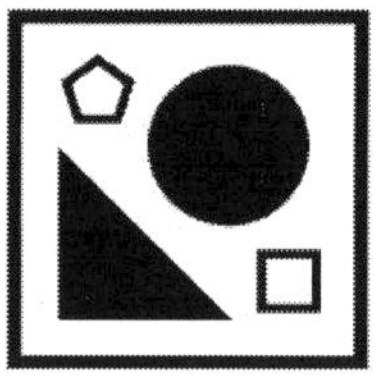

C) 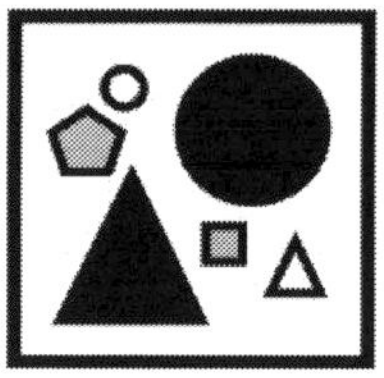

D) 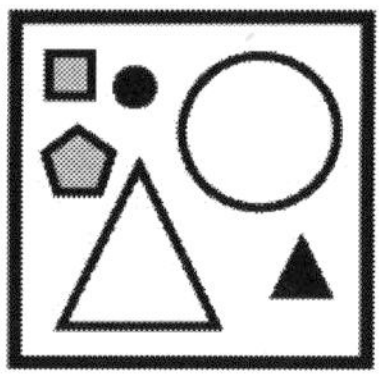

Q256

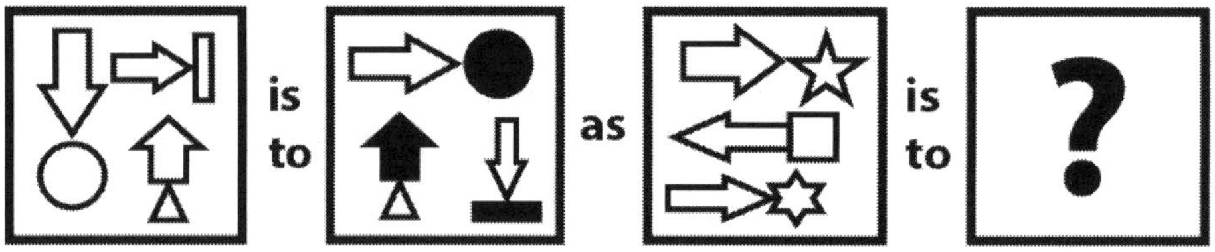

A) 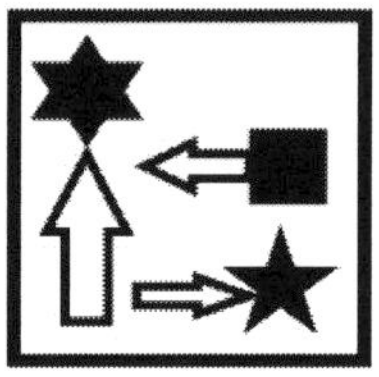

B) 

C) 

D) 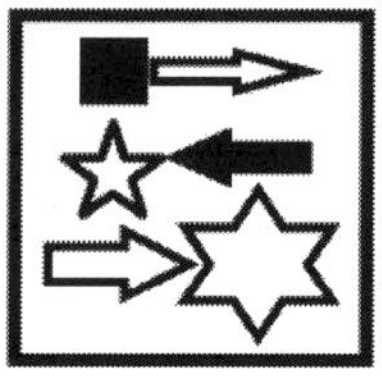

Q257

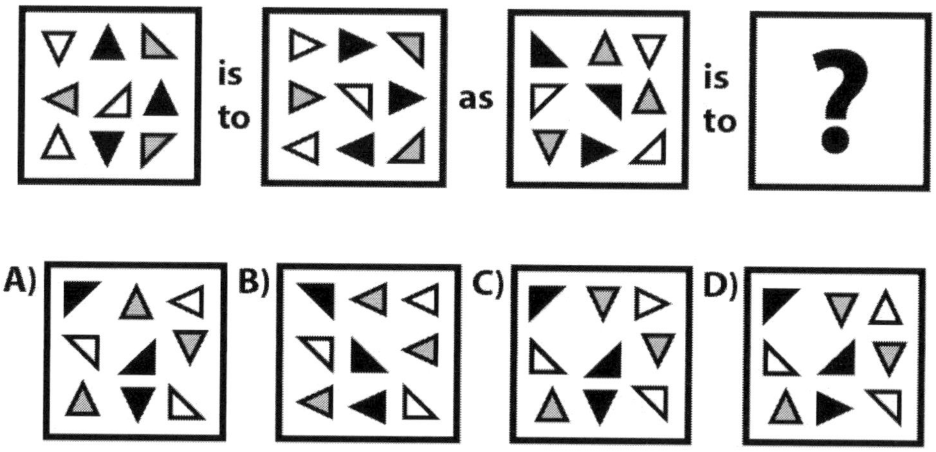

Q258

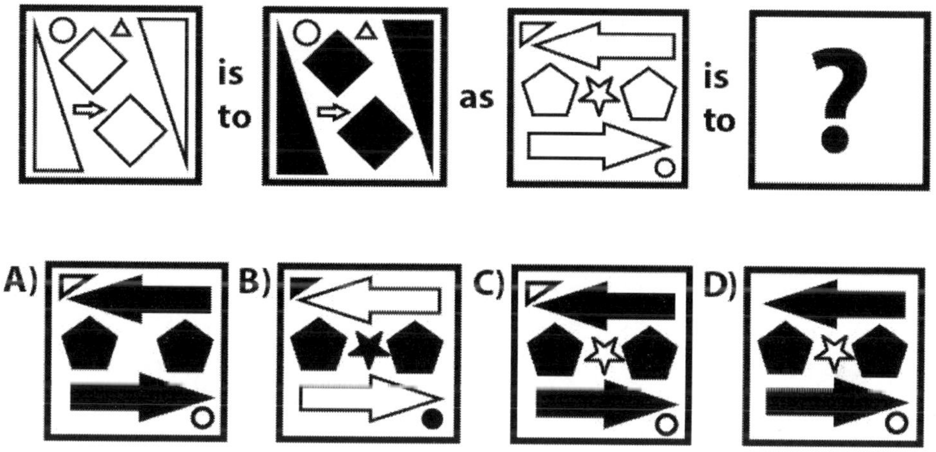

Q259

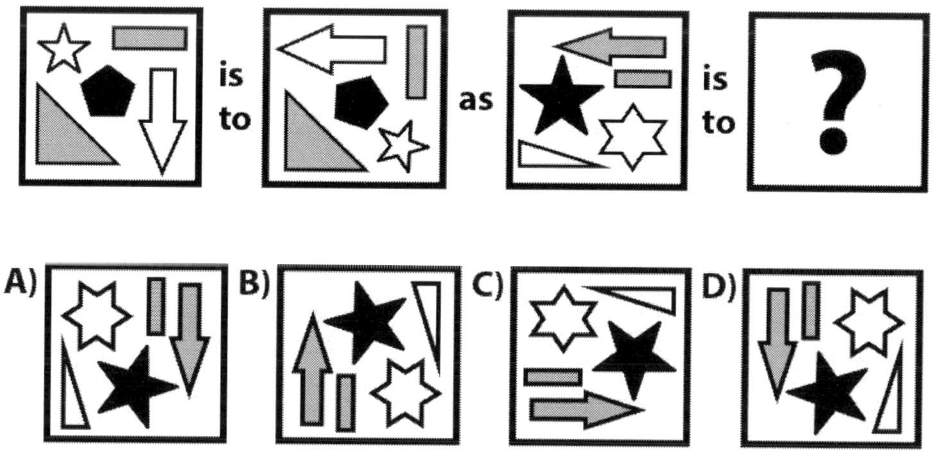

Q260

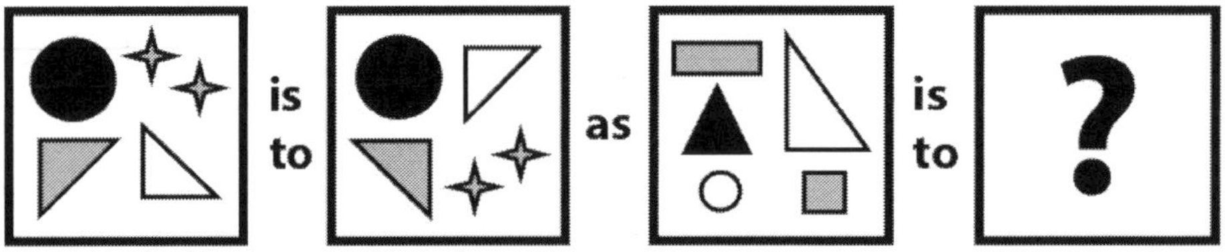

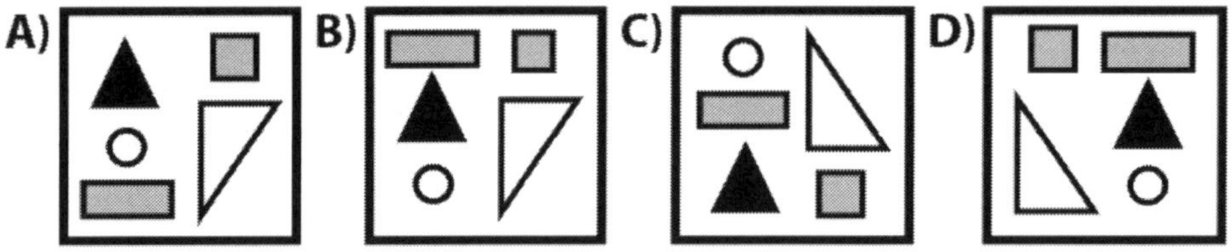

Q261

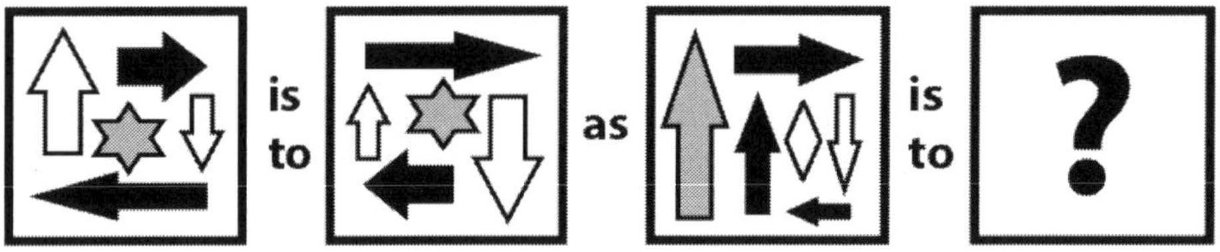

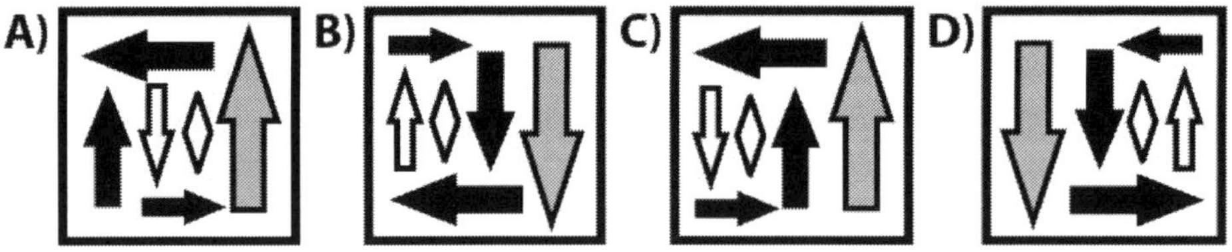

Q262

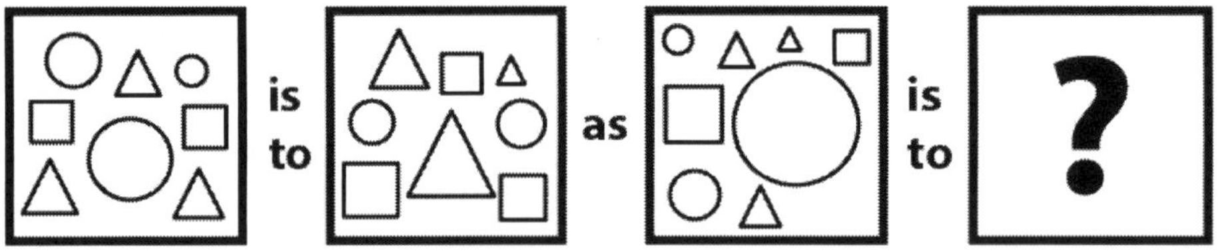

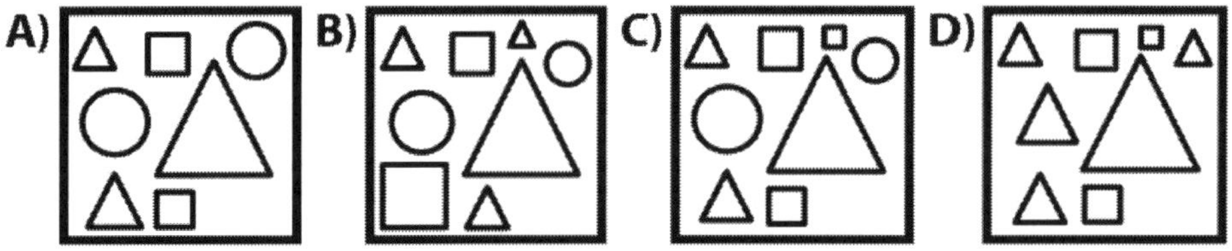

Q263

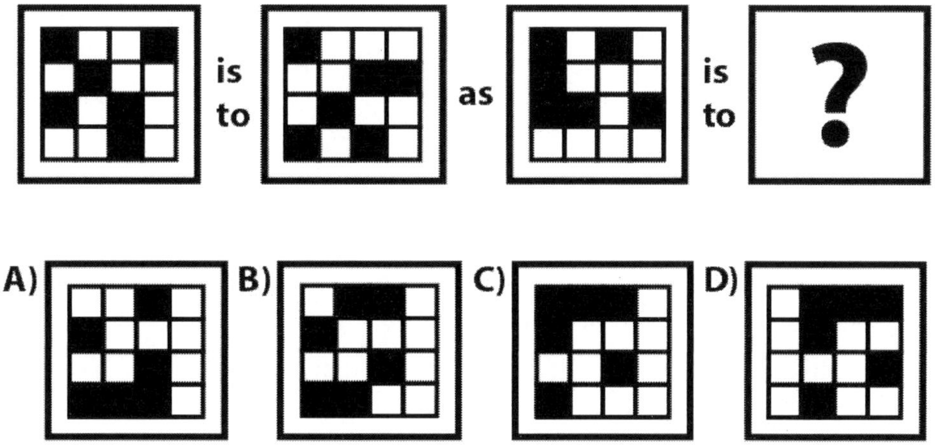

Q264

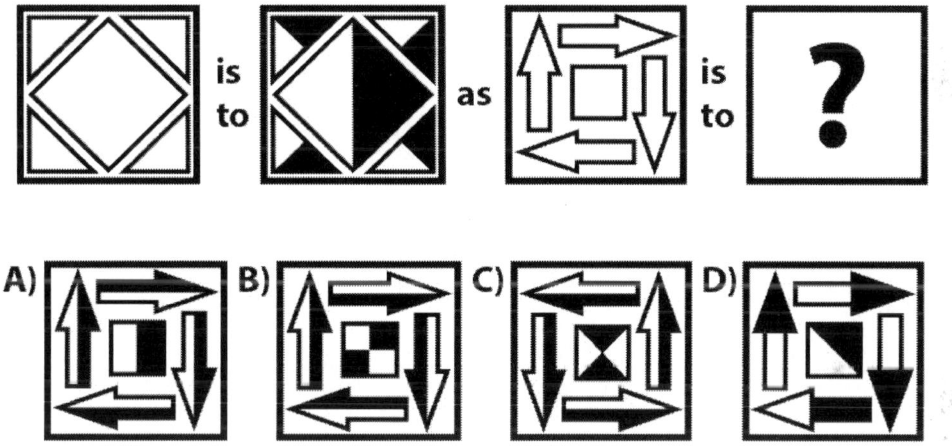

Q265

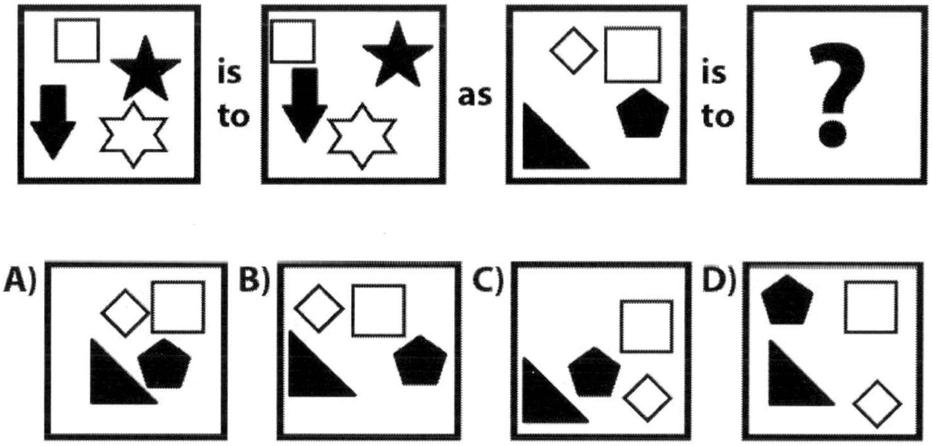

Q266

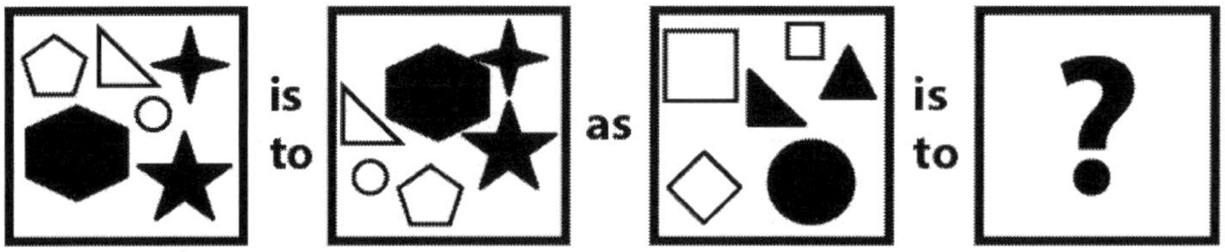

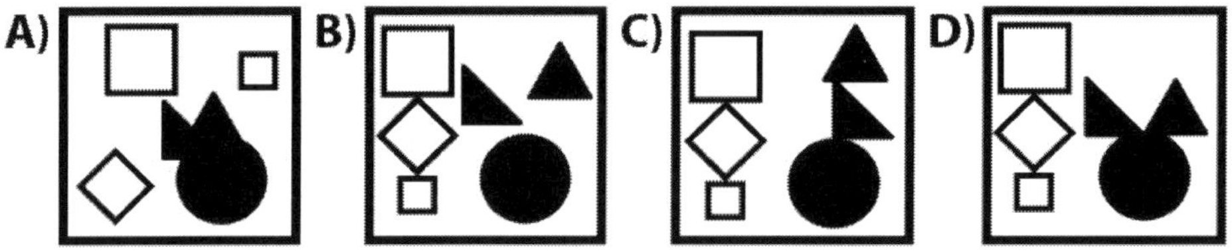

Q267

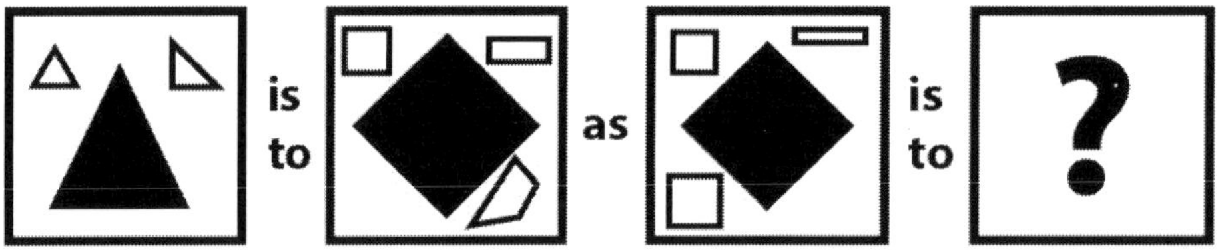

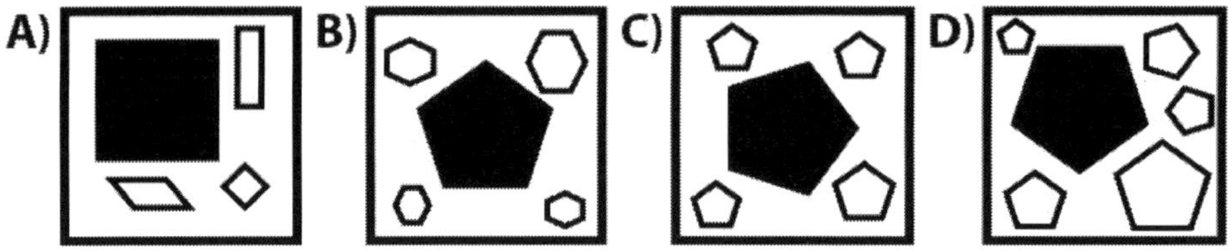

Q268

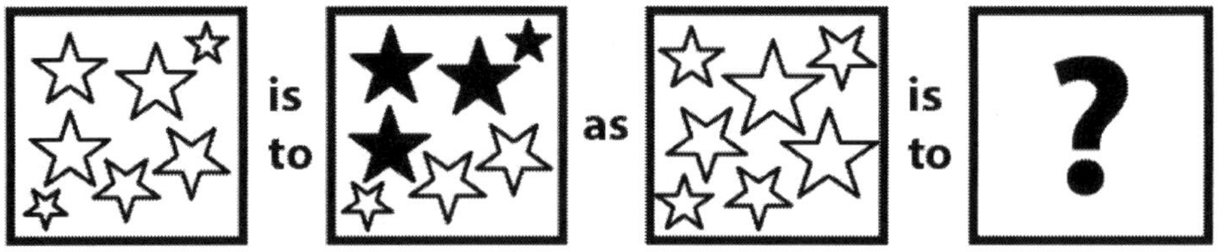

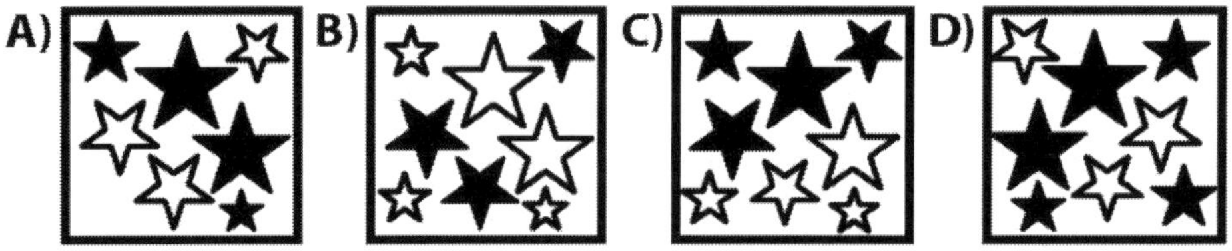

Q269

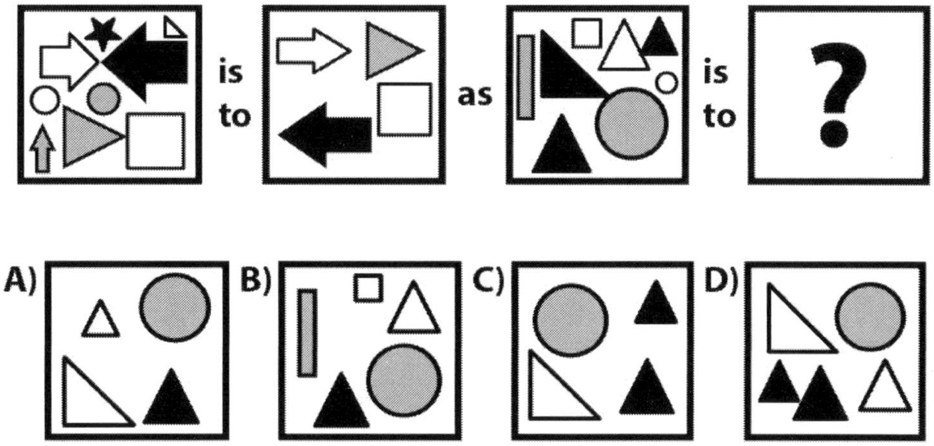

Q270

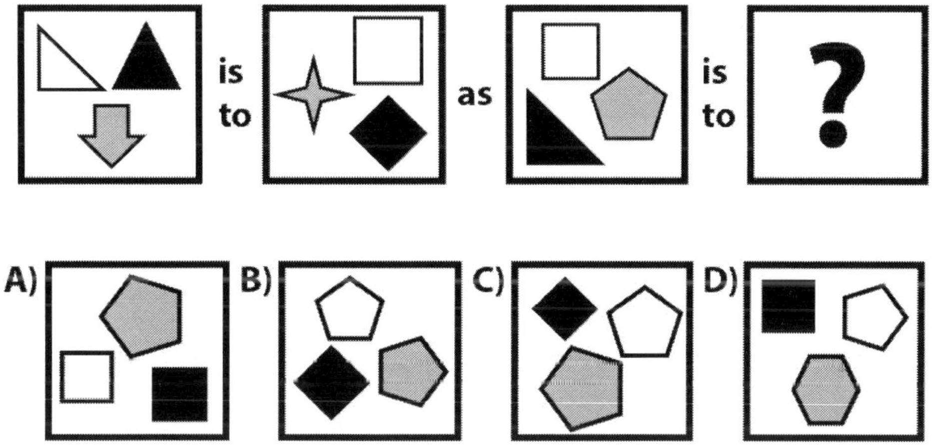

Q271

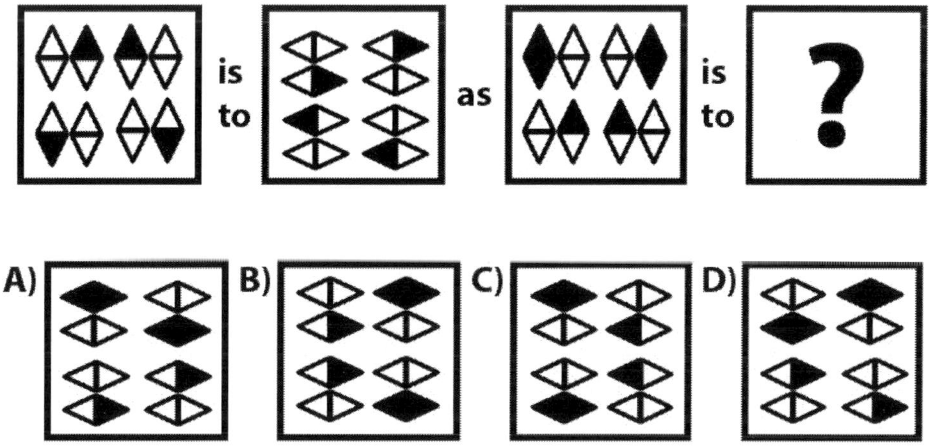

Q272

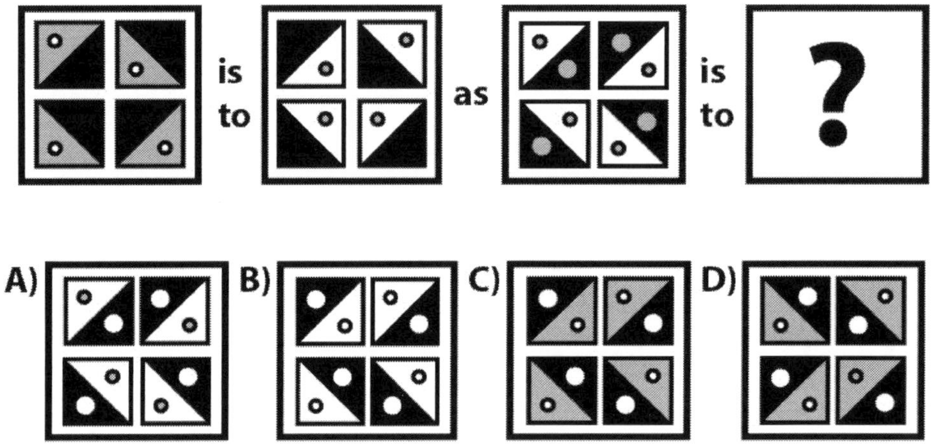

Q273

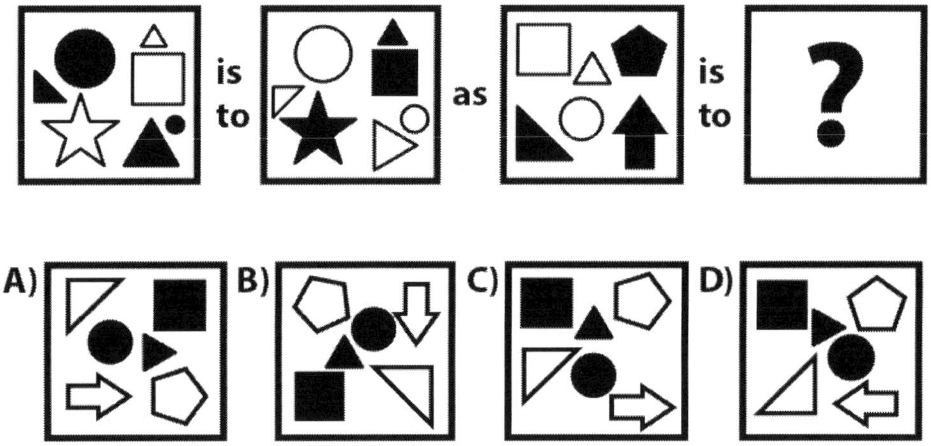

Q274

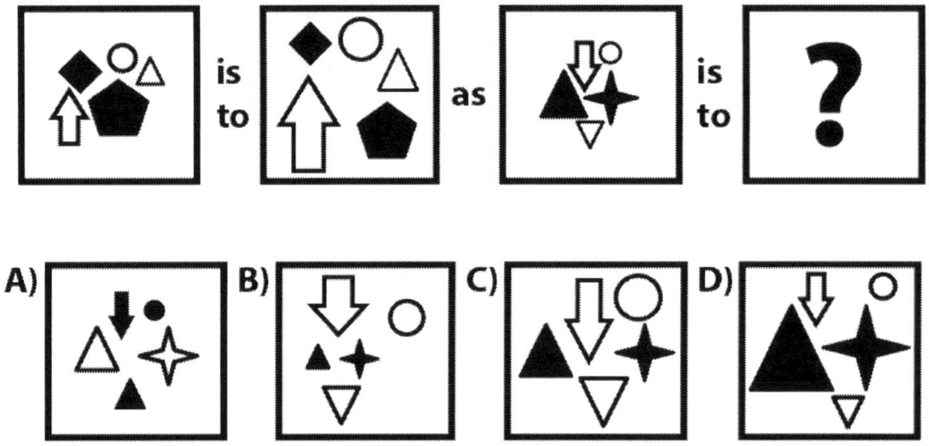

Q275

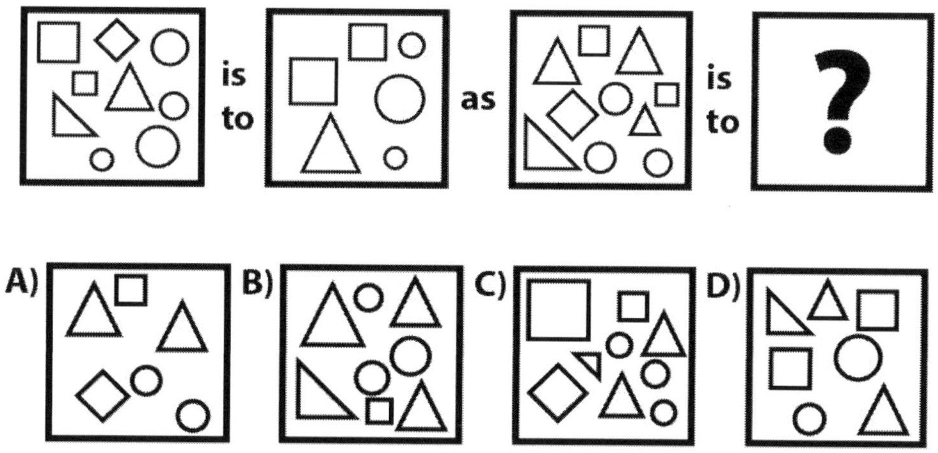

Q276

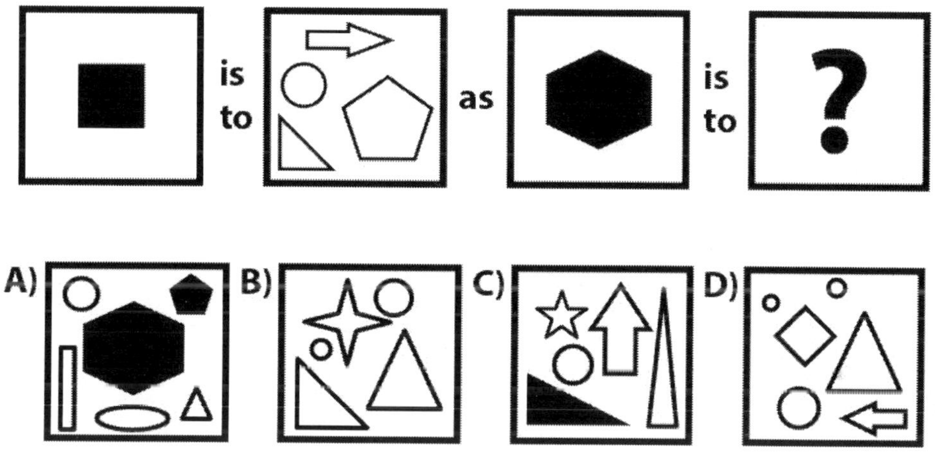

Q277

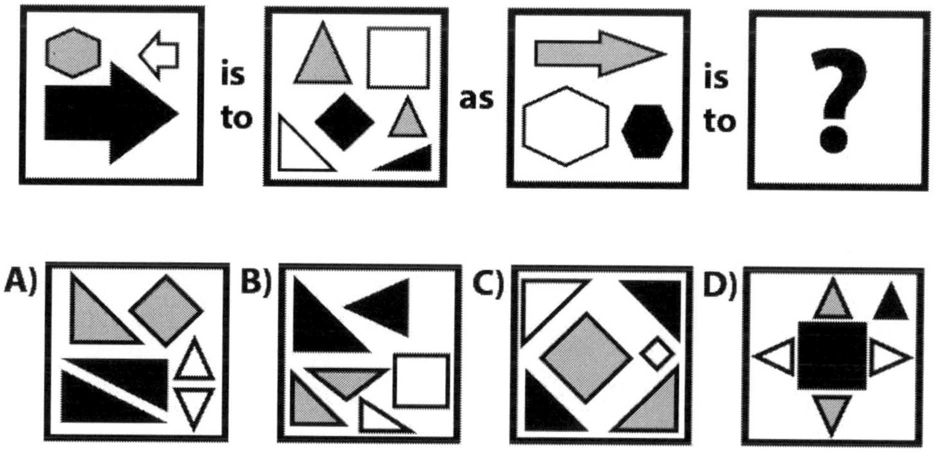

Q278

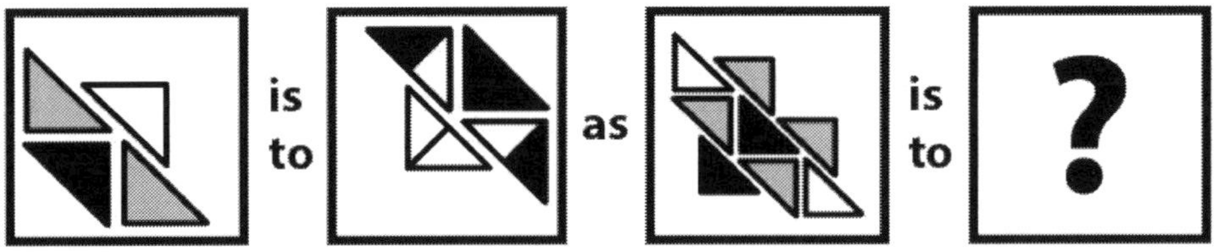

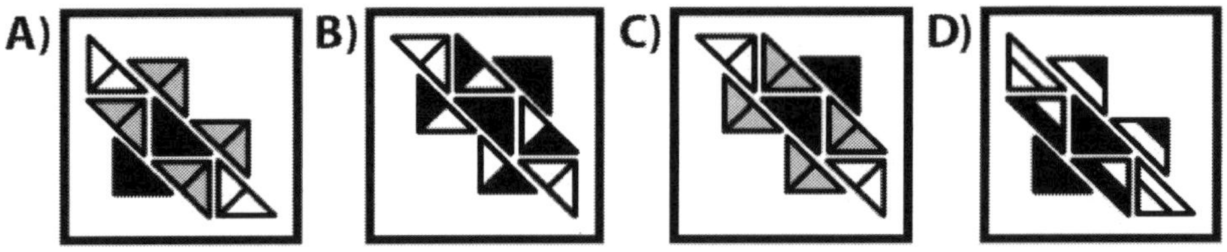

Q279

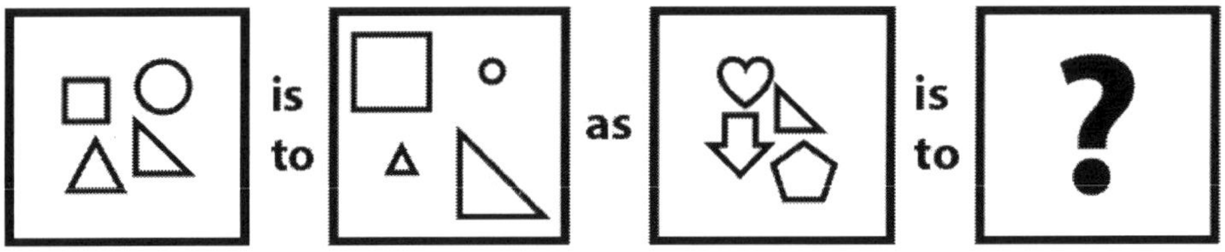

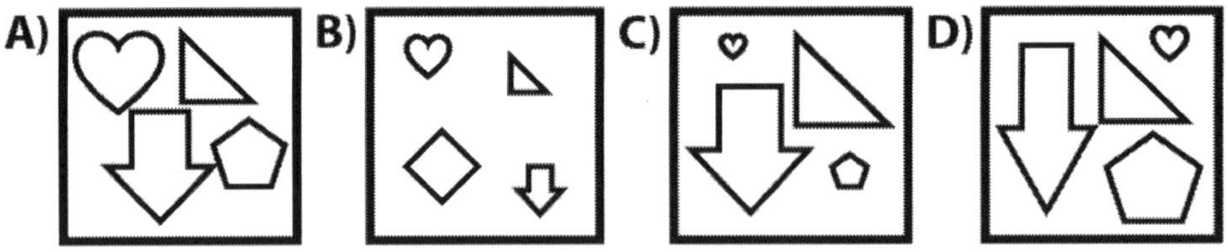

Q280

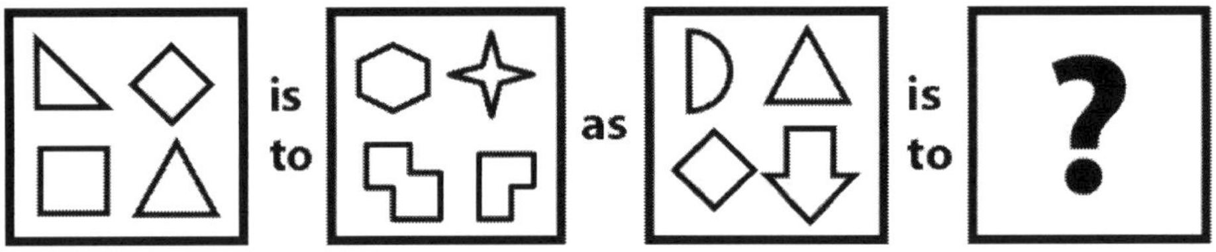

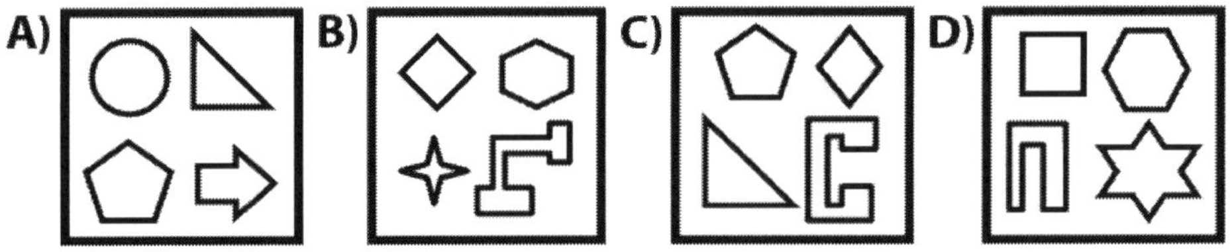

Q281

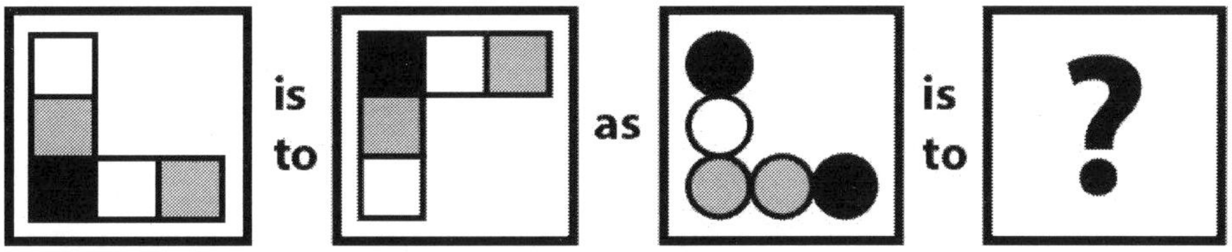

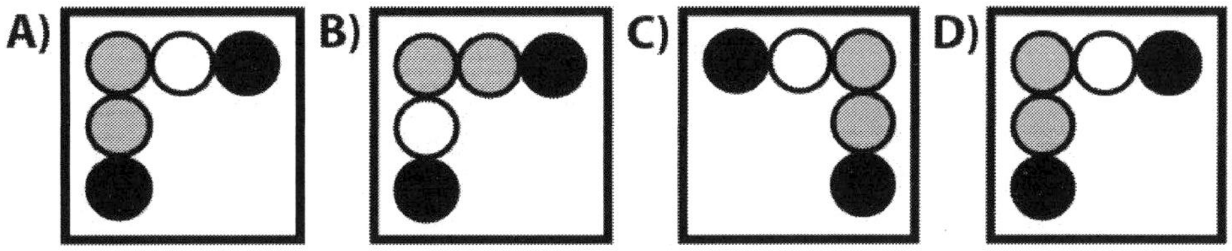

Q282

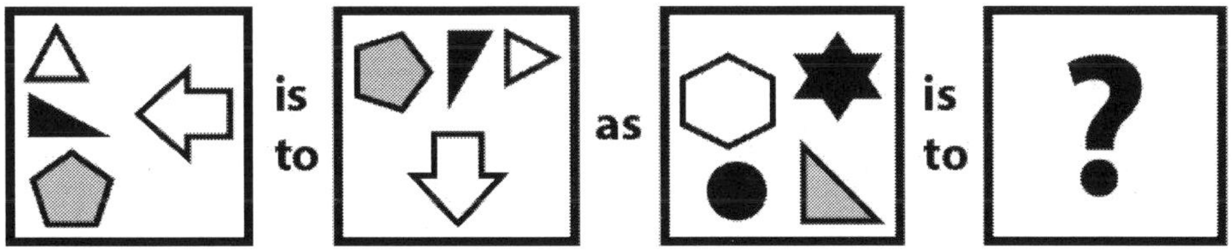

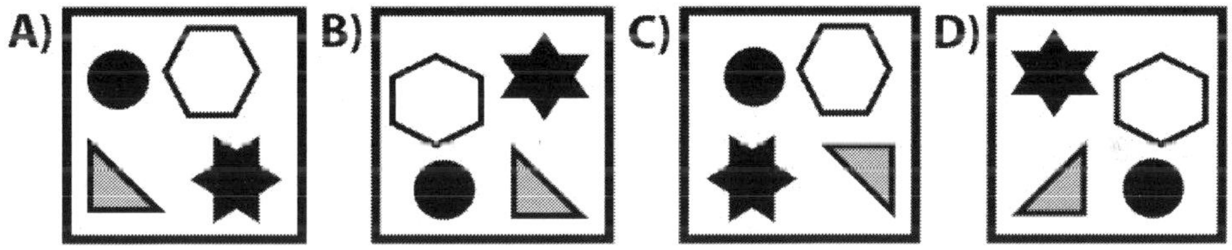

Q283

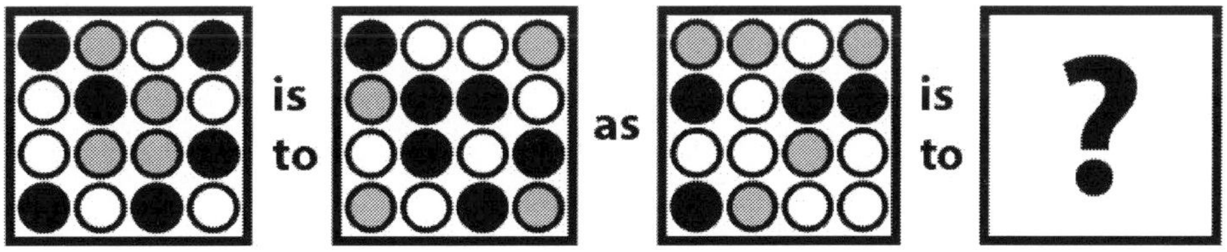

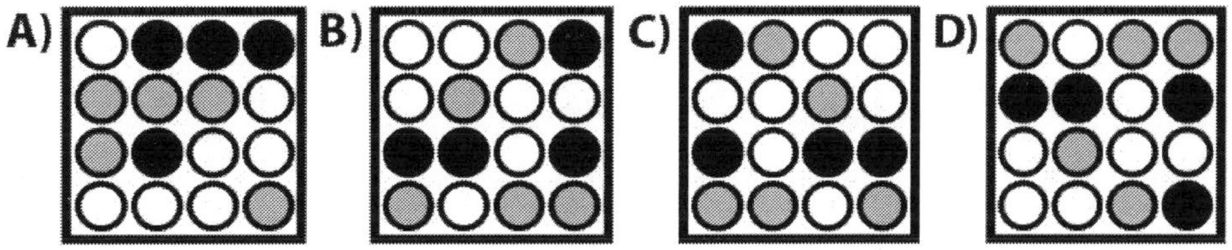

Q284

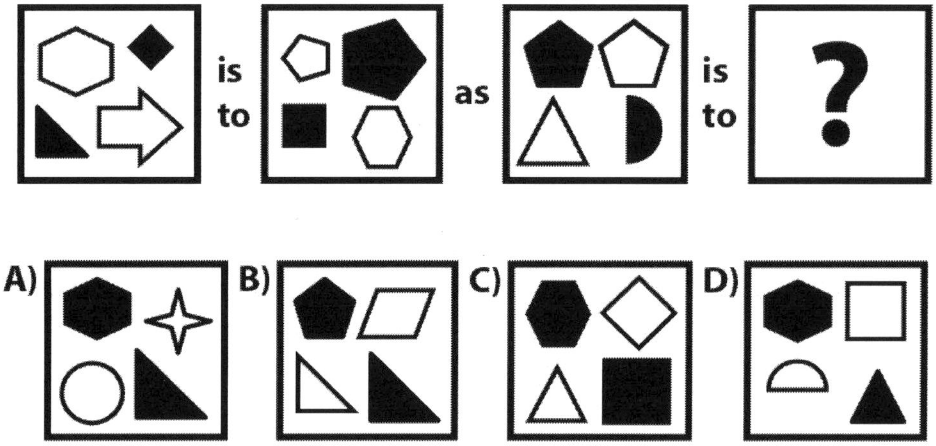

Q285

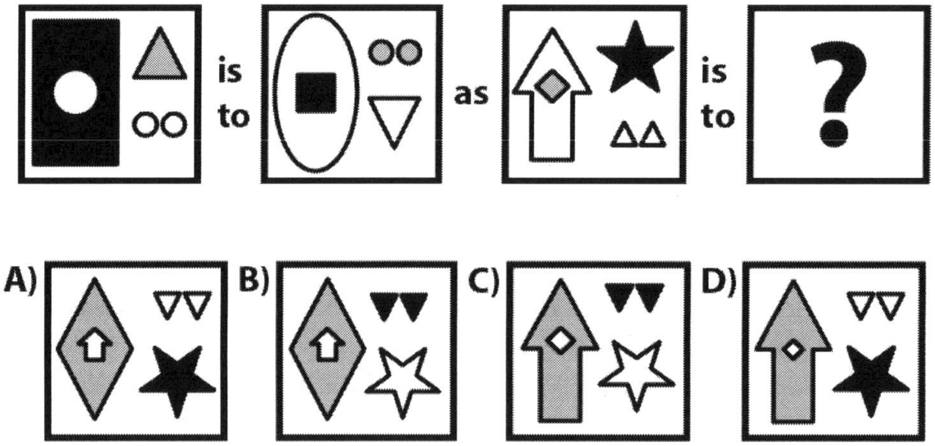

Q286

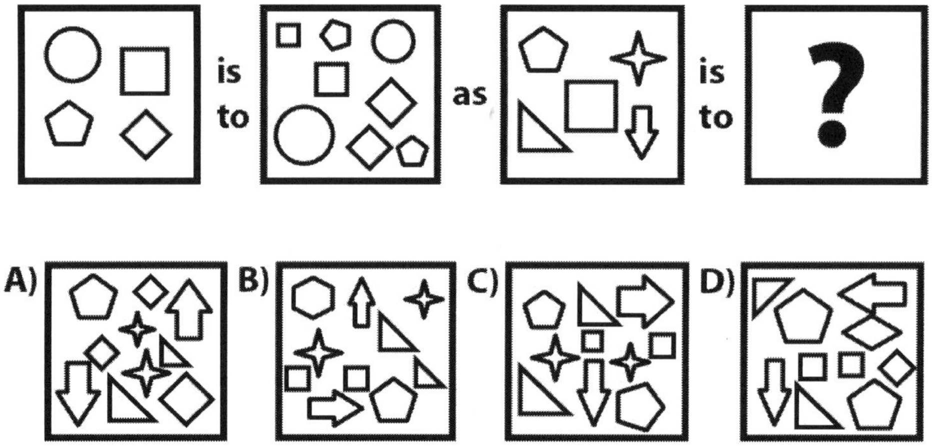

Q287

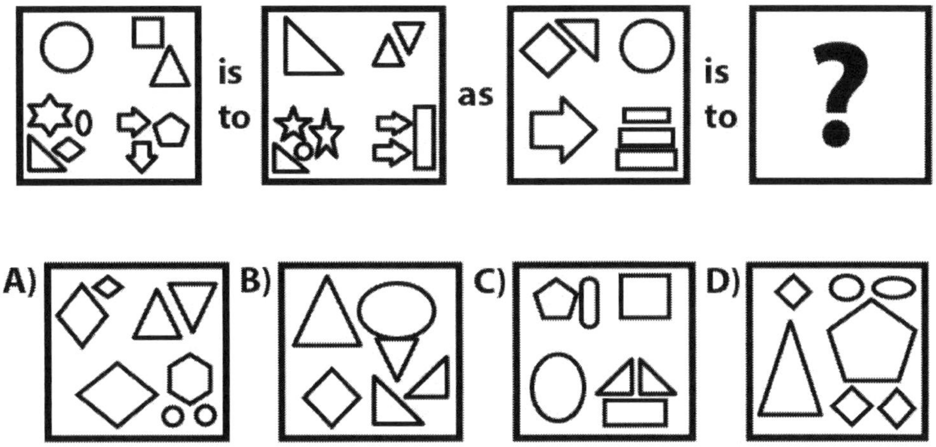

Q288

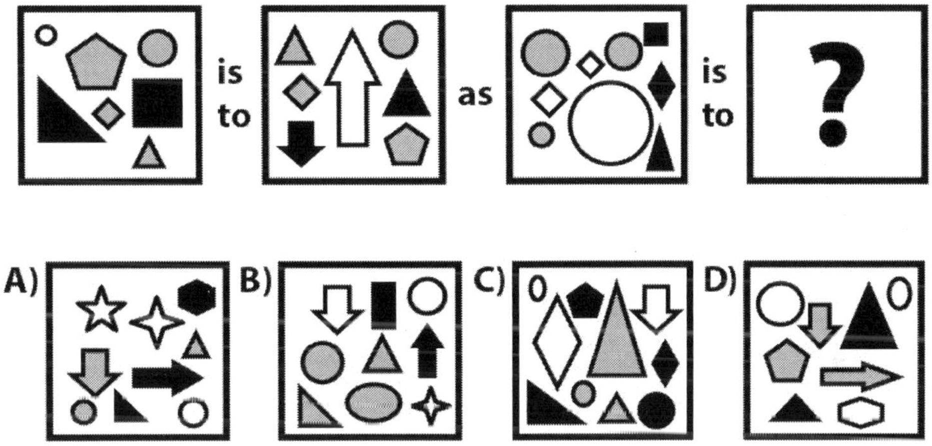

Q289

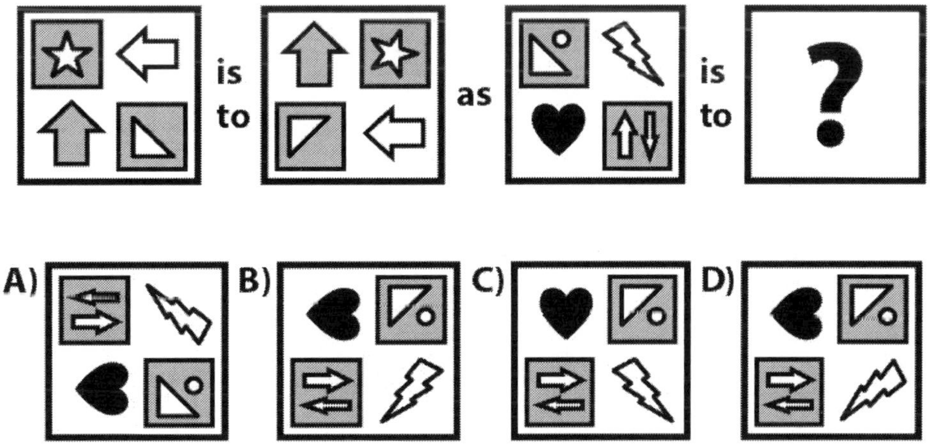

Q290

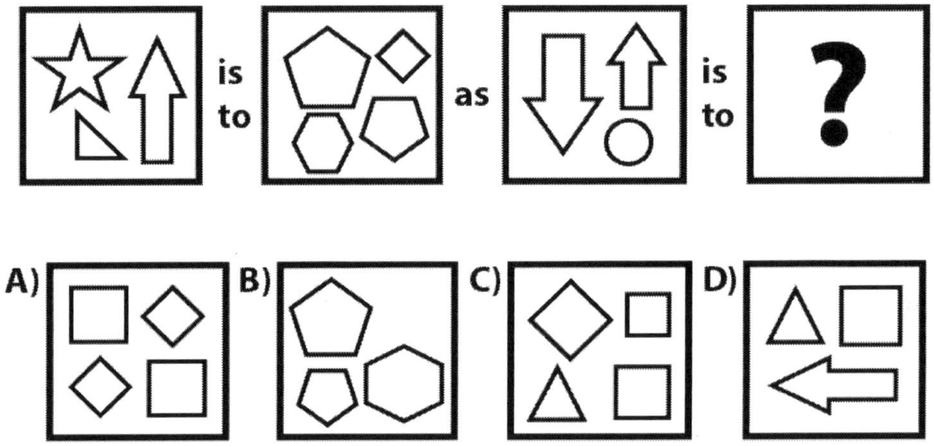

Q291

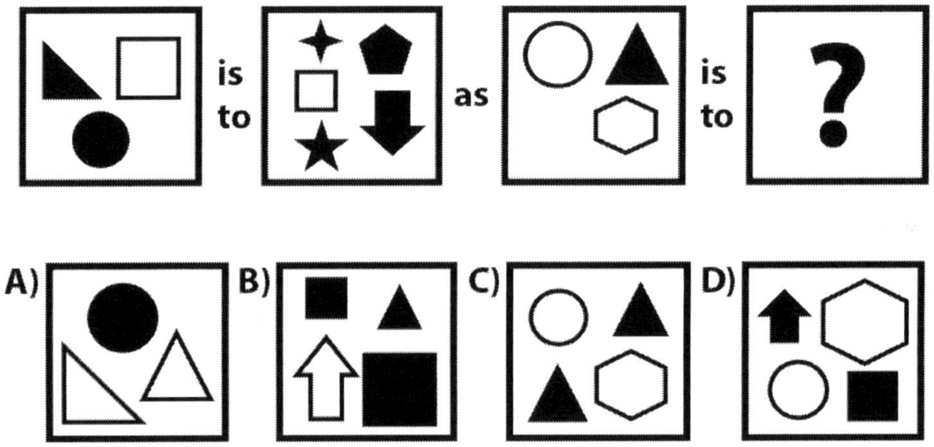

Q292

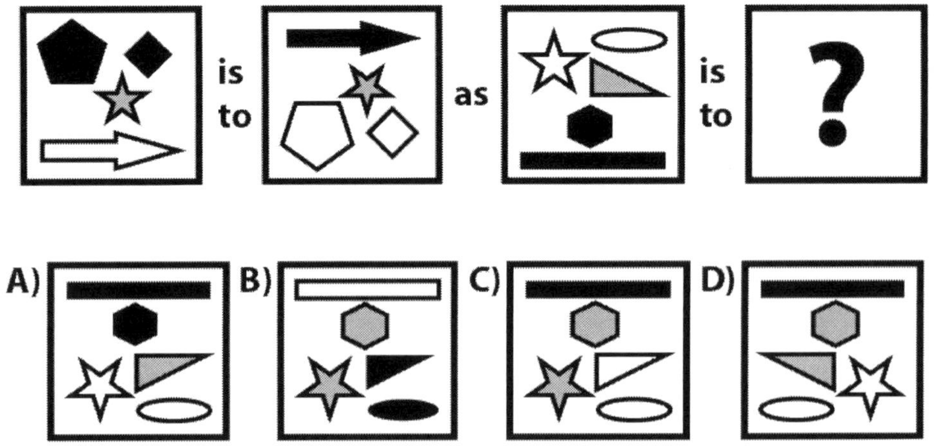

Q293

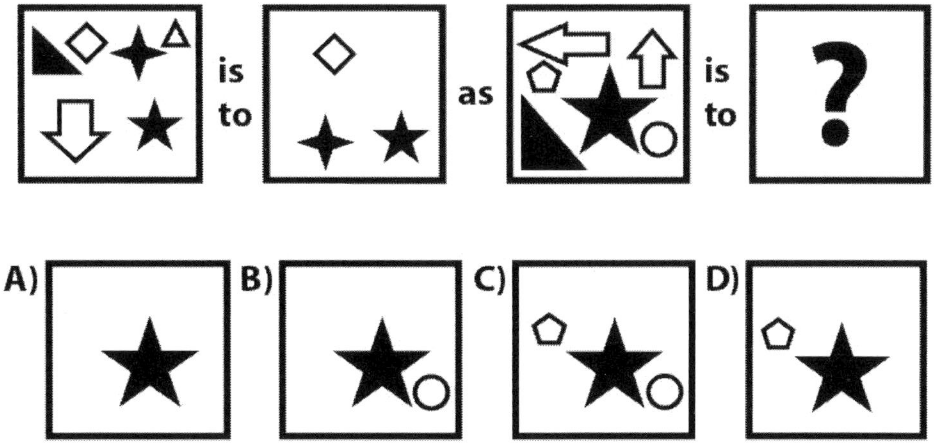

Q294

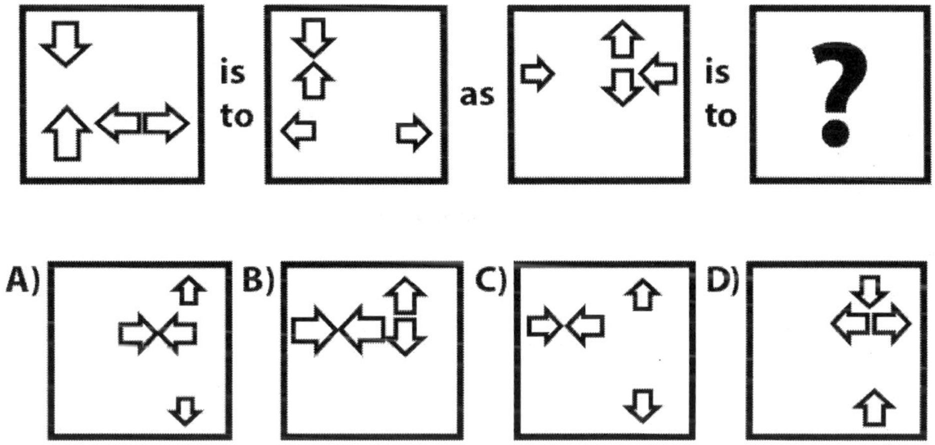

Q295

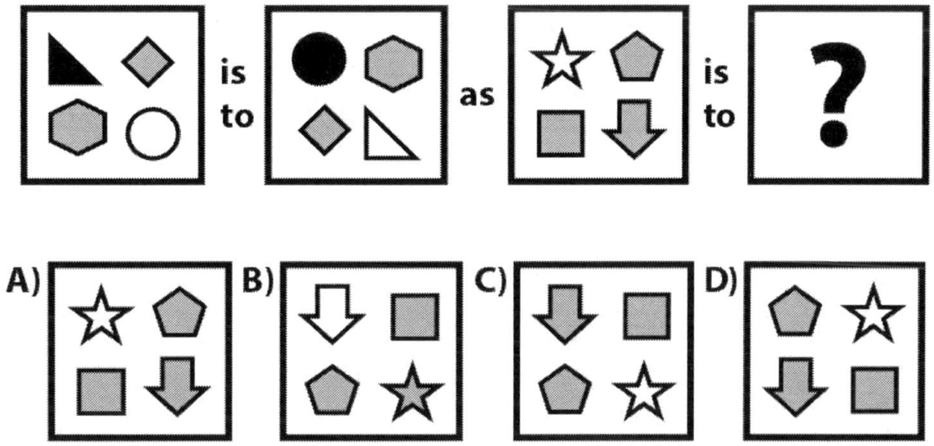

Q296

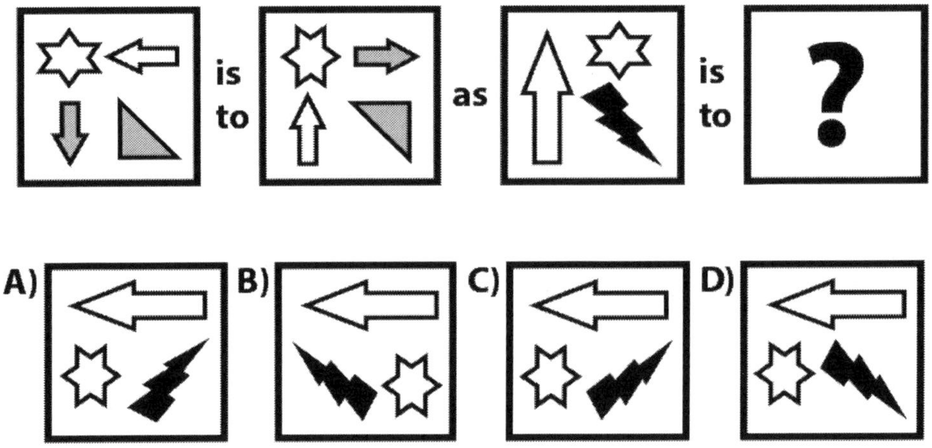

Q297

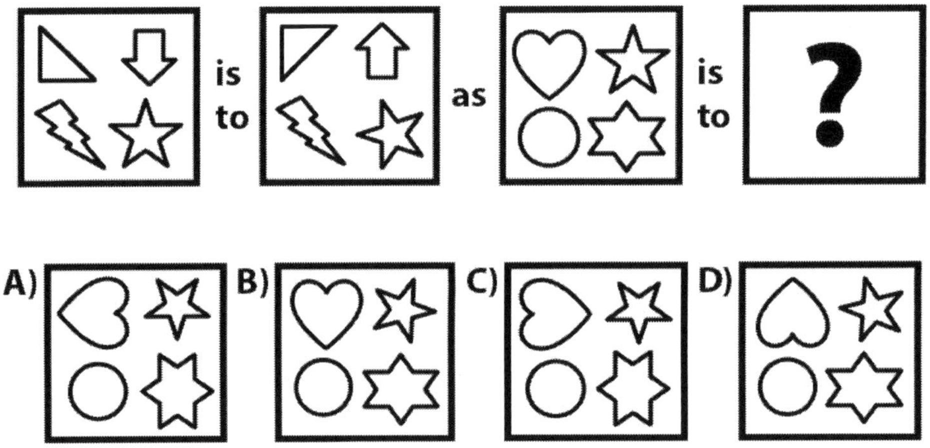

Q298

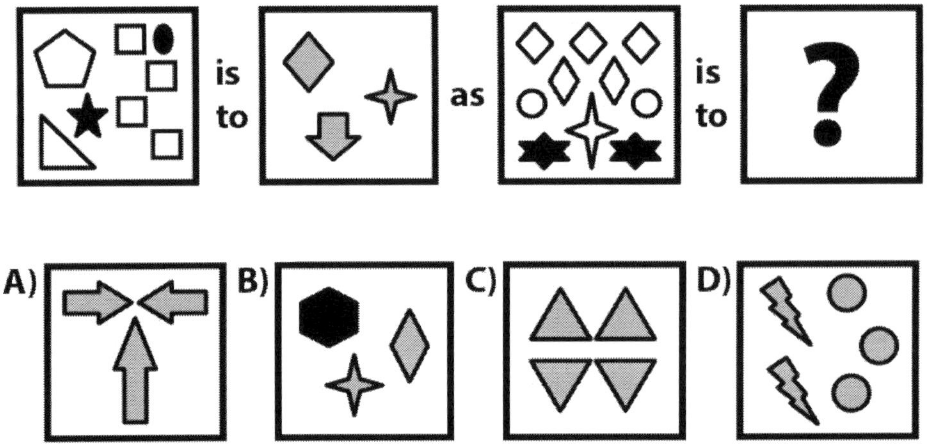

Q299

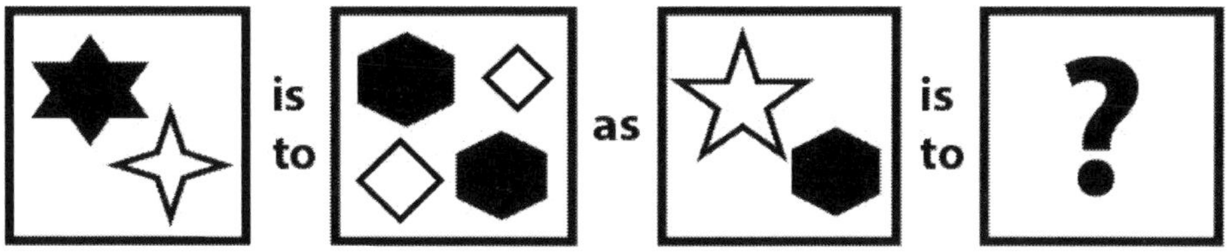

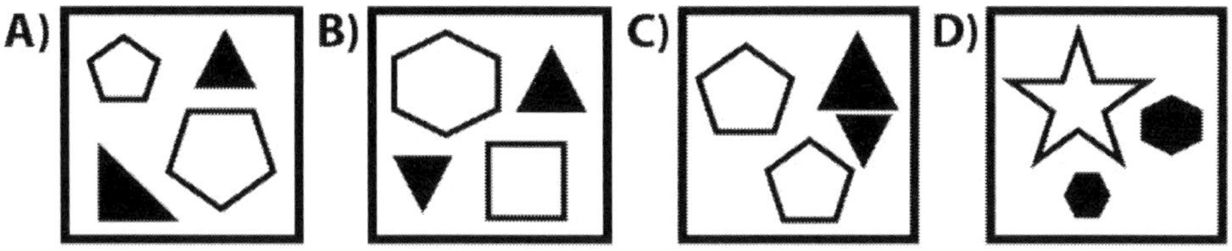

Q300

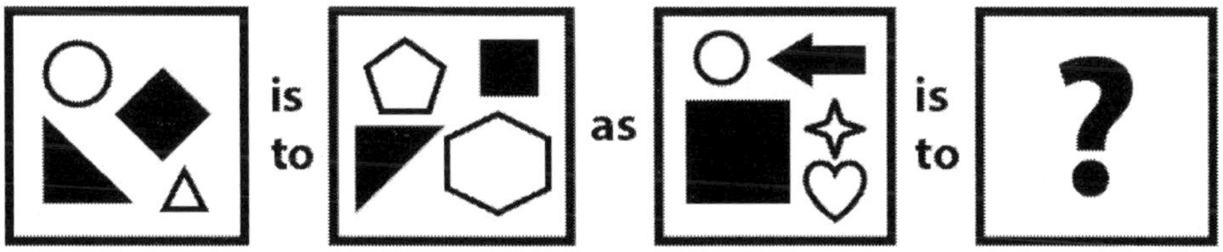

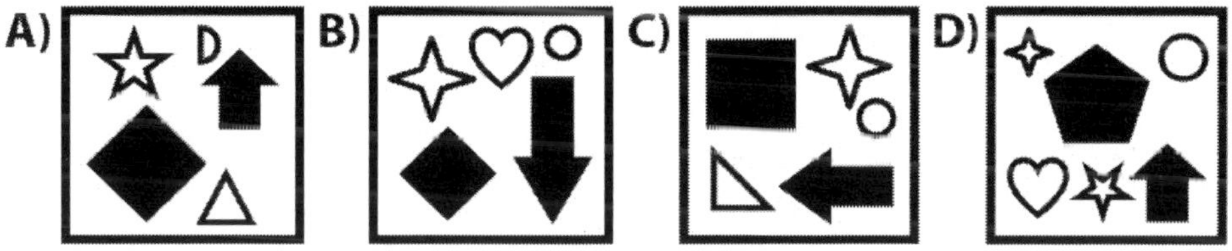

Situational Judgement

The Basics

Situational judgment is a psychological aptitude test; it is an assessment method used to evaluate your ability in solving problems in work-related situations. Situational Judgement Tests (or SJTs) are widely used in medicine as one of the criteria when deciding on applicants; it is used for the Foundation Programme and GP applications.

The aim of the situational judgment section is to assess your ability to understand situations that you could encounter as a medical student or doctor and how you would deal with them. It is a method to **test some of the qualities required in a healthcare professional** (e.g. integrity and ability to work in a team).

In the UCAT, the situational judgment section consists of 20 scenarios with 67 items. Each scenario will have 3-6 items. You will have 26 Minutes to complete this section, which translates to approximately 22 seconds per item. As with all UCAT sections, you have one additional minute to read the instructions at the start. Ensure you're careful to mark your intended answers when working at this pace.

This is the last section of your exam, you are almost near the end- only twenty seven more minutes to go. You still need to stay focused; it might seem obvious, but make sure you read the whole scenario and understand it prior to answering. When answering, imagine you are the person in the scenario. The majority of the scenarios will be about medical students, imagine you are in their shoes.

The series of scenarios include possible actions and considerations. Each scenario is comprised of two sets of questions. In set one you will be asked to assess the "appropriateness" of options in relation to the scenario.

The four possible appropriateness choices are:

- ***A very appropriate thing to do*** – This is an ideal action.
- ***Appropriate, but not ideal*** – This option can be done but not necessarily the best thing to be done.
- ***Inappropriate, but not awful*** – This should not be done, but if it does occur the consequences are not terrible.
- ***A very inappropriate thing to do*** – This should not be done in any circumstances, as it will make the situation worse.

In set two, you will be asked to assess the "importance" of options in relation to the scenario,

The four possible importance options are:

- ***Very important*** – something that is essential to take into account.
- ***Important*** – something you should take into account but is not vital.
- ***Of minor importance*** – something that may be considered, but will not affect the outcome if it is not taken into account.
- ***Not important at all*** – something that is not relevant at all.

Section E includes non-cognitive abilities and so is marked differently to the other sections. You will be awarded full marks if your response completely matches the correct answer. If your answer is close but not exactly right you will receive partial marks, and if there are no correct answers you will receive no marks. Your score is then calculated and expressed in one of four bands, band 1 being the highest and band 4 being the lowest. The band resembles how close your responses were to the assessment panel's agreed answers.

Things you MUST NOT do as a medical student:

- Write or sign drug charts.
- Sign or authorise anything that a doctor should do (operation consent forms, death certificates etc).
- Make any decisions that affect treatment.
- Change any treatment regime for any reason.
- Perform practical procedures without supervision.
- Break patient confidentiality or do anything that places confidentiality at risk.
- Behave dishonestly in any way.

Things you MUST do as a medical student:

- Raise any concerns regarding patient safety with an appropriate person.
- Report any inappropriate behaviour you witness to an appropriate person.
- Attend all scheduled teaching and training.
- Take responsibility for your learning and seek opportunities to learn.
- Dress and present yourself in a clean and smart way.

Things you CAN do as a medical student:

- Speak to patients.
- Examine patients.
- Write in patient notes (but must indicate your name and role).
- Perform simple practical procedures like taking blood, inserting cannulas or catheters (if you are trained to and with adequate supervision).
- Help doctors with more complex procedures according to their strict directions.
- Attend meetings where patients are discussed.
- Do things you have been trained to do.

Question Answering Strategy

Treat every option as independent – the options may seem similar, but don't let the different options confuse you, read each option as if it is a question on its own. It is important to know that responses should **NOT** be judged as though they are the **ONLY** thing you are to do. An answer should not be judged as inappropriate because it incomplete, but only if there is some actual inappropriate action taking place. For example, if a scenario says "a patient on the ward complains she is in pain", the response "ask the patient what is causing the problem" would be very appropriate, even though any good response would also include informing the nurses and doctors about what you had been told.

There might be multiple correct responses for each scenario, so don't feel you have to answer each stem differently. Thus an answer choice may be used once, more than once or not at all for all scenarios.

If you are unsure of the answer, mark the question and move on. Avoid spending longer than 30 seconds on any question, otherwise you will fall behind the pace and not finish the section.

As with every other section, if you are completely unsure of the answers, answer the question anyway. There is no negative marking and your initial instinct may be close to the intended answer.

- If there are several people mentioned in the scenario make sure you are answering about the correct person.
- Think of what you 'should' do rather than what you necessarily would do.
- Always think of **patient safety** and acting in the patient's best interests.

Read "Tomorrow's Doctors"

This is a publication produced by the GMC (General Medical Council) which can be found on their website. The GMC regulate the medical profession, ensuring standards remain high. This publication can be found on their website, and it outlines the expectations of the next generation of doctors – the generation of doctors you are aspiring to join. **Reading through this will get you into a professional way of thinking** that will help you judge these questions accurately.

Step into Character

When doing this section, imagine you're there. Imagine yourself as a caring and conscientious medical student a few years from now, in each situation as it unfolds. What would you do? What do you think would be the right thing to do?

Hierarchy

The patient is of primary importance. All decisions that affect patient care should be made to benefit the patient. Of secondary importance are your work colleagues. So if there is no risk to patients, you should help out your colleagues and avoid doing anything that would undermine them or harm their reputation – but if doing so would bring detriment to any patient then the patients priorities come to the top. Finally of lowest importance is yourself. You should avoid working outside hours and strive to further your education, but not at the expense of more important or urgent priorities. Remember the key principles of professional conduct and you cannot go far wrong. **Of first and foremost importance is patient**

safety. Make sure you make all judgements with this in mind.

Top tip! Read the GMC publication "*Tomorrow's Doctors*" – this will help you think the right way.

Medical Ethics

There tend to be a few ethical questions in each SJT paper so it is well worth your time to learn medical ethics. Whilst there are huge ethical textbooks available– you only need to be familiar with the basic principles for the purposes of the UCAT. These principles can be applied to all cases regardless what the social/ethnic background the healthcare professional or patient is from. In addition to being helpful in the UCAT, you'll need to know them for the interview stages anyway so they're well worth learning now rather than later. The principles are:

Beneficence

The wellbeing of the patient should be the doctor's first priority. In medicine this means that one must act in the patient's best interests to ensure the best outcome is achieved for them i.e. 'Do Good'.

Non-Maleficence

This is the principle of avoiding harm to the patient (i.e. Do no harm). There can be a danger that in a willingness to treat, doctors can sometimes cause more harm to the patient than good. This can especially be the case with major interventions, such as chemotherapy or surgery. Where a course of action has both potential harms and potential benefits, non-maleficence must be balanced against beneficence.

Autonomy

The patient has the right to determine their own health care. This therefore requires the doctor to be a good communicator, so that the patient is sufficiently informed to make their own decisions. 'Informed consent' is thus a vital precursor to any treatment. A doctor must respect a patient's refusal for treatment even if they think it is not the correct choice. Note that patients cannot <u>demand</u> treatment – only refuse it, e.g. an alcoholic patient can refuse rehabilitation but cannot demand a liver transplant.

There are many situations where the application of autonomy can be quite complex, for example:

- **Treating Children**: Consent is required from the parents, although the autonomy of the child is taken into account increasingly as they get older.
- **Treating adults without the capacity** to make important decisions. The first challenge with this is in assessing whether or not a patient has the capacity to make the decisions. Just because a patient has a mental illness does not necessarily mean that they lack the capacity to make decisions about their health care. Where patients do lack capacity, the power to make decisions is transferred to the next of kin (or Legal Power of Attorney, if one has been set up).

Justice

This principle deals with the fair distribution and allocation of healthcare resources for the population.

Consent

This is an extension of Autonomy- patients must agree to a procedure or intervention. For consent to be valid, it must be **voluntary informed consent.** This means that the patient must have sufficient mental capacity to make the decision, they must be presented with all the relevant information (benefits, side effects and the likely complications) in a way they can understand and they must make the choice freely without being put under pressure.

***p tip!* Consent is only valid** if it is given:

- On the basis of full information.
- With sufficient mental capacity.
- Freely without pressure.
- Communicated unambiguously.

Confidentiality

Patients expect that the information they reveal to doctors will be kept private- this is a key component in maintaining the trust between patients and doctors. You must ensure that patient details are kept confidential. Confidentiality can be broken if you suspect that a patient is a risk to themselves or to others e.g. Terrorism, suicides.

When answering a question on medical ethics, you need to ensure that you show an appreciation for the fact that there are often two sides to the argument. Where appropriate, you should outline both points of view and how they pertain to the main principles of medical ethics and then come to a reasoned judgement.

Situational Judgement Questions

Scenario 1

A conversation is taking place between a midwife Kate and the senior Dr Herbert: Jacob, the medical student, is observing. Dr Herbert is being rude to the Kate and is acting superior. When Dr Herbert leaves, Jacob overhears Kate talking to the other midwives about his behaviour, and how it happens frequently, and makes both the midwives and the patients feel uncomfortable.

How appropriate are the following actions from Jacob?

1. Tell Kate that you will help to file a complaint against Dr Herbert.
2. Make Dr Herbert aware that perhaps he should be kinder the next time he speaks to Kate and patients.
3. Ignore the situation and do nothing.
4. Alert his supervisor as to what he saw, and to get advice on what to do.
5. Tell Dr Herbert that his behaviour was making patients and midwives feel uncomfortable.

Scenario 2

A medical student, George, is sitting in a foot clinic with Dr Walker. George notices that Dr Walker hasn't been washing his hands between patients, despite examining the feet of all of his patients without gloves. In his training George was told that he must wash his hands properly before and after touching each patient to prevent the spread of infections.

How appropriate are each of the following responses by George in this situation?

6. Alert Dr Walker that he ought to wash his hands more after the current consultation has finished.
7. Wash his hands before and after each patient in the hopes that Dr Walker will follow by example.
8. Do nothing because Dr Walker is an experienced consultant.
9. Tell the nurse in charge of the foot patients after the clinic has finished.
10. Write in the patient notes that Dr Walker didn't wash his hands before examining them.

Scenario 3

A medical student, Linh, is working on a project with a small group of other students. The students have to examine real skull bones, which were provided by the medical school's museum, and are very valuable. One of the students in Linh's group accidentally drops the skull and some of the smaller delicate bones shatter.

How appropriate are the following responses by Linh?

11. Ignore what happened, throw the skull remains away, and borrow another group's skull to finish the project.
12. Alert the museum curator about what happened as a group, and write a letter of apology together.
13. Pretend that the skull was stolen.
14. Tell the museum curator in private about who dropped the skull.
15. Tell her supervisor.

Scenario 4

A medical student, Henry, is living in a set of halls with students that study many different subjects. The other students find it funny to joke about Henry's work. Henry is finding it difficult to keep up with his work, and silently takes offense every time the other students joke with him. The night before one of Henry's exams, the other students make a joke that really affects Henry, and he is unable to concentrate on finishing up his revision.

How appropriate are each of the following responses by Henry?

16. Speak to his personal tutor about how he can organise himself and tackle his work in the future.
17. Retaliate by insulting the other students.
18. Do nothing because he doesn't want to offend anyone and is embarrassed about not being able to cope with the workload.
19. Move out of the halls.
20. Speak to his medical student friends about how annoying he finds his flat mates.

Scenario 5

Mark, a medical student, is working with a group of nursing and physiotherapy students to learn about integrated care. Mark is mistaken for a junior doctor, as he is not in uniform, and is asked to test the urine of an elderly patient on the ward using a dipstick. Mark is familiar with the patient, and knows exactly how to do the test. Unfortunately, the doctor that asked him to do the test has left, and there are no other members of staff that are able to do the test for another 5 hours. The results of the test will determine the patient's management.

How appropriate are the following responses by Mark?

21. Get the most senior student in his study group to perform the test and write the results in the patient's notes.
22. Do the test himself and write the results in the patient's notes.
23. Bleep the doctor that is in charge of the patient to alert him about his mistake.
24. Pretend that the doctor never asked him to do the test.
25. Try to find another member of staff that would be capable of performing the test.

Scenario 6

A medical student, Adele, is studying for her first year exams. She has started to panic, and does not feel as though she will be able to complete her revision before the exams start. If Adele fails the exams she would have to resit them in her holidays, which she has come to terms with. She is embarrassed of the possibility of failing, and would rather tell her friends and family that she was ill and unable to take the exams than face the embarrassment of failure. It is against the Medical School rules to opt out of an exam without a medical reason and a Doctor's letter.

How appropriate are the following actions for Adele to take?

26. Fake an illness and postpone her exams.
27. Speak to her parents and her personal tutor about her struggle to get through the revision.
28. Speak to the other medical students to see if they all felt the same way about their work.
29. Refuse to turn up to the exams on the day and pretend that she had food poisoning.
30. Make an efficient revision plan for her remaining days before the exams and attempt to do the exams as best as she can.

Scenario 7

Rohan, a final year medical student, notices that Dijam, one of the medical students on his ward who had been drinking a lot the previous night is on call.

How appropriate are the following actions by Rohan?

31. Advise Dijam to go home.
32. Ignore the situation because Dijam wasn't actually treating any of the patients.
33. Inform the doctors that are on call with Dijam.
34. Joke with Dijam about how he managed to make it into work on time.
35. Inform the Doctor that is in charge of Dijam and Rohan's attachment about Dijam's state.

Scenario 8

Patrick is a medical student, and is working with another group of students on a project that they will receive a joint mark for. Patrick has noticed that there are a couple of loud dominating people in the group, and that the rest of the group are very shy and quiet, and rarely contribute to the conversations. Jina is one particularly loud student that is involved, however she has been making some excellent points and is happy to do a lot of the work.

How appropriate are the following responses by Patrick?

36. Ignore the situation and allow Jina to do the majority of the work.
37. Ask his personal tutor for advice on how he should tackle the situation.
38. Ask the quieter members of the team about what they think of Jina.
39. Subtly hint to everyone to try to contribute more during the sessions so that it is a more even contribution from everyone.
40. Confront Jina and tell her to be less dominating during the sessions.

Scenario 9

Nazia, a medical student, has been working on busy hospital ward. She has been writing up notes from the patient's notes into her notebook so that she can construct a presentation on the case for her study group. No-one is allowed to remove the patient's notes from the hospital. However, she has noticed that one of her friends, Joshua, has a set of patient's notes sticking out of his bag. He has an appointment to get to, and has no time to write the notes up whilst at the hospital. Joshua says that he will return the notes first thing in the morning after he completes the work at home.

How appropriate are the following responses from Nazia?

41. Tell Joshua to do the presentation the next day instead when he has more time.
42. Ignore what he is doing.
43. Tell the ward nurses after Joshua leaves with the notes.
44. Seek advice from your clinical supervisor.
45. Tell Joshua that you will write the notes for him so he doesn't have to take the notes away from the hospital.

Scenario 10

Mr. Marshall has been seeing Dr Kelly regularly for years to check up on his diabetes. Recently, Mr Marshall has been seen by a different specialist doctor, Dr O'Brien. Dr O'Brien runs a test that shows that Mr. Marshall has cancer. He is then booked to see Dr O'Brien the following week who will break the diagnosis. Mr. Marshall is currently in clinic with Dr Kelly and asks her "is everything okay?"

How appropriate are the following responses by Dr Kelly?

46. Tell Mr. Marshall that everything is fine.
47. Reassure Mr. Marshall that Dr O'Brien will be able to answer his question better.
48. Tell Mr. Marshall that she is not allowed to discuss that information with him yet.
49. Look away and say nothing to try to express the seriousness of the situation.
50. Tell Mr. Marshall that he has cancer.

Scenario 11

Mary, a patient, has been in hospital for a long time whilst she recovers from a leg wound, and is desperate to return home. One day, Dr Anil is speaking to her on the ward. He has to leave urgently to answer his bleep call. Mary is left with a junior medical student, Julia. She asks Julia why she is still in the hospital, and wants to know if she can leave that day.

How appropriate are the following responses by Julia?

51. Explain to Mary that she is unable to answer her question, and that the doctor will be back soon.
52. Tell Mary that in most cases people wouldn't be able to leave the hospital at her stage of recovery.
53. Tell Mary that she can self-discharge from hospital if she is very keen to leave, but that it might be against medical opinion.
54. Tell Mary that she will find out and let her know.
55. Answer Mary's questions directly.

Scenario 12

Daniel, a first year medical student, is visiting a hospital for the first time since he started medical school. The doctor supervising them asked Hannah, another student to let the group know that they would be having a hand washing assessment consisting of practical and theoretical aspects. Unfortunately, Daniel was not been about the assessment, and doesn't know how to wash his hands properly.

How appropriate are the following responses by Daniel?

56. Ask to have his turn once a few of his colleagues had been so he can observe.
57. Confront Hannah and ask her why she didn't tell him about the assessment.
58. Tell the doctor that it was Hannah's fault.
59. Ask the group to see how many people were prepared for the assessment.
60. Ask the doctor if he can have his assessment another day so he can learn the skill and the theory properly.

Scenario 13

Helen, a medical student, is waiting for her exam results. She was very worried because she didn't feel as though she was ready for them. When the results come out, she realises that she has to retake her exams. She had booked to go travelling with a friend in South America over the summer holidays, but the resit exams are during the holidays and she is now worried that she will be unable to go, or that if she goes she will not have enough time to revise for the exams. She is also worried that her friend will be left to travel by herself if she doesn't go.

How appropriate are the following responses by Helen in this situation?

61. Call her friend and cancel the holiday.
62. Go travelling but take her revision with her and revise every day.
63. Go for part of the holiday and come home early to revise for the exams.
64. Go travelling and cram in the revision in the few days between coming back and taking the exams.
65. Try to get another friend to replace her so she can stay at home and revise but without leaving her friend to fend for herself.

Scenario 14

Celia, a medical student, is living at home instead of at halls because she doesn't live far away from the medical school. She found it hard to make friends in first year, and wants to move out for her second year or she fears that she will be further isolated from everyone. Unfortunately, that would depend on financial support from her parents. Celia's parents are unable to provide much financial aid, and Celia doesn't have time to take up another job.

How appropriate are the following responses by Celia?

66. Confront her parents and demand the money because they are 'denying her a student experience'.
67. Live at home but join a sports team so she can meet more people and join in with the student lifestyle a little more.
68. Start spending every night at her friend's room in halls.
69. Live at home in resentment and isolate herself from her university friends.
70. Come to an agreement with her parents that if she can move out for a couple of years and then live at home for the rest of medical school.

Scenario 15

Xun, a medical student, is due to hand in an essay the following day at 8AM but is only half way to finishing it at 9PM. The essay will contribute 20% to his final grade and he is beginning to panic.

How appropriate are the following responses by Xun?

71. Stay up late and finish the essay so that he doesn't miss the deadline.
72. Call the head of the assessments and explain his situation to them, in the hope that there will be some leniency.
73. Give up and hand in the essay half-complete.
74. Copy out a similar essay that a friend has written.
75. Fake an illness and ask for an extension.

Scenario 16

Nahor, a medical student, has always enjoyed having creative hairstyles. He is starting his rotations in the hospitals next week, and is worried that he will be unable to express himself through his hair anymore.

How appropriate are the following responses by Nahor in this situation?

76. Cut his hair and get a professional looking colour and style.
77. Start his hospital rotations with his pink long hair, and refuse to change it if he is asked to.
78. Start his hospital rotations with his pink long hair, and only change it if he is asked to.
79. Keep his hair a little quirky but make it look more professional that it has previously been.
80. Request permission from the clinical dean to keep his hair as it is.

Scenario 17

Charles, a medical student, was on call with Dr Patel in a busy hospital. Dr Patel told Charles to wait for the doctor that is going to handover to arrive before he leaves. The doctor isn't due to arrive for another 30 minutes. Charles has a sports match in 15 minutes, and needs to leave before then. Unfortunately Dr Patel is busy with a patient and is not answering his bleep.

How appropriate are the following responses by Charles?

81. Leave and email Dr Patel with a letter of apology.
82. Call up the captain of the sports team to apologise, and promise that you will make the second half of the match.
83. Leave the on call room and try to find Dr Patel to talk to him in person.
84. Leave a message with one of the nurses in the on call room to tell the doctor that is meant to be taking over.
85. Try to call up the doctor that is taking over to explain the situation to him.

Scenario 18

Archie, a medical student, is in clinic with Dr Coombe. Dr Coombe explains to the patient that her medication isn't working and that will have to try something else. Dr Coombe has to take an urgent call and walks out of the room- leaving Archie and the patient in the room. The patient then starts to ask Archie lots of questions about her medication.

How appropriate are the following responses by Archie?

86. Explain that he is unable to say, but that the patient should direct her questions towards Dr Coombe when he returns.
87. Try to answer the questions to the best of his ability.
88. Tell the patient that they should 'Google' the answers.
89. Tell the patient that he will 'Google' the answers.
90. Excuse himself and walk out of the room to leave the patient in there by herself until Dr Coombe returns.

Scenario 19

Matthias, a medical student, has hurt his knee whilst playing hockey. He will need to wear a full leg brace which will prevent him from walking around the hospital. Matthias is concerned that it will affect his studies adversely. He will have to take at least 6 weeks off.

How appropriate are the following responses by Matthias?

91. Write to the medical school and his personal tutor for advice as soon as possible.
92. Try to go to the hospital for 2 days to see if he can cope.
93. Do all of his book work whilst he is unable to walk around the hospital, so that he can focus on clinical training when he's better.
94. Stop going into hospital without letting anyone know.
95. Stop going into hospital and ask his friends to let the medical school know.

Scenario 20

Jessie, a medical student, has a friend called Gemma. Jessie suspects that Gemma has an eating disorder. Gemma was very stressed at medical school, and Jessie is uncertain with how to proceed.

How appropriate are the following responses by Jessie in this situation?

96. Ignore the situation and hope that someone else will notice.
97. Try to talk to Gemma and bring up her eating disorder.
98. Chat to Gemma about her stress and ask if she is coping. Allow her to bring up the disorder on her own account.
99. Speak to Gemma's parents about it, without consulting her.
100. Speak to your personal tutor for advice.

Scenario 21

Helen, a medical student, is has to retake her end of year exams because she failed them the first time. She had booked to go travelling with a friend in South America over the summer holidays, but the resit exams are during this period. She is worried that she will be unable to go and therefore, her friend will be left to travel by herself. If she goes she won't have enough time to revise for the exams.

How appropriate are the following responses by Helen in this situation?

101. Call her friend and cancel the holiday.
102. Go travelling but take her revision with her and revise every day.
103. Go for part of the holiday and come home early to revise for the exams.
104. Go travelling and cram in the revision in the few days between coming back and taking the exams.
105. Transfer her holiday booking to another mutually good friend so she can stay at home and revise but without leaving her friend to fend for herself.

Scenario 22

Daniel and Sean are medical students who are working together on a project. They get into a heated argument in the hospital lobby because Daniel has been prioritising his social life recently which is frustrating Sean.

How important are the following factors for Sean in deciding on what to do?

106. Sean can generally produce better work than Daniel anyway.
107. The mark that they get will be recorded in their log books.
108. Daniel and Sean have to work together for the rest of the year.
109. Daniel has recently broken up with his girlfriend.
110. Sean usually does most of the work when they have to do projects together.

Scenario 23

A medical student Tanya is invited to attend a clinic with Dr Garg who is in charge of Tanya's grade for the whole term. On the morning of the clinic, Tanya realises that she has not finished her essay that is due the next day.

How important are the following factors for Tanya to consider in deciding on what to do?

111. The importance of the essay towards her final mark for the year.
112. Tanya's friend did not find the clinic very educational.
113. Tanya's reputation with Dr Garg.
114. Whether or not Tanya will be able to attend a different clinic with Dr Garg.
115. How long it will take to finish the essay.

Scenario 24

Caroline, a final year medical student, is teaching first year medical students. She notices that they frequently arrive looking untidy and has noticed that some of the doctors have started to comment on how badly dressed the first year students are. She is worried that she will offend the students if she asks them to dress more appropriately, because 2 of the students are on her sports team.

How important are the following factors for Caroline in deciding on what to do?

116. Caroline's reputation with the doctors.
117. The first year students are only in hospital for 2 hours every week.
118. The first year students have direct contact with the patients and the hospital staff.
119. 2 of the students are on her sports team.
120. The first year students don't have their professionalism exams until third year.

Scenario 25

A medical student, Albert, is in his third year and is captain of the hockey team. He has noticed that his hockey training on Wednesday afternoons always clashes with his consultant teaching sessions. The consultant will be responsible for his final grade for the year.

How important are the following factors for Albert in deciding on what to do?

121. His hockey team needs him this year to win the championships.
122. Albert is on a sports scholarship at medical school.
123. His grade will determine if he can progress to his fourth year.
124. The consultant is free on Wednesday mornings.
125. This is the only teaching he will get on this particular topic this year.

Scenario 26

A patient is in a consultation with Dr Davison and Sybil, a medical student is observing. The doctor swears a number of times during the consultation, and Sybil notices that the patient is getting uncomfortable.

How important are the following factors for Sybil in deciding on what to do?

126. Dr Davison is marking one of Sybil's assessments.
127. The patient appears to be uncomfortable with Dr Davison swearing.
128. How often Dr Davison swears during other patient consultations.
129. If other members of staff are aware of Dr Davison's swearing.
130. If the patient has seen Dr Davison before.

Scenario 27

Marco and Alex are medical students on their surgical placement. They are invited to observe surgery with Mr. Daniels and told not to touch the sterile equipment. Before the operation begins, Marco sees Alex accidentally touch the sterile trolley with the operating equipment on it. Alex doesn't tell anyone, and Marco thinks that he should inform someone.

How important are the following factors for Marco in deciding on what to do?

131. The risk to the patient who is about to have the operation.
132. The inconvenience for all of the theatre staff to have to bring out a new sterile trolley.
133. Alex would be embarrassed because he touched something that he wasn't meant to.
134. Alex only briefly touched the trolley.
135. Mr Daniels would be disappointed in Marco and Alex.

Scenario 28

A medical student, Freddie, is on a busy hospital ward. A patient is addicted to pain medication and constantly bullies staff, so that they are reluctant to see her. Freddie has noticed that the doctors and nurses have been attending to her less frequently than before. One day, after she has been reviewed by the doctors and nurses, she starts to verbally abuse Freddie. She demands that he gets her more pain medication.

How important are the following factors for Freddie in determining what he should do?

136. The patient might be in pain.
137. The patient is being avoided by staff.
138. Freddie is not authorised to administer pain medication.
139. The patient may have already had her regular pain medication.
140. The patient has recently been reviewed by the doctors and nurses.

Scenario 29

Jenny is a junior doctor who is training under Mr. Gupta. Her sister, Claire, is due to be operated on by Mr. Gupta to correct a hernia. Claire is nervous about the operation and asks Jenny what she thinks about Mr. Gupta. Jenny knows that Mr. Gupta is a very good surgeon but he is often late when seeing patients on the wards. Therefore, he always appears to be rushing, flustered, and a little sweaty when speaking to them before their operations, which can make them lose confidence in him. Jenny must decide on what to say to her sister Claire.

How <u>important</u> are the following factors for <u>Jenny</u> in deciding on what to do?

141. Mr. Gupta is very competent.
142. The surgeon is often flustered when speaking to patients.
143. Mr. Gupta recently reprimanded Jenny for filling in a drug chart incorrectly.
144. Claire is already quite anxious about having an operation.
145. Patients usually do better if they are confident and at ease before an operation.

Scenario 30

A medical student, Alex, is on the university rugby team. He has been given model answers for various written assessments from older members of the rugby team. His friend, Annabel, realises that the Medical school often repeats their questions, and that it is against the rules to pass down previous papers from year to year.

How <u>important</u> are the following factors for <u>Annabel</u> in deciding on what to do?

146. Alex and Annabel dated for the first year, until he broke up with her.
147. Alex is a hard working student.
148. In this particular year, most of the questions won't be the same as in previous years.
149. Annabel isn't part of a team where information from older members is readily available.
150. The answers are not available to all students.

Scenario 31

Matthew, a medical student, is running late for his teaching session. He missed his bus and the next one doesn't come for another hour. His class was warned yesterday that if they were late for another session without a good reason, then they would not get a good grade for professionalism at the end of the term.

How <u>important</u> are the following factors for <u>Matthew</u> in deciding on what to do?

151. His marks for professionalism are not included in his final grade for the year.
152. Public transport information updates are readily available online.
153. The rest of his class is usually late.
154. Matthew is usually on time for most classes.
155. His teacher will be involved in his studies for the next year.

Scenario 32

Michaela, a medical student, is shadowing doctors on the intensive care unit of a busy hospital. Unfortunately Michaela becomes unwell during the week. She was told on her first day to stay at home if she becomes ill to minimise the risk of spreading infection to the patients. She is reluctant to remain at home because she this is her first and only week on the intensive care unit.

How <u>important</u> are the following factors for <u>Michaela</u> in deciding on what to do?

156. Michaela cannot spend another week on the intensive care unit.
157. Michaela's illness is just a mild cold and is unlikely to cause serious harm.
158. The illness doesn't affect her ability to interact with patients.
159. Michaela was told by the doctors not to come in if she became unwell.
160. Michaela's friend told her that she would learn a lot during her time on the intensive care unit.

Scenario 33

Jenny, a 4th year medical student, has booked and paid to go on the university ski trip. Unfortunately, she finds out that she has the option to sit a set of mock practical exams during the week of the ski trip. Jenny will lose the full amount of money if she pulls out of the ski trip. One of Jenny's friends has their mock exam the day after Jenny gets back. Jenny wants to try and swap their exam dates.

How important are the following factors for Jenny in deciding on what to do?

161. How useful the mock exams will be.
162. The cost of her ski trip.
163. The mock exams are optional.
164. The university's policy on swapping dates of exams.
165. Jenny has performed well on all exams in medical school so far.

Scenario 34

Luke, a medical student, has wanted to do a particular project for months. He has already spoken with the project's supervisor and planned it with him. He has also put it as his top choice for a project, although he knows that of other people also want to do the same project. Later next week, Luke finds out that he has been allocated to his second choice project instead. His friend, Architha, has been allocated the project that he wanted even though it was her last choice. Based, on this, Luke wants to make an official appeal.

How important are the following factors for Luke in deciding whether to appeal?

166. Luke has spoken to the project supervisor.
167. Architha didn't want to have the project.
168. The project grade will count for Luke's final grade at the end of the year.
169. Luke finds it difficult to invest time in a project that he doesn't care about.
170. Luke was allocated his second choice of project.

Scenario 35

Lucinda, a medical student, has been performing very well in her exams so far. She has been in a relationship with Andy (who is also in her year) for 6 weeks. Unfortunately, Andy will need to repeat the year as he has been struggling with the workload. Lucinda is desperate to stay in his year. Andy suggests that she fail her exams on purpose so that she can stay in his year.

How important are the following factors for Lucinda in deciding on what to do?

171. If Lucinda fails her exams the mark will be on her university transcript when she graduates.
172. Jobs as a junior doctor are partially determined based on your grades at medical school.
173. Lucinda and Andy have only been in a relationship for 6 weeks.
174. Lucinda's friends are performing very well and will progress onto the next year.
175. Andy has asked her to fail her exams on purpose.

Scenario 36

Shiv, a medical student, is nearly at the end of his rotation. He really wants to go to Australia for the Christmas holidays to see his girlfriend who is on her elective there. The flights are much cheaper if he skips the final day of his rotation. Most of his medical friends have already finished for the holidays because the doctors that were in charge of them finished their final assessments early. However, Shiv has a very strict doctor who insists that their final assessments will be on the final day of term, and no sooner. The doctor is due to retire after Christmas.

How important are the following factors for Shiv in deciding on what to do?

176. Shiv must pay for his own flights with the money he has saved up.
177. Shiv's final assessment involves the doctor asking him how the term has gone for him, and then signing his log book.
178. Shiv has been punctual and has produced impressive work throughout the rotation.
179. Shiv's doctor will be retiring after Christmas.
180. Shiv's girlfriend is in Australia.

Scenario 37

Jazzmynne, a medical student, is a talented vocalist and is offered the chance to go on a prestigious singing tour for a month with her choir. Unfortunately, this would mean missing a month of classes.

How important are the following factors for Jazzmynne in deciding on what to do?

181. Her choir has never been on an international tour before and this might be Jazzmynne's only chance to go.
182. Jazzmynne would end up missing half of one of her clinical rotations.
183. Jazzmynne's parents get anxious when she misses class.
184. Jazzmynne sometimes struggles to keep up with her workload.
185. Jazzmynne's friends are also going on the tour with her.

Scenario 38

Ellen, a medical student, has been writing for the university newspaper since her first year. She likes to focus on stories that are topical for the students. Recently, the new principal of the medical school has created a ban on stories that involve student bars and social lives. Ellen wants to start a petition to change this rule.

How important are the following factors for Ellen in deciding on what to do?

186. Ellen is in her final year of medical school.
187. The university has a good reputation for responding positively to student petitions.
188. 90% of the university newspaper readers are medical students.
189. The principal wants to encourage more stories about the health press, the world, and academics, rather than gossip at the bars.
190. Ellen doesn't like the new principal very much.

Scenario 39

Guy, a medical student, works at the student bar during the week. The recent change in the university's health and safety policy imposes a maximum number of students that can enter the bar at any time. This means that on popular nights, there is usually an hour-long queue to get into the bar. Guy thinks that this is unfair, and drafts a letter to the university, asking them to expand the student bar.

How important are the following factors for Guy in deciding on what to do?

191. Students are being denied access to their own bars.
192. Guy will get more work and therefore money if the bar expands.
193. The university has dropped in student satisfaction league tables.
194. The bar is very expensive.
195. The university is having financial troubles.

Scenario 40

Olivia, a medical student, wants to run for president of the student union. She has been involved for many years, and is very dedicated to the union. Her friend, Phil, also wants to run for president. Phil is very popular, although he has not contributed as much to the union as Olivia.

How important are the following factors for Olivia in deciding on what to do?

196. Olivia and Phil were previously in a relationship.
197. Phil is in his final year but Olivia is in her penultimate year.
198. Olivia has worked for the student union for a lot longer than Phil has.
199. Neither Phil nor Olivia are happy to run for any other position on the committee.
200. Olivia gave up the presidency of the student union last year because her friend who was in his final year wanted it.

Scenario 41

Annie, a final year medical student, is in the library. She notices George, another final year student, rushing out of the library and accidentally leaving some of his papers by the photocopying machine. She later finds out that they are copies of the upcoming final year exam.

How appropriate are each of the following responses by Annie in this situation?

201. Tell George she found the exam and won't inform anyone else as long as she can have a copy of the exam herself.
202. Copy the exam and distribute it to all the final year medical students so it is fair for everyone.
203. Ignore the situation and do nothing.
204. Alert her supervisor as to what she saw, and get advice on what to do.
205. Alert the medical school as to what she saw.

Scenario 42

Kate is a medical student on a ward round. A patient calls her and complains that a small amount of money has disappeared from her bedside table.

How appropriate are each of the following responses by Kate in this situation?

206. Call the police on the patients behalf, stealing is a criminal offense.
207. Tell the patient that she should have been more careful and you will see what you can do.
208. Tell the patient that she should not be making false accusations.
209. Ask the patient for further details about the theft, reassure her you will see what you can do and alert the nurse in charge of the ward.
210. Send an e-mail out to all other medical students to alert them of the theft.

Scenario 43

During a discussion with a fellow medical student, Andrew, in the student common room, Sam notices that a bag of marijuana falls out of Andrew's bag.

How appropriate are each of the following responses by Sam?

211. Accuse Andrew of drug possession and tell him he will be informing his supervisor.
212. Seek information from Andrew about why he has the marijuana in his bag, and tell him he will ignore the situation if he gets rid of it.
213. Discuss the incident with his own supervisor.
214. Offer support to Andrew and recommend he seek professional help.
215. Pretend he did not see anything and do nothing.

Scenario 44

Anna is a final year medical student attached to a medical team.. One morning, a junior doctor from the team arrives very drunk. The junior doctor is about to start his ward duties.

How appropriate are each of the following responses by Anna?

216. Alert a more senior member of the team to the situation at hand.
217. Do nothing as she is only a medical student.
218. Allow the junior doctor to carry out his ward duties and accompany him to make sure he is not making any mistakes.
219 Reflect on the situation later that evening.
220. Advise the junior doctor to inform the team and go home.

Scenario 45

Sean is a medical student working on a group project with three other students. One of the students, Sarah, is consistently arriving late and is not contributing her fair share of work to the group project.
How appropriate are each of the following responses by Sean?

221. Tell the group's supervisor about Sarah's tardiness and contribution.
222. Discuss the problem with other members of the group.
223. Approach Sarah and tell her that her attitude and poor contribution are causing problems and she needs to pull her weight. .
224. Ask Sarah if there is a reason for her lateness and lack of contribution and if there is anything Sean can do to help.
225. Ignore the situation. The rest of the group is working well and you can work harder to complete the group project.

Scenario 46

Mary is a medical student who is attending a placement on the wards. One day she sees a nurse pick antibiotics out of a drug trolley and place them in her handbag for personal use.
How appropriate are each of the following responses by Mary?

226. Approach the nurse and inform her that this is not best practice.
227. Inform the nurse in charge.
228. Report the matter to the Consultant supervising her.
229. Pretend she did not see anything as the nurse probably needs the antibiotics.
230. Write a reflective piece on the nurse's practice.

Scenario 47

Alan is a medical student who is having a bedside teaching session. During the session the Consultant asks Alan a range of questions, some of which he struggles to answer. At the end of the session Alan feels that the Consultant was rude and has embarrassed him in front of the patient.
How appropriate are each of the following responses by Alan in this situation?

231. Complain about the incident to a senior nurse.
232. Arrange a meeting with the Consultant to discuss the incident.
233. Argue with the Consultant at the bedside so he knows he is being rude.
234. Arrange a meeting with his medical school supervisor to discuss the incident.
235. Once the session is over apologise to the patient about the consultant's behaviour.

Scenario 48

Harry is a medical student doing a placement on a medical ward. One of the nurses comes up to Harry and complains to him about one of his colleagues, Joe's, body odour and is asking if he could have a quiet word with him.
How appropriate are each of the following responses by Harry in this situation?

236. Tell the nurse that this is really an issue for the ward Consultant to deal with and she should go and talk to him,
237. Raise the issue in confidence with Joe.
238. Tell the nurse he will speak to Joe about it, but then ignore the issue. Harry does not want to hurt Joe's feelings.
239. Send an anonymous note to Joe.
240. Raise the issue at a student group meeting with Joe present.

Scenario 49

Helen is a final year medical student. She has written a case report for publication and her Consultant has recently reviewed the final draft. When he gives her the case report back with comments, he has added two names to the list of authors. Helen enquires and the Consultant explains that it is his wife and his Registrar who are currently applying for jobs and need publications on their CVs.

How appropriate are each of the following responses by Helen in this situation?

241. Tell the consultant that she can't publish the case report with the two names added and will only publish it under her name.
242. Agree to add the names as it's only a case report and not a research paper.
243. Discuss the matter with her medical school supervisor.
244. Discuss the matter with the consultant in a private meeting.
245. Choose not to publish the case report at all.

Scenario 50

The medical school library has sent out a notice for a few missing books. John and Clare, both medical students, are studying at her home. Whilst they are studying, John sees a pile of books on her shelf which suspiciously look like the ones from the library.

How appropriate are each of the following responses by John in this situation?

246. Accuse Clare of stealing the books from the library.
247. Ask Clare if these are actually the books from the library and tell her to return them if they are the missing books.
248. Contacting the police, theft is a crime.
249. Inform the medical school library of his suspicions.
250. Discussing the situation with his supervisor.

Scenario 51

Nadia, a fifth year medical student, is currently on a four week rotation on the neonatal wards. She has been assigned to shadow one of the consultants, Anne. During her first week, whenever Nadia approaches Anne, she is told that 'there is not much going on today, why don't you head home early'. This continues for a week and Nadia is starting to feel like she hasn't learnt anything whilst shadowing Anne.

How appropriate are each of the following responses by Nadia in this situation?

251. Speak to Anne about her feelings of being ignored, and find a solution with Anne.
252. Watch and wait- there is still three weeks left to her attachment and things may improve.
253. Discuss the situation with her supervisor.
254. Stop coming to the ward and go to the library instead.
255. Find another doctor on the ward who she can shadow.

Scenario 52

Dean,a third year medical student, is currently on a placement in hospital with a group of three other students. During their placement they have to get their attendance and some clinical skills signed off by doctors. On the last day of their placement, one of the other students, Laura, approaches Dean and asks him to sign off some of her attendance and two of her skills.

How appropriate are each of the following responses by Dean?

256. Reprimand Laura for delaying signing the book until now, refuse to sign the book and give her tips of how to be more organised.
257. Agree to sign the missing boxes for Laura, Dean knows she attended everyday.
258. Suggest she finds one of the junior doctors to sign her book.
259. Ask Laura to demonstrate the skills and then sign them.
260. Report Laura to the medical school.

Scenario 53

Emma is shadowing a junior doctor, Steven, on the wards. He is trying to cannulate a patient and after three failed attempts, he stops and leaves the patient's bedside flustered without an explanation. Emma is still stood by the patient's bedside.

How appropriate are each of the following responses by Emma in this situation?

261. Try to cannulate the patient herself, she was successful in inserting one yesterday.
262. Speak to the nurse in charge about Steven.
263. Excuse herself from the patient's bedside and go and find Steven.
264. Speak to Steven's consultant.
265. Complain about Steven to the patient.

Scenario 54

Jill is a medical student. She is shadowing a registrar in surgery, who is currently clerking a patient who needs an operation. The registrar leaves Jill with the patient and goes to get the operation consent forms. While he is away the patient makes a racist comment about the registrar.

How appropriate are each of the following responses by Jill in this situation?

266. She should retaliate and call the patient a racist idiot.
267. Pretend she didn't hear the patient's comment.
268. Politely tell the patient that this language is not tolerated in the hospital.
269. Discuss the matter with the consultant in charge.
270. Report the matter to the registrar.

Scenario 55

John is a first year medical student, he is working with four other medical students on a group project. Hannah, one of the other students, is dominating the group discussions and is doing a large amount of the work.

How appropriate are each of the following responses by John in this situation?

271. Discuss the issue with the other members of the group.
272. Speak to Hannah and tell her she is not allowing others to contribute ,and if she doesn't change she has to leave the group.
273. Allow Hannah to continue to dominate the group discussions and to do the majority of the work.
274. Speak to his supervisor.
275. Speak to Hannah and tell her it would be good if all members of the group contributed equally to the project.

Scenario 56

Jenny, a medical student, hears that one of her colleagues has recently lost their grandmother. They are both at hospital on their rotation, when her colleague bursts into tears.

How appropriate are each of the following responses by Jenny in this situation?

276. Advise her colleague to go home for the day.
277. Offer her colleague support.
278. Discuss this with her supervisor.
279. Tell her colleague it is inappropriate to cry on the wards and to stop.
280. Give her colleague some time alone.

Scenario 57

Maya, a sixth year medical student, is out with a group of her friends from medical school. They are all out at a restaurant for an evening meal. The students start discussing some of the interesting patients they had seen over the last few weeks. Some of the patients' names are being mentioned in the conversation, and other diners could certainly overhear.

How appropriate are each of the following responses by Maya in this situation?

281. Maya should join in the conversation and speak about a particularly interesting patient she had seen.
282. Maya should warn her friends that they are in a public place and should not be talking about patients using their names.
283. Maya should try to change the subject of the conversation.
284. Maya should report her friends to the medical school
285. Excuse herself from the table and leave.

Scenario 58

Michael is a medical student; one of his colleagues Simon confides in him that he is suffering from depression and feels it is affecting their work. He asks Michael not to tell anyone.

How appropriate are each of the following responses by Michael in this situation?

286. Speak to his own supervisor without telling Simon.
287. Advise Simon to speak to his supervisor.
288. Mock him and tell him he should get over it.
289. Tell other students in the medical school so they can offer some support.
290. Offer any help he can, and advise him to see his GP or a counselor.

Scenario 59

Mark is a medical student, he walk into the doctor's mess and sees one of the doctors watching adult pornography on one of the hospital computers.

How appropriate are each of the following responses by Mark in this situation?

291. Pretend he didn't see anything and leave the doctor's mess immediately.
292. Speak to his supervisor.
293. Confront the doctor about the issue.
294. Spread the news in the hospital that there was a doctor watching pornography during working hours.
295. Contact the hospital IT services.

Scenario 60

Alice has arranged to go out for dinner with her boyfriend tonight. Just before leaving medical school she receives an e-mail which informs her that tomorrow morning's seminar has been moved to this evening and starts in the next 30 minutes.

How appropriate are each of the following responses by Alice in this situation?

296. Tell another student to apologise to the seminar leader for her absence.
297. Leave as planned, and hope her absence goes unnoticed.
298. Find out what the seminar is about and speak to the seminar leader and explain that she had prior arrangements.
299. Call her boyfriend and tell him that the dinner needs to be cancelled, as she must attend an important teaching session.
300. Write a rude email to the seminar leader complaining about the short notice.

ANSWERS

Verbal Reasoning Answers

Q	A	Q	A	Q	A	Q	A	Q	A
1	False	51	False	101	False	151	B	201	D
2	False	52	False	102	True	152	A	202	D
3	True	53	True	103	False	153	A	203	C
4	Can't tell	54	True	104	False	154	C	204	B
5	Can't tell	55	Can't tell	105	False	155	C	205	A
6	False	56	False	106	Can't tell	156	B	206	A
7	False	57	True	107	B	157	A	207	C
8	Can't tell	58	False	108	C	158	D	208	A
9	Can't tell	59	False	109	B	159	B	209	C
10	True	60	True	110	B	160	A	210	A
11	False	61	False	111	D	161	C	211	A
12	False	62	Can't tell	112	C	162	C	212	C
13	Can't tell	63	False	113	B	163	B	213	A
14	False	64	True	114	D	164	B	214	C
15	Can't tell	65	False	115	C	165	A	215	D
16	False	66	False	116	D	166	D	216	B
17	Can't tell	67	False	117	A	167	A	217	B
18	True	68	False	118	C	168	C	218	A
19	Can't tell	69	Can't tell	119	C	169	D	219	A
20	True	70	True	120	A	170	C	220	C
21	Can't tell	71	False	121	C	171	C	221	True
22	Can't tell	72	False	122	C	172	A	222	D
23	True	73	False	123	D	173	B	223	C
24	False	74	False	124	B	174	A	224	C
25	True	75	False	125	A	175	A	225	B
26	False	76	False	126	D	176	C	226	C
27	True	77	False	127	B	177	B	227	D
28	False	78	True	128	C	178	C	228	A
29	Can't tell	79	False	129	C	179	B	229	C
30	False	80	False	130	D	180	D	230	D
31	Can't tell	81	Can't tell	131	C	181	C	231	C
32	False	82	Can't tell	132	D	182	C	232	A
33	False	83	Can't tell	133	B	183	B	233	B
34	False	84	Can't tell	134	C	184	A	234	D
35	False	85	False	135	C	185	B	235	C
36	False	86	True	136	C	186	C	236	False
37	Can't tell	87	Can't tell	137	B	187	A	237	C
38	Can't tell	88	True	138	B	188	C	238	A
39	False	89	False	139	D	189	D	239	C
40	True	90	Can't tell	140	A	190	A	240	A
41	True	91	False	141	B	191	A	241	True
42	Can't tell	92	False	142	C	192	C	242	False
43	False	93	False	143	C	193	D	243	Can't tell
44	False	94	False	144	C	194	A	244	Can't tell
45	True	95	True	145	C	195	C	245	False
46	Can't tell	96	Can't tell	146	C	196	A	246	False
47	False	97	True	147	A	197	B	247	Can't tell
48	True	98	True	148	C	198	C	248	Can't tell
49	True	99	False	149	C	199	C	249	True
50	Can't tell	100	True	150	B	200	B	250	True

Set 1:

1. **False** -In paragraph 2, the passage says that only the countries that signed the protocol were legally bound.
2. False -In 2004, the condition that over 55% of emissions were accounted for was met without Australia and the US.
3. **True** -in paragraph 2: 'each country that signed the protocol agreed to reduce their emissions to their own specific target'.
4. **Can't tell** -We know this is when the Kyoto Protocol was enforced but there is no information to suggest whether emissions actually decreased.
5. **Can't tell** -Paragraph 4 says that a 60% emission reduction would have a 'significant impact', but we cannot tell if the remaining effects would be harmful or not. The passage is also talking about a global reduction of 60% - there is no mention of each individual country needing reduce their emissions by 60%.

Set 2:

6. **False** -From paragraph 1, we can see that the Soviets were mainly concerned with showing off their economic power and technological superiority.
7. **False** -Paragraph 3 says that Project Apollo was tasked with landing the first man on the moon.
8. **Can't tell** -The passage does not tell us why the Soviets did not land a man on the moon.
9. **Can't tell** -We do not know the state of the American space efforts prior to the launch of Sputnik – we just know that its launch 'prompted urgency'.
10. **True** -The Soviets had just sent Yuri Gagarin into space and it wasn't expected that the US would beat the Soviets in landing a man on the moon; therefore the US was behind the Soviets at this stage.

Set 3:

11. **False**- Paragraph 1 says Pheidippides was the fastest runner
12. **False**-Paragraph 2 says that they were standardised from 1921 but using the 1908 distance
13. **Can't tell**-Paragraph 1 says the Greeks were not expecting to beat the Persians, but we do not know if the Persians were expecting to beat the Greeks, despite their larger army
14. **False**- Paragraph 2: to be an IAAF marathon the distance must be 26.2 miles. The original route was 25 miles
15. **Can't tell** -We know that the Persian soldiers outnumbered the Greeks and had superior cavalry, but we are not told about their training

Set 4:

16. **False**- From paragraph 1, we can see that birds would not survive if they did not migrate
17. **Can't tell**-Whilst there is only mention here of migrating in flocks, nowhere does it specifically state that either all migrating birds do so or that any migrating birds do not
18. **True**- Although the leading bird does not benefit at the time, they continually change position within the flock according to paragraph 3
19. **Can't tell** -Paragraph 3 shows that the Northern bald ibis does not behave in this way so it is not known what would happen
20. **True** -Paragraph 1 states they migrate north in the spring, and south in the winter

Set 5:

21. **Can't tell** -We know the amount of wild flowers has decreased by this amount but we can't tell if the bee population fell by a proportional amount. The 50% reduction mentioned in Paragraph 1 only refers to honey bees
22. **Can't tell**-Whilst the UK have experienced a significantly greater decline than the European average, there is no data from the rest of the world.
23. True -Paragraph 2 tells us modern techniques produce more food.
24. **False** -As well as pollination, bees are also involved in complex food chains and cannot be replaced
25. **True** -From paragraph 1 we see that pesticides are one of the causes of bee population decline. Therefore, reducing pesticide usage would reduce this rate of decline.

Set 6:

26. **False** -This would affect the thinking distance, not the braking distance.
27. **True** -From paragraph 2 we see that the increased traction of winter tyres is because the softness of their material allows better traction.
28. **False**- From paragraph 4, we are told it is not safe to run the engine when the exhaust pipe is blocked because of the risk of carbon monoxide production.
29. **Can't tell**-There is not sufficient information in the passage to suggest whether the softer tyres are dangerous to use in hot conditions.
30. **False**- Paragraph 3 says it is safer to steer out of the way than to brake.

Set 7:

31. **Can't tell** -In Paragraph 1, we are told the method is named after Socrates, but we are not told whether he was the first person to use it or whether he simply adapted and/or popularised the Socratic method.
32. **False** -The Socratic method challenges the statements and opinions that a person makes, not their wisdom.
33. False -Although Socrates was trialled with these charges, the Socratic method as described was not the cause.
34. **False** -We can see from the final paragraph that he chose to die defending knowledge and wisdom, rather than fleeing in fear.

35. **False** -From paragraph 2 we see that Socrates did not provide answers to these difficult questions.

Set 8:
36. **False** -Paragraph 1 says the dialects of the Saxon, Angle and Jute tribes formed the Anglo-Saxon language.
37. **Can't tell**-Paragraph 2 says English speakers would struggle to understand Old English, but we do not know about German speakers.
38. **Can't tell**-The story of Beowulf only mentions that he kills Grendel and his mother, not about his strength compared to other warriors.
39. **False**-The Friesian dialect is similar to Old English but they are not the same.
40. **True** -The Celtic Britons were originally living in England before being forced into Wales.

Set 9:
41. **True**-Paragraph 1 says that stars in the constellation Cassiopeia are visible only in the northern hemisphere; therefore they are not visible in the southern hemisphere.
42. **Can't tell** -The passage does not tell us if Cassiopeia rises and falls in the sky or not.
43. **False**-Paragraph 3 says the star sign represents the position of the sun, not the visible constellations.
44. **False** -Paragraph 2 says Polaris is used for navigation as its position is constant in the sky.
45. **True**-Paragraph 1 mentions different constellations being visible from different places on the Earth.

Set 10:
46. **Can't tell**-The passage tells us about maple tree sap but we don't know about other trees.
47. **False** -He was angered because of the laziness of the village people.
48. **True** -Paragraph 1 says that the process is similar although different equipment is used.
49. **True**-Paragraph 1 says the sap is only harvested during March.
50. **Can't tell** -Although the laziness associated with drinking maple syrup suggests hunting is harder than syrup drinking, the people may just have not hunted because they did not need to – not because it was harder.

Set 11:
51. **False**-Paragraph 1 says Stockholm syndrome happens sometimes, not always.
52. **False** -The passage suggests that the hugging and kissing occurred due to the positive relationship formed between the captors and hostages.
53. **True** -Paragraph 4 says the FBI is willing to devote resources to understanding Stockholm syndrome in order to aid crisis negotiation.
54. **True**-The explanation given in paragraph 3 suggests that the hostages fearing for their life is a step in the development of Stockholm syndrome.
55. **Can't tell** -Although this incident is the origin of the name 'Stockholm syndrome', it is not mentioned whether this phenomenon has happened before

Set 12:
56. **False**-It is this mucous layer that offers protection from the anemone tentacles
57. **True**- Paragraph 2 mentions that the bright colour of the clownfish lures in fish which the anemone eventually stings and eats.
58. **False**-Paragraph 3 mentions that anemones increase the lifespan of clownfish but are not essential for clownfish to live.
59. **False**- Paragraphs 1 and 3 mention that only certain anemone form this mutually beneficial relationship.
60. **True** -Paragraph 2 says the anemone sting protects the clownfish from predators.

Set 13:
61. **False**-Paragraph 2 indicates he was opposed to the death penalty.
62. **Can't tell**-The passage only tells us that the guillotine was commonly used during the French Revolution, it doesn't tell us what was used for execution before the French Revolution.
63. **False** -Although it can cause death by asphyxiation, the common cause of death is snapping of the neck.
64. **True**- This was Joseph Guillotin's explanation.
65. **False** -Paragraph 1 tells us the guillotine was the common form of execution as it was the only legal method of execution.

Set 14:
66. **False** -The Gherkin is famous for its distinctive shape, and although this forms part of a cooling system it is not famous for that reason.
67. **False** -The City of London governing body wanted redevelopment to restore the old historic look – implying the Baltic Exchange had this look before the bombing.
68. **False** -The Gherkin was bought for £630m and sold for £700m, so a profit was made on the sale.
69. **Can't tell** -We are told the building is damaged by bombs, but we are not told what the intention of the attack was.
70. **True**- It is stated in paragraph 1 that Norman Foster is famous for this.

Set 15:
71. **False** -The passage tells us London is significantly more expensive.
72. **False** -There are no legal implications for paying below the living wage as it is the minimum wage that is legally binding.
73. **False**-This individual would be earning less than the living wage and so would not be able to live comfortably according to the definition in paragraph 1.

74. **False** -Some employees will be fired and others would have to work harder; some employees may already be earning more than the living wage and so would not benefit.
75. **False** -The family of that individual will also benefit from the living wage, as well as the company they work for.

Set 16:
76. **False** -Although a country with more people will likely have a greater ecological footprint, it is through their increased usage of resources, not a direct consequence of the population. There can be significant discrepancies.
77. **False**- This is the bio-productive capacity of the Earth, not the total space available.
78. **True** -The final paragraph mentions that reducing use of unsustainable resources will reduce the ecological footprint.
79. **False** -The final paragraph says that a global effort is needed.
80. **False** -The final paragraph says that we can increase the bio-productive space available.

Set 17:
81. **Can't tell** -Paragraph one states that some believe them to be 'one of the most important', which does not necessarily mean they are the most influential.
82. **Can't tell** -The passage states it started the UK punk movement, but this does not necessarily mean it began the global movement.
83. **Can't tell** -The passage states that there were lyrics written about abortion, but they do not state the moral stance these lyrics took.
84. **Can't tell** -The passage tells us that some songs attacked the music industry and that controversial topics such as the Holocaust were commented on, however we do not know if these two topics were said to be related.
85. **False** -They attacked 'blindly accepting royalty as an authority', and so attacked a royalist standpoint.
86. **True** -Not at the same time, but The Sex Pistols had two individual bassists over the course of their existence.

Set 18:
87. **Can't tell** -The passage doesn't mention what proportion of people exposed to asbestos will get mesothelioma.
88. **True** -As breast cancer is the most common cancer in the UK and very rare in men, it must be very common in women.
89. **False** -The success rates of tumour removal procedures were improved by surgical hygiene.
90. **Can't tell** -The passage doesn't mention the relative success rates between the two methods.
91. **False** -Some tumours are able to metastasise, meaning that there are also tumours that do not.

Set 19:
92. **False** -The land was claimed because the British people did not believe that anybody actually owned the land.
93. **False** -Not all of the 517,000 Aborigines are living in cities and towns.
94. **False**-They were only able to reclaim the land that they could prove they originally owned.
95. **True** -Only a few Aborigines lack the education to integrate with modern Australian life.
96. **Can't tell** -We do not know what the south-east Asian lifestyle involved.

Set 20:
97. **True** -It was discovered that chilli peppers had similar taste to black peppercorn and so became valuable around the world.
98. **True** -Paragraph 2 says that spicy food allows people to sweat.
99. **False** -Paragraph 1 says 'most' peppers are spicy, but not all.
100. **True**-The capsaicin receptor is responsible for the pain associated with spicy chillies.
101. **False** -The description of labelled line coding says these different methods of activating this receptor will cause the same sensation.

Set 21:
102. **True**- Dropping out of school will affect the level of education, which is a social determinant of health.
103. **False** -They can also be measured by the quality of life.
104. **False** -Although this would prevent the described mechanism from happening, many other mechanisms are acting at the same time. This was just one example of many possible mechanisms.
105. **False** -The final paragraph says we are reducing the gap between those more privileged and those who are more disadvantaged.
106. **Can't tell** -The life expectancy described in paragraph 2 is an average and so can't reliably be used in specific examples.

Set 22:
107. **B**- The passage suggests that the critics suppose 'human beings to be capable of no pleasures except those of which swine are capable', and so suggest the potential of higher pleasures. They do not call their critics degraded, but suggest that the critics degrade human nature, nor do they accuse critics of being either miserable or indulgent.
108. **C**- This action does not see happiness as its justification, but conforming to social norms. It does not seek to increase pleasure or reduce pain, just follow dogma, which is not according to the principle of utility.
109. **B**- Mill does not describe the religious views of his critics, or explicitly call them reactionary, and in fact describes them 'some of the most estimable in feeling and purpose'. He does mention the countries of origin for some of his critics, and they are all in Europe.
110. **B**- The passage also states 'desirable things' could be 'means' to pleasure.

111. **D**-Utility is defined as the foundation of the system, and a belief that the increasing of happiness/decreasing of happiness is good. The passage specifically states that it has not given an exhaustive definition of things that are pleasurable/painful, and it does not specifically define Epicureans, simply suggests a link between them and utilitarian's - which is not an exhaustive explanation of the term.

Set 23:

112. **C**-Though sandstone is made from sand, the passage does not state that ALL rocks are made from this material.
113. **B**-The passage discusses the valley when implementing the wall-building analogy.
114. **D**- 'Some ancient source' is all we are told, and so the source is undisclosed (Paragraph 3).
115. **C**- This rock is said in paragraph 2 to be found 'everywhere', so not 'nowhere'.
116. **D**- Paragraph 3: The grains are said to be sorted in groups 'of a size', i.e. measurements. They are all described as 'worn and rounded', and no mention is made of differentiation through age/shape.

Set 24:

117. **A**- Though the flowers smell pleasant, no mention is made of this scent being used to manufacture perfumes.
118. **C**- The passage states that the flower could bloom more than once a century, precluding 'D', but that it is thought to only do so in a century, providing evidence for 'C'.
119. **C**- The statement claims that Narcissus plants are 'prized by many' over Lilies, but this does not mean that all people - or even the majority of people - think the former is more attractive/better than the latter, or that all homeowners enjoy the plant.
120. **A**- It is actually a substance 'very similar to rum', not rum itself.
121. **C**- The genus 'belongs' to the family, as stated in paragraph 1.

Set 25:

122. **C**-Women in Illinois, not across USA, were subject to the law, and the passage does not state either a change in fashion or actual arrests, only the potential for arrests.
123. **D**- The pulling out of feathers from live birds was seen as the negative to using osprey feathers.
124. **B**- They could be possessed only 'in their proper season'.
125. **A**- The problem cited is that the article was already in use in the clothing of numerous military men. The authority of the princess/sexist politics does not feature in the passage, and 'D' is patently false
126. **D**- None of those are precluded, as only 'harmless' and 'dead' birds (in their entirety) were prohibited. Wearing a living bird was not explicitly banned.

Set 26:

127. **B**- Nothing in the above passage provides evidence for 'C', 'D' or 'A' - in fact, the 'indie' description of Pope opposes the idea of him working for a games company at all. 'B' is supported by the fact the game is available on a number of devices and system operators.
128. **C**- The immigration officer's job is to process people correctly - not to grow or limit the number of immigrants, as in 'A' and 'B'. 'D' is vague, as 'to stamp passports' does not necessarily mean to stamp them correctly, and false stamps would be counter to the purpose of the border guard's position.
129. **C**- Though the game player may perform either a body scan or finger print check when something is amiss is the candidate's documents, they will not necessarily do either of these - first, they will 'enquire', which is synonymous with 'C', 'asking…for further information'. The only one of the statements that will be universally true for discrepancies therefore is c.
130. **D**- The game-player may accept 'bribes', so 'A' is not true. The game player 'may' arrest candidates, but the passage does not state he or she must, so 'B' is false. The game-player is allowed two mistakes, so to an extent, can be forgiven - making 'C' incorrect. As further mistakes will lead to being 'pecuniarily punished', 'D' is the only accurate statement.

Set 27:

131. **C**- The head of LA NAACP is a civil rights' activist.
132. **D**- The other aspects may appear in films, but only racial slurs were cited as a 'common' element without specifying location of setting of sub-type.
133. **B**- 'Primarily' means the same as 'predominately' in this case, and the cast has been described as 'predominately' black - meaning most, but not all, cast members are black.
134. **C**- Original intended audiences were black city-dwellers: 'B' is too broad and 'A' is too narrow. 'D' is not at all supported in the passage. 'C' describes the growing audience, and how the genre is now 'not exclusive to any race' (Paragraph 2)
135. **C**- It is possible, but nothing in the statement suggests the potentially racy titles are a nod towards sexploitation genre. The innuendo may be incidental, or the choice of words completely divorced from the pornographic films of the past.

Set 28:

136. **C**- It would be a massive assumption to state that just because two characters in a book are 'vicious', all of them will be, so 'A' is not necessarily correct. 'B' also believes in a despair that is described to belong to the Comedian, but not Rorscach. The argument of the passage is that 'D', which Moore may believe, is not the case - the beloved character is not simply worshipped for his violence, but for his belief in justice. 'C' is correct, as Moore describes how he wished Rorschach not to be a favourite character, but a warning.
137. **B**- False. The fact he finds things a 'joke' is what makes him the Comedian. He may not be all that funny, but the joke is still there.

138. **B**- He does not mention madness ('D'), or invoke shame ('C'), or simply state it is good to be good ('A') - specifically, he states we must act as if the world is 'just', even when not, to attain dignity.
139. **D**- No value judgment is made comparing violent actions or on the Comedian's jokes so 'A' and 'B' are false. The passage also acknowledge Rorschach's violence, showing 'C' is wrong, but does state that his actions are due to the fact he believes he is acting in the name of justice, which lends him an ethical justification to his actions.
140. **A**- The lack of meaning in anything is what leads him to treat everything as a joke - it is not hatred, but the inability to see 'purpose' in himself or his fellow man.

Set 29:

141. **B**- The passage's explanation of The Bechdel Test does not state that the test is used to show 'sexism', so a failed film does not equate to a sexist one.
142. **C**- This is the only film that shows a female-female conversation not on a man. 'A' and 'B' only feature conversations focused on males and 'D' does not have two women speaking to one another.
143. **C**- Though of the two horror films mentioned in the extract one passes it and another one fails, the passage does not make use this to make any claims on the genre as a whole.
144. **C**- Her comment that it is 'strict' shows she has a reservation, but her general agreeing that it is a 'good idea' shows she approves of the notion. Her statement is too qualified to be described by 'A', too positive to be understood by 'B', and contains a judgement precluding 'C' as a correct statement.
145. **C**- The two women are not named within the comic strip - though two women are behind the idea (one in suggesting it, the other in illustrating it), that is not to say that the two depicted women are the same.

Set 30:

146. **C**- The possible 'idea' that repetition is funny is inherently funny is mentioned, but neither confirmed nor denied.
147. **A**- This is the only statement actually mentioned above. Laughing twice at the same joke does not make it 'twice as funny', that is a logical fallacy; it does not state that all relationships dictate that the two parties find themselves funny (this is too vague) and being 'comfortable' is not cited as encouraging laughter.
148. **C**- There is no mention of a humour requirement for the first joke.
149. **C**- Though the call-back here is described as a comic trope, this does not necessarily preclude the same device being used in something un-comic: in the same way word-play or alliteration can be used to achieve a multitude effects, not all humorous.
150. **B**- Though 'A' is a potential, it is not a requirement of the call back, and 'C' is not supported through the passage's material. At no point is the call-back named significant, compared to other tropes: it is simply one that the passage focuses on. It does however state that it can be used by a comedian, and used for comedy, so 'B' is correct.

Set 31:

151. **B**- She was the fourth, after Catherine, Mary and her namesake Harriet Elizabeth, who died as an infant.
152. **A**- He was a 'Rev', a reverend, and a 'divine'. She was born in the USA, not UK, and in the 19th century. Her town is said to be 'characteristic', and so not 'average'.
153. **A**- She is said to have 'veneration' in all who knew her.
154. **C**- It is only described as the 'most sad' and 'most tender' memory of her childhood, not her life. It is, however, described as 'the first memorable incident' and thus the earliest one of her life.
155. **C**- She wrote her Charles, so at least wrote one letter. The autobiography mentioned belonged to her brother, not her, and she had five brothers and sisters waiting for her when she was born, not only brothers. She was actually four when her mother died, as the narrator tells us, and her remembering being between 'three and four' is a false memory.

Set 32:

156. **B**- He thought it was 'a pity that only rich people could own books', and from this he 'finally determined to contrive' of a new way of printing. The passage does not state that he wished to make money, found books too expensive to get a hold of or was impatient himself when it came to the production of books.
157. **A**- The need to be careful is mentioned, as is the fact that the process takes a long time both in creating the block and due to the fact one block can only print one page. That it may tire a carver to make the block is possible, but it is not cited in the passage.
158. **D**- The statement says it is 'very likely' he was taught to read, but is not definite. That his father comes from a 'good family' does not mean he is a member of the aristocracy, necessarily. Though block printing was used as the boy grew up, it does not state this was the most popular process. The mention of Gutenberg's family's 'wealthy friends' indicates they were sociable.
159. **B**- The paper was laid on top of the block, not underneath.
160. **A**- There is nothing written in the passage praising the craftsmanship of manuscripts. The appropriateness of the titles for both book production processes is explained, and the 'wealthy friends' are described as a source to borrow books from, thus a way of expanding your reading.

Set 33:

161. **C**- In both examples given above, Apollo is the giver - but these are only two of 'several' versions, and it is possible others exist.
162. **C**- The gift of prophecy is supernatural, therefore this is the best answer. There is no evidence to suggest that she knew chastity would lead to her tragic fate, that she is 'often' seen as a home wrecker (though she is killed by Clytemnestra, this does not prove Cassandra, the slave, is perceived as a vindictive 'other woman') or that parents use the name to express hate – they may just like the sound, and not care about its history, or not know the history at all.

163. **B-** Nothing is said about the state of Cassandra's childhood, but it is mentioned that plays are written about her and that Homer has written about her, showing 'C' and 'D' are true. The fact her father was a king proves she was from a royal line.
164. **B-** The passage states the 'presentation of her character alters'.
165. **A-** It is not said that she ignores or refuses to accept the gift, or demands more presents, even in the first story, just that she refuses to sleep with him. Only the broken promise, as described in the second version of the myth, is mentioned above.

Set 34:

166. **D-** The passage attacks a generalisation, and shows an example that refutes one given to the 'musical' genre. Nothing is mentioned of Sondheim's talents, or what his role was in creating the musical, nor are their claims made to Wheeler's literary tastes (he may just like ONE penny dreadful). This musical may deal with morbid themes, but that's not to say that most do - it could be only a select few that do.
167. **A-** The pies make the crimes 'culinary' in nature, the mention of revenge shows Todd's illegal acts to be 'vengeful' and the judge's rape is a 'sexual' crime. There is nothing explicitly suggesting the crimes of any party are funny, or to be considered funny.
168. **C-** Though the original title 'A String of Pearls: A Romance' may appear to suggest a romantic relationship within the narrative, nothing in the passage states the two are a couple.
169. **D-** Is essentially synonymous is the quoted belief, 'we all deserve to die', which include both bad and good people and makes no significant reference to gender exclusion/inclusion.
170. C- There are four mentioned themes, but that does not mean there are only four themes, nor does 'legal corruption' get named as the central theme. As the entirety of Sweeney Todd is not discussed in the passage, only a central plot line, one could not exclude the potential of something positive happening in the play - even a minor incident. The themes mentioned are, however, indeed macabre.

Set 35:

171. **C-** The above passage is about WWII trains, not WWI ones.
172. **A-** The soldier makes a chair by using a tipped-up suitcase. It is a marine, not a sailor, learning on the back of a chair, and the passage states 'some', not 'many' queue for two hours to go to the diner car, whilst similarly 'some' (not necessarily 'many') go hungry.
173. **B-** The passage discourages mothers from going on trains with a baby, stating they should only do it as a necessity.
174. **A-** 'At every stop' more people come on the train.
175. **A-** The passage does not insult anyone, but it does say the railroads are doing their job 'well'.

Set 36:

176. **C** The passage states the slice of bread is an ounce, and contains 3/4 ounce of flour, making it 75% flour.
177. **B-** It says it is possible that they do, but also possible that they don't. There is no emphatic claim.
178. **C-** It is over a million loaves a day, 319 million pounds - not bushels - a year and 365,000 loaves - not over - a year.
179. **B-** False. It may seem unimportant, but the passage goes on to explain how a single slice of bread has value.
180. **D-** The government have researched waste, but not taken responsibility for it, nor is it said they should do more to combat this. The final sentence confirms that housekeepers are responsible for their own food wastage.

Set 37:

181. **C-** Fourteen women and three men are described to be arrested.
182. **C-** She was the only woman, but it does not state whether either man was brought to trial.
183. **B-** The majority ultimately rule, but Hall 'dissented', or disagreed, with the other two originally.
184. **A-** It is said that it was proved upon trial that she was informed of a right to vote and had no doubt over her entitlement at the time of voting.
185. **B-** They were charged independently.

Set 38:

186. **C-** Nowhere does it state that all European countries have similar creatures (though certain types can be found in both British Isles and Norway) nor does it state the array of animals is limited to this one nation. Sharing animals and birds does not necessitate sharing geographical features, but it is said a country with forest and moorlands is likely to have a variety of birds and animals, so one can see the link between forests and creatures.
187. **A-** There was a time when the English dreaded wolves and bears, but that indicates the past, or at least does not include the present. Norwegians being superior is not suggested here.
188. **C-** Bears are called destroyers, which is sufficient to conclude they cause damage.
189. **D-** They are ruthlessly hunted by farmers in country districts, but numerous only in the forest tracts in the Far North.
190. **A-** The word fortunately implies that it is good the wolves are no longer central. The children are under no threat, as the threat of wolves belongs to a bygone time, there is no mention of regret that such a time is gone and Norsemen are not demonstrated in the above passage to have respect for Nature, but instead they are said to interfere with it through hunting and driving wolves farther afield from their current homes.

Set 39:

191. **A-** They were seen as the 'friendly or hostile manifestation of some higher powers, demonical and Divine.' The 'manifestation' of the 'Divine' could be interpreted as a religious quality.
192. **C-** A small minority believe that dreams are not the dreamer's own psychical act, meaning the majority believe that they are.

193. **D-** There is incongruity between feelings and images, suggesting a lack of a logical link between the two. Waking thoughts are said to find some dreams repugnant, and though dreams are described as forgotten, that is not necessarily due to them being dull.
194. **A-** It asks can sense be made of each single dream.
195. **C-** A link between the psychical sleeping and waking self is suggested, but not definitively proved. Pre-scientific communities, according to the passage, had a hypothesis that left them with 'no uncertainty'. The 'origin of the dream' remains a question in Freud's writing that has been left without a satisfactory answer. That 'our reminiscences' may 'mutilate' a dream is mentioned, leaving 'C' the only statement with support from the passage.

Set 40:
196. **A-**"Most" requires over half by definition, and "most" of the people living in this area were the descendants of immigrants who moved to the country a "full century ago".
197. **B-** Hall only makes a claim for New England, not the entirety of America, being the descendants of 20,000 immigrants. The 'one million' figure comes from Franklin, not Hall. Less than 80,000 ("under" 80,000) people led to the population boom of one million. One million is over ten times (under) 80,000, so "b" is correct.
198. **C-** It is said to be "distinct" to older aristocracy "of the royal governor's courts". It is not similar to any European aristocracy. There is no specific reference to it not being a system based on lineage.
199. **C-** It says that these were the texts read by the most people, but that does not mean they were the most plentiful – other books may have outnumbered the bibles, even if they received fewer readers.
200. **B-** "A", "c" and "d" are cited in the passage (the journey took 'the better part of the year', it was 'hazardous' and 'expensive'), whereas 'B' is not referenced at all.

Set 41:
201. **D** – Paragraph 2 states that the "main thing" which must be considered when assessing Russia's role is the sapping of the German, Austro-Hungarian and Turkish resources.
202. **5** – America, Italy, Romania and Britain are mentioned at the end of paragraph 1, and France in paragraph 3.
203. **C** – Russia certainly had a greater role when compared to America, Italy, Romania & Britain (paragraph 1). However, there are no details of France's efforts throughout the war.
204. **B** – A & C contributed, but the final catastrophe of the Central Powers was the direct consequence of the offensive of the Allies in 1918 (paragraph 2). Thus, as this was the final catastrophe, this can be concluded to be what won the war.
205. **A** – The final paragraph states that both Russia's and France's efforts were required to stop Germany from the winning the war, which they came very close to.

Set 42:
206. **A** – At the end of paragraph 4, the passage says 'Journalists did some of their finest work and made me proud to be one of them'.
207. **C** – Paragraph 3 states magazines offered perspective, rather than necessarily the facts.
208. **A** – Paragraph 4 states that the internet was responsible for allowing the former audience to write the news.
209. **C** – In paragraph 3 it states 'people gathered around the radio for the immediate news'.
210. **A** – A or B are the 2 most likely answers, as paragraph 2 states about a fallen leader. However, since paragraph 2 only mentions D Roosevelt as being a president (and not John F. Kennedy) this is the best answer.

Set 43:
211. **A** – Paragraph 2 states inhabitants defended their own territory. While paragraph 3 states towns drew up formal treaties with other boroughs, which may include laws of protection, indicating they did, in fact, draw up treaties to defend each other, in addition to defending their own territory.
212. **C** – Paragraph 2 states that inhabitants elected their own rulers and officials in whatever way they themselves chose to adopt.
213. **A** – The first sentence concludes that the 15th century town life is nothing like England today. The last sentence in the second paragraph states there is some comparison with modern America. Therefore, this statement is correct.
214. **C** – The final paragraph states that 'often their authority stretched out over a wide district, and surrounding villages gathered to their markets and obeyed their laws'.
215. **D** – There is mention of war (arming soldiers), of banning trading between boroughs (shutting down privileges of commerce) and treaties in the text.

Set 44:
216. **B** – The second sentence states that male power has risen and thus has not always occurred.
217. **B** – At the end of paragraph 1, it is stated that the Jewish God has attributes of power, thus, D is wrong. There is no mention of the Christian God, therefore, C & A cannot be the answer.
218. **A** – The final sentence talks about how faiths may give an insight into past society.
219. **A** – The first sentence states that 'nowhere is the influence of sex more plainly manifested than in the formulation of religious conceptions and creeds'. Answers B and D could have been right if the question was not *most clearly*.
220. **C** – There is never any mention of the author's own beliefs, there are only discussions of others' beliefs.

Set 45:
221. **True** – The writer says that a "novel with a purpose" constitutes a violation of the unwritten contract tactility existing between writer and reader.
222. **D** – At the end of the first paragraph, the passage states a novel may conduce to delectation (pleasure and delight) during hours of idleness in man. All the other statements the passage states the opposite

223. **C** – The author does not agree with novels which portray the author's views on socialism, religion or divorce laws. However, there is no indication to which the author dislikes the most.
224. **C** – The only plausible answers are C and D (the author argues against A & B). It states that the unwritten contract is a novel should be an 'intellectual artistic luxury', which is earlier described as being able to delectate (to please) – a synonym of amusement. There is no mention of a good novel needing to be fiction.
225. **B** – C and D are beliefs of the author. A novel should instruct the reader is the opinion, while "novel with a purpose" is the answer ('realisation') to this opinion. Therefore, the answer is B rather than A.

Set 46:

226. **C** – While the first paragraph talks of these happy memories, all are asked as questions rather than being presented as fact.
227. **D** – The passage is based on different opinions on what patriotism is, thus, it cannot be deduced that the author can quantify how many American's are patriotic without an agreed definition.
228. **A** – Paragraph 3 states that one proposed definition of patriotism is the training of wholesale murders, i.e. mass killing. There is not mention of depression or workplaces. Children fantasising about having wings to fly to distant lands is not a sufficient reason for D to be the correct answer over A.
229. **C** – While paragraph 1 talks of wonderful tales of great deeds and conquests, this is insinuated to be of the past. The author then in paragraph 2 says that the stories mothers tell today are those of sorrow, tears, and grief.
230. **D** – This is the only answer where the author specifically says children wonder. The others could be inferred but are not as factually correct.

Set 47:

231. **C** – The start of paragraph 2 states that a good man can receive a gift well.
232. **A** – In paragraph 1, it states "we wish to be self-sustained" when referring to some men's opinions.
233. **B** – In paragraph 2, the author states that he can rejoice (i.e. like) to receive gifts as well as sometimes grieving upon the presentation of a gift. He later goes on to say he is ashamed of being pleased by gifts. However despite this, for certain periods, he does sometimes like gifts.
234. **D** – In paragraph 1, it states "we can receive anything from love, for that is a way of receiving it from ourselves".
235. **C** – Paragraph 2 states "if the gift pleases me overmuch, then I should be ashamed that the donor should read my heart, and see that I love his commodity, and not him." I.e. in this situation, the author feels bad that he does not appreciate the unique effort and insight of the giver as much as the physical gift. Answer B could be inferred, however, the answer C is stated. A is not true and so D cannot be the answer.

Set 48:

236. **A** – False. The final sentence states that mathematics was a science which Goethe was imperfectly acquainted with.
237. **C** – Having writers speak about a paper indicates this is the most popular (the first sentence). But it is specific parts of this paper (prismatic spectrum and refraction) which were mostly spoke about. Therefore, C rather than A is correct.
238. **A** – The translator was aware of the opposition which the theoretical views alluded to conflict with and wanted to first select the experiments which showed evidence to support Goethe's view. It says this was incompatible with the author's view.
239. **C** – "Doctrine of Colours" and two short essays entitled "Contributions to Optics" are mentioned.
240. **A** – This is stated in the first sentence. While his views are different from the received theories of Newton, it does not say it disproves Newton's theories.

Set 49:

241. **True** – In paragraph 2 the passage says "gradually" (but surely) the thoughts of money takes over the thoughts of a girl so that income is the most important thing – therefore, based on the information solely in the passage, this is true.
242. **False** – In paragraph one, the passage states that this is the view of stereotypical Philistine's and therefore not the author's view.
243. **Can't tell** – Nowhere does the passage mention Nora's opinion of wanting a child (be it with anyone).
244. **Can't tell** – The first paragraph states every twelfth marriage ends in divorce, but nowhere does it say what population of people this statistic was calculated from. In paragraph 6, it talks of American life but this does not necessarily mean the statistic is from America.
245. **False** – In the second paragraph, it states that over time, a married woman's mind strays from these thoughts.

Set 50:

246. **False** – In paragraph 1, it states a series of temporary measures were initiated (somewhere in the 1960s/70s). However, in paragraph 2 it says the Terrorism Act 2000 was passed as a definite measure following twenty years of temporary measures, therefore, the temporary measures in Ulster could not have been implemented in the 60s, as this would be over thirty years.
247. **Can't tell** – Nothing stated anywhere in the text of legislation actively replacing it.
248. **Can't tell** – Paragraph 2 would suggest so, but there is no definitive description of why the acts were passed like there is in paragraph 1.
249. **True** – Paragraph 3 states that the ATCSA marked a more firm move towards the 'management of anticipatory risk' which was to characterize the counter-terrorism legislation of the 21st century.
250. **True** – The second paragraph states that the 2000 Terrorism Act was passed "following twenty years of temporary measures."

Decision Making Answers

Question	Answer	Question	Answer	Question	Answer	Question	Answer
1	D	26	D	51	C	76	B
2	B	27	B & D	52	B	77	A
3	B	28	A & D	53	D	78	C
4	B & C	29	A	54	A	79	A
5	D	30	C	55	A	80	A
6	C	31	B	56	D	81	A
7	C	32	A & C	57	C	82	B
8	B	33	B & D	58	A	83	C
9	C & E	34	C	59	A	84	All false
10	B	35	D	60	D	85	B, C & D
11	C	36	D	61	C	86	C
12	B	37	C	62	C	87	D
13	B	38	B	63	B	88	A
14	B	39	A	64	D	89	B & D
15	C	40	A	65	C	90	B
16	C	41	C	66	D	91	B
17	A	42	A	67	C	92	C
18	D	43	D	68	D	93	A
19	E	44	D	69	A	94	B
20	C	45	A	70	D	95	B
21	D	46	B	71	B	96	C
22	D	47	A	72	D	97	A
23	C	48	B	73	D		
24	D	49	D	74	D		
25	B	50	C	75	D		

Question 1: D

The easiest thing to do is draw the relative positions. We know Harrington is north of Westside and Pilbury. We know that Twotown is between Pilbury and Westside. Crewville is south of Twotown, Westside and Harrington but we do not know but its location relative to Pilbury.

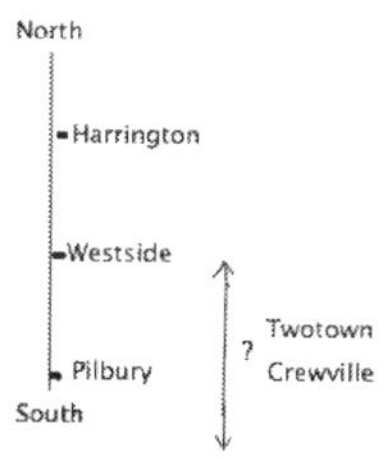

Question 2: B

By making a grid and filling in the relevant information the days Dr James works can be deduced:

	Sunday	Monday	Tuesday	Wednesday	Thursday	Friday	Saturday
Dr Evans	X	√	X	X	√	√	√
Dr James	X	√	√	√	√	X	√
Dr Luca	X	X	√	√	X	√	√

- No one works Sunday.
- All work Saturday.
- Dr Evans works Mondays and Fridays.
- Dr Luca cannot work Monday or Thursday.
- So, Dr James works Monday.
- And, Dr Evans and Dr James must work Thursday.
- Dr Evans cannot work 4 days consecutively so he cannot work Wednesday.
- Which means Dr James and Luca must work Wednesday.
- (mentioned earlier in the question) Dr Evans only works 4 days, so cannot work Tuesday.
- Which means Dr James and Luca work Tuesday.
- Dr James cannot work 5 days consecutively so cannot work Friday.
- Which means Dr Luca must work Friday.

Question 3: B

All thieves are criminals. So the circle must be fully inside the square, we are told judges cannot be criminals so the star must be completely separate from the other two.

Question 4: B and C

Using the information to make a diagram:

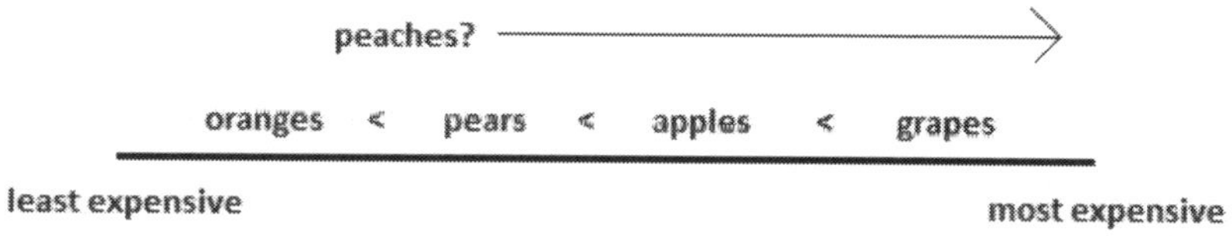

Hence **A** is incorrect. **D** and **E** may be true but we do not have enough information to say for sure. **B** is correct as we know peaches are more expensive than oranges but not about their price relative to pears. Equally we know **C** to be true as grapes are more expensive than apples so they must be more expensive than pears.

Question 5: D

Using Bella's statements, as she must contradicted herself with her two statements, as one of them must be true, we know that it was definitely either Charlotte or Edward. Looking to the other statements, e.g. Darcy's we know that it was either Charlotte or Bella, as only one of the two statements saying it was both of them can have been a lie. Hence it must have been Charlotte.

Question 6: C

Work through each statement and the true figures.

A. Overlap of pain and flu-like symptoms must be at least 4% (56+48-100). 4% of 150: 0.04 x 150=6

B. 30% high blood pressure and 20% diabetes, so max percentage with both must be 20%. 20% of 150: 0.2*150 = 30

C. Total number of patients – patients with flu-like symptoms – patients with high blood pressure. Assume different populations to get max number without either. 150 – (0.56 x 150) – (0.3 x 150) = 21

D. This is an obvious trap that you might fall into if you added up the percentages and noted that the total was >100%. However, this isn't a problem as patients can discussed two problems.

Question 7: C

We know that Charles is born in 2002, therefore in 2010 he must be 8. There are 3 years between Charles and Adam, and Charles is the middle grandchild. As Bertie is older than Adam, Adam must be younger than Charles so Adam must be 5 in 2010. In 2010, if Adam is 5, Bertie must be 10 (states he is double the age of Adam). The question asks for ages in 2015: Adam = 10, Bertie = 15, Charles = 13

Question 8: B

In this question it is worth remembering it will take more people a shorter amount of time.

Work out how many man hours it takes to build the house. Days x hours x builders

12 x 7 x 4 = 336 hours

Work out how many hours it will take the 7man workforce: 336/7 = 48 hours

Convert to 8 hour days: 48/8 = 6 days

Question 9: C & E

The easiest way to work this out is using a table. With the information we know:

2nd		
3rd	Jaya	
4th		

Ellen made carrot cake and it was not last. It now cannot be 1st or 3rd as these places are taken so it must be second:

2nd	Ellen	Carrot cake
3rd	Jaya	
4th		

Aleena's was better than the tiramisu, so she can't have come last, therefore Aleena must have placed first

2nd	Ellen	Carrot cake
3rd	Jaya	
4th		

And the girl who made the Victoria sponge was better than Veronica:

2nd	Ellen	Carrot cake
3rd	Jaya	Victoria Sponge
4th	Veronica	Tiramisu

Question 10: B

After the first round; he knocks off 8 bottles to leave 8 left on the shelf. He then puts back 4 bottles. There are therefore 12 left on the shelf. After the second round, he has hit 3 bottles and damages 6 bottles in total, and an additional 2 at the end. He then puts up 2 new bottles to leave 12 – 8 + 2 = 6 bottles left on the shelf. After the final round, John knocks off 3 bottles from the shelf to leave 3 bottles standing.

Question 11: C

Remember that pick up and drop off stops may be the same stop, therefore the minimum number of stops the bus had to make was 7. This would take 7 x 1.5 = 10.5 minutes.

Therefore the total journey time = 24 + 10.5 = 34.5 minutes.

Question 12: B

The time could be 21:25, if first 2 digits were reversed by the glass of water (21 would be reversed to give 15). **A** cannot be the answer, because this would involve altering the last 2 digits, and we can see that 25 on a digital clock, when reversed simply gives 25 (the 2 on the left becomes a 5 on the right, and the 5 on the right becomes a 2 on the left). **C** cannot be the answer, as this involves reversing the middle 2 digits. As with the right two digits, the middle 2 digits of 2:5 would simply reverse to give itself, 2:5. **D** could be the time if the *2nd* and *4th* digits were reversed, as they would both become 2's. However, the question says that 2 *adjacent* digits are reversed, meaning that the 2nd and 4th digits cannot be reversed as required here. **E** is not possible as it would require all four numbers to be reversed. Thus, the answer is **B**.

Question 13: B

To answer this, we simply calculate how much total room in the pan will be taken up by the food for each guest:

- 2 rashers of bacon, giving a total of 14% of the available space.
- 4 sausages, taking up a total of 12% of the available space.
- 1 egg takes up 12% of the available space.

Adding these figures together, we see that each guest's food takes up a total of 38% of the available space.

Thus, Ryan can only cook for 2 guests at once, since 38% multiplied by 3 is 114%, and we cannot use up more than 100% of the available space in the pan.

Question 14: B

The trains come into the station together every 40 minutes, as the lowest common multiple of 2, 5 and 8 is 40. Hence, if the last time trains came together was 15 minutes ago, the next time will be in 25 minutes.

Question 15: C

Tiles can be added at either end of the 3 lines of 2 tiles horizontally or at either end of the 2 lines of 2 tiles vertically. This is a total of 10, but in two cases these positions are the same (at the bottom of the left hand vertical line and the top of the right hand vertical line). So the answer is 10 – 2 = 8.

Question 16: C

Georgia is shorter than her Mum and Dad, and each of her siblings is at least as tall as Mum (and we know Mum is shorter than Dad because Ellie is between the two), so we know Georgia is the shortest. We know that Ellie, Tom and Dad are all taller than Mum, so Mum is second shortest. Ellie is shorter than Dad and Tom is taller than Dad, so we can work out that Ellie must be third shortest.

Question 17: A

Danielle must be sat next to Caitlin. Bella must be sat next to the teaching assistant. Hence these two pairs must sit in different rows. One pair must be sat at the front with Ashley, and the other must be sat at the back with Emily. Since the teaching assistant has to sit on the left, this must mean that Bella is sat in the middle seat and either Ashley or Emily (depending on which row they are in) is sat in the right hand seat. However, Bella cannot sit next to Emily, so this means Bella and the teaching assistant must be in the front row. So Ashley must be sat in the front right seat.

Question 18: D

We can see from the fact that all the possible answers end "AME" that the letters "AME" must be translated to the last 3 letters of the coded word, "JVN", under the code. J is the 10th letter of the alphabet so it is 9 letters on from A (V is the 21st letter of the alphabet and M is the 13th, and N is the 14th letter of the alphabet and E is the 5th, therefore these pairs are also 9 letters apart). Therefore P is the code for the letter 9 letters before it in the alphabet. P is the 16th letter of the alphabet, therefore it is the code for the 7th letter of the alphabet, G. Therefore from these solutions the only possibility for the original word is GAME.

Question 19: E

To find out whether many of these statements are true it is necessary to work out the departure and arrival times, and journey time, for each girl.

Lauren departs at 2:30pm and arrives at 4pm, therefore her journey takes 1.5 hours
Chloe departs at 1:30pm and her journey takes 1 hour longer than 1.5 hours (Lauren's journey), therefore her journey takes 2.5 hours and she arrives at 4pm
Amy arrives at 4:15pm and her journey takes 2 times 1.5 hours (Lauren's journey), therefore her journey takes 3 hours and she departs at 1:15pm.
Looking at each statement, the only one which is definitely true is **E**: Amy departs at 1:15pm and Chloe departs at 1:30pm therefore Amy departed before Chloe.

D *may* be true, but nothing in the question shows it is *definitely* true, so it can be safely ignored.

Question 20: C

For the total score to be odd, there must be either three odd or one odd and two even scores obtained. Since the solitary odd score could be either the first, second or third throw there are four possible outcomes that result in an odd total score. Additionally, there are the same number of possibilities giving an even score (either all three even or two odd and one even scores obtained), and the chance of throwing odd or even with any given dart is equal. Therefore, there is an equal probability of three darts totalling to an odd score as to an even score, and so the chance of an odd score is ½.

Question 21: D

A. Not appropriate as it is highly judgemental towards the abilities of nurses. Nurses already play an important role in care delivery and in many cases already make important decisions. The NHS would not be able to deliver care efficiently without the input of specialty nurses.
B. Worse version of statement a). Same reasons why this is inappropriate.
C. In general, not completely wrong, but the fact that it places the ability of nurses over these of doctors without limitation is the flaw of this argument. Nurses and doctors work together to deliver care with different areas of responsibility.
D. Correct answer. True and less restrictive than the version in c). Nurses input valuable and it would definitely be helpful to give nurses more freedom for decision making.

Question 22: D

a) is wrong because the text specifically states that he sees many squirrels. B) is wrong because the birds fly off as soon as James approaches. C) is an assumption not backed by the text resource and therefore must be wrong.

Question 23: C

A. Incorrect. This is not about being all-knowing and infallible. It is about the assumption of do no harm.

B. Training is not mentioned in the quote at all, therefore this answers is incorrect. It can be further assumed that for a physician to be able to tell the present and future, he must have undergone some degree of training.

C. Correct. Non-maleficence means do no harm.

D. In some cases techniques of the past are valuable and still used today, in some cases they are not. In any case this quote is not about techniques, but about the moral background of actions.

Question 24: D

A. Incorrect. This would solve the problem but ignore all ethical basis we use for medical decision making.

B. Incorrect. This would cause a significant impact to the everyday life of the families of the patients making it a highly unethical decision.

C. Incorrect. The entire idea of the NHS is based on the notion that there is no discrimination between the rich and the poor. It is for that reason unacceptable to charge patients for extended hospital stays unless they get different care.

D. Correct. All other answers are incorrect per descriptions above.

Question 25: B

The relationship of goats and pigs to cows is 4:1 meaning that in every 5 animals, 1 has to be a cow. The value of the individual animals is a distraction that is not needed for the calculation of this question. 5 = 40

Question 26: D

A. Incorrect. Young apes mingle with any group as it says in the text.

B. Incorrect. The widest range of social interactions is displayed by the youngest apes which mingle freely with any group of monkeys.

C. Incorrect. Has nothing to do with the actual question.

D. Correct. There seems to be a separation between adolescent male and female apes as their preferred groups of social interaction are separated. It says specifically in the text that adolescent female apes mingle exclusively with young and older female apes.

Question 27: B & D

A. No. This conclusion cannot be drawn as no information is given regarding the friend. He/she could simply be of smaller statue. Also, it is unknown what mount of cooking equipment the two are taking.

B. Yes. They both carry equipment that is important for them having a good time.

C. No. Similar to a) the simple fact that there is a chance that Steve's load may be heavier than his friends does not provide enough information to deduct his friend to be female.

D. Yes. Due to the amount of kit the two are carrying, most importantly the tent and sleeping equipment suggests that the two want to stay wherever they are going at least for one night.

Question 28: A & D

Order of seats from left to right: Sophie – Maria – Anna – Louise – Jenny

A. True. The only unallocated seat is between Sophie and Anna, therefore Maria must sit on the second seat from the left.

B. False. Sophie sits at the edge with regards to the row occupied by the 5 girls, the text never suggests that she mat sit at the edge of the hall. As a matter of fact, since the text specifically states that they sit in front of the stage, it is unlikely that Sophie sits at the edge of the concert hall.

C. False. Jenny sits at the far right.

D. True. Louise sits between Jenny and Anna.

Question 29: A

A. True. Sven plants salad, carrots and courgettes, making it three. Tomatoes are strictly speaking fruits, so they are not counted.

B. False. Carrots are orange.

C. False. The text does not deliver any data regarding the prevalence of tomato allergies. All we know is that Sven has a tomato allergy.

D. False. Conclusion a) is true.

Question 30: C

A. False. Rome is the most Southern city.

B. False. According to the travel organisation, Amsterdam must be further South than Berlin.

C. True. They will start in the UK, move on to German, then the Netherlands, then France, then Italy.

D. False, c) is true.

Question 31: B

A. False. The text clearly states that computer technology firms are heavily involved in military contracts.
B. True. The only food producing industry branch that is involved in military contracts according to the text is the beef industry.
C. False. This conclusion cannot reasonably be made as the data in the text passage is insufficient.
D. False. This uses information not mentioned in the text source at all.

Question 32: A & D

Order of houses: Austin – Peter – Steve – David – Mark

A. True. Steve lives in the middle of the row of houses.
B. False. There is no information about the size of the town.
C. True. Peter must live between Steve and Austin as this is the only available house that is not allocated by the description.
D. False. David lives between Steve and Mark.

Question 33: B & D

A. False. Whilst it is true that baldness can affect women as well, the study only focuses on men.
B. True. Both anabolic steroid consumption as well as type 2 diabetes can be linked to life style choices, therefore there is a connection between hair loss and life style changes.
C. False. The majority of cases are due to a genetic predisposition and independent of external factors. It can therefore be assumed that shampoo will not help with hair loss.
D. True. The link is directly mentioned in the text.

Question 34: C

A. False. The forest also contains fruit trees.
B. False. False. There are needle trees, oaks, beeches and fruit trees..
C. True. Christmas trees are needle tress which represent the majority of trees in the forest.
D. False. We can't answer that question as no actual size of the forest is given.

Question 35: D

A. True. Since they spend 50% of their life in the ocean, the other 50% must be on land since they are flightless.
B. True. Penguins life in large groups making them herd animals.
C. True. Says so specifically in the text.
D. False. Penguins live in various climate regions as it says in the text.

Question 36: D

A. False. Fossil fuel technology has constantly been improved in efficiency and has not been overcome to this day.
B. False. Import of fossil fuels such as coal and oil is expensive, but not expensive enough to make it economically unsound as it forms an essential part of most industrial productions steps.
C. False. Fossil fuels are limited.
D. True. Due to our huge energy demand, an immediate switch to non-fossil fuels is difficult. Also, there are less developed countries where fossil fuels represent the primary source of energy sue to technological constraints regarding energy generation.

Question 37: C

A. False. There are some parts of the population that are not allowed to vote as they have not yet reached the legal voting age.
B. False. This is only in part responsible for the decision not to vote.
C. True. Voters must be of a certain age and also be allowed to vote based on other criteria.
D. False.

Question 38: B

A. False. Older parents are more likely to have genetically abnormal children.
B. True. Due to the accumulative mutagenic effect the risk of genetic alteration due to environmental mutagens is lower in younger parents.
C. False. Sperm cells are constantly regenerated. It is egg cells that are present at birth.
D. False. Answer b is correct.

Question 39: A

A. True. Peter is 3 seconds faster than Felix, who is 5 seconds faster than Lucas.
B. False, Dorian finishes second, and according to the text the top 3 places are separated by 1 second.
C. False. Dorian finishes second.
D. False. Answer a) is correct.

Question 40: A

The sum of each circle must represent the amount of people with the specific preferences.
Gummi bears: 5, of which 2 like chocolate and 2 like biscuits.
Chocolate: 6, of which 2 also like gummi bears and 2 like biscuits. 2 only like chocolate.
Biscuits: 3, of which 1 also likes gummy bears and 2 also like chocolate.

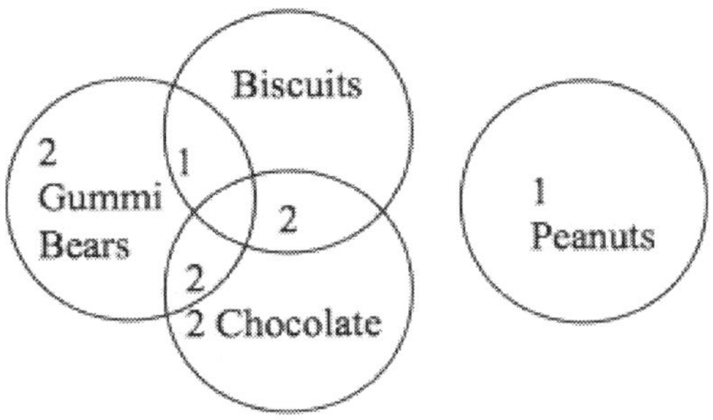

Question 41: C

As the all the batches have the same value and the company has sold less candy. The previous year the company sold 38 322 tons of candy and this year they only sold 32 500 tons of candy.
Calculations:
Product 1: 10 000 = 110% of last year's sales => last year: 9091
Product 2: 500 = 5% of last year's sales => last year: 10000
Product 3 12 000 = 130% of last year's sales => last year: 9231
Product 4 and 5 are unchanged.

Question 42: A

The assumption that the surgeon only does private work is not supported by the resource as he only lists his 4 main procedures. It should not be assumed that this is the only work he does.

Question 43: D

Since there is a 50% chance of one of the two being a smoker, there is a 25% chance of both f of them being smokers.

Question 44: D

The question does not address issues such as income or relationships of power. Whilst indirectly, answers a) and c) may well be true, there is no factual information in the question to back up that claim.

Question 45: A

50% of cases due to respiratory problems. 25% of cases due to cardiovascular causes, 15% of cases due to abdominal disease, 5% due to traffic accidents, 5% due to work accidents.

Question 46: B

65% of 15% equates to 10%. 15% does not represent a large proportion, therefore answer a) must be incorrect. Nuts are not the most common source of allergies according to the text, in general food intolerances represent the most common cause for allergies, therefore c) is wrong. The question is specifically about children and for this reason, answer d) is incorrect too.

Question 47: A

The fact that chimpanzees continuously use tools shows that they understand their effect, this makes b) true and therefore the wrong answer. With regards to answer c), using tools in itself represents a form of environmental manipulation making c) true and therefore the incorrect answer for this question.

Question 48: B

Carl weighs 50kg, Luke weighs 45kg, Ben and Alex weigh 40kg and Peter weighs 35kg. In total, they weigh 210kg, meaning the house structure will weigh 15kg according to their calculation.

Question 49: D

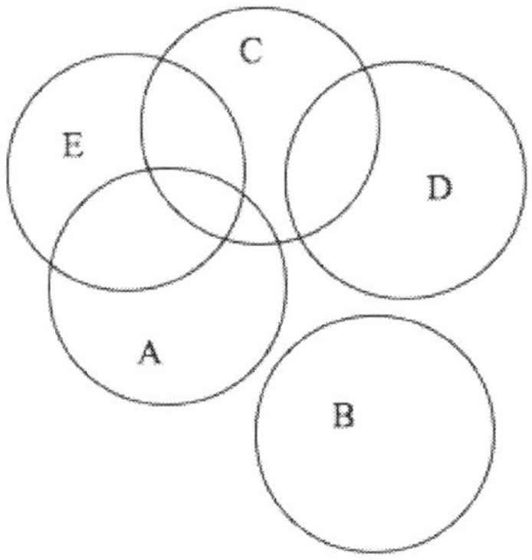

Question 50: C

Ants do not compete amongst individuals for resources but amongst colonies of the same species, therefore a) is incorrect. For similar reasons, b) must be incorrect as different species may have different food preferences meaning that there is no interspecies competition. D) is incorrect as the text specifically states that some species of ants live of plant material, whilst others live off animal material.

Question 51: C
Many pesticides carry health risks for the consumer and are present in the food we consume every day, which carries significant health risks.

Question 52: B
False – True – False – False.

Question 53: D
Answer a) is true as I mentioned in the text. Answer b) is true as farming formed the basis to feed a population restricted to one location. C) is true as crops need time to grow and harvest which is not conducive to a nomadic lifestyle.

Question 54: A
All of the conclusions are true. Since the goal of school is the intellectual development of children, increasing exercise may help improve performance. A sedentary life style ins marked by a lack of exercise, therefore this may contribute to poorer school performance. C) is basically the original statement, but rephrased.

Question 55: A
The mere fact that these plants stand in a similar constellation to their sun, as Earth does to our sun is only one part of the equation. This is relevant because it increases the likelihood of liquid water anywhere near the surface of the plant, which, next to air is one of the most essential points. The other assumptions are largely irrelevant for questions of habitability.

Question 56: D
The fact that species C lives of berries when available but then falls back to seeds or insects means that they can find food in any season. Answer a) Is incorrect as only species C eats berries, answer b) is incorrect as there is no mention of their beaks in the text, answer c) is incorrect as Species A will also eat sunflower seeds.

Question 57 C
Whether health-care professionals are role-models for society or not may be debatable, but they represent important points of contact between the public and the healthcare system giving them certain responsibilities, therefore a) is incorrect. B) is incorrect as it is not related to the question. D) is true, but irrelevant to the question and therefore is false.

Question 58: A.

A. Correct as per the final sentence of the passage
B. incorrect as per text
C. Incorrect as the text is about young men and women are not mentioned anywhere.
D. Incorrect as option (a) is correct.

Question 59: A

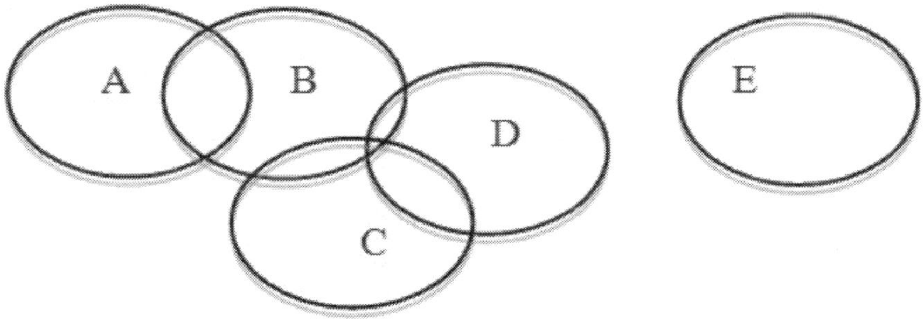

Population A: Applicants with excel skills
Population B: Applicants with excel and Photoshop skills
Population C: Applicants with excel, Photoshop and language skills
Population D: Applicants with excel, Photoshop, language and communication skills.
Population E: Applicants with only one language but experience.

Question 60: D
The overall order is: Tom - Richard - Anthony - Steve - Tony
The text describes that Richard finished joint bottom in section C, therefore he did not finish well in the section.

Question 61: C

A. Incorrect. The new cigarette blend releases twice as much CO.
B. False. The new cigarette contains less tar.
C. True. The new cigarette contains twice as much nicotine than the competition meaning one has to smoke two competitor cigarettes for every on to reach the same level of nicotine.
D. Incorrect. In all aspects mentioned, except for the tar, the new blend is worse than the competitions product.

Question 62: C

Elmsworth to Eastwich:		30 minutes
Waiting time at Eastwich:	5 minutes	
Eastwich to Northtown:		45 minutes
Waiting time at Northtown:	5 minutes	
Northtown to Southwarf:		30 minutes
Stop at Northtown station:	5 minutes	
Total:		120 minutes

Question 63: B

Team A: 7 points.
Team B: 3 points.
Team C: 4 points.
Team D: 12 points.
Team E: 1 point.

A. False. Since team D is unbeaten and each team plays each opponent only once, they achieve the most points.
B. True. Since team B finishes with 3 points they must draw three times, with team A, C and E.
C. False. Team C will collect fewer points than team D.
D. Irrelevant therefore false.

Question 64: D

A. Incorrect. Whilst the war is over. Resource conservation makes sense none the less.
B. Incorrect. Not a strong enough argument.
C. Possibly true, but not a big problem.
D. Correct. An issue that demonstrates both urgency as well necessity.

Question 65: C

The progression of the race is as follows: Start -15km- Chris -10km- Philip -6km- Anne -5km- Tara -4km- Peter -2km- finish. Therefore the distances between stops progressively reduce through the race

Question 66: D

Whilst all other options are valid, the last is the by far strongest issue when it comes to quality research.

Question 67: C

Stephanie – Sophie – Patricia – Tina – Annette

Question 68: D

A. The text states that there is a high degree of variability in decision making.
B. The text states that there is no regard for social background.
C. Similar reason as statement b.

Question 69: A

Cambridge – Imperial – Sheffield – Southampton – Cardiff

Question 70: D

A. Very superficial, delivers no actual argumentative value.
B. True, but not the strongest argument.
C. Similar to a). Also leads in a different direction than the argument itself.
D. True and the most basic and most central argument in support of the problem as described by the statement.

Question 71: B

A. False. The passage is about Tim, not Tom.
B. True. The passage says this is his favourite method.
C. Possibly true, but no comparison of strategies is made.
D. False.

Question 72: D

A. False. This statement only investigates small fish.
B. False. Water temperature is never mentioned.
C. False. The statement directly mentions that worse eyesight improves individual survival chances.
D. True. In cases of impaired visual function such as through dirt in murky water or through worse eye sight of the predator, the individual seems to be better protected.

Question 73: D

A. Incorrect. Since 50% of people consider healthcare to be the number one issue, there is clearly a problem with heath care provision.
B. Incorrect. Only because 10% consider defense the most important issue does not mean the population feels very secure. It just means they consider other points more important.
C. False. Irrelevant to the question.
D. Correct. Healthcare = 50%, education = 25%, infrastructure = 15%, defense = 10%

Question 74: D

A. Correct. Health care accounts for 22% whereas public cleanliness is 16%.
B. Correct. Housing accounts for 24% whereas healthcare is at 22%
C. Correct at 11%.
D. Incorrect. Since education accounts for 28% and housing for 5% less, this makes it 23%.

Question 75: D

A. Incorrect. The text specifically states that this happens.
B. Incorrect. Whilst this might be true in reality, it is not supported by the text.
C. Incorrect. According to the text, males attract females with their mating calls.
D. Correct.

Question 76: B

A. Incorrect. The groups are led by females.
B. Correct. The purpose of the group is to protect the young.
C. Incorrect. The groups are led by an individual according to the text.
D. Incorrect.

Question 77: A

A. Correct.
B. Incorrect. They eat two colours of fruit.
C. Incorrect. We only know that monkeys don't like to eat them.
D. Incorrect as irrelevant.

Question 78: C

A. Incorrect. Whilst without members, there can be no group, this presents little with regards to support for the statement.
B. Irrelevant – not mentioned in question.
C. Correct a strong and plausible rationale.
D. Incorrect.

Question 79: A

A. Correct.
B. Incorrect. Since C and B are the same, they both sold 2000 units.
C. Incorrect. The text does not address price.
D. False. Set D is the second to last most commonly sold handset.

Question 80: A

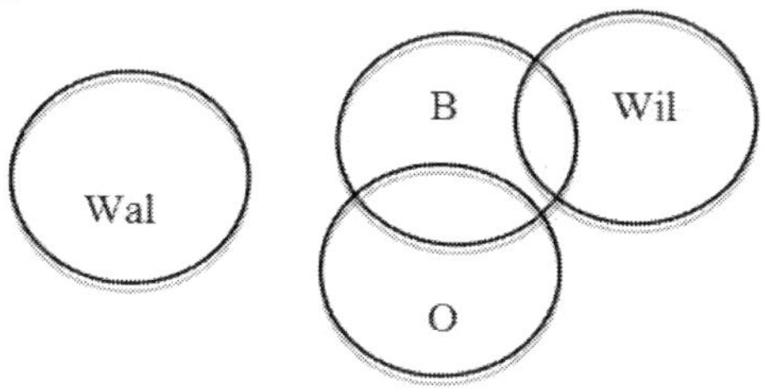

Walnut tree cannot grow around other trees due to the poison. The other trees both grow with Beech but Oak and Willow do not grow well together.

Question 81: A

A. Correct. 80% of 5 represent 4.
B. Incorrect. There are no vegan dishes in the order.
C. Incorrect. Whilst this might be true, there is no evidence to support this.
D. Incorrect.

Question 82: B
A. False. Since only gold medals are considered, Group A falls behind group B
B. True, it must have more gold medals to rank in top position
C. False as per text.
D. False.

Question 83: C
A. Incorrect. The statement is true.
B. Incorrect as the statement is true.
C. Correct as climate change causes increased temperatures in the normal breeding grounds rather than in the South.
D. Incorrect as the statement is true.

Question 84: All false
A. False – the passage describes coloured clothes
B. False – no red clothes are described
C. False – he owns sports clothes
D. False – some are but we cannot conclude that most are

Question 85: B, C & D
Peter - Eugene – John – David – Anthony.
Therefore (a) = false, (b) = true, (c) = true, (d) = true.
Question 86: C
A. True, but not the strongest argument.
B. False.
C. True, strongest argument.
D. False, as it replaces one unfair restriction with another.

Question 87: D
A. False. Per the text bears do not hunt.
B. False. Bears prefer berries over any other food source.
C. False. Bears attack if their cubs are in danger.
D. True.

Question 88: A

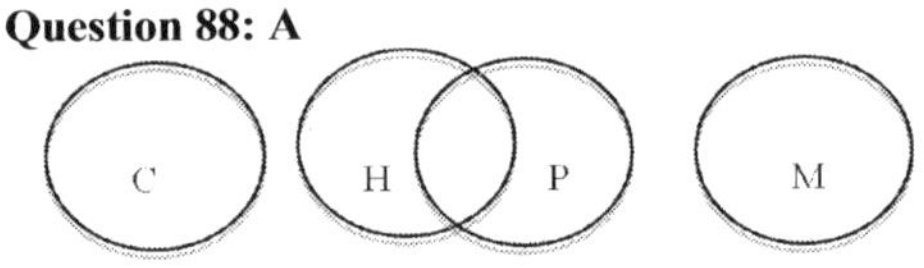

Because some ants are exclusively dedicated to construction work, and male ants are exclusively for reproduction, the correct option shows both of these independently.

Question 89: B & D
A. False – there are cherry trees.
B. True – all the described plants are trees.
C. False – her husband plants cherry trees.
D. True – raspberry bushes are all she planted; the other plants were either there before or planted by her husband

Question 90: B
A. Partially true, certainly not the strongest argument.
B. Correct. The term "unhealthy foods" is not well enough defined and can vary greatly.
C. False. Obesity is not mentioned in the argument.
D. False.

Question 91: B
A. Incorrect. This is not an actual quantitative value.
B. Correct since the text states that using nails will make the wardrobe more likely to collapse.
C. Incorrect. The text specifically states, that Walnut is darker than pine.
D. Incorrect. Peter does not play a role in the question.

Question 92: C
A. Incorrect.
B. Incorrect. At no point is the material named specifically.
C. True. As material C contains a significant proportion of the expensive material B, it must be purchased making material C expensive.
D. Incorrect. They must interact in order to produce material C which has different properties than its basic components.

Question 93: A

A. Correct.
B. False. Company B makes $50,000, Company C makes $90,000
C. False. The text specifically states, that it is the smallest company.
D. False. The text only says that this company has the smallest income which does not mean that it is going bankrupt.

Question 94: B

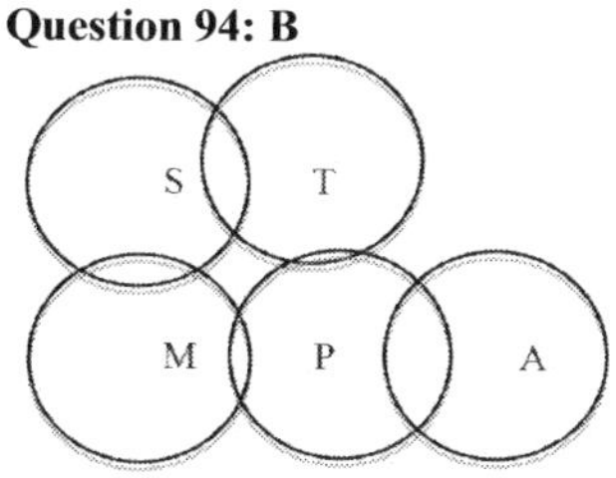

This is quite a complex one, so it may help to draw a 5x5 table to compare everyone's relationships. Identify the people who get on well to work out which people should overlap on the Venn diagram. Notice that Sarah gets on with Tina and Marylin only. Peter gets on with everyone except Sarah. These two pieces of information are enough to make option B the clear choice.

Question 95: B

A. Incorrect and irrelevant. Not addressed in the statement.
B. Correct. As population continues to grow newspaper numbers reduce.
C. False. This is a matter of opinion.
D. False.

Question 96: C

A. Incorrect. The same number of children want to be actors as well as politicians, 20 children.
B. Incorrect. Since 80 children don't know what they want to be yet, this is the majority.
C. True.
D. False. Since the same number of children want to be actors and politicians (20), more children want to be teachers than politicians.

Question 97: A

A. True – as per text
B. False – neither score
C. False – information not in passage
D. False – information not in passage, we only know he scores fewer goals

Quantitative Reasoning Answers

Q	A	Q	A	Q	A	Q	A	Q	A	Q	A
1	C	51	A	101	A	151	C	201	E	251	C
2	D	52	E	102	E	152	B	202	B	252	B
3	D	53	C	103	A	153	C	203	C	253	A
4	D	54	E	104	C	154	B	204	D	254	C
5	C	55	C	105	B	155	B	205	C	255	C
6	B	56	A	106	C	156	D	206	B	256	D
7	A	57	D	107	C	157	D	207	C	257	C
8	A	58	D	108	B	158	C	208	A	258	A
9	B	59	C	109	B	159	B	209	C	259	D
10	A	60	D	110	C	160	A	210	C	260	D
11	D	61	C	111	C	161	B	211	B	261	A
12	B	62	A	112	C	162	B	212	C	262	D
13	A	63	E	113	C	163	A	213	D	263	A
14	B	64	E	114	A	164	B	214	B	264	A
15	B	65	D	115	A	165	A	215	D	265	C
16	D	66	B	116	B	166	D	216	A	266	D
17	B	67	C	117	C	167	A	217	B	267	A
18	D	68	D	118	A	168	B	218	C	268	D
19	B	69	E	119	B	169	B	219	A	269	A
20	B	70	B	120	D	170	C	220	B	270	D
21	B	71	C	121	B	171	B	221	C	271	E
22	B	72	E	122	C	172	C	222	B	272	A
23	C	73	D	123	C	173	B	223	E	273	D
24	B	74	A	124	A	174	B	224	B	274	B
25	B	75	E	125	B	175	D	225	D	275	E
26	B	76	C	126	A	176	D	226	C	276	D
27	D	77	E	127	B	177	B	227	E	277	B
28	B	78	D	128	C	178	D	228	C	278	E
29	B	79	D	129	C	179	D	229	B	279	A
30	B	80	D	130	D	180	C	230	D	280	A
31	C	81	A	131	C	181	D	231	D	281	C
32	B	82	C	132	A	182	A	232	C	282	C
33	B	83	E	133	C	183	D	233	E	283	E
34	D	84	B	134	B	184	C	234	D	284	C
35	B	85	D	135	C	185	B	235	C	285	A
36	D	86	E	136	B	186	A	236	B	286	D
37	C	87	D	137	C	187	C	237	C	287	C
38	D	88	B	138	A	188	D	238	C	288	E
39	E	89	B	139	B	189	A	239	B	289	E
40	C	90	B	140	B	190	C	240	D	290	C
41	C	91	C	141	D	191	B	241	A	291	A
42	A	92	D	142	C	192	D	242	B	292	D
43	E	93	C	143	B	193	B	243	E	293	E
44	A	94	E	144	D	194	C	244	B	294	A
45	E	95	E	145	B	195	A	245	D	295	D
46	C	96	B	146	C	196	D	246	A	296	C
47	A	97	D	147	B	197	D	247	B	297	D
48	D	98	C	148	B	198	C	248	B	298	B
49	D	99	D	149	B	199	C	249	B	299	D
50	C	100	A	150	D	200	A	250	C	300	E

SET 1

Question 1: C
We can work out that the tax rates must fit in the following equation:
($50 x Food tax rate) + ($30 x Clothes tax rate) + $80 = $88. Only the tax rates in Casova fit correctly in this equation.

Question 2: D
To answer this question, we calculate how much the supplier will make for selling the items, by considering the tax rate in each state, and deducting it from the price accordingly.

Thus, in Bolovia, each year the supplier makes 250 x ($40/1.20 + $40/1.15 + $40/1.10 + $40/1.15) = $34,812 a year. In Asteria, each year the supplier makes 250 x ($40/1.10 + $40/1.15 + $40/1.10 + $40/1.15) = $35,572. (Note that in the case of an item being applicable to 2 tax rates, the higher rate will be charged. Thus, in Bolovia, imported clothes will be charged at the clothes tax rate of 15%, since this is higher than the imports rate.)
Thus, by moving to Asteria, the supplier will make $760 more each year. Therefore it will take 26.3 years to recover the purchase cost of $20,000.

Question 3: D
If John spends $88, he will spend £12 on tax. Thus, the tax rate is 12/88 = 13.6%.
If John shops in Asteria, the maximum tax rate he would have to pay is 10%; at Casova it would be 10%. If he spends at least $50 on food in Derivia, he pays no tax on it. Thus, he can spend a maximum of $38 on imported goods (at a maximum tax rate of 15%). This equates to a tax of $5.70 (not $12). Finally, if John spends $10 on imported goods in Bolovia – he would pay $0.50 in tax. Thus, he can spend up to $78 on clothes taxed at 15%. The tax on the clothes is therefore $11.70, giving $12.20 tax in total as the maximum. Since he pays $12 dollars tax, he shops in Bolovia.

Question 4: D
The sum of the basic prices is 100+30+10+100 = $240. Now the highest tax rate on the board is 20% (for imports to Asteria), thus the maximum tax is $240 x 1.20 = $288. However, this is impossible to attain (since if we bought everything in Asteria, the ham would be cheaper, as it is not imported and would only be taxed at the food rate). Therefore no option allows the overall price to be as high as $288, so this is the answer. Answer A) is possible if all products were bought in the state they are produced in. Answer C) is the correct answer if all products were bought in Asteria (and accounting for the reduced tax rate for the ham, which is not an import). Answer B) is possible if the ham was bought in Asteria, the caviar and orange juice were bought in Casova and the dress was bought in Bolovia.

SET 2

Question 5: C
Firstly, find the pressure it can withstand in Pascals: 200 pounds per square inch x 7,000 Pascals per pound per square inch = 1.4 million Pascals.
Then divide this by 1,000 Pa to get the depth the probe can withstand (we can see from the question that the pressure increases by 1,000 Pa for every metre depth increase):
1,400,000/1,000 = 1,400 metres into the ocean, which is 1.4 km.

Question 6: B
Calculate that the probe can drop 300,000 Pa/1,000 Pa per metre = 300 metres into the ocean before breaking.
Now rearrange the equation in the question, to make t the subject, as follows:
$2d = \sqrt{(t^3)}$
$(2d)^2 = t^3$
$t = \sqrt[3]{(2d)^2}$
Then substitute the depth into this supplied equation:
$t = \sqrt[3]{(2d)^2} = \sqrt[3]{(2x300)^2} = 71$ seconds.

SET 3

Question 7: A
Calculate the amount of drug taken for each disease:
Black Trump Virus = 4 mg x 80 kg x 3 times a day x 28 days = 26.88 g
Swamp Fever = 3x80x1x7 = 1.68 g
Yellow Tick = 1x80x2x84 – 13.44 g
Red Rage = 5x80x2x21 = 16.80 g
At a quick glance, the swamp fever dosage is much lower than all the others – you can discount this and use that to save a little time if you need to.

Question 8: A
First calculate that Carol took 20.16 grams of the drug during the two courses for Yellow Tick, using the same method as for John, but using Carol's weight of 60kg. Therefore 20.16 grams (the amount left over) corresponds to the dosage for the unknown disease:
4x60x3x28 = 20.16 g, therefore the unknown disease was Black Trump Virus.

Question 9: B
The first time he takes 3 x 80 x 1 x 7 = 1.68 grams, and the second time he takes 4 x 110 x 3 x 28 = 36.96 grams. Thus the ratio is 1.68 : 36.96 = 1:22.

Question 10: A
By calculating the dose required in each of the cases, we see that the only one that is above 15.5 grams over 4 weeks is the dosage for Red Rage:
5 x 75 x 2 x 21 = 15.75 g – therefore Danny must be suffering from Red Rage.

Question 11: D
Heavier people need a higher dose. To find the maximum weight, we use the equation: 5 x weight x 2 x 21 = 10 g, where "weight" represents the maximum weight requiring a dosage of less than 10 g.

So the maximum weight to not need a dosage exceeding 10 g is = 10,000 mg/(21 days x 2 daily doses x 5 mg/kg) = 47.62 kg.

SET 4

Question 12: B
To solve this, divide the flour content by the overall mass. A quick inspection might show you that this is likely to be Madeira, which is confirmed by the calculation (250/825 = 0.3). Thus, 30% of the Madeira's total weight is flour, which is a higher percentage than for any other cake

Question 13: A
In this question, there must be one cake where: (2,600/mass of cake) = (625/mass of flour in cake). Thus, there is a number that both the mass of the cake and the mass of flour can be multiplied by, in order to get these numbers respectively.
We can see that if we multiply the mass of the sponge cake by 5, we get 2,600 g. Equally, if we multiply the mass of flour in the sponge cake recipe (125g) by 5, then we get 625 g. Thus, Sponge cake is the answer. No other cake recipe can be multiplied by a given number to get an overall weight of 2,600 g and 625 g of flour.

Question 14: B
We use 1.50+1.25+1.10+1 times the ingredients for one cake, so the wedding cake will use 4.85 times as much of the ingredients listed for one cakes. We can use this to find which of the possible answers can be the amount of sugar in the cake, i.e. the sugar called for in one recipe multiplied by 4.85.
The quickest way to do this is to divide each possible answer by 4.85, and see if the result matches the weight of sugar in any of the cakes. We see that 970 g/4.85 = 200 g, which is the amount of sugar in the chocolate cake. None of the other amounts are possible. Thus, B is the answer.

Question 15: B
A kilogram of flour costs 55 x 2/3 pence and we are using 0.25 kg, so 9.167 p worth of flour goes into a Madeira cake. For sugar, we have 0.175 kg x 70 p per kg = 12.25 p worth of sugar going into the cake.
The ratio is thus 9.167:12.25 = approx 0.75:1 = 3:4

Question 16: D
As before, the flour costs: 55 p per 1.5 kg x 2/3 x 0.2 kg = 7.3 pence.
The milk costs: 44 p per kg x 150 g/1000 g per kg = 6.6 pence.
Thus the ratio is 7.3:6.6 = 1:0.9 = 10:9.

SET 5

Question 17: B
In total, 108 people out of the 200 tested have the disease; this is 108/200 = 0.54. Thus, the answer is 54%.

Question 18: D
As the infection rate is different for men and women, the infection rates must be calculated separately and combined:
(231,768 x 0.53 women x 0.63) + (231,768 x 0.47 men x 0.45) = 126,406 to the nearest whole person.

Question 19: B
There are 45 men and 63 women in the test group who have the Kryptos virus. Thus 15 of the men and 45 of the women have visited Atlantis. As we now know that 60 people have visited Atlantis, we can see that 108 – 60 = 48 have not visited. Now we simply calculate 48 as a percentage of 108. 48/108 = 0.44. Thus, 44% of people testing positive for the Virus in Test A have *not* visited Atlantis.

Question 20: B
We can see that 20/45 men testing positive in Test A have also tested positive in Test B, so we assume that the rest were false positives stemming from the inaccuracies of Test A. We are told to assume the same proportion of false positives in the women tested, so we simply apply this fraction to the number of women testing positive in Test A. Thus, we simply calculate 63 x (20/45) = 28. Thus, we expect that 28 women actually have Kryptos Virus.

Question 21: B
In total 108 people tested positive under test A, and 49 of these tested positive under test B (using the data given in the last question). Therefore the percentage of people positive in Test A also testing positive in Test B is 49 out of 108, which is 45.4%.

SET 6

Question 22: B
The cost of the plan is 190 + 600 + 140 = £930 per day

Question 23: C
Firstly we need to find the two options that save the most money, aside from the one already stated. The two best options are to send material from Plant A to Store 1, and material from plant B to store 2. We can see from the table that these 2 options will be £30 per day cheaper than sending from Plant A to store 2, and plant B to store 1 (as with the current business plan).

The new total cost is 100 + 180 + 450 = £730. Thus the saving is (930 – 730) = £200. £200 is 22% of £930, so the percentage saving is 22% (to the nearest whole number).

SET 7

Question 24: B
The shop sold 512 books outside of the visit event (sum of sales in the table), and 106 at the event.
Thus the percentage at the event was 106/(512+106) = 17%.

Question 25: B
Firstly calculate the different revenues:
Non-fiction revenue = (12+30) x£10 = £420
Fiction revenue = (50+45+23+90+103+159) x£6 = £2,820
Then calculate the non-fiction percentage: 420/(2,820+420) = 13%.

Question 26: B
The weekly revenue is seven times the daily revenue.
Daily revenue from Fiction: (50+45+23+90+103+159) x£6 = £2,820.
Daily revenue from Non-fiction 2x(12+30) x£10 = £840.
Therefore weekly revenue is 7x(£28.20+£840) = £25,620.

Question 27: D
The shop's revenue is now £6 x (100+90+23+90+103+159) + £10 x (12+30) per day. This income equates to £3,810 per day and £26,670 per week.

Therefore the percentage difference is 26,670/25,620 = 1.04, giving a 4% increase on the previous week.

SET 8

Question 28: B
2 nights in Venice in a 3 star hotel, 1 room (the children are exempt) = 2x1x3 = 6 euros
2 nights in Rome in a 3 star hotel, 3 people paying (the child aged 9 is exempt) = 2x3x5 = 30 Euros
2 nights in Padua in a 3 star hotel, 2 people paying (both children exempt) = 2x2x2 = 8 euros
2 nights in Siena in the high season, 3 paying (child aged 9 exempt) = 2x3x2 = 12 euros
So the entire cost is the sum of these costs = 6+30+8+12 = 56 euros.

Question 29: B
In Rome he pays 6 euros x 7 nights = 42 Euros. In Padua he pays 3 euros x 8 nights = 24 Euros. 42:24 = 7:4.

Question 30: B
A 3 star hotel in Venice for 2 days costs Alice 6 Euros. 3 days in a 4 star hotel in Padua costs 9 Euros. This is 50% more in Padua than in Venice.

Question 31: C
The maximum cost of tax in a 4 star hotel in Rome is 6 euros x 10 nights = 60 EUR. Up until this point it will always be cheaper in Padua. In Padua the cost for a 4 star hotel is 3 euros a night, therefore after 20 days the cost of the Padua hotel is equal to the cost of a stay of equivalent duration in Rome.

SET 9

Question 32: B
First find the wall length: 15m x 0.6 = 9m. Therefore, the area of the room is 9m x 9m = 81 m^2

Question 33: B
The area of the house is 100 + 4 + (10 x 20) + (3 x 10) + (15 x 15) + 81 = 640 m^2.
The area of the master bedroom is 225 m^2, so the percentage area is 225/640 = 35%.

Question 34: D
The extra wall that is needed is the amount to extend both walls plus the new end wall.
The 20m wall is extended to 25m, and it is of height 3m, thus 5 x 3 = 15 m^2 is required.
Then the same amount of wall is needed for the other side, thus 2 x 15 = 30 m^2.
Then the back wall must be rebuilt, size = 10m x 3m = 30 m^2.
Sum these areas to a total of 60 m^2.

Question 35: B
Builder 1 costs: (15 x 300) + 200 = £4,700
Builder 2 costs: (16 x 300) = £4,800.
Therefore the requested ratio is 47:48, which is 1:1.02, to 3 s.f.

SET 10

Question 36: D
200 SMSs are free, so he pays for 7. £5 monthly fee + 7 SMSs x £0.20 + 15 minutes x £0.20 = £9.40

Question 37: C
Plan A SMSs cost 10p each. Plan B minimum cost is £5 monthly fee, but then provides 200 free SMSs. 51 SMSs at £0.10 each cost £5.10, which is more than £5. Thus, sending 51 SMSs would be cheaper on Plan B (sending 50 would be the same price on each plan).

Question 38: D
To answer this question, work out the cost of each plan.
5 minutes x 30 days = 150 minutes. 150 minutes cost: 150 x £0.10 = £15 on Plan A, 150 x £0.20 = £30 on

Plan B, (150-100 free minutes) x £0.20 = £10 on Plan C and 150 x £0.00 = £0 on Plan D.
Including the monthly fee, the cost to call becomes A: £15, B: £35, C: £20 and D: £15. All SMSs cost on Plan A but not D, so D is cheapest.

Note that we did not have to calculate the cost of texts in order to get the answer. If you like, you could work out the cost of the SMSs on each plan too, but if you notice that after calculating the cost of calls and monthly fees Plan A and Plan D come out at the same price, it is apparent that Plan D will be cheaper as SMSs are free, and this will save time.

Question 39: E
They each send 223 SMSs and make no calls. Option E is cheaper for Evan than Chris: For Plan B (223 SMSs – 200 free SMSs) x £0.20 = £4.60, so with the £5 monthly fee the total cost is £9.60. For Plan C all 223 SMSs are within the free limit, but the monthly fee is £10, so Chris pays more.

In option A, Evan pays £10.80, whilst Chris pays just the £10 monthly fee.
In option B, Evan pays £10.20, whilst Chris still just pays the monthly fee of £10.
In option C, Evan pays £36.80, whilst Chris still pays only the monthly fee of £10 (this is the biggest saving Chris makes relative to Evan out of all the options).
In option D, Evan pays between £27.40 and £29.80, depending on which month (and whether there are 28, 30 or 31 days in it), whilst Chris pays between £12.40 and £14.80, again dependent on which month.

Question 40: C
100 minutes are free on Plan C. Plan D has unlimited minutes and costs £5 more than C per month. At 20p a minute, Rachel can call for 25 minutes for £5, so can exceed her free minutes by 25 %, at which point Plan D is the same price. If she exceeds the free minutes allowance by any more than this, then plan D would be cheaper.

SET 11

Question 41: C
4 tablespoons is 4 x 15 ml = 60 ml. 250 ml is 1 cup, so 4 tablespoons is 60 ml/250 ml = 0.24 cups. 2 cups + 1 cup + ½ cup + 0.24 cups = 3.74 cups.

Question 42: A
First calculate the weight of butter called for by the recipe:
4 tablespoons = 60 ml = 0.06 litres = 0.06 dm^3 (the question states that 1dm^3 = 1 litre).
Weight of butter: 950 grams/dm^3 x 0.06 dm^3 = 57 grams.

Next, calculate the weight of milk called for by the recipe:
½ cup = 1.25 dl = 0.125 litres = 0.125 dm^3.
Weight of milk: 1050 grams/dm^3 x 0.125 dm^3 = 131.25 grams.

Question 43: E
Any whole number multiple of flour, sugar or milk can be measured with a ½ cup.

4 tablespoons is 60 ml, ½ cup is 125 ml. The least common multiple of 60 and 125 is 1500, representing the smallest possible amount of butter that can be measured with half-cup measures.

1500 grams of butter makes 25 batches of muffins, which would require 25 x 2 cups = 50 cups of flour.
Thus, the weight ratio of Milk:Butter is 131.25/57:1 = 2.3:1.

Question 44: A
The recipe will have:
2 cups of milk = 500 ml = 0.5 dm^3
1 cup of sugar = 250 ml = 0.25 dm^3
½ cup of flour = 125 ml = 0.125 dm^3
4 tablespoons of butter = 60 ml = 0.06 dm^3.
Therefore the volume of the batter is 0.5 dm^3 + 0.25 dm^3 + 0.125 dm^3 + 0.06 dm^3 = 0.935 dm^3.

Now, to calculate the density of the batter, multiply the density of each ingredient by the proportion of the batter it makes up, and then add up these figures, as follows:
(1050 grams/dm^3 milk x 0.5/0.935) + (850 grams/dm^3 sugar x 0.25/0.935) + (600 grams/dm^3 flour x 0.125/0.935) + (950 grams/dm^3 butter x 0.06/0.935) = 561.5 grams/dm^3 + 227.3 grams/dm^3 + 80.2 grams/dm^3 + 61.0 grams/dm^3 = 930 grams/dm^3

Question 45: E
10 muffins x 100 grams = 1,000 grams batter required.

The recipe calls for:
2 cups flour = 5 dl = 0.5 dm^3 flour. Weight of the flour is 0.5 dm^3 x 600 grams/dm^3 = 300 grams.
1 cup sugar = 2.5 dl = 0.25 dm^3 sugar. Weight of the sugar is 0.25 dm^3 x 850 grams/dm^3 = 212.5 grams.
From question 42 we remember that the weight of the milk as called for by the recipe is 131.25 grams and weight of the butter is 57 grams.

Thus the overall weight of the batter is 300 + 212.5 + 131.25 + 57 = 700.75 grams.
700.75/1,000 grams batter = 57/B grams butter, where B is the amount of butter required in 1,000g batter. B = 81.3 grams butter.

Question 46: C
700.75/1,000 grams batter = 300/F grams flour, where F is the amount of flour required to make 1,000 grams of muffin. F = 428.11 grams. 428.11 grams/1000 grams = 0.428 = 43 % to the nearest whole number.

SET 12

Question 47: A
The trend shows a 10 km^2 decrease in thickness for every 100 °C decrease in temperature. 10 km^2 thickness is 1,300 °C, so extrapolating the trend gives 0 km^2 thickness at 1,200 °C.

Question 48: D
Spreading rate is not affected by temperature, it is an independent variable. This question is designed to test your attention to detail and reinforce the importance of reading questions properly. Ensure you constantly pay attention to what the question is asking.

Question 49: D
Crustal volume per year = 20 km^2 crustal thickness x 20 mm/year spreading rate x 1 year = 20,000,000,000,000 mm^2 x 20 mm = 400,000,000,000,000 mm^3 = 400,000 m^3

Question 50: C
In answering this question, it is not necessary to use the same units for crustal thickness and spreading rate, as long as we use the same units for the crustal thickness *from both locations*, and likewise for the spreading rate.

Location A = 10 x 100 = 1,000. Location C = 30 x 150 = 4,500. A:C = 1:4,500/1,000 = 1:4.5

Question 51: A
Crustal volume per time = crustal thickness x spreading rate.
Crustal thickness at E is 10 km^2 and at F is 25 km^2.
Crustal volume per time is equal, so 10 km^2 x spreading rate E = 25 km^2 x spreading rate F. Therefore the spreading rate at E = 2.5 the spreading rate at F. Thus, it is 250 % faster.

Question 52: E
Temperature at D is 1,600 °C, decreased by 10 % it would be 1440 °C. From the trend in temperature and crustal thickness this corresponds to a crustal thickness of 24 km^2. Crustal volume per 3 years = 24 km^2 crustal thickness x 50 mm/year x 3 years = 24,000,000,000,000 mm^2 x 150 mm = 3,600,000,000,000,000 mm^3

SET 13

Question 53: C
A: 9/25, B: 6/23, C: 7/22, D: 8/24. (9+6+7+8)/(25+23+22+24) = 30/94 = 32 % to the nearest whole number.

Question 54: E
In Group A, drug-takers visual accuracy is 36%/27% = 33.33% improved.
In Group C, drug-takers visual accuracy is 31%/29% = 6.90% improved.
A:C = 33.33%/6.90%:1 = 4.83:1.

Question 55: C
10 women and 15 men have 45 % and unknown (P %) accuracy, respectively.
All 25 have an average of 36 % accuracy.
(10/25 x 45) + (15/25 x P) = 36.
P=30.

Question 56: A
Diabetics with vision problems correspond to Group A. In Group A, 15 of 25 volunteers reported better vision after taking the drug, but 9 of 25 volunteers taking a placebo also reported vision improvement. This suggests only 6 of 25 had reported improvements in their vision thanks to the effects of the drug.
6/25 x 100,000 people = 24,000 people.

Question 57: D
The placebo group showed no change, so only the volunteers being affected by the drug compound will see greater improvements to their vision.
15 – 9 = 6 volunteers affected by drug originally.
200% of the dose gave (18-9)/6 = 1.5 = 150 % the number of people with drug-related improvements.
300% of the dose will thus give 300 % / 200 % x 150 % = 225 % the number of people.
6 volunteers x 225% = 13.5 volunteers. (9+13.5)/25 volunteers = 22.5/25 volunteers = 90.0 % of volunteers.

Question 58: D
D is supported, because in all groups taking the placebo, there was an increase in accuracy with reading letters, suggesting better vision, and in many cases this was equivalent to the increase in those taking the drug.

The data suggest that A) and B) are incorrect. Only one group showed a higher increase in accuracy amongst the placebo group, in all other groups the people taking the drug had a larger % increase in accuracy. In healthy volunteers, there was as much of an increase in accuracy amongst those taking a placebo, suggesting the drug does not have as much of an effect in healthy volunteers. Options C) and E) are relatively meaningless statements which are not supported by the data.

SET 14

Question 59: C
5 calories x 200 pounds x 1 hour = 1000 calories running.
Cycling burns 50 calories + (5 calories x -5) for each mile = 25 calories per mile. Cycling 5 miles gives a total burn 125 calories, which is less than the amount burned running.

Thus, the maximum calorie burn comes from running, which will burn 1000 calories.

Question 60: D
Losing 10 pounds requires a 35 000 calorie deficit.
30 min run: 200 pounds x 0.5 hours x 5 calories = 500 calories.
20 mile cycle at 20 mph: 50 calories + (5 calories/mph x 10 mph) = 100 calories/mile for 20 miles = 2,000 calories. Daily burn is 2500 calories. 35,000/2,000 calories per day = 14 days taken to lose 10 pounds.

Question 61: C
Both their weight loss goal and calories burned running are linearly proportional to weight. Thus, they need to run for the same amount of time in order to achieve their goals.

Question 62: A
10% of 140 pounds is 14 pounds of weight, thus this is how much weight she wishes to lose.
At 3,500 calories/pound she needs a 14 pounds x 3500 calories/pound = 49,000 calorie deficit.

Her BMR is 1500 calories and she eats 400+500+250+200=1,350 calories per day, so her daily calorie deficit is 1,500 calories-1,350 calories = 150 calories.

It will take her 49 000 calories/150 calories per day = 326.67 days to reach her goal (327 to the nearest day).

Question 63: E

10 miles at 10 mph: 50 calories + (5 calories x 0 mph) = 50 calories/mile for 10 miles = 500 calories.

She requires a 49,000 calorie deficit, as worked out in the previous question. Previously she had a daily deficit of 150 calories, now she has a daily deficit of 650 calories. Thus, she now has a calorie deficit which is 4.33 times the previous deficit, so she will reach her goal 4.33 times faster.

Question 64: E

1 chocolate is the least she can eat, which means she eats 3 pieces of chicken and 6 bowls of cereal.
1x350 calories + 3x250 calories + 6x400 calories = 3,500 calories.

The lowest calorie arrangement of the 3 other foods is 1 lasagna, 3 vegetables and 6 apples.
1x700 calories + 3x200 calories + 6x100 calories = 1,900 calories.

She has a 3,500 calories per day – 1500 calorie BMR = 2,000 calorie surplus before and 400 calorie surplus after. 2,000 calories:400 calories = 5:1.

SET 15

Question 65: D

Price during day with single tickets is 4 coupons x £1 = £4.
Price at night with 10% off coupons is 3 coupons x £0.90 = £2.70.
Thus the saving is £1.30
Hence, the % saving is £1.30/£4.00 = 0.325 = 32.5 %.

Question 66: B

Price without a wristband is £1 per coupon x 120 % = £1.20 per coupon.
The number of coupons required is: 10 coupons entrance + 40 coupons for roller coaster + 6 coupons for candy floss + 1 coupon for the games + 4 coupons for the fun house + 3 coupons for the swings = 64 coupons.
64 coupons x £1.20 = £76.80.
Price with a wristband: £70 and 6 coupons for candy floss + 1 coupon for the games x £1.20 = £8.40. Thus the total price with a wristband is £78.40.

Therefore, the ratio is 1:£76.80/£78.40, which is 1:0.98.

Question 67: C

Andy rode the swings 20 % more times than he played games. The smallest number of times he could have gone on the swings is 6 times (since he can't have gone on the swings a non-integer number of times) so he played 5 games and went on the rollercoaster 9 times.
At night rates, rollercoaster 9 times x 3 coupons = 27 coupons and swings 6 times x 2 coupons = 12 coupons.
39 coupons at £1 each are worth £39, which is less than the £70 wristband.

If he had played 10 games, ridden the swings 12 times and rollercoaster 18 times, the wristband would have been more cost effective. This is the second cheapest possibility whilst still going on the swings an integer number of times (since 10 is the next multiple of 5). Thus, we know Andy must have played 5 games, been on the swings 6 times and the rollercoaster 9 times.

39 ride coupons + 5 game coupons + 5 entrance coupons = 49 coupons = £49.

Question 68: D

They got 69 coupons each for £69 pounds. They each must have spent 10 coupons at the entrance.
Together the roller coaster and fun house cost 6 coupons, so Anna took 59/6 = 9 rides on each and had 5 coupons left over, since the question states she went on each ride for *half* her rides, we assume she did not use any of the remaining coupons, since she could only have gone on one more ride, and thus it would not have been exactly half.

The fun house and swings cost 5 coupons together, so James took 59/5 = 11 rides on each and had 4 coupons left which he spent on 1 last ride on the swings.

Anna took 18 rides and James 23 rides. Anna: James = 1:23/18 = 1:1.28.

Question 69: E

First we calculate how much candyfloss Erik buys each weekend, using the 100% increase for the first 4 weeks, and the 50% increase thereafter as detailed in the question.
Week 1: 1, 2: 2, 3: 4, 4: 8, 5: 16, 6: 24, 7: 36, 8: 54, 9: 81, 10: 0. Thus, he bought a total of 226 lots of candy floss.
226 candy floss x 2 coupons x £1 pound each = £452.

Cost with season pass = £1000.
Cost without pass = £700 + £452 = £1,152.

SET 16

Question 70: B
2 x (£14.00 + £2.00 + 2x£2.00) + 1 x (£8.00 + 3x£1.00) + 3 x (£10.00) = £40.00 + £11.00 + £30.00 = £81.00.
50% off orders over £50 means he pays £81.00/2 = £40.50.
Ratio of cost Without:With is £1152/£1000:1 = 1.15:1.

Question 71: C
£35 is 50% of £70.
£70 buys £70/£14 = 5 large cheese pan pizzas.
Large pizzas have 10 slices: 10 slices x 5 pizzas = 50 slices.

Question 72: E
£60 is 50% off £120.
£120 is evenly divisible by all prices of plain cheese pizzas except the large pan. Dividing £120 by the price of the large pan gives 8.571. Since Joey cannot have bought a non-integer number of pizzas, he cannot have bought this type of pizza which costs £14.00.

Question 73: D
30 slices is 3 large pizzas or 5 small pizzas.
3 large pan pizzas with 2 toppings and stuffed crust cost: 3 x (£14.00 + (2x£2.00) + £2.00) = £60.00.
5 small pan pizzas with 2 toppings and stuffed crust cost: 5 x (£10.00 + 2x£0.50 + £1.00) = £60.00.
Large:Small ratio is 1:£60.00/£60.00 = 1:1.00

Question 74: A
The lowest price order over £31 is 2 small pizzas and 1 medium pizza costing £32 total. 30% off £32 = £22.40. They get 20 slices with this order, but we know that they got 25% more than they could eat. Thus, if we treat 20 slices as 125%, then 100% is the amount that they ate. 20/1.25 = 16, so this is the amount that they could eat.

SET 17

Question 75: E
1 hour at Job A = £10 starter - £5 travel + £10 per hour = £15.
1 hour at Job B = £5 starter - £0 travel + £15 per hour = £20.
1 hour at Job C = £5 starter - £10 travel + £20 per hour = £15.
A:B:C = £15:£20:£15 = 1:1.33:1.

Question 76: C
In her first 50 hours she worked 25 2-hour jobs: 25 x (£10 - £5 + 2x£10) = 25 x £25 = £625.
Her hourly wage was then increased to £10 + £5 = £15.

She then worked 4 1-hour jobs: 4 x (£10 - £5 + 1x£15) = 4 x £20 = £80.
Then she worked 1 4-hour job: 1 x (£10 - £5 + 4x£15) = 1 x £65 = £65.

Her total earnings were £625 + £80 + £65 = £770.00

Question 77: E
For Job A, for the first 50 hours she would earn £10 an hour. Thus, for the first 25 2-hour jobs she would earn 25 x (£10 - £5 +2x£10) = £625. After 50 hours, her hourly wage would increase to £15 an hour. Thus, for the second lot of 25 2-hour jobs she would earn 25 x (£10 - £5 + 2x£15) = £875. Thus, in total she would earn £1,750.
For Job B, for the 50 2-hour jobs, she would earn 50 x (£5 + 2x£15) = £1,750. She does not get the pay increase because she does not work any hours after the pay rise at 100 hours.
For Job C, for the 50 2-hour jobs, she would earn 50 x (£5 - £10 + 2x£20) = £1,750.
Thus, B and C are the same.

Question 78: D
Average job length for Job C is 4 hours.
1 4-hour job earns: £5 starter - £10 travel + 4x£20 per hour = £75 per job.
Maximum earnings £1250/£75 = 17 jobs.
17 jobs x 4 hours = 68 hours.

Question 79: D
Hourly wage has risen twice by £5 to £30 per hour (since it rises £5 for each 100 hours worked).
100 hours/4 hour jobs = 25 jobs.
For a 4 hour job she earns: £5 starter - £10 travel + 4x£30 per hour = £115 per job.
25 jobs x £115 per job = £2,875.

10% of £2,875 = £287.50. This is the amount she pays in income tax.

Question 80: D
Working 50 hours for Job B earns 50 times the hourly rate plus 50 times the fixed starter wage, as jobs average 1 hour in duration. Therefore the income = (50x£15) + (50x£5) = £1,000.00.
The extra 50 hours can be worked at either Job A, B or C (note that Jobs A and B have travel expenses).
The same calculation for Job A gives (10x50) + (10 x 25) – (5x25) = £625.00.
The same calculation for Job C gives (50x20) + (5x12.5) – (10x12.5) = £937.50.

Therefore she earns most by working 100 hours for Job B.

SET 18

Question 81: A
Monday has the 2nd highest number of passengers, so this will be the 2nd highest grossing day. On Monday the revenue is £5 x 2346 underground passengers = £11,730.00.
On Wednesday the revenue is 3,103 x 0.85 x £5 = £1,3187.75. £13,187.75 - £11,730.00 = £1,457.75

Question 82: C
Total number of weekday underground passengers = 2346 +1798 +3103 + 2118 + 1397 = 10,762
Total number of weekday car passengers = total passengers – number of drivers =
Monday: 1873-1517=356
Tusesday: 2421-1632=789
Wednesday: 1116-987=129
Thursday: 2101-1465=636
Friday: 2822-2024 =798
356+789+129+636+798 = 2708

The average ratio is 10,762 : 2,708 = 1:3.97

Question 83: E
Tuesday: 2,421/1,632= 1.48
Weekend: 1,339/478= 2.80.
Ratio of Tuesday to Saturday = 1.48/2.8 = 1:1.89

Question 84: B
This is straightforward: 2,346/576 = 4.07:1 = 1:0.25

Question 85: D
There are 4,219 commuters each day (as seen by adding the total car passengers and underground passengers on any given day). For every 1 car there are 1.7 passengers and 2 underground riders. Thus, by dividing 1.7 by 3.7 and multiplying this by the total number of passengers (4219), we can calculate how many people are in cars:
1.7/3.7 x 4,219 = 1,938 people drive (to the nearest whole number, obviously there cannot be a non-integer number of people driving).
Now, by dividing the number of people driving (1938) by the number of passengers, we can calculate the number of cars: 1938/1.7 = 1,140 cars.
1,140 cars x £4 = £4,560. £4,560 + 1,938x£1 = £6,498. 80% of £6,498 is £5,198.40.

SET 19

Question 86: E
First calculate the Superior room cost at night: 3hrs x £26.00/hr = £78.00. Now add 10%: £78 x 1.1 = £85.80

Question 87: D
Total cost minus deposit = 12hrs x £30/hr = £360
Deposit = £460 - £360 = £100

Question 88: B
Total deposit = £10 + £25 = £35
6hrs in Standard room = 6hrs x £18/hr = £108
6hrs in Basic Room = £221 – (£108 + £35) = £78
Basic room hourly rate (2-6hrs) = £78 ÷ 6hrs = £13/hr

Question 89: B
1.5hrs in Superior room (night session) = 1.5hrs x £30/hr = £45
Decreased by 5% = £45 x 0.95 = £42.75
Total cost = £50 deposit + £42.75 = £92.75

Question 90: B
Basic room all day cost = 18hrs x £8/hr = £144
All week = 7 days x £144 = £1,008
Three weeks = £1,008 x 3 = £3,024
Deducting the VAT = £3,024/1.25 = £2,419.20

SET 20

Question 91: C
Total number of people aged under 22 = sum of first two columns = 62
Number aged <22 who spotted >10 differences = 11 + 8 + 3 + 2 = 24
Percentage = 24/62 = 38.7%

Question 92: D
Valid results for 5-10 spots for ages 16-22 = 0.25 x 12 = 3
Total number of valid results for 16-22 = 10 + 3 + 8 + 2 = 23
Percentage of over 15 spots for 16-22 = 2 ÷ 23 = 8.7%

Question 93: C
Total who spotted over 10 = sum of bottom two rows = 52. 25% of 52 = 13

Question 94: E
Total 48+ who spotted <5 = 15 + 19 = 34
Total aged 48+ = sum of final two columns = 66
Percentage of 48+ who spotted <5 = 34 ÷ 66 = 52% (2 s.f.)
52% of 10,000 = 0.52 x 10,000 = 5,200

Question 95: E
50% increase in 16-34s who spot 11-15 = 1.5 x (8 + 6) = 21
New total who spot 11-15 = 11 + 21 + 2 + 8 + 9 = 51
Ratio = 21:51

SET 21

Question 96: B
Number that play Football = 22% of 1300 = 286
Number that play Hockey = 8 % of 1300 = 104
Thus, the difference = 286-104 = 182 Boys + Girls; Therefore, 182/2 = 91 Boys

Question 97: D
22% of 350 = 77 students
77 ÷ 11 people per team = 7 teams

Question 98: C
Number of basketball boys = 0.05 x 1,300 = 65. 80% of 65 = 52
Number of netball girls = 0.08 x1, 300 = 104
Total number of netball-players = 104 + 52 = 156
Male proportion = 52 ÷ 156 = 33% (2 s.f.)

Question 99: D
Number of *Other* students = 0.12 x 1,300 = 156
Other ball sports = 0.25 x 156 = 39
Total non-ball sports (swimming & athletics) = (0.06 + 0.03) x 1300 = 117
Total "other" non ball sports = 156 – 39 = 117
Total ball sports = 1,300 – 117 – 117 = 1,066

Question 100: A
Girls who play hockey = 0.07 x 1,300 = 91
Boys who play cricket = 0.1 x 1,300 = 130
Difference = 39. *Note the tennis info makes no difference (50:50 split)*

SET 22

Question 101: A
Total apples processed in 1998 = 1,100,547 + 2,983,411 = 4,083,958
Total apples processed in 2003 = 1,931,784 + 2,439,012 = 4,370,796
Ratio = 4,370,796 ÷ 4,083,958 = 1.07 (i.e. 7% increase)

Question 102: E
Number of No Goods in worst year = 571,221
Total number of No Goods = sum of bottom row = 2,823,732
Percentage = 571,221 ÷ 2,823,732 = 20.2% (3 s.f.)

Question 103: A
2004 total No Goods = 3 x 571,221 = 1,713,663
70% of edible apples are processed, as are all passable apples.
Difference = (0.7 x 1,931,784 + 2,439,012) – 1,713,663 = 2,077,598

Question 104: C
Total number of edibles 1998-2003 = sum of top row = 9,201,790
20% increase = 1.2 x 9,201,790 = 11,042,148
30% of these are sold as they come = 0.3 x 11,042,148 = 3,312,644

Question 105: B
Apples processed for cider = (1,931,784 x 0.7) + 2,439,012 = 3,791,260.8
Litres of cider = 3,791,260.80 ÷ 20 = 189,600 litres (4 s.f.)

SET 23

Question 106: C
Decreased average speed = 0.92 x 5 mph = 4.6 mph
Miles covered = 4.6 x (40 ÷ 60) = 3.07 miles
Km covered = 1.6 x 3.07 miles = 4.9 km

Question 107: C
Distance per session = 26 miles ÷ 4 = 6.5 miles
Time per session = 6.5 miles ÷ 5 mph = 1.3 hrs = 1hr 18mins

Question 108: B
New wet average speed = 0.92 x 4.6 mph = 4.232 mph
12 km in miles = 12 km ÷ 1.6 = 7.5 miles
Time taken = 7.5 miles ÷ 4.232 mph = 1.77 hrs = 1hr 46mins

Question 109: B
Distance of second jog = 4 km x 1.5 = 6 km
Distance of third jog = 6 km x 1.5 = 9 km
Distance of last jog = 9 km x 1.5 = 13.5 km
13.5 km in miles = 13.5 km ÷ 1.6 = 8.4375 miles
Time = 8.4375 miles ÷ 5 mph = 1.69 hrs = 1hr 41mins

Question 110: C
3hrs 42mins = 3.7 hrs
Average speed = 26 miles ÷ 3.7 hrs = 7.027 mph
7.027 mph ÷ 5 mph = 1.405 (i.e. 41% increase)

SET 24

Question 111: C
Standard price = (£325 + £100) ÷ 2 = £212.50
For two people for one week = £212.50 x 2 = £425
Deducting 20% due to discount = 0.8 x £425 = £340

Question 112: C
Four weeks rent per person = 4 x £480 = £1,920
Total group rent = 12 x £1,920 = £23,040
Booking fee per person = 0.1 x £480 = £48
Total booking fee = 12 x £48 = £576
Total cost = £23,040 + £576 = £23,616

Question 113: C
One person for 10 days = £80 x (20÷7) = £228.57
Two people for 10 days = 2 x £228.57 = £457.14
Booking fee = £492.89 - £457.14 = £35.75

Question 114: A
Total rent = £220 x 2 weeks x 4 people = £1,760
Total discount = £1,760 x 0.2 = £352
Total cost = £1,760 - £352 = £1,408

Question 115: A
Booking fee = 0.1 x £19,500 = £1,950
Total rental charge = £19,500 - £1,950 = £17,550
Number of people = £17,550 ÷ £325 = 54
Number in each palazzo = 54 ÷ 3 = 18 people.

SET 25

Question 116: B
The price of the food is £3.95 + £2.95 + £3.95 = £10.85. Orders between £10 and £15 are charged £1.50 for delivery. Including delivery, the cost is £12.35. We then add 20%, so multiply this by 1.2. Hence the cost of the takeaway is £14.82.

Question 117: C
The total price is (3 x £2.95) + (2 x £4.95) + £3.95 = £22.70. Delivery is free above £15. We then add 20%, hence the total cost is £27.24.
A promotional offer is introduced whereby customers receive a 10% discount for orders over £9 (not including delivery).

Question 118: A
The total price is (2 x £2.95) + £3.95 = £9.85. Add £3 for delivery under £10: 9.85 + 3 = 11.865. Add 20% for VAT: 11.865 x 1.2 = £15.42

Question 119: B
The total is £3.95 + (3 x £2.95) + £3.95 = £16.75. Delivery is free over £15. We then add 20% for VAT: 16.75 x 1.2 = £20.10

Question 120: D
The total price is (2 x £2.95) + (2 x £4.95) + £3.95 = £19.75 (price of only two noodles because of offer)
Delivery is free over £15. We then add 20% for VAT: 19.75 x 1.2 = £23.70

SET 26

Question 121: B
Divide the profits earned by MediCo by the total profits earned by all suppliers: (15,000 + 30,000 + 25,000 + 35,000) = £105,000. 30,000/105,000 = 28.6%.

Question 122: C
Divide the profits earned by MediCo and Lifecare combined by the total profits earned by all suppliers: (15,000 + 30,000 + 25,000 + 35,000) = £105000. (30,000 + 35,000)/105,000 = 61.9%.

Question 123: C
Increase the profit of PillPlus by 15% and use this value when calculating the new total profit earned by all suppliers: 25,000 x 1.15 = 28,750. 28,750/(15,000 + 30,000 + 28,750 + 35,000) = 26.4%.

Question 124: A
As all profits across suppliers decrease by an equal amount, this is irrelevant and cancels in the division. 0.9(35,000 + 15,000)/0.9(35,000 + 28,750 + 30,000 + 15,000) = 46%.

Question 125: B
Take account of the first fall in profits of 10% and then a further fall of 5%: (15,000 + 35,000) x 0.9 x 0.95 = £42,750.

SET 27

Question 126: A
The total value for the Stuntman is £12500 + £345 + £145 + £295 = £13,285.
Adding 20% VAT, this is £13,285 x 1.2 = £15,942.

Question 127: B
Remember to include tax in all calculations:
Saloon: (£21500 + £495 + £245 + £445) = £22,685. £22,685 x 1.2 = £27,222.
Pod: (£18000 + £445 + £395 + £495) = £19335. £19335 x 1.2 = £23,202.
£27,222 - £23,202 = £4020

Question 128: C
Racer: (£15,000 x 1.2) = £18,000.
Stuntman: (£12500 + £345 + £145 + £295) = £13,285. £13,285 x 1.2 = £15,942.
£18,000 - £15,942 = £2,058

Question 129: C
The Pod with no optional extras is £18000 x 1.2 = £21,600.
The Racer with all optional extras with a 10% discount is (£15000 + £395 + £195 + £395) x 0.9 x 1.2 = £17,263.80.
£21,600 - £17263.80 = £4,336.20

Question 130: D
Saloon with leather seats and easy-park technology = £21500 + £495 + £445 = £22440.
Add 20% = £22,440 x 1.2 = £26,928. Reduced by 20% = £26928 x 0.8 = £21,542.40.
Pod = £18,000 x 1.2 = £21600.
£21,600 - £21,542.40 = £57.60

SET 28

Question 131: C
Emissions increased by 1,000 tonnes from 1,000 to 2,000 tonnes over 5 years, therefore the rate of increase was 200 tonnes per year

Question 132: A
If there had been no crash, 2,010 emissions would have been 3,000 Tonnes, as calculated by applying an increase in emissions of 200 Tonnes/year from 2005 to 2010.
With the economic crash, 2010 emissions were 2500 Tonnes:
3,000 – 2,500 = 500 Tonnes less in 2010 due to the economic crash.

Question 133: C
Percentage increase = (new amount – old amount)/old amount x 100
= (3,000–2,000)/2,000 x 100 = 50%.
Note that you are asked for the percentage INCREASE. (New amount/old amount) x100 = percentage CHANGE.

Question 134: B
2015 – 2020 the amount would increase from 3,000 tonnes to 3,500 tonnes without any action. This equates to a rate of increase of 100 tonnes per year. With the new act, this is reduced by 50% to 50 tonnes per year, thus over 5 years: Overall saving = 50 x 5 = 250 Tonnes

Question 135: C
The emissions in 2020 = projected – rate reduction (50% of the difference between projected total and current total). Rate reduction = 50 tonnes per year. Projected rate = current emissions (3,000 tonnes) + projected increase without the act (5 x 100, which is 500).
= (3,000+500) – (5 x 50) = 3250 Tonnes

SET 29

Question 136: B
For between 10 and 100 units, single sided black and white printing costs £0.07 per page. 74 x 7p = £5.18.

Question 137: C
£100 will clearly buy more than 100 sheets as all prices are under £1, therefore use the 100+ price:
The price for double sided colour printing over 100 sheets is £0.25.
£100/0.25 = 400 sheets

Question 138: A
For over 100 sheets of double sided black and white, the cost per sheet is £0.10 each. Hence the total non-discounted price for 150 sheets is 150 x £0.10 = £15. If this is discounted by 10%, this is £15 x 0.9 = £13.50.

Question 139: B
Price for buying separately = 150 x 0.15 = £22.50
Price buying together = 150 x 0.10 x 0.9 (discount) = £13.50
Difference = £9
Number of sheets could buy with £9 = 9/0.15 = 60 sheets

Question 140: B
The price for 227 sheets of double sided black and white printing is £0.10 each, so the total is £22.70.
The price for 34 sheets of double sided colour printing is £0.30 each, so the total is £10.20.
The total for all the sheets is £32.90.
If this is discounted by 10%, this is £32.90 x 0.9 = £29.61.

SET 30

Question 141: D
We can calculate the number of people who reacted positively in each group and then add up the total:
75% of 300 is 225
65% of 300 is 195
70% of 300 is 210
55% of 300 is 165
225 + 195 + 210 + 165 = 795

Question 142: C
In group 2, 30% reacted negatively: 30% of 300 is 90.
In group 3, 15% reacted negatively: 15% of 300 is 45.
Therefore the difference is 45; 45 more people in group 2 reacted negatively than people in group 3.

Question 143: B
We can calculate the number of people who reacted negatively in each group and then add up the total:
20% of 300 is 60
30% of 300 is 90
15% of 300 is 45
25% of 300 is 75
60 + 90 + 45 + 75 = 270. 270 as a percentage of the total, 1200, is 22.5%, which rounds to 23%.

Question 144: D
The overall success rate of the first four groups was = (75 + 65 + 70 + 55)/4 = 66.25%
Therefore increase in success rate = 82/66.25 = 23.77% increase.

Question 145: B
In the answer to question 143 we calculated that in the first 4 groups, 270 people reacted negatively. In group 5, 15% of 300 people, which is 45 people, reacted negatively. Hence the negative reactions total 315 people.

SET 31

Question 146: C
The total number of views of The Last Chase is 20,000 + 20,000 + 15,000 + 20,000 = 75,000.
The total number of views of The Final Frontier is 15,000 + 20,000 + 25,000 + 35,000 = 95,000.
Hence the difference is 95,000 – 75,000 = 20,000

Question 147: B
The difference in viewers is 20,000. If £2,500 is earned per 1,000 viewers, then the difference in advertising revenue will be £2,500 x 20 = £50,000.

Question 148: B
Growth rate is 5,000 per quarter between Q1 and Q3 of 2014. Therefore the total growth during 2015:
35,000 + (5,000 x 4) = 55,000

Question 149: B
Growth rate is 5,000 per quarter between Q1 and Q3 of 2014. Therefore the total growth during 2015:
Q1: 35,000 + 5,000 = 40,000
Q2: 40,000 + 5,000 = 45,000
Q3: 45,000 + 5,000 = 50,000
Q4: 50,000 + 5,000 = 55,000
Thus, the total number of views = 40,000 + 45,000 + 50,000 + 55,000 = 190,000.

Question 150: D
Without the show cancellation, there are 35,000 Final Frontier views and 20,000 Last Chase views. With the cancellation, half of the Last Chase views transfer over to Final Frontier, this equates to 10,000 views. Therefore the Final Frontier now has 45,000 views in this scenario.

SET 32

Question 151: C
55% + 25% = 80% of Scottish patients wait less than half an hour. 80% of 50,000 patients = 40,000, therefore 40,000 patients waited for less than half an hour for an appointment.

Question 152: B
We can work out how many patients had to wait more than half an hour for an appointment in each part of the UK then find the total:
In England, 10% of 100,000 patients = 10,000 patients had to wait longer than half an hour.
In Scotland, 20% of 50,000 patients = 10,000 patients had to wait longer than half an hour.
In Wales, 25% of 25,000 patients = 6,250 patients had to wait longer than half an hour.
In Northern Ireland, 15% of 25,000 patients = 3,750 patients had to wait longer than half an hour.
The total number of patients that had to wait longer than half an hour is 10,000 + 10,000 + 6,250 + 3,750 = 30,000.
30,000/200,000 = 15%

Question 153: C
In the previous question we found that 30,000 patients had to wait longer than half an hour, so 40% of 30,000 people complained = 12,000.

In England, 30% of 100,000 patients = 30,000 patients had to wait 11-30 minutes.
In Scotland, 25% of 50,000 patients = 12,500 patients had to wait 11-30 minutes.
In Wales, 25% of 25,000 patients = 6,250 patients had to wait had to wait 11-30 minutes.
In Northern Ireland, 25% of 25,000 patients = 6,250 patients had to wait 11-30 minutes.
The total number of patients that had to wait 11-30 minutes is 30,000 + 12,500 + 6,250 + 6,250 = 55,000.
If 20% of 55,000 patients complain, this is 11,000.
Hence the total number of complaints is 11,000 + 12,000 = 23,000.

Question 154: B
Use the total survey size to calculate the proportion: 23,000/200,000 = 11.5%.

Question 155: B
We worked out in question 153 that 30,000 people had to wait longer than 30 minutes and 55,000 people had to wait between 11 and 30 minutes. If the targets are met, 15,000 people will have to wait longer than 30 minutes and 41,250 will have to wait between 11 and 30 minutes. If 20% of these 41,250 people complain, this is 8,250 complaints. If 40% of the 15,000 people complain this is 6,000 complaints. Hence there are a total of 14,250 complaints. The previous number of complaints was 23,000, hence the percentage decrease is (23,000-14,250)/23,000 = 0.38 = 38%.

SET 33

Question 156: D
The decrease in the price of crude oil between January and March is $150-$100 = $50, as can be seen in the graph. This fall has occurred over a 2-month period, giving a decrease in price of $25 per month.

Question 157: D
This is a question of estimation. The average production across the year is at least 7 million barrels per day. Multiplying this by 365 gives around 2,550 million barrels per year. All other options require less than 7 million barrels daily production, and it is clear there are at least 7 million barrels per day. Therefore the answer is 2,700 million.

Alternatively, we can estimate using 30 days per month, and multiplying the amount of barrels produced per day in each month by 30 (this is more accurate but more time consuming). 6+7+7+7.5+7.5+7+7.5+8+8.5+8.5+8+9 = 91.5, multiplying by 30 gives just over 2,700 million barrels per year.

Question 158: C
Use both graphs. For July, multiply the oil price by the amount sold in the month, and then multiply by the number of days in the month.
July = 7.5 million barrels x $75 per barrel x 31 days = $17,400 million = $17.4 billion

Question 159: B
If the costs are 40%, the gross profit is 60%.
Oil sales in June 2014 totalled 7 million barrels x $100 per barrel x 30 days = £21,000 million = $21 billion.
Therefore gross profit was 0.6 x $21 billion = $12.6 billion.

Question 160: A
You are given the total sales value of $204 billion, so work with this. Work clearly in stages and this question is not hard.
The profit is 60% of this, which is $122.4 billion.
This is split 5:2 between the oil companies and the oil-producing nation. Thus, the profit for the oil companies is 5/7 of $122.4 billion is profit for the oil companies, which is $87.43 billion.
Corporation tax is then 30% of this profit, which is $26.23 billion.

SET 34

Question 161: B
Calculate the total people with no asthma, then take it away from the total number of people which is 250:
80% of the 50 people aged 0-5 have no asthma, which is 40.
75% of the 50 people aged 5-10 have no asthma, which is 37.5.
85% of the people aged 10-21 have no asthma, which is 42.5.
95% of the people aged 21-30 have no asthma, which is 47.5.
95% of the people aged 30+ have no asthma, which is 47.5.
Hence the total people who have no asthma is 215.
Hence the total people with asthma is 250 – 215 = 35.

Question 162: B
Of children aged 0-5, 15% have mild asthma which is 7.5. Hence 3.75 will develop respiratory problems.
Of children aged 0-5, 5% have severe asthma which is 2.5. Hence 2.25 will develop respiratory problems.
Of children aged 5-10, 20% have mild asthma which is 10. Hence 5 will develop respiratory problems.
Of children aged 5-10, 5% have severe asthma which is 2.5. Hence 2.25 will develop respiratory problems.
Hence 13.25 children per 100 will develop respiratory problems, so the answer is 13.25%.

Question 163: A
(15%+20%)/2 = 17.5% diagnosed. 17.5% x 0.35 = 6.125% Incorrect diagnoses.

Question 164: B
Taking into account that only 65% of children diagnosed with mild asthma were diagnosed correctly:
17.5% diagnosed (mild) ➔ 11.375% correctly diagnosed ➔ 5.69% complications
5% diagnosed (severe) ➔ 4.5% complications (all are correct diagnoses)
Therefore 5.69 + 4.5 = 10% overall respiratory complication rate.

Question 165: A
False diagnoses: (0.15x0.35x0.07x50,000,000) 0-5 year olds + (0.2x0.35x0.1x50,000,000) 5-10 year olds = 533,750
Cost per diagnosis: £50 per year = £250 over 5 years
Total money wasted: 533,750 x £250 = £133 million

SET 35

Question 166: D
Total value of company A = (price per share x number of shares) = £60 x 10 million = £600 million
Government holding = 75% of 600 million = £450 million
Disinvestment (50%) = 0.5 x 450 = £225 million
Hence £225 million is raised from the disinvestment.

Question 167: A
Total value of company B = (price per share x number of shares) = £20 x 50 million = 1,000 million
Government holding = 50% of 1,000 Million = £500 million
Disinvestment (25%) = 0.25 x 500 = £125 million

Question 168: B
Government holds 1/3 of the 30 million shares, which is 10 million shares.
It sold each share for £35, £5 less than the £40 market price. Hence the additional revenue for selling at the market price would have been £5 per share x 10 million shares = £50 million.

Question 169: B
Government holds 25% of 40 million shares, which is 10 million shares.
The price of each share fell from £30 to £35, so fell by £5 per share.
If the price of 10 million shares fell by £5, the total fall was £50 million.

Question 170: C
Government holds 12.5% of 50 million shares, which is 6.25 million.
The price has risen by £5 per share, so the total rise is £31.25 million.

Question 171: B
Total value of option A = £10 x 60 million x 75% = £450 Million
Total value of option B = £20 x 50 million x 50% = £500 Million
Hence they will fetch difference values, with B fetching more.

SET 36

Question 172: C
In 2011-2012, food grain production was 100, and this was a 25% increase on 2010-2011.
If 100 is 125%, then 100% = 80. Hence food production in tonnes in 2010-2011 was 80 tonnes.

Question 173: B
Target production (2011-12) = 60 tonnes
Actual production (2010-11) = 50/125% = 40 tonnes
Difference = 60 - 40 = 20 tonnes

Question 174: B
Difference = Target - Actual = 50 - 40 = 10 tonnes

Question 175: D
Cotton production (2010-11) = 30/120% = 25 tonnes
Jute production (2010-11) = 20/125% = 16 tonnes
Combined = 25 + 16 = 41 tonnes

Question 176: D
Food grain production (2010-11) = 100/125% = 80 tonnes
Oil seeds production (2010-11) = 50/125% = 40 tonnes
Difference = 80 - 40 = 40 tonnes

Question 177: B
Total production (2011-12) = 100+50+40+30+20 = 240 tonnes
Cotton as a percentage of total = 30/240 = 12.5%

SET 37

Question 178: D
Sales of product B in Feb = 7,000
Total sales of all products in Feb = 10,250 + 7,000 + 3,750 + 3100 = 24,100
Percentage of product B's sales = 7,000/24,100 = 29%

Question 179: D
Percentage increase:
Product A = (11,000-10,500)/10,500 = 4.76%
Product B = (7,500-7,250)/7,250 = 3.45%
Product C = (4,250-4,000)/4,000 = 6.25%
Product D = (4,000-3,500)/3,500 = 14.29%

Hence product D witnessed highest percentage growth.

However to answer this question more quickly, look at the numbers – the numbers are giving you a clue. You can visually see that product D's sales' values have gone up the equal maximum amount of £500. But it is also apparent that the absolute value of sales is the lowest, therefore you can deduce that D is the largest percentage increase without actually doing any sums!

Question 180: C
Sales of product C in May = 4,250 x 1.2 = 5,100
Therefore sales of product D in May = 5,100
Percentage increase in sales of D from April to May = (5,100 – 4,000)/4,000 = 27.5%

Question 181: D
Sale of products (A+C) in January = 13,000
Sale of products (A+C) in April = 15,250
Percentage increase in combined sale from January to April = (15,250 – 13,000)/13,000 = 17.31%

Question 182: A
Sale of product (A+B) in May = 1.2 x (11,000+75,00) = 22,200
Sale of product (C+D) in May = 1.3 x (4,250+4,000) = 10,725
Total sales in May = 32925

Question 183: D
Sale of product A in May = 1.2 x 11,000 = 13,200
Sale of product (B+C+D) in May = 1.1 x (7,500+4,250+4,000) = 173,25
Total sales in May = 13,200+17,325 = 30,525
Percentage of sales of A over total sales = 13,200/30,525 = 43.24%

SET 38

Question 184: C
Overall profit is 30% of revenue. Since profit = £2.5 million, overall revenue = 2.5/30 x 100 = £8.3 Million

Question 185: B
Let us assume cost per article = C; Total number of articles = N
Cost per consignment:
Rail = 25C/30N = 0.83C/N
Road = 25C/45N = 0.56C/N
Air = 50C/25N = 2C/N
Hence road has the lowest cost per consignment.
However if you look at the figures, a shortcut is apparent. Road occupies by far the greatest number of consignments, but the cost is the equal lowest in the business. Therefore at a glance you can see the answer is road, even before you open the calculator and start doing unnecessary sums.

Question 186: A
The ratio will be the same for any number of consignments as the proportions are preserved.
Ratio of total revenue to total cost = £20:£5 = 4:1

Question 187: C
From the table it is given that 50% of the total costs are associated with air transportation, so 50% of the total costs are due to air travel.
50% x £54,000 = £27,000

Question 188: D
From the table it is given that 30% are delivered by rail and 45% by road, so 75% of consignments are delivered by rail and road taken together.
75% x 17,145 = 12,859

SET 39

Question 189: A

This is a difficult question that would be worth "flagging for review". Set the percentage of lead in alloy A to a, and the percentage of tin in alloy C to b. We can then find the percentage of copper in each as a function of a and b.

Alloy	Zinc	Tin	Lead	Copper	Nickel
A	10%	40%	a%	(40-a)%	10%
B	25%	15%	50%	5%	5%
C	15%	b%	20%	(30-b)%	35%

The key thing here is to use the composition of Alloy G. We can find the composition of Alloy G in terms of a and b and then set the amounts of tin, lead and copper equal to each other to find a and b:

For Alloy G, the percentages will be weighted according to the proportion A:B:C = 2:1:3:
2/6 (40) + 1/6 (15) + 3/6 (b) = 2/6 (a) + 1/6 (50) + 3/6 (20) = 2/6 (40-a) + 1/6 (5) + 3/6 (30-b)

80 + 15 + 3b = 2a + 50 + 60 = 80 -2a + 5 + 90 -3b
Solving above equation, we will get values:
95 + 3b = 2a + 110
2a + 110 = 175 – 2a – 3b
3b = 65 – 4a
2a = 95 – 110 + 65 – 4a
6a = 50
a = 50/6
b = 95/9
Percentage of Lead in alloy A = a = 50/6% = 25/3% = 8.33%

Question 190: C

Using our solution from the previous question, we found that the percentage of Tin in alloy C, b, was:
b = 95/9
Percentage of Tin in alloy C = 95/9 = 10.6%

Question 191: B

Zinc percentage in alloy X is equal to the average of the percentages of the composite alloys, as they are present in equal proportions. This can be found by adding together and dividing by 3.
X = (10+25+15)/3 = 50/3 = 16.67%

Question 192: D

To solve, subtract the amounts of the known metals to find the remaining metal, which is equal to the percentage of Tin and Copper combined in alloy C. We know there are no other components as this is stated in the question.

(100% – 15% – 20% – 35%) = 30%

Question 193: B

We know the percentages of tin in each of the alloys which make up Alloy G, and the composition of Alloy G. Alloy G is made up of alloys A:B:C in the ratio 2:1:3. Alloy A has 40% tin, alloy B has 15% and alloy C has 95/9% tin. Hence the percentage in Alloy G is (2/6 x 40)+(1/6 x 15)+(3/6 x 95/9) = 21.11%.

Question 194: C
Percentage of elements in alloy G:

We know that Alloy G has 21.11% Tin from the last question. We also know from the initial explanation that it has the same concentration of tin, lead and copper. This is 3 elements with the same concentration. We then need to work out how much nickel and zinc there is to check whether there is a 4th.

Alloy G is made up of alloys A:B:C in the ratio 2:1:3. Alloy A has 10% nickel, alloy B has 5% and alloy C has 35% nickel. Hence the percentage in Alloy G is ((2x10)+(1x5)+(3x35))/6, = 21.6666.

We can also work out from the fact that these 4 elements plus Zinc are 100% of the total that Zinc is 15%.

Zinc = 15%
Tin = 21.11%
Lead = 21.11%
Copper = 21.11%
Nickel = 21.67%

SET 40

Question 195: A
Number of persons who voted in favour of Hilary Clinton = 60% of 17% of 11,500 = 0.6x0.17x11, 500 = 1173.

Question 196: D
We cannot find the number of people living in New York, as we do not know the proportion of citizens of New York who voted for people other than Robert Guiliani. We can only say that there was a minimum of 460 New York citizens. We cannot determine the actual number.

Question 197: D
0.39 x 11,500 = 44,85 votes for Bush.
Therefore 4,485/(11,500 x 0.8) gives the proportion of US citizens who voted for Bush.
This equals 48.8%.

Question 198: C
10% of 40% of people surveyed are in favour of Rumsfield and employees of the federal government, so 10% of 40% of 11,500 = 460 people.
Also from the table, Rumsfield has 5% of 11500 votes = 575 people who are in favour of him in total.
Hence the number of people who are in favour of Rumsfeld who are not employees of the federal government is 575-460 = 115.

Question 199: C
The number of people polled was constant. The decrease in percentage is from 16% to 2%, i.e. 14 % of 11,500 = 1,610 people.

Question 200: A
The number of people polled was constant. The decrease in percentage is from 40% to 39%, i.e. 1% of 11,500 = 115 people.

SET 41

Question 201: E
15% indicates that only 85% of the total price is to be paid.
50p is the price per unit for premium mugs for quantity below 49 units.
20p is the price per unit for basic mugs for quantity below 49 units.
5p is the price per unit for logo on basic mugs for quantity below 49 units.
Using this information, we can work out:
0.85x(5x50p+4x(20p+5p)) = 297.5p = £2.975 rounded up to £2.98
Therefore the company will have to pay £2.98

Question 202: B
20p is the price per unit for premium mugs for quantity above 500 units.
10p is the price per unit for basic mugs for quantity between 100 and 499 units.
3p is the price to add logos to those mugs.
4p is the price per unit for black and white flyers for quantity between 10 and 99 units.
Combining this information together gives the equation:
750x20p +130x(10p+3p)+80x4p=17010p = £170.10 rounded down to £170
So, the company will have to pay £170.

Question 203: C
Step I.
£250 equals 25,000p
25,000p – 50x10p = 24,500p
10p is the price per unit for colour flyer between 10 and 99 units.
Step II. 24,500p/(10p+2p)=2041.667. Therefore she can buy 2041 medium mugs.
Once you bought the flyers you are left with 24,500p and you want to know how many medium mugs with logo you can buy.
10p is the price per unit for medium mugs above 500 units.
2p is the price per unit for logo on medium mugs above 500 units.

Question 204: D
Step I.
2014: 70x(26p+4p)+150x5p= 2850p
26p is the price per unit for medium mugs below 99 units in 2014.
4p is the price per unit for logo on medium mugs below 99 units in 2014.
5p is the price per unit for colour flyers above 100 units in 2014.
Step II.
2015: 70x(26p+3p)+150x4p=2630p
26p is the price per unit for medium mugs below 99 units in 2015.
3p is the price per unit for logo on medium mugs below 99 units in 2015.
4p is the price per unit for colour flyers above 100 units in 2015.
Step III.
1-(2630/2850)=0.077 = 8%

Question 205: C
£325,750/(1.012^(3)) =£314,298.9 rounded down to £314,299
1.2% equals 0.0012
3 years between 2012 and 2015.

SET 42

Question 206: B
The easiest way to solve this problem is using a Venn diagram. The Venn diagram below shows all possible combinations of the three devices each student can have as well as the number of students with a combination of devices. The sum of the numbers in the Venn diagram must be equal to the total number of students.
Using the information given in the graphs, we know there are:

- 30 students with all three devices
- 50 students with smartphone only
- 40 students with tablet only
- 50 students with laptop only
- 180 students with smartphone
- 190 students with tablet
- 200 students with laptop

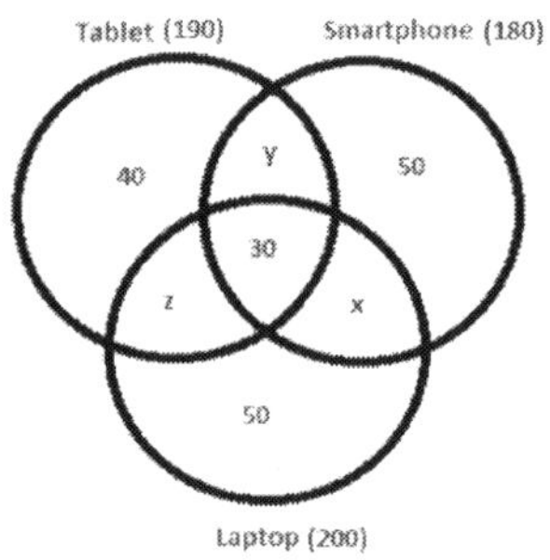

Therefore we can construct the following Venn diagram:

Laptop: 200=50+30+z+x → z=120-x
Smartphone: 180 =50+30+x+y → y=100-x
Tablet: 190=40+30+y+z → y=120-z

So, we see that y=100-x and y=120-z and thus z=20+x
Then, we see that z=20+x and z=120-x and thus x=50
Plug it in to see, z=20+x=70 and y=100-x=50

Now, the total number of students is the sum of the numbers in the Venn diagram.

Question 207: C
Using the previously constructed Venn diagram, we can see the total number of students with a smartphone and a laptop is 50.

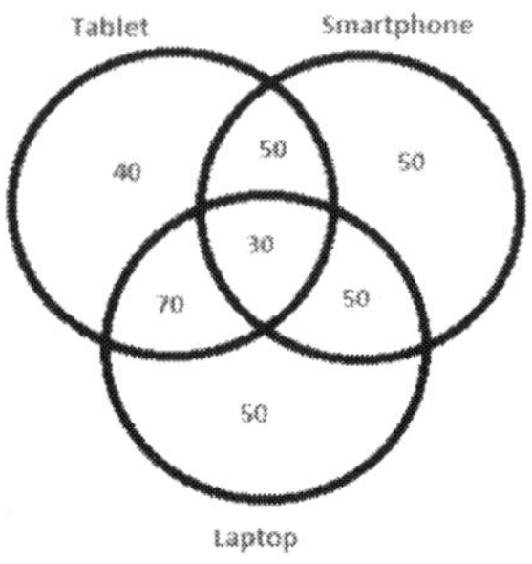

Question 208: A
180 students have smartphone
100 students have both tablet and laptop
So, 180-100=80, 80 students.

Question 209: C
Total number of students: 340
80 students have both smartphone and laptop.
80/340=0.25 → 23.5%

Question 210: C
185/345=0.536 → 54%
185 – no of students with smartphone (AFTER)
345 – total no of students (AFTER)

BEFORE

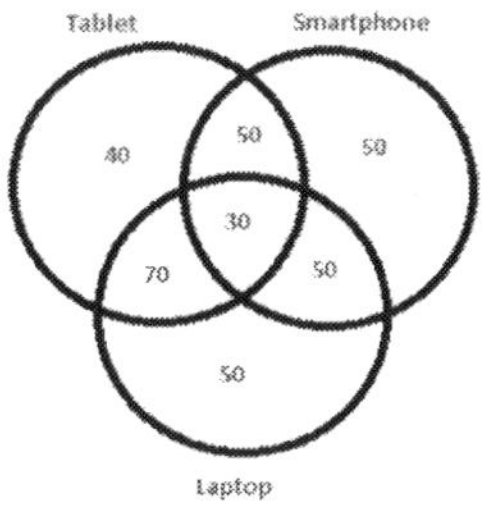

AFTER

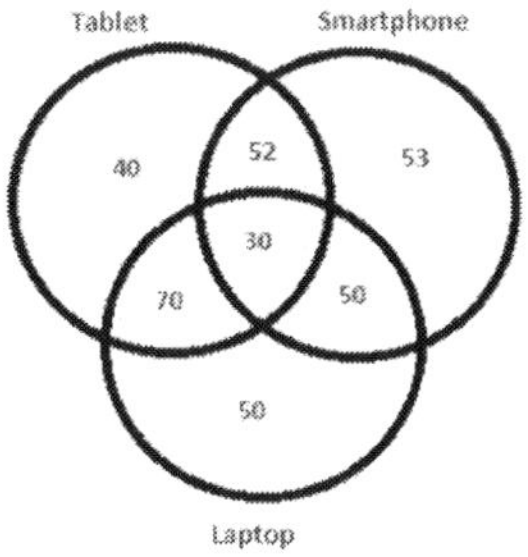

SET 43
Question 211: B
From 7.10am, trains run in every 20 minutes and hence the first one after 2pm will depart at 2.10pm - in every 20 minutes. This gives us three trains per hour from 2.10pm which would come to 12 trains before 6.15pm.

Question 212: C
From 8.18am, trains run in every 20 minutes and hence the first one Antonia can catch is the 2.58pm train. As it takes 21 minutes to get to London Liverpool Street station, she can arrive by 3.19pm.

Question 213: D
There are three trains in the morning before 7.10am. Thereafter, 3 trains per hour and the last one departs at 23.10pm. There are 16 hours between 7.10am and 23.10pm, so 3+16x3=51. 51 trains run all day.

Question 214: B
The first train after 3pm departs at 3.10pm from Cambridge Station and arrives at Tottenham Hale by 4.28pm.

Question 215: D
Using the equation: velocity = distance/time
7 minutes = 7/60 hour from Audley End to Bishops Stortford
10.5 miles between Audley End and Bishops Stortford
10.5 miles / (7/60) hour = 90 miles per hour

SET 44
Question 216: A
The top five rivers in the table are the longest.
Take the length in miles from column 2 and add them together.
Sum: 220+215+185+143+134=897 miles

Question 217: B
Firstly, you add the drainage area of all seven rivers from column C. Then you add the increase in drainage area of River Thames (1345.5 square mile). Finally, you can calculate the percentage increase, dividing New by Old.
Old: 4,409+4,994+4,029+3,236+1,597+560+431=19256
New: 1345.5+4,409+4,994+4,029+3,236+1,597+560+431=20601.5
Percentage: 20601.5/19256=1.06987 → 7%

Question 218: C
River Thames: 4,994 square mile
River Wye: 1,597 square mile
Percentage:
4,994/1,597=3.127 → 313%

Question 219: A
Lowest average discharge: River Tay – length: 117 miles
Highest average discharge: River Trent – length: 185 miles
Difference: 185-117=68

SET 45
Question 220: B
Remember that only the SIX longest rivers shall be included in the calculation.
Use the figures from column 3 to obtain the equation:
(4,409+4,994+4,029+3,236+1,597+560)/6=3137.5

Question 21: C
The largest section on the pie chart for Scottish GDP is Government and Other Services – it accounts for 29% of total Scottish GDP.

Question 222: B
Using the figures we are given: 4,2tn pounds and 5% (1.05) growth, we can plug them into the equation: GDP_{2014} x 1.05 = 4.2tn
This can be arranged as: → GDP_{2014}=4,2/1,05=4

Question 223: E
This requires a simple subtraction.
Manufacturing in Scottish GDP 14%
Business Services and Finance in UK GDP 28%
Difference: 28-14=14 → 14%

Question 224: B
We can use the figures given us to formulate the following equation:
£1.2tn (GDP in 2014) x 1.03 (3% GDP increase) x 0.01 (1% share of Agriculture, Forestry and Fishing) = 0.01236tn

Question 225: D
The three largest sections of the UK GDP pie chart are:
Distribution, Hotels and Catering 15%
Business Services Finance 28%
Government and Other Services 24%

SET 46
Question 226: C
The most-watched TV show is Geordie shore
Year 1 divided by Year 2
9.2/12.5=1.35869 → 36%

Question 227: E
The Voice: 3.4 and 4.1 in year 1 and 2 respectively
Britain's got talent: 5.2 and 5.6 in year 1 and 2 respectively
Year I: 5.2+3.4=8.6
Year II: 5.6+4.1=9.7
Difference: 9.7-8.6=1.1

Question 228: C
The show that the fewest percentage of males watched in year 2 was The Voice.

Question 229: B
Year 2 (all five TV show) / year1 (all five TV show) = (4.1+5.6+1.4+12.5+3)/(5+9.2+1.3+5.2+3.4) = 1.1037 → 10%

Question 230: D
Total population of females in year 2: 30 million
Number of females who watched Geordie Shore: 30x0.21=6.3 million
Number of males who watched Geordie Shore: 12.5-6.3=6.2 million

SET 47
Question 231: D
Basic plan: £45.29 + £7.50 = £52.79
250 free texts – more than 75 free minutes: (300-250) x15 = £7.50
Premium plan: £47.89
More than 300 free texts – more than 75 free minutes
£52.79 - £47.89 = £4.90

Question 232: C
Premium plan: £47.89
£60 - £47.89 = 12.11, so he has £12.11 left
Cheapest calls: Standard Calls – 6p
12.11/0.06= 201.83=201 minutes.

Question 233: E
45 texts free, 125 mins same network free, 100 minutes free with other network → 225 mins other network in both options.
Before → 225 x 0.15 = 33.75
After → 225 x 0.16 = 36. Difference is £2.25

Question 234: D
Basic plan: £45.29 + £58.50 = £103.79
(800-150) x9p= £58.50 – 150 minutes for free
Premium plan: £47.89 + £45.00 =£92.89
(800-500) x15p= 4500p = £45.00 – 500 minutes for free
Difference:
£103.79- £92.89 = £10.90

Question 235: C
Basic plan: £45.29x1.15 + (450-250)x £0.15 = £52.08+£30.00=£82.08
Premium plan: £47.89x1.15=£55.07
Difference: £82.08 - £55.07=£27.01

SET 48
Question 236: B
Davos: 15cm, 15cm, 15cm and 10cm in November, December, January, February respectively
Chamonix Mont-Blanc: 5cm, 40cm, 15cm, 20cm in November, December, January, February respectively
We can use these figures to create the equation:
(15+15+15+10)+(5+40+15+20)/8=16.875 cm

Question 237: C
Davos: 15cm, 15cm, 15cm and 10cm in November, December, January, February respectively
Average snowfall in Davos: (15+15+15+10)/4 = 13.75
Chamonix Mont-Blanc: 5cm, 40cm, 15cm, 20cm in November, December, January, February respectively
Average snowfall in Chamonix Mont-Blanc: (5+40+15+20)/4 =20
Cortina d' Ampezzo: 50cm, 50cm, 40cm and 5cm in November, December, January, February respectively
Average snowfall in Cortina d' Ampezzo: (50+50+40+5)/4=36.25
Garmisch Partenkirchen: 10cm, 15cm, 35cm, 20cm in November, December, January, February respectively
Average snowfall in Garmisch Partenkirchen: (10+15+35+20)/4=20
So the highest average snowfall was in Cotine d'Ampezzo.

Question 238: C
Inserting figures from all of the places into an equation:
December/February = (15+15+50+40)/(35+10+40+20)=120/105=1.14

Question 239: B
We are told that in November 2014 there is 30cm of snowfall (in all four areas)
To work out November 2015, we need to add all the areas: - Garmisch-Partenkirchen: 10cm, Davos: 15cm, Cortina d'Ampezzo: 5cm, Chamonix Mont-Blanc: 5cm
This gives us 35cm for November 2015
This gives us the equation: 35/30=1.1667

Question 240: D
We need to add the values for November and February for both of these places.
Cortina d' Ampezzo 5 + 40 = 45
Garmisch Partenkirchen 35 + 10 = 45
Sum: 45 + 45 = 90

SET 49
Question 241: A
Remember that two expenses relate to HSBC:

Mileage to and from presentation in Cambridge	£16.80

Sum: £35.90+£16.80=£52.70
Check: Sum is greater than any other item on the list.

Question 242: B
Add all of the expenses from each company together.
£35.90+£16.80+£15.40+£20.00+£49.50=£137.60

Question 243: E

HSBC	Breakfast with client	£35.90	Meal
Black Rock	Return ticket – Train journey to meeting in London	£20.00	Train
MKB	Lunch with client	£49.50	Meal

Meal/Train: (£35.90+£49.50)/(£15.40+£20.00)-1=1.413 → 141%

Question 244: B
Mileage paid at £0.25 per mile for the first 100 miles each month and £0.10 thereafter
Paid: £16.80
100 miles x £0.25 per mile = £25 → this is higher than £16.80 that Kevin actually paid, so the £0.25 per mile applies. → £16.80/£0.25=67.2

Question 245: D

Single ticket - Train journey to meeting in London	£15.40	Travel
Breakfast with client	£35.90	Meal
Return ticket – Train journey to meeting in London	£20.00	Travel
Lunch with client	£49.50	Meal

The total sum of travel expenses - £16.80+£15.40+£20.00=£52.2
75% of travel expenses - £52.2 x 0.75 =£39.15
Difference - £52.2-£39.15= £13.05
Accommodation and meal expenses - £35.90+£49.50=£85.40
90% of accommodation and meal expenses - £85.40x0.9=£76.86
Difference - £85.40--£76.86=£8.54
Sum of differences: £13.05+£8.54=£21.59

SET 50
Question 246: A
£30 per hour and Total cost £50 → £50-£30=£20

Question 247: B
Gamma for 6 hours = £25 deposit + (£115 x 6 hours) = 25 + 690 = £715
Beta for 6 hours = £20 deposit + (£90 x 6 hours) = 20 + 540 = £560
Difference = 715 – 560 = **£155**

Question 248: B
Using the information from the table:
Alpha: £50
Gamma: £140
Beta: £110
Delta: £250
Aron can afford to rent Alpha, Beta and Gamma for one hour (£300).
Alpha, Beta, Gamma and Delta would cost £550 which is out of his budget.

Question 249: B
Alpha: £30 per half an hour → £90 for three hours plus deposit of £20 → £110
Gamma: 3hours x £115 (cost per hour) + £25 (deposit) = £370
Sum: £110+£370=£480

Question 250: C
Old: Deposit £100 + (£150x8) = £1300. New: (£100 x 1.05) + (£150x8) = £1305

SET 51
Question 251: C
Remember to convert all of the prices into £
Around the World offers a price of 400 €.
Every 1.5€ equals the value of 1£. 400/1.5 = 266,67 rounded up to £267.
This is cheaper than the other options available.

Question 252: B
The differences from the European price in pounds are 190, 175, 180 and 200.
The average of the differences is (190+175+180+200)/4 = 186.25 rounded up to 186.3

Question 253: A
The discounted price of Take Me There is 560-50=510$, in pounds 510/2=255
This discounted ticket is £5 more expensive than the original price of In The Air (£250).
In percentages, this difference is 5/250x100 = 2%

Question 254: C
The total revenue of Around The World is 10x450+5x300=€6000, in pounds 6000/1.5=£4000
The total revenue of Good Fly is 25x100+12x300= £6100
The difference between revenues is £2100, which is 2100/6100x100=34.42….% of the higher revenue, rounded up to 34.43%

Question 255: C
The original price in pounds is 610/2=£305, the new price is 610/2.5=£244.
The difference is 305-244=£61

SET 52
Question 256: D
Looking at the pie chart for Indian GDP, the largest section is for manufacturing, which accounts for 24% of total Indian GDP.

Question 257: C
UK: Government and Other Services (24%) / Business Services and Finance (28%) = 86%
India: Government and Other Services (9%) / Business Services and Finance (15%) = 60%
UK – India = 26%
Question 258: A
The three largest sections of the pie chart for Indian GDP are:
Distribution, Hotels and Catering 20%
Business Services Finance 15%
Manufacturing: 24%

Question 259: D
Bottom two performing sector in the UK: Agriculture, Forestry and Fishing (1%), Other Production (4%)
Contribution: £4.2tn (total GDP) x 0.05 (1%+4%) = £210Bn
Bottom two performing sector in India: Other Production (3%), Construction (6%)
Contribution: £2tn (total GDP) x 0.12 (9%+3%) = £180Bn
UK minus India: £210Bn - £180Bn = £30Bn

Question 260: D
Largest sector in the UK: Business Services and Finance: £4.2tn x 0.28 =£1.176tn
Largest sector in India: Manufacturing: £2tn x 0.2 =£400Bn
Size of the UK economy: £4.2tn
Size of Business Services and Finance in the UK is £1.176tn, which is the largest

SET 53
Question 261: A
1500 JPY at 1 JPY = 0.013 USD → 1500 x 0.013 = 19.50

Question 262: D
I JPY = 0.022 GBP
1 JPY = 0.015 USD
GBP/USD = 0.022 / 0.015 = 1.47

Question 263: A
% increase: ((JPY/CAD) 2012 / (JPY/CAD) 2011) - 1 = 0.119 / 0.115 = 0.0348. → 3.5%.

Question 264: A
USD 1300 at USD/JPY rate of 0.010 in 2010 → JPY 130,000
USD 1300 at USD/JPY rate of 0.015 in 2013 → JPY 86,667
Difference: JPY 130,000 - JPY 86,667 = 43,333

Question 265: C
Looking at the table it is easy to notice that EUR exchange rate is near constant over the given time period except for one change in 2011 by 0.001. This is smaller than all the other currency changes

	2010	2011	2012	2013
GBP	0.021	0.020	0.019	0.022
USD	0.010	0.013	0.013	0.015
EUR	0.015	0.016	0.015	0.015
CAD	0.123	0.115	0.119	0.125

SET 54
Question 266: D
Boston: 4.4 – 4 = 0.4 million
Chicago: 3.3 – 3.5 = -0.2 million
Denver: 2.1 – 2 = 0.1 million
El Monte 1.5 – 0.8 = 0.7 million
El Monte has the highest growth in population

Question 267: A
Boston: 542,000– 235,675 = 306,325
Chicago: 350,685 – 345,526 = 5159
Denver: 249,990 – 231,456 = 18534
El Monte 62,044 – 54,000 = 8044

Question 268: D
Boston: 542,000/4.4 million = 0.123
Chicago: 350,685/3.3 million = 0.106
Denver: 249,990/2.1 million = 0.119
El Monte 62,044/1.5 million = 0.041

Question 269: A
2014:
Boston: 542,000/4.4 million = 0.123
Chicago: 350,685/3.3 million = 0.106
Denver: 249,990/2.1 million = 0.119
El Monte 62,044/1.5 million = 0.041
2009:
Boston: 235,675/4 million = 0.059
Chicago: 345,526/3.5 million = 0.099
Denver: 231,456/2 million = 0.116
El Monte 54,000/0.8 million = 0.068
Difference:
Boston: 0.123 - 0.059 = 0.064
Chicago: 0.106 - 0.099 = 0.007
Denver: 0.119 - 0.116 = 0.003
El Monte: 0.041 - 0.068 = -0.027

Question 270: D
2009: Boston: 235,675/4 million = 0.059
2014: Boston: 542,000/4.4 million = 0.123
Difference: Boston: 0.123 - 0.059 = 0.064

SET 55
Question 271: E
Starting rate: 15 % of 2,450 → £367.5
Basic rate: 25% of 2,450 – 33,500 so 25% of £31,050 → £7762.50
Higher rate: 40% of 33,500 – 37,000 → 40% of £3500 → £1400
Overall: £367.5 + £7762.25 + £1400 =£9530

Question 272: A
They earn the same salary.

Question 273: D
Starting rate: 15 % of 2,450 → £367.5
Basic rate: 25% of 2,451 – 33,500 so 25% of £31,049 → £7762.25
Higher rate: 40% of 33,500 – 42,000 → 40% of £8500 → £3400
Monthly average: (£367.5+ £7762.25+ £3400)/12 =£960.80

Question 274: B
Adam's income tax with £37,000 salary
Starting rate: 15 % of 2,450 → £367.5
Basic rate: 25% of 2,451 – 33,500 so 25% of £31,049 → £7762.25
Higher rate: 40% of 33,500 – 37,000 → 40% of £3500 → £1400
Overall: £367.5+ £7762.25+ £1400 =£9529.75

Adam's income tax with £41,000 salary
Starting rate: 15 % of 2,450 → £367.5
Basic rate: 25% of 2,451 – 33,500 so 25% of £31,049 → £7762.25
Higher rate: 40% of 33,500 – 41,000 → 40% of £7500 → £3000
Overall: £367.5+ £7762.25+ £3000=£11129.75
Difference: £11129.75 - £9529.75= £1600

Question 275: E
2014-15: £2,450
2015-16: £2,730
Difference: £2,730 - £2,450 = £280 increase

SET 56
Question 276: D
Follows from the table.

Question 277: B
£654,150,000 (total sales) / 7 (number of projects) = 93,450,000

Question 278: E
£45,000,000 x 1% + £180,000,000 x 4% = 450,000 + 7,200,000 = 7,650,000

Question 279: A
Follows from the table.

Question 280: A
Sum: £45,000,000 + £150,453,000 + £180,000,000 +£654,150,000 = £1,029,603,000

SET 57
Question 281: C
Previous day share price x (1 + change from previous day) = current share price
Change from previous day is +0.13%
Current share price is £134.432
£134.432 / (1-0.0013) = £134.257

Question 282: C
British Land highest: 54.934
British Land lowest: 54.914
Difference: 54.934 - 54.914 = 0.02

Question 283: E
Calculate previous day share price first, then calculate market capitalisation
HSBC current share price: 25.432
HSBC volume: 7,345,321
Market capitalisation: 25.432 x 7,345,321 = 186,806,203.672
Change from previous day: -0.03%
25.432/(1-0.0003) = 25.4396318896
Therefore, the market capitalisation previous day was 186,806,203.672 / (1 + 0.03) =186,750,178.618
25.439 etc. x 7,345,321 = 186, 862, 262.351

Question 284: C
Follows from the table.

Question 285: A
BP market cap: 286.123 (share price) x 4,431,748 (volume) = 1,268,025,033.004
British Land market cap: 54.923 (share price) x 4,999,432 (volume) = 274,583,803,736
Difference: 1,268,025,033.004 - 274,583,803,736 = 993,441,229.268

SET 58
Question 286: D
Psychology: 10/6 = 1.66
To determine the course with a similar ratio of men to women as psychology, we need to calculate the ratios for all of the other courses
Mathematics: 8/7 =1.14 Physics: 10/15 = 0.66 Programming: 4/5 = 0.8 Literature: 12/8 = 1.5
History: 7/7 =1
From these figures, we can see that Literature has the most similar ratio.

Question 287: C
Physics: 10/15 = 0.66
Similarly to the previous question, we need to calculate the ratios for all other courses
Psychology: 10/6 = 1.66 Mathematics: 8/7 =1.14 Programming: 4/5 = 0.8 Literature: 12/8 = 1.5
History: 7/7 =1

Question 288: E
Can't tell because students can take more than one course.

Question 289: E
As one student can take more than one course and we do not have any information about the total number of students we cannot say.

Question 290: C
Before ratio: 10:6 = (10/6):1 = 1.66:1. After ratio: 13:6 = (13/6):1 = 2.16:1
Difference: 2.16-1.66 = 0.5

SET 59
Question 291: A
Women in employment: 85.5% (employed) + 5% (self-employed) + 2.7% (employed other) = 93.2%
Men in employment: 81.3% (employed) + 8% (self-employed) + 4.5% (employed other) = 93.8%
Difference: 93.8% - 93.2% = 0.6

Question 292: D
Women self-employed: 5% - Women unemployed: 6.8% → sum: 11.8%
Men self-employed: 8% - Men unemployed: 6.1% → sum: 14.1%
Ratio men to women: 14.1% / 11.8% = 1.2

Question 293: E
21 million (women employed) x 0.05 (5% self-employed) = 1.05 million
If there are 21 million women in employment → 21 million are either employed, self-employed or employed other – so 21 million women is (85.5+5+2.7) 93.2% of the country. This means 6.8% of the country is 1532189 so country population is 22,532,189. 5% of this is 1,126,609 so answer should be 1.13 million

Question 294: A
Men unemployed: 6.1% → 31 million x 0.061 = 1.891
Women unemployed: 6.8% → 32 million x 0.068 = 2.176
Difference 2.176 – 1.891 = 0.285

Question 295: D
Women in employment (as defined above): 93.2. Unemployed women: 6.8. 93.2/6.8 = 13.7

SET 60
Question 296: C
Energy cost: electricity plus gas. Note that Gas and Electricity together add up to ¼ of the total area. And therefore, 360 pounds x ¼ = 90 pounds

Question 297: D
Household purchases, travel and gas costs – ½ of the total area → 180 pounds. Energy costs – ¼ of the total area → 90 pounds. Ratio: 180 / 90 = 2

Question 298: B
The largest section of the pie chart is for 'Travel'

Question 299: D
Household purchases, travel and gas costs – ½ of the total area → 180 pounds
Energy costs – ¼ of the total area → 90 pounds

Question 300: E
The smallest section of the pie chart is for 'TV subscription'

Abstract Reasoning Answers

Q	A	Q	A	Q	A	Q	A	Q	A	Q	A
1	B	51	Neither	101	A	151	A	201	C	251	A
2	Neither	52	B	102	A	152	Neither	202	A	252	D
3	A	53	A	103	Neither	153	A	203	A	253	D
4	A	54	Neither	104	B	154	B	204	D	254	D
5	Neither	55	B	105	Neither	155	A	205	D	255	C
6	B	56	A	106	A	156	Neither	206	A	256	B
7	A	57	Neither	107	Neither	157	A	207	C	257	C
8	A	58	B	108	A	158	A	208	B	258	C
9	Neither	59	Neither	109	B	159	Neither	209	B	259	A
10	Neither	60	A	110	B	160	B	210	A	260	B
11	A	61	A	111	B	161	B	211	D	261	B
12	B	62	A	112	Neither	162	A	212	A	262	C
13	Neither	63	B	113	Neither	163	A	213	C	263	A
14	A	64	B	114	B	164	B	214	A	264	A
15	A	65	A	115	A	165	A	215	D	265	B
16	B	66	A	116	A	166	A	216	D	266	A
17	B	67	A	117	A	167	B	217	A	267	C
18	A	68	B	118	Neither	168	Neither	218	C	268	A
19	A	69	Neither	119	B	169	A	219	D	269	A
20	A	70	Neither	120	Neither	170	B	220	C	270	D
21	A	71	B	121	Neither	171	Neither	221	A	271	A
22	A	72	A	122	Neither	172	B	222	D	272	C
23	B	73	Neither	123	A	173	B	223	D	273	C
24	B	74	Neither	124	A	174	A	224	B	274	C
25	Neither	75	A	125	B	175	Neither	225	C	275	D
26	B	76	A	126	Neither	176	B	226	B	276	D
27	A	77	A	127	A	177	Neither	227	D	277	A
28	A	78	B	128	Neither	178	D	228	C	278	B
29	B	79	A	129	Neither	179	B	229	A	279	C
30	B	80	Neither	130	B	180	A	230	A	280	B
31	B	81	B	131	Neither	181	Neither	231	A	281	B
32	Neither	82	Neither	132	Neither	182	Neither	232	D	282	A
33	Neither	83	Neither	133	Neither	183	A	233	A	283	A
34	A	84	A	134	A	184	A	234	C	284	D
35	A	85	A	135	B	185	Neither	235	B	285	B
36	B	86	B	136	A	186	Neither	236	C	286	C
37	A	87	A	137	B	187	Neither	237	C	287	C
38	Neither	88	B	138	Neither	188	A	238	C	288	A
39	A	89	Neither	139	Neither	189	B	239	D	289	C
40	Neither	90	B	140	B	190	A	240	A	290	C
41	B	91	Neither	141	A	191	Neither	241	A	291	D
42	Neither	92	A	142	Neither	192	A	242	D	292	A
43	A	93	Neither	143	B	193	Neither	243	B	293	A
44	B	94	A	144	A	194	B	244	A	294	C
45	Neither	95	A	145	B	195	Neither	245	A	295	B
46	B	96	B	146	Neither	196	B	246	D	296	D
47	Neither	97	B	147	B	197	Neither	247	C	297	A
48	A	98	A	148	Neither	198	B	248	C	298	C
49	B	99	B	149	A	199	Neither	249	D	299	A
50	Neither	100	B	150	A	200	B	250	B	300	A

	Set A Rule	Set B Rule
Set 1	**3** Shapes are white **2** Shapes are black	**2** Shapes are white **3** Shapes are black
Set 2	**2** Shapes are white **1** Shape is black	**1** Shape is white **2** Shapes are black
Set 3	There is always a **triangle** in the **top left corner**	There is always a **quadrilateral** in the **bottom right corner**
Set 4	There are an **even** number of rectangles	There are an **odd** number of rectangles
Set 5	Each circle has at least one tangential line.	At least one circle is **intersected** by a line.
Set 6	**None** of the shapes intersect with each other.	At least **one** of the shapes intersects with another shape/line.
Set 7	The total number of dots is **10**	The total number of dots is **9**
Set 8	The four-sided shapes are in **different** section of the box.	The four-sided shapes are in the **same** section of the box.
Set 9	All boxes have a **five-pointed star** in the **Centre**	All boxes have a **triangle** in the **bottom left corner**
Set 10	The black **circle** is always in the **bottom left corner**	The two small **dots** are always in the **top right corner**
Set 11	The circles **are all tangential to** each other	The circles **intersect** each other
Set 12	There are always **three squares, two triangles** and one circle	There are always **three triangles, two squares** and one circle
Set 13	The sum of the edges is **odd**	The sum of the edges of is **even**
Set 14	The sum of the edges is **twelve**	The sum of the edges is **fourteen**
Set 15	Each box contains **4** right angles	Each box contains **6** right angles
Set 16	Each black shape has a **larger** white counterpart	Each black shape has a **smaller** white counterpart
Set 17	Number of Dots = Number of **Stars**	Number of Dots = Number of **Diamonds**
Set 18	Even-sided polygons are **black** Odd-sided polygons are **white**	Even-sided polygons are **white** Odd-sided polygons are **black**
Set 19	Number of Stars = Number of **Triangles**	Number of Stars = Number of **Diamonds**
Set 20	There are **no** right angles	There is at least **one** right angle

Set 21	There is a **horizontal** line for each rectangle and a **vertical** line for each square	There is a **vertical** line for each rectangle and a **horizontal** line for each square
Set 22	One shape has **2** more edges than the other	One shape has **3** more edges than the other
Set 23	Even-sided polygons are **black** Odd-sided polygons are **white**	Even-sided polygons are **white** Odd-sided polygons are **black**
Set 24	The number of triangles + circles = **3**	The number of triangles + circles = **2**
Set 25	The vector sum of the arrows is **left/right**	The vector sum of the arrows is **up/down**
Set 26	There are **nine** corners in total	There are **ten** corners in total
Set 27	There is one **more** shape outside the circle than inside the circle	There is one **less** shape outside the circle than inside the circle
Set 28	The arrows only form **acute** angles	The arrows only form **obtuse** angles
Set 29	Shapes are made up of arrows all pointing at the same corner	Shapes are made up of arrows all pointing at different corners
Set 30	A central shape is intersected by an **even** number of other shapes	A central shape is intersected by an **odd** number of other shapes
Set 31	There is an **odd** number of corners in total	There is an **even** number of corners in total
Set 32	All **white** shapes are located on the left side	All **black** shapes are located on the left side
Set 33	The number of edges is a prime number	The number of edges is **not** prime number
Set 34	There are an even number of **black** shapes	There are an even number of **white** shapes
Set 35	All shapes contain right angles	All shapes **don't** contain any right angles
Set 36	Every shape is a quadrilateral	Every shape is **not** a quadrilateral
Set 37	There is always a **circle** in the top left hand corner	There is always a **triangle** in the top left hand corner
Set 38	**Two** corners are occupied by shapes	**Three** corners are occupied by shapes
Set 39	There is only **one** black shape	There are only **two** black shapes
Set 40	There are always three members of the same colour and shape, **but** different sizes	There are always three members of the same colour, shape **and** size

Question 201: C
As the sequences progresses, the number of objects within each frame increases by two.

Question 202: A
The total number of objects in each panel totals seven. In the bottom half, the number of white circles increases by one each panel. In the top half, the number of black circles alternates between one and three between each panel with the grey circles making up the remainder to total seven.

Question 203: A
The sequence alternates between a 3-edged and 4-edged zig-zag. Within each zig-zag will be a black circle and a grey shape.

Question 204: D
The circle and triangle begin at the bottom-left corner and rotate clockwise throughout the panels and cycle between the colours white-grey-black. Each panel also contains two white stars and a square.

Question 205: D
The top-right and bottom-left shapes are both the same colour and alternate between white and black. The top-left and bottom-right shapes are also both the same colour and alternate between black and white.

Question 206: A
Whilst the curve rotates 180° with each progressing frame, the total number of sides increases by 1. The colours are distracting factors.

Question 207: C
As the sequence progresses, the difference between the number of squares and circles increases by one.

Question 208: B
The shapes within the smaller white squares rotate 90° clockwise within each frame. The total number of white shapes is greater than the total number of black shapes by one.

Question 209: B
The total number of right-angles in each frame increases by one.

Question 210: A
There are a number of distractors in this series – pay attention to only the arrows. Each frame has an arrow that rotates in both the direction it faces (up-right-down-left) and the quadrant in which it is located. The arrow alternates between the colours white and black.

Question 211: D
The total number of sides for white shapes increases by one each frame. This is the same as the number of black shapes

Question 212: A
Each of the circles in the top row moves to the left once, each of the circles in the bottom row move to the right once. The circles in the middle row flip in the horizontal axis.

Question 213: C
The total number of edges increases by five each time.

Question 214: A
As the sequence progresses, the number of black circles subtract the number of white circles increases by two (6-8-10-12-14).

Question 215: D
The five-pointed start rotates clockwise by 90° in each frame. One of these points will face either up-down-left-right. If the arrow is pointing in the same direction as this, it will be coloured black.

Question 216: D
The total number of sides of all the shapes increases in the sequence 6, 9, 12, 15… When the total number of sides is odd the shapes are black, when the total is even the shapes are white.

Question 217: A
The number of shapes with right-angles increases by one.

Question 218: C
As the sequence progresses, the quadrant in which the black shape sits rotates. The two closest shapes are always grey and the furthest shape is always white.

Question 219: D
Each shape is rotated 90° clockwise, however their position is random.

Question 220: C
The number of arrows pointing directly at another shape alternates between one and three.

Question 221: A
All circles move closer towards each other and the circles in the bottom row cycle between white-grey-black. The other two circles are the same colour as the circle in their column.

Question 222: D
Each frame contains a two or three-sided 'container' that rotates. Shapes with right angles can only be placed within the container whilst shapes without right angles can only be placed outside the container.

Question 223: D
The difference between the number of the most abundant shape subtract the least abundant increases by one each frame.

Question 224: B
As the sequence progresses, the number of edges outside the central square increases by the number of edges within the central square. The colour of all the shapes outside the central square is the same as that of the shape within the central square in the previous frame.

Question 225: C
Every square alternates its colour between white and grey. New squares that are added are grey.

Question 226: B
Each shape is replaced by another shape with one more edge. Instead of a six-sided shape, two triangles are created instead. If there is another shape with the same number of edges, the shape is coloured black.

Question 227: D
As the sequence progresses, an increasing number of circles are added to the frame. Every circle cycles between the colours white-grey-black.

Question 228: C
Every arrow splits into two arrows pointing in opposite directions, the whole frame then rotates 90°. After pointing in both the up/down and left/right direction the arrows change colour.

Question 229: A
As the sequence progresses, every shape is moved to a random location in each subsequent frame. If the shape was intersecting another shape, it alternates colour between white and grey. All collisions are coloured black.

Question 230: A
The number of stars in the top right corner increases by one and alternates colour between black-grey-white. The circle-triangle pair rotates clockwise 90° but remains in the bottom left corner and alternates between colours white-grey-black.

Question 231: A
Every square/triangle is split into two right-angled triangles. The circles alternate between being white and outside the rectangle, and being black and inside the rectangle.

Question 232: D
The entire frame rotates by 90° clockwise. The triangles alternate between white and grey.

Question 233: A
The central grey shape alternates between a four-point and six-point star. The total number of other shapes will be the same as the number of points on the star. All arrows are coloured black.

Question 234: C
The overall pattern flips vertically every frame. As the pattern progresses, two more triangles are coloured in.

Question 235: B
The total number of circles increases by one each frame. All circles are coloured grey.

Question 236: C
The total number of intersections that are coloured black increases by one each frame. The colours of the large circle alternate between white and grey.

Question 237: C
The arrows in each frame point in different directions. As the series progresses, the direction that is missed rotates between left-up-right-down

Question 238: C
The pentagon rotates 90° anti-clockwise and alternates between white and grey.

Question 239: D
The black central shape alternates between a square and a pentagon. The number of triangles present in the frame is equal to the number of sides of the central shape.

Question 240: A
Black shapes rotate clockwise 90° whilst white shapes rotate anti-clockwise 90° each frame.

Question 241: A
Every circle moves one space to the right.

Question 242: D
The number of circles in the top half increases by one whilst the number in the bottom half decreases by one. The colour of the circles within each half alternates between white and black.

Question 243: B
The triangles in the outer section rotate anti-clockwise every frame whilst the central diamond rotates clockwise.

Question 244: A
The colours in the central diamond alternate between black and white. The triangles in the outer segment rotate their colours clockwise between grey-black-white.

Question 245: A
Each quadrant of the frame is rotated 90° clockwise.

Question 246: D
The black shapes rotate clockwise within the bottom-left quadrant. The white shapes flip vertically.

Question 247: C
Each frame has an increasing number of intersections. All shapes that touch another shape are coloured grey.

Question 248: C
As the sequence progresses, every large shape is converted into a small shape and one new large shape is added to the frame.

Question 249: D
The large square cycles between the colours grey-white-black. The large triangle cycles between black-white-grey. The smaller shapes in the top-left quadrant rotate clockwise whilst the smaller shapes in the bottom-right rotate anti-clockwise.

Question 250: B
The total number of sides for black shapes increases by one each frame.

Question 251: A
The left half of the image is flipped vertically whilst the right half is flipped horizontally. Any shape that is found in the same area in the same orientation is coloured black.

Question 252: D
Shapes with right-angles are rotated by 90° clockwise whilst those without right-angles are coloured black.

Question 253: D
White shapes increase their number of edges by one black shapes are flipped horizontally.

Question 254: D
All triangles are removed. The other shapes move to a random position

Question 255: C
The white shapes gain a larger black shape.

Question 256: B
If an arrow points at a shape it turns black, if the arrow points away from the shape then the arrow itself turns black. The orientation / organisation of shapes is not significant.

Question 257: C
White shapes rotated 90° anti-clockwise. Grey shapes are rotated 180°. Black shapes are rotated 90° clockwise.

Question 258: C
Shapes that have an identical pair (regardless of rotation) are coloured black.

Question 259: A
The entire image is rotated 90° clock-wise and then flipped vertically.

Question 260: B
The left half of the image is flipped horizontally whilst the right half is flipped vertically.

Question 261: B
The entire image is rotated 180°.

Question 262: C
Circles become triangles, triangles become squares and squares become circles. All shapes keep the same size and position.

Question 263: A
The entire image is rotated 90° anti-clockwise.

Question 264: A
Each shape is split in half along one line of reflection with one half being coloured black.

Question 265: B
Black shapes are moved upwards whilst white shapes are moved towards the left.

Question 266: A
Black shapes are moved such that they all touch each other whilst white shapes are moved such that they do not touch.

Question 267: C
The number of edges of the large black shape increases by one. The rest of the shapes are white and each have the same number of sides. The total number of shapes is equal to this same number.

Question 268: A
The stars that are pointing upwards are coloured black whilst the others are kept white.

Question 269: A
Only the shapes touching another shape remain.

Question 270: D
The colours rotate clockwise whilst the number of sides for each shape increases by one.

Question 271: A
Each individual quadrant is rotated 90° clockwise.

Question 272: C
Each quadrant is rotated 180° and the colours grey and white are switched.

Question 273: C
Every black shape is rotated 90° clockwise and coloured white whilst every white shape becomes black.

Question 274: C
Black shapes move away from each other whilst white shapes get bigger.

Question 275: D
For every shape with the same number of sides, the total decreases by one.

Question 276: D
The total number of white shapes is equal to the number of sides of the large black shape.

Question 277: A
Each shape is split into two shapes of the same colour with the same total number of edges.

Question 278: B
Every triangle is split in half through its right-angle. Grey triangles are placed by two smaller white and black triangles. The frame is rotated 180°

Question 279: C
Shapes with right-angles get larger. Shapes without right-angles get smaller.

Question 280: B
The shape in each quadrant has twice as many sides as that of the original shape.

Question 281: B
The shape is flipped diagonally and rotated 90°

Question 282: A
The entire image is rotated 90° to the right and then the new bottom half of the image is flipped vertically

Question 283: A
Each quadrant is rotated 180°.

Question 284: D
Increase the number of sides of black shapes by one and decrease the number of sides of white shapes by one.

Question 285: B
The left half of the image swaps between the shapes. The right half is rotated 180° and the colour of the shaped inverted.

Question 286: C
For every shape, there will be another shape that is not necessarily the same size or rotation.

Question 287: C
The total number of shapes within each quadrant are identical

Question 288: A
Same number of white, grey and black shapes.

Question 289: C
All objects move quadrant in a clockwise direction. Objects within squares also rotate 90° clockwise.

Question 290: C
The total number of sides is the same

Question 291: D
Every black shape becomes two different black shapes.

Question 292: A
The entire image is flipped vertically but the colours remain the same.

Question 293: A
All shapes with an odd number of sides are removed.

Question 294: C
For arrows pointing towards each other, one arrow will move next to the other. For arrows pointing away from each other, one arrow will move away from the other.

Question 295: B
The top-left and bottom-right shapes swap whilst the top-right and bottom-left shapes swap. The location of the colours remains the same

Question 296: D
The image is flipped in the diagonal axis (top-left to bottom-right)

Question 297: A
The shape in the top-left is rotated 90° clockwise; top-right 180°; bottom-right 90° anti-clockwise.

Question 298: C
The number of black shapes to calculate the number of grey shapes displayed divides the number of white shapes.

Question 299: A
Each shape is split into two shapes with half the number of sides as the original shape.

Question 300: A
Shapes with right-angles are rotated. Those without right-angles are replaced by other shapes.

Situational Judgement Answers

Q	A	Q	A	Q	A	Q	A	Q	A	Q	A
1	D	51	A	101	C	151	C	201	D	251	A
2	B	52	D	102	B	152	B	202	D	252	B
3	D	53	C	103	A	153	D	203	D	253	A
4	A	54	A	104	D	154	A	204	A	254	C
5	B	55	C	105	A	155	A	205	A	255	B
6	A	56	A	106	C	156	A	206	D	256	B
7	B	57	C	107	B	157	C	207	B	257	D
8	D	58	D	108	B	158	D	208	D	258	A
9	C	59	A	109	C	159	A	209	A	259	D
10	D	60	B	110	A	160	B	210	B	260	C
11	D	61	D	111	A	161	A	211	C	261	D
12	A	62	C	112	D	162	C	212	D	262	B
13	D	63	A	113	C	163	B	213	A	263	A
14	C	64	D	114	A	164	A	214	A	264	A
15	B	65	A	115	A	165	C	215	D	265	D
16	A	66	D	116	B	166	A	216	A	266	D
17	D	67	A	117	D	167	A	217	D	267	D
18	D	68	C	118	A	168	D	218	D	268	A
19	C	69	A	119	C	169	C	219	C	269	A
20	C	70	A	120	D	170	A	220	A	270	B
21	D	71	A	121	D	171	A	221	A	271	A
22	B	72	B	122	A	172	A	222	B	272	D
23	A	73	D	123	A	173	B	223	C	273	D
24	D	74	D	124	B	174	C	224	A	274	A
25	A	75	D	125	A	175	C	225	D	275	A
26	D	76	A	126	D	176	A	226	B	276	B
27	A	77	D	127	B	177	D	227	A	277	A
28	A	78	C	128	B	178	B	228	A	278	A
29	D	79	A	129	C	179	D	229	D	279	D
30	A	80	B	130	A	180	C	230	B	280	C
31	A	81	D	131	A	181	A	231	D	281	D
32	D	82	A	132	D	182	A	232	A	282	A
33	B	83	A	133	C	183	C	233	D	283	C
34	D	84	C	134	C	184	A	234	A	284	B
35	B	85	A	135	C	185	D	235	D	285	D
36	C	86	A	136	B	186	C	236	C	286	B
37	A	87	D	137	D	187	A	237	A	287	A
38	B	88	C	138	A	188	A	238	D	288	D
39	B	89	D	139	A	189	C	239	C	289	C
40	C	90	C	140	A	190	D	240	D	290	A
41	A	91	A	141	A	191	A	241	B	291	D
42	D	92	C	142	B	192	C	242	D	292	A
43	B	93	A	143	D	193	A	243	A	293	B
44	A	94	D	144	A	194	D	244	A	294	D
45	B	95	C	145	A	195	B	245	C	295	B
46	D	96	D	146	C	196	D	246	D	296	B
47	A	97	B	147	B	197	A	247	A	297	C
48	B	98	A	148	B	198	B	248	D	298	A
49	D	99	B	149	D	199	A	249	B	299	B
50	C	100	D	150	A	200	A	250	A	300	D

How appropriate is...? Scenarios: 1-21 and 41-60	A	A very appropriate thing to do
	B	Appropriate, but not ideal
	C	Inappropriate, but not awful
	D	A very inappropriate thing to do
How important is...? Scenarios: 22-40	A	Very important
	B	Important
	C	Of minor importance
	D	Not important at all

Scenario 1:

1. **Very inappropriate** because Jacob didn't know the entire story and this could be resolved by having a simple conversation instead. There is no need at his stage to get more people involved, especially as the doctor's behaviour has not directly affected the patient's safety or treatment.
2. **Appropriate but not ideal**, because the medical student would not be telling the doctor anything specific.
3. **Very inappropriate** because as a medical student you are a member of the health care team as well, so if there is something that is affecting the rest of the staff and patients, then it should not be ignored.
4. **Very appropriate** because the supervisor would be able to advise the student as to what they should do.
5. **Appropriate but not ideal**, whilst it makes Dr Herbert aware of the issue, it is quite confrontational and Dr Herbert may become defensive.

Scenario 2:

6. **Very appropriate**, because Dr Walker could have gotten into a bad habit and may be unaware that he hasn't been washing his hands.
7. **Appropriate but not ideal,** because Dr Walker may not pick up on the hint, although it might save George some awkwardness in having to ask Dr Walker directly.
8. **Very inappropriate** because hospitals function as a team. If George is aware of something that could potentially cause patients harm, he must try to solve the issue.
9. **Inappropriate but not awful**, because it is not addressing the situation and could make it a bigger problem than it actually is. In general, problems with doctors should be escalated to more senior doctors; problems with nurses should be escalated to more senior nurses.
10. **Very inappropriate** because Dr Walker would not have been informed and the fact that George would have witnessed it without trying to correct the problem could back fire onto him and get him into trouble if any harm were to arise.

Scenario 3:

11. **Very inappropriate** because the medical school museum would have to account for the missing bones. The bones are very valuable, and even the remains of bones could be useful as they would make them into slides or as cut sections.
12. **Very appropriate** because it acknowledges the respect to both the bones and the museum. The bones came from a real human, so cannot be treated as though they are any old piece of waste.
13. **Very inappropriate** because this would prompt an investigation and would waste a lot of money from the medical school. It would also mean that future classes may be banned from performing such projects, hindering their educational experience.
14. **Inappropriate but not awful,** because despite the fact that the curator would be informed of what occurred, it could get your colleague into trouble that could have been avoided.
15. **Appropriate but not ideal,** because the supervisor can give advice as to what to do, but it does not directly address the problem.

Scenario 4:

16. **Very appropriate** because his tutor can give him proper advice and will also be aware of any reasons behind a potentially disappointing exam mark.
17. **Very inappropriate** because it will increase tensions and result in a more stressful environment, which would hinder his progress even more.
18. **Very inappropriate** because he will end up feeling very isolated and lonely and anxious, which will also ruin both his friendships and his work progress.
19. **Inappropriate but not awful,** because he will lose out on friendships as well as go through the difficulty of finding another place to live. This could end up as a lonely option with no support network.
20. **Appropriate but not ideal** because he may find that everyone is having similar problems. It doesn't directly address the problems but Henry might find it helpful to discuss the situation with someone else.

Scenario 5:

21. **Very inappropriate** because Mark was only asked because he was mistaken for a doctor. Therefore exchanging one student for another would be an inappropriate action. Also, the other student wasn't asked.
22. **Appropriate but not ideal,** because Mark could document the results as a student and write exactly who he was. Students are allowed to perform tests, just not to administer medication.
23. **Very appropriate** because it will alert the doctor as to his mistake, and the student can be advised appropriately.
24. **Very inappropriate** because the test needs to be done, and the doctor would assume that the test had been done. Therefore the patient could be left waiting for a long time.
25. **Very appropriate** because they might be better qualified to do the test.

Scenario 6:

26. **Very inappropriate** because it is dishonest and if the truth were to emerge, she could be expelled from the medical school for such an act.
27. **Very appropriate** because they can support her and help her organise the rest of her revision.
28. **Very appropriate** because it can reassure her and give her more confidence as most people would probably feel similar.
29. **Very inappropriate** because this is also dishonest and therefore, unprofessional.
30. **Very appropriate** because she might just pass her exams and surprise herself.

Scenario 7:

31. **Very appropriate** because Dijam should not be in the hospital and is not employed to be in the hospital so can go home to recuperate.
32. **Very inappropriate** because Dijam still has contact with the patients and it is against the rules to be hungover or have alcohol in your system as a student on the wards. Dijam could get asked to do certain tasks and must make sure that he is mentally and physically competent.
33. **Appropriate** because they might send Dijam home as well, or could allow him to stay but restrict what he was allowed to do for the day.
34. **Very inappropriate** because this is a very serious violation of professionalism and joking about it is not addressing the problem.
35. **Appropriate but not ideal** because Dijam could get into more trouble than he probably ought to. That doctor also may not have witnessed Dijam in his state anyway, so it is better to inform the doctors that Dijam is shadowing than the one that is in charge.

Scenario 8:

36. **Inappropriate but not awful** as the work should be a joint effort from everyone but it won't be confrontational.
37. **Very appropriate** because Patrick's personal tutor can advise him accordingly.
38. **Appropriate but not ideal** - it will allow them to speak up but the conversation wouldn't involve Jina.
39. **Appropriate but not ideal** because the group members may not pick up on the hinting.
40. **Inappropriate** because the confrontational approach could offend Jina and not achieve what Patrick was hoping for.

Scenario 9:

41. **Very appropriate** because Joshua should never be allowed to breach confidentiality and take the patient's notes away from the hospital.
42. **Very inappropriate** because Nazia has a duty to not allow any serious breaches of confidentiality if she is aware of them.
43. **Appropriate but not ideal** because although people have been made aware, the notes have already left the hospital.
44. **Very appropriate** because your clinical advisor can give you the best advice when it is unclear what is best to do.
45. **Appropriate but not ideal** because it prevents Joshua from taking the notes away from the hospital but will cost Megan her time.

Scenario 10:

46. **Very inappropriate** as this is a clear lie and therefore grossly unprofessional.
47. **Very appropriate** because Dr Kelly cannot really explain much to Mr. Marshall without breaking the bad news to him.
48. **Appropriate but not ideal** because this may damage their relationship.
49. **Very inappropriate** because this may create confusion and being unnecessarily cryptic.
50. **Inappropriate but not awful** because although it will address his concerns, Dr Kelly is not the best person to break the news.

Scenario 11:

51. **Very appropriate** because Julia is unable to advise Mary.
52. **Very inappropriate** because Julia isn't experienced enough to assess when Mary will be able to go home.
53. **Inappropriate but not awful** because whilst technically true, it is not Julia's responsibility to advise Mary on anything without the permission of her doctor.
54. **Very appropriate** as she would then be giving correct information and also addressing Mary's concerns.
55. **Inappropriate** because Julia is not qualified and cannot answer Mary's questions.

Scenario 12:

56. **Very appropriate** because it shows that Daniel is trying his best to learn the skill with minimal fuss.
57. **Inappropriate but not awful** because Hannah needs to know that she missed someone out, but it won't solve the immediate problem.
58. **Very inappropriate** because it could have been a genuine mistake on Hannah's part, and will not make the current situation better.
59. **Very appropriate** because it might have been an issue that affected lots of people, instead of just Daniel.
60. **Appropriate but not ideal**. This shows that Daniel cares about his assessment but also means extra hassle for the doctor.

Scenario 13:

61. **Very inappropriate** because her friend will have spent a lot of money on the flights and will be left to fend for herself or not be able to go.
62. **Inappropriate but not awful** because the holiday will not be enjoyable for Helen's friend, and Helen will also not benefit from having a fun experience.
63. **Very appropriate** because Helen also needs a break and being able to go for part of the holiday will be rewarding without having to miss out completely, and will leave enough time to prepare for the exams too.
64. **Very inappropriate** because Helen will be jeopardizing her chances of remaining in medical school.
65. **Very appropriate** because she will not be disappointing her friend as much, and will still be able to do her revision.

Scenario 14:

66. **Very inappropriate** because Celia's parents have not chosen to isolate her on purpose.
67. **Very appropriate** because Celia can meet new people without having to worry about insulting her parents.
68. **Inappropriate but not awful** as although she will be closer to her friends, she may turn into an unwelcome guest quite quickly.
69. **Very inappropriate** because this will affect her mental health and her relationships, and will probably lead to underperformance in her studies as well
70. **Very appropriate** because it shows that she understands her family's situation whilst attempting to address her own predicaments.

Scenario 15:

71. **Very appropriate** – Xun should try to do it to the best of his ability in the remaining time.
72. **Appropriate but not ideal**– it is unlikely that the deadline will be unchanged but there is always space for honesty and he might just be lucky.
73. **Very inappropriate** because this action will affect his final grade.
74. **Very inappropriate** because this is plagiarism and both Xun and his friend would be penalised for it.
75. Very inappropriate because he would be lying to the assessment office and could get into a lot of trouble for it.

Scenario 16:

76. **Very appropriate** because he will be showing that he respects the hospital, infection control, and the patients.
77. **Very inappropriate** because this will set a bad first impression to his patients and colleagues – made worse by his refusal.
78. **Inappropriate but not awful.** Nahor may set a bad first impression but there is a small chance that he might be allowed to keep it.
79. **Very appropriate** because he can still enjoy keeping his hair in an individual style without looking unprofessional.
80. **Appropriate but not ideal.** Whilst this is a proactive approach, it is such a minor issue that it is not worth wasting the dean's time about. In addition, the answer is very likely to be 'no'.

Scenario 17:

81. **Very inappropriate** because Dr Patel will not receive the email until he has handed over to the doctor that they are waiting for and it could affect patient safety if Charles leaves.
82. **Very appropriate** because Charles knew he was going to be on call. If the doctor was running late then it would be different, but as this was planned Charles should wait for his commitment to finish first.
83. **Very appropriate** because it addresses the problem directly and Dr Patel would then know that Charles was leaving.
84. **Inappropriate but not awful** because Charles should not rely on messengers as they aren't as reliable as telling Dr Patel himself.
85. **Very appropriate** because the doctor that is taking over will be aware of the situation and can brief Dr Patel appropriately.

Scenario 18:

86. **Very appropriate** because Archie is being truthful and professional without ignoring the patient and still addresses her concerns.
87. **Very inappropriate** because Archie is not qualified to answer questions regarding management from a patient.
88. **Inappropriate but not awful** because whilst Archie is not giving any harmful information directly, the patient is unlikely to find his advice useful and it doesn't really address the problem.
89. **Very inappropriate** because Archie doesn't have the expertise necessary to give medical advice – with or without the use of Google.
90. **Inappropriate but not awful** because it is doesn't address the problem directly but at least isn't going to make the situation worse.

Scenario 19:

91. **Very appropriate** because they can advise Matthias on the best possible care.
92. **Inappropriate but not awful** because it may slow his recovery and may be dangerous. However, he would at least know if he was able to cope with the activity.
93. **Very appropriate** because it shows that he is being proactive and does not want to waste time.
94. **Very inappropriate** because the medical school might assume that he is being lazy and not going to hospital as he isn't committed.
95. **Inappropriate but not awful** because the medical school should find out from Matthias- not his friends.

Scenario 20:

96. **Very inappropriate** because Jessie may be the only person who notices this and is therefore in a position to address it. If nothing is done, Gemma may become very isolated.
97. **Appropriat**e but not ideal because Gemma will probably not want to talk about her eating disorder and avoid the topic in the future.
98. **Very appropriate** because it shows that Jessie can be trusted and is there for Gemma, without being confrontational.
99. **Appropriate but not ideal** as whilst it may make Gemma's parents aware – it is likely to strain their friendship.
100. **Very appropriate** because they will have seen this scenario before, and will know how to respond to it.

Scenario 21:

101. **Inappropriate, but no awful** – although this will allow her to revise for her exams, her friend will have spent a lot of money on the flights and will be left to fend for herself or not be able to go.
102. **Appropriate but not ideal-** Helen would be addressing both issues but given the circumstances, her revision may suffer or her friend may not enjoy the holiday as much.
103. **Very appropriate** because Helen also needs a break and being able to go for part of the holiday would be rewarding and shouldn't affect her revision as long as she comes back early enough.
104. **Very inappropriate** because Helen will be jeopardizing her chances of remaining in medical school.
105. **Very appropriate** because she will not be disappointing her friend as much, and will still be able to do her revision.

Scenario 22:

106. **Of minor importance** because the task should be joint effort.
107. **Important,** because this means that their grade is significant, and Sean will want to do as well as possible.
108. **Important** because they should learn how to work together to prevent future problems with their group work.
109. **Of minor importance**- although this might be troubling Daniel, he shouldn't let his social life affect his work life.
110. **Very important** because Daniel maybe used to not pulling his weight, and will have to be informed that he needs to contribute more.

Scenario 23:

111. **Very important**, because if the essay counts towards Tanya's final mark for the year then she would want to do very well.
112. **Not important at all** – different people learn in different ways and every clinic is different.
113. Of minor importance, because Dr Garg will be assessing her at the end of the term.
114. **Very important**, because if this opportunity is available at another time, then missing this particular clinic is not particularly disastrous for Tanya's learning.
115. **Very important,** because Tanya can complete the essay in time for the clinic, then she would not be compromising her learning.

Scenario 24:

116. **Important**, because the doctors that will be assessing Caroline will associate her with the dishevelled looking first year students and it may look unprofessional.
117. **Not important at all**, because they will still be representing the medical school and as such have a duty towards acting properly.
118. **Very important,** because the first year students are therefore expected to dress appropriately and professionally.
119. **Of minor importance,** because if she needs to ask them to dress more appropriately, they shouldn't get offended.
120. **Not important at all** – the students are representing the medical profession and must appear appropriately presentable regardless of when their examinations are.

Scenario 25:

121. **Not important at all** – timetabled clinical commitments should always come first (without extenuating circumstances).
122. **Very important**, because he may have to show a sports contribution to the medical school if he is on a scholarship. If this is the case, his firm head might understand, and rearrange the teaching sessions.
123. **Very important,** because he may not be allowed to finish his degree if he chooses to miss the sessions and not inform the consultant.
124. **Important** because this might allow him to rearrange the teaching sessions.
125. **Very important** because if he is missing invaluable teaching then this will affect his training and disadvantage him in the long run.

Scenario 26:

126. **Not important at all** – patient satisfaction in important and challenging bad practice does not reflect badly on students.
127. **Important** because the patient might be reluctant to ask questions or comply with the treatment if they are uncomfortable.
128. **Important** because if it is not a regular thing, then perhaps it is because Dr Davison is particularly stressed one day and might not be aware that he is swearing.
129. **Of minor importance** because whether or not they are aware of his swearing, it still makes the patient feel uncomfortable.
130. **Very important** because that means that the patient was either comfortable with the doctor previously, or that they were uncomfortable from before.

Scenario 27:

131. **Very important** because the patient could be subjected to avoidable infections, which could be life threatening.
132. **Not important at all** because the risk of the patient receiving an infection is worth the time required for the theatre staff to get more equipment ready.
133. **Of minor importance,** because he is only a medical student so can be forgiven for making mistakes. The repercussions of not saying anything could be far more serious.
134. **Of minor importance** because there is still a risk of infection if he is not sterile but the trolley is. He could still transmit infections.
135. **Of minor importance** because it is still important to protect the patient first and foremost.

Scenario 28:

136. **Important** because if the patient really is in pain then action should be taken. However, given that the patient is addicted to pain medication, it becomes less important.
137. **Not important at all** because her demands for pain medication are irrelevant to the staff, especially since she has just been reviewed by the doctors and nurses.
138. **Very important** because Freddie cannot administer any medications.
139. **Very important** because this means that the pain medication is not working or she is asking for it unnecessarily.
140. **Very important** because the patient has been reviewed and is therefore unlikely to need anything else so soon.

Scenario 29:

141. **Very important** because this is the key issue and the most important one for patient outcomes.
142. **Important** because letting Claire know this would put Claire at ease but it is not an essential piece of information to convey.
143. **Not important at all** as it is irrelevant to Claire's operation.
144. **Very important,** because her anxiety could affect her recovery if she is not completely comfortable with the surgeon.
145. **Very important** because if this is true, it will help Claire's recovery.

Scenario 30:

146. **Of minor importance** because Annabel should respond according to the situation, not because of who is involved. However, she should be wary that her actions are not in revenge.
147. **Important** because it will show that he usually works hard, whether or not he receives the help.
148. **Important** because the help from his rugby friends would not count as cheating.
149. **Not important at all** – Annabel might be jealous that she doesn't have this support network, but that should not influence her actions.
150. **Very important** because it severely disadvantages students who don't have access to the answers.

Scenario 31:

151. **Of minor importance** – whilst it won't stop him progressing with his degree, professionalism is a very important thing, and the medical school might want to investigate it further.
152. **Important,** because Matthew would have evidence of the public transport being delayed.
153. **Not important at all,** because the punctuality of the rest of his class does not reflect on Matthew at all.
154. **Very important,** because if Matthew can prove that his punctuality is usually satisfactory, then he can be more readily forgiven or excused for being late on the one occasion.
155. **Very important,** because Matthew should maintain a good rapport with his teacher if they are to see each other regularly for the next year.

Scenario 32:

156. **Very important,** because the week will be a vital part of her learning experience, and she will miss out if she misses the opportunity.
157. **Of minor importance** because whilst it may not cause seriously harm healthy people, it could seriously harm ill patients.
158. **Not important at all** because the issue here is of infection control – not if Michaela can function in the hospital.
159. **Very important** because if a patient became ill, Michaela would be unable to say that she had not been instructed appropriately.
160. **Important,** as it'd be a useful opportunity but not very important because the information is just her friend's opinion.

Scenario 33:

161. **Very important,** as this may be Jenny's only attempt to see what the exams are going to be like.
162. **Of minor importance** – Jenny's education is more important than losing out on money for a ski trip. However, it is still important, especially depending on what her financial situation is, but is not as relevant when deciding on how important the exams are.
163. **Important,** as Jenny would not have to worry about missing them or swapping her exam dates.
164. **Very important,** because if the university agrees to swap their exam dates then the issue would be resolved.
165. **Of minor importance**, although she has done well on exams so far, there is no guarantee that it would be the same for this set of mocks. It is still something to bear in mind whilst making her choice.

Scenario 34:

166. **Very important**, because it shows that he was very interested and proactive in the subject. It can also be used as evidence that Luke should be reconsidered for the project.
167. **Very important** because Architha may be willing to help Luke in his appeal as she could also gain from it.
168. **Not important at all,** because Luke should try to achieve the best grade possible with whichever project he was given.
169. **Of minor importance,** although Luke will find it difficult to concentrate on the project that he was allocated, personal preferences should not hinder his overall performance.
170. **Very important,** because the medical school can show that took his preferences into account.

Scenario 35:

171. **Very important,** because the mark will reflect on her ability for the rest of her life.
172. **Very important,** because this act might prevent Lucinda from getting the job she wants later on in her medical career.
173. **Important,** because it is a short period of time and if their relationship ends then Lucinda would have waster a year.
174. **Of minor importance**- although she is used to being with people that do well, they shouldn't affect her decision.
175. **Of minor importance**, although they are in a relationship, she needs to make the decision herself rather than be pressured into it.

Scenario 36:

176. **Very important,** because Shiv will save a lot of money if he skips the last day.
177. **Not important at all**, because the content of the assessment is not the issue but rather its timing.
178. **Important,** because this shows that Shiv is a good student. It also means that the doctor may have already formed an opinion for Shiv, and might be more likely to be lenient if he misses the final assessment.
179. **Not important at all,** because it will have no impact on Shiv's grade.
180. **Of minor importance** – although Shiv would like to meet with his girlfriend, he will be able to see her eventually so this isn't important in deciding **when** to leave.

Scenario 37:

181. **Very important** because if Jazzmynne won't get another chance to go on tour then it may be worth considering if she can miss classes.
182. **Very important,** because her learning is also important, and if she misses this rotation then she may not necessarily get the chance to catch up again.
183. **Of minor importance,** because Jazzmynne is an adult and if she feels as though she can handle the workload then she should be able to make her decisions herself. However, she should still keep her parent's concerns in mind.
184. **Very important**, because if Jazzmynne sometimes struggles to keep up with her workload without having any help, then with the extra stress of missing lots of work, she might struggle a lot.
185. **Not important at all** as Jazzmynne should not make the decision based on how much she would gain from the tour not because of what her friends decide.

Scenario 38:

186. **Of minor importance.** The changes may not come into action for Ellen to see but if she still feels strongly about the paper then it shouldn't change her actions.
187. **Very important**, as this shows that the university will take the opinions of the students into account.
188. **Very important,** because if the general stories are changed completely, then the majority of student readers may stop reading the papers. This could impact the newspaper's finances adversely.
189. **Of minor importance,** because the principal's stories can still be incorporated into the newspapers without abolishing the papers on the students' social lives.
190. **Not important at all** as this isn't a personal issue and should be handled professionally instead.

Scenario 39:

191. **Very important,** because the student bars should be safe, controlled spaces for the students to enjoy themselves.
192. **Of minor importance** – whilst extra money would be useful, the decision to appeal should be based on the needs of the student body rather than serving a selfish agenda.
193. **Very important**, because this is another factor that could bring their satisfaction ratings down further.
194. **Not important at all** – the issue is not about the cost but about the waiting times.
195. **Important,** because expanding the bar could bring in more money for the university.

Scenario 40:

196. **Not important at all,** because this should be handled amiably rather than making it personal.
197. **Very important,** because Phil does not have a chance of running again, but Olivia does.
198. **Important,** because it shows that Olivia is dedicated to the student union. It is not very important as there will be other factors that will differentiate Olivia and Phil.
199. **Very important,** because this excludes any chance of compromise with position allocation.
200. **Very important,** because it shows that Olivia has already compromised with the position previously, and will be unlikely to want to compromise again

Scenario 41:

201. **Very inappropriate-**This shows a lack of honesty and integrity and it is unfair to other students.
202. **Very inappropriate-** Although this appears to be a fair process as all the students are receiving the exam, it undermines the exam process and displays a lack of integrity in practice.
203. **Very inappropriate-** As a medical student you should take initiative and escalate situations appropriately. When you see that there is something that can affect the rest of the students and the medical school, you should involve those at a senior level
204. **Very appropriate-** The supervisor would be able to advise the student on what to do and would be able to help them in escalating the issue if required.
205. **Very appropriate-** The medical school will have a protocol for reporting situations such as these, and can deal with the situation accordingly.

Scenario 42:

206. **Very inappropriate-** Kate does not know the circumstances surrounding the missing money. It would be inappropriate to involve the police without the patient's permission and without exploring other avenues such as asking the senior nurses or look for the money herself.
207. **Appropriate but not ideal-** Kate needs to be careful not to sound patronising, as the patient will know that the wards are very exposed. However, it is good she offers them reassurance.
208. **Very inappropriate-** This is very patronising to the patient. Kate is accusing them of lying without understanding the full story. Also she has not provided any re-assurance that she will follow this up with more senior members of the department.
209. **Very appropriate-** Kate has taken some further details, she has re-assured the patient and has escalated the issue to the right person. Also the nurse in charge will be aware of the hospital processes and would be able to provide the patient with more information and assurance.
210. **Appropriate but not ideal-** Alerting other students of the theft is appropriate so they can keep their possessions safe and be on the lookout for the money, however it does not deal with the patient's alleged theft.

Scenario 43:

211. **Inappropriate but not awful-** Sam should not accuse Andrew of possession before he clarifies the situation. However, escalating the problem to his supervisor is appropriate.
212. **Very inappropriate-** Ignoring the situation, especially when Andrew may need help and support is inappropriate. There are also future implications to consider. Agreeing with Andrew to get rid of the drugs may lead Andrew to feel that taking drugs is ok.
213. **Very appropriate-** The supervisor would be able to provide advice to Sam on what he should do next.
214. **Very appropriate-** Offering support to Andrew would provide reassurance and a possibility to confide in a friend. Recommending professional help means that Sam recognises his own limitations and has signposted Andrew down the correct pathway.
215. **Very inappropriate-** Doing nothing is totally inappropriate. Seeing patients under the influence of drugs may put patient safety at risk and totally undermines a doctor's position of trust.

Scenario 44:

216. **Very appropriate:** Anna has recognised her limitations, informing someone who is senior who has more experience will ensure that the situation is dealt with more promptly and effectively. Patient safety is also maintained, and will ensure that the junior doctor receives professional help if he needs it.
217. **Very inappropriate-**Anna should not ignore the situation, the doctor is obviously drunk and he may put patients in danger. As a medical student if she sees there is something wrong in medical practice she needs to act on it.
218. **Very inappropriate-** Anna needs to recognise the limitations of her expertise and allowing the doctor to carry out his duties under the influence of alcohol can place patient safety at risk.
219. **Inappropriate but not awful-** It is good to reflect on difficult situations in practice, however this has not provided a solution to the current situation.
220. **Very appropriate -** Anna has recognised that the doctor is drunk and won't be able to carry out his duties. Advising him to inform the team so they are aware of the situation is very appropriate. More senior members of the team will be able to follow this up and ensure that the ward is appropriately staffed. .

Scenario 45

221. **Very appropriate-** Escalating the problem to the supervisor will enable the supervisor to provide solutions to the problem, support the group and encourage Sarah.

222. **Appropriate but not ideal-** Seeing how other group members feel about the current situation is appropriate, however it may lead to spreading gossip about Sarah.
223. **Inappropriate but not awful-** Informing Sarah that he has noticed her lateness and lack of contribution is an appropriate course of action. However the approach used is very patronising, furthermore there may be an underlying reason for her lateness that Sean should have asked about.
224. **Very appropriate-** Clarifying the situation with Sarah and making her aware that her lateness and contribution have not gone unnoticed allows her to increase her contribution and change her behaviour. Providing support may mean that he is able to remedy the current situation.
225. **Very inappropriate-** This is unfair to the other group members, in addition Sarah may be going through personal problems that she needs support for.

Scenario 46

226. **Appropriate but not ideal-** The nurse may not be aware of whom Mary is and Mary may come across as patronising, so the nurse may not be inclined to listen to her.
227. **Very appropriate-** Reporting the situation to a senior member is appropriate. The best person to report it to is the nurses immediate senior.
228. **Very appropriate-** Reporting the situation to the consultant is appropriate as they would be able to provide Mary with advice on what to do, or take it to the nurse's immediate senior themselves.
229. **Very inappropriate-** The nurse has acted unprofessionally, taking medications from the ward may put patients at risk, therefore the nurse needs to be made aware of the effects of her actions, and her need to uphold professional values.
230. **Appropriate but not ideal-** Reflecting on situations at medical placements is integral, as it will allow Mary to become a better future doctor. However, she has not dealt with the current situation of the nurse taking the medication.

Scenario 47

231. **Very inappropriate**- This is a matter between the consultant and Alan. Involving the nurse is inappropriate as she may inform the consultant, but this would involve an unnecessary party and may erode trust between the consultant and Alan.
232. **Very appropriate-**Alan's issue is with the consultant, so directly discussing it with him may allow Alan to gain a good relationship with the consultant and allow them to come to a joint decision regarding the remaining sessions.
233. **Very inappropriate-** This will only inflame the situation. The consultant may not realise that he is being harsh on Alan and therefore openly arguing in front of the patient is unprofessional and only sour their relationship.
234. **Very appropriate-** Alan is involving the relevant authority. It is his supervisor who is responsible for his educational needs, and his supervisor is in a position to provide advice at an appropriate level.
235. **Very inappropriate-** In this case, Alan is involving a patient in a conflict which is really none of their concern Alan is also undermining the Consultant's credibility behind their back.

Scenario 48

236. **Inappropriate but not awful** The nurse has specifically asked Harry if he could have a word with his fellow student, because she may have felt that it is a situation that could be solved at the student level without involving doctors. Harry may feel that this is not his responsibility.
237. **Very appropriate-** Addressing the issue with the colleague in question avoids public humiliation and a solution to the problem may be reached without involving someone else such as the consultant.
238. **Very inappropriate-** Harry is being dishonest to the nurse especially when he has promised to speak to Joe.
239. **Inappropriate but not awful-** Harry is not publically humiliating Joe and he has not ignored the issue, but sending him an anonymous note is very cowardly and may upset Joe.
240. **Very inappropriate-**This action will achieve nothing other than publicly humiliating Joe in front of other students.

Scenario 49

241. **Appropriate but not ideal-** It is appropriate to be honest to the consultant and to refuse to add the names unless they have contributed to the report.
242. **Very inappropriate-** This is dishonest and unprofessional, it doesn't matter what type of publication; it is a matter of personal ethics that Helen has to her patients and society.
243. **Very appropriate-**Escalating the problem to the medical student supervisor is appropriate as he would be able to support and provide Helen with the advice needed.
244. **Very appropriate-** Helen could clarify if the added names have actually contributed to the report and to discuss her concerns.
245. **Inappropriate but not awful-** This does not solve the situation; not publishing avoids being an accessory to fraudulent activity, however Helen is losing a chance to add an achievement to her own CV.

Scenario 50

246. **Very inappropriate-**John is being presumptive here, the books may be Clare's own, and Clare may have borrowed the books from the library and forgot to return them.
247. **Very appropriate-** John has clarified the situation with Clare and has asked her to return the books, so has provided a solution. Medical school library books are a resource for all students so now other students would be able to use the missing books.
248. **Very inappropriate-** There is no need to contact the police in this situation, John would be wasting their time and resources.

249. **Appropriate but not ideal-** The medical school library would now know that they do not need to purchase more copies of the missing books, and they may follow it up independently, but John has not ensured that Clare would return them.
250. **Very appropriate-** If John is not sure of how to tackle the situation it would be best to discuss it with his supervisor as he would give him the advice needed.

Scenario 51

251. **Very appropriate-** Speaking to Anne is the best approach to take as Anne may not be aware of how Nadia is feeling. Anne and Nadia may also be able to find an arrangement of providing teaching sessions when the ward is quite.
252. **Appropriate but not ideal-**Nadia needs to take initiative for her own learning. If she feels she is not making the most of her experience then she needs to inform someone, and speaking sooner rather than later would obviously be better for her, as the situation may not improve on its own. However she may feel that it is too early and the situation may improve on its own as she is new to the ward.
253. **Very appropriate-** Her supervisor would be a good person to speak to, to get advice and help
254. **Inappropriate but not awful-** Nadia needs to spend time on the wards during her medical school years, as this will give her invaluable patient experience, However, she may feel that her time is spent more efficiently in the library.
255. **Appropriate but not ideal-** Nadia has taken initiative for her learning, however Anne may be offended if she has not discussed this with her prior to finding another doctor. Also the other doctors may have other students assigned or other commitments to attend to.

Scenario 52

256. **Appropriate but not ideal-** Reprimanding Laura is patronising, however refusing to sign the book is the right thing to do. Students should not be signing each other's books as it undermines the value of the clinical experience. However, offering tips for the future is a way of being supportive.
257. **Very inappropriate-** Despite seeing Laura attending the sessions, this is dishonest. It would be considered forgery as doctors are required to sign.
258. **Very appropriate-** Directing Laura to the right person who is meant to be signing the book is appropriate as they know the appropriate steps to take.
259. **Very inappropriate-** Even if she has demonstrated the skill, students should not be signing assessments each another.
260. **Inappropriate but not awful-** Reporting Laura to the medical school without clarifying the situation or trying the solve it is a bit extreme, however forgery is a great academic offence.

Scenario 53

261. **Very inappropriate-** There must be a reason why it took Steven three attempts to cannulate the patient, Emma should work within her limitations.
262. **Appropriate but not ideal-** It would be best to clarify the situation with Steven before escalating, and it would be best to escalate to his direct senior. However, alerting the nurse in charge about Steven's behaviour may avoid the situation escalating to a complaint by the patient.
263. **Very appropriate-**Steven has left Emma in an awkward position. It's best to go and find him and check everything is okay- he may have gone to get more cannulation equipment and was planning to come back.
264. **Very appropriate-** Escalating the situation to a more senior doctor is appropriate, they would be able to provide Emma with advice on what to do.
265. **Very inappropriate-** Emma is undermining Steven as a doctor, and this would affect patient-doctor trust.

Scenario 54

266. **Very inappropriate-** Jill should remain professional in her manner even if the patient has said something offensive, and retaliating could make the situation worse.
267. **Very inappropriate-** As a medical student Jill is part of the team. Ignoring the situation shows she is not a good team player. The patient may also view her silence as an excuse to continue to make these racist remarks.
268. **Very appropriate-** Racist comments are not tolerated in any workplace, so speaking to the patient politely maintains professionalism and shows that Jill has taken initiative.
269. **Very appropriate-** Discussing the matter with the consultant in charge is appropriate, he will provide Jill with the right advice and can help in de-escalating the situation.
270. **Appropriate but not ideal-** Reporting the matter straight to the registrar is appropriate as he would know the hospital protocol, especially since he is the one treating the patient. However it may be better to report it to someone else in case he takes offense.

Scenario 55

271. **Very appropriate-** Depending on how the other members of the group feel, he could then get a better understanding of the group dynamics and the appropriate steps to take.
272. **Very inappropriate-** This is being very patronising and unfair to Hannah, she needs to contribute to the group project as well.
273. **Very inappropriate-**All the group members need to contribute equally to the project. This would also be unfair to the other members of the group.
274. **Very appropriate-** The supervisor would be able to provide advice and he would usually know the appropriate steps to take in regards to involving Hannah.
275. **Very appropriate-** Speaking to Hannah directly to let her know of how you are feeling and maybe offer both support and guidance.

Scenario 56

276. **Appropriate but not ideal-** It would be best for her colleague to go home. She may become more distressed, and won't be able to do her work effectively, however she will need to notify her supervisor as she may need a few more days off.
277. **Very appropriate-** Offering support to a colleague who is going through a difficult time would be appropriate.
278. **Very appropriate-** This is very appropriate as he would be able to provide Jenny with advice and provide her colleague with support.
279. **Very inappropriate-** Jenny is not being supportive at all, this may cause her colleague to become more distressed.
280. **Inappropriate but not awful-** Jenny may have thought that leaving her colleague and giving her a few minutes will help her to calm down, but her colleague may feel alone and unsupported.

Scenario 57

281. **Very inappropriate** - This is a breach of patient confidentiality. Patient details should not be discussed in public places.
282. **Very appropriate-** Maya is within a group of friends and she should remind her friends of patient confidentiality and their duty to protect it.
283. **Inappropriate but not awful-** Maya is trying to changing the subject of the conversation, however she may not be successful and she has not highlighted to her friends that what they are doing is wrong.
284. **Appropriate but not ideal-** Maya's friends need to made aware of their actions at this stage, not saying anything means her friends will continue breaching patient confidentiality until they are called by the medical school. This would also cause unnecessary worry for her friends, and suspicion of her, especially when the matter could have been solved between friends.
285. **Very inappropriate-** By excusing herself she has taken no action to make her friends aware that they are breaching patient confidentiality, so they will continue discussing patient cases, which is not acceptable.

Scenario 58

286. **Appropriate but not ideal-** The supervisor would be able to provide Michael with advice on how to proceed, but Simon may not have wanted anyone else to know.
287. **Very appropriate-** Simon has been advised to speak to his supervisor so that the supervisor could provide him with the support he needed. He will also be aware of the medical school procedures so he would be able to assist Simon directly.
288. **Very inappropriate-** Simon has confided in Michael seeking support, mocking him may make him feel worse about himself.
289. **Inappropriate but not awful-** Simon has confided in Michael and has asked him not to tell anyone. Michael feels if more people know then they might help him, but he has broken Simon's confidence and lost his trust.
290. **Very appropriate-** Advising him to seek help from the right channels is the right thing to do. Seeking medical advice is also a duty of all students and doctors if they feel their physical or mental health has an impact on their work.

Scenario 59

291. **Very inappropriate-** The doctor is in breach of hospital regulations and his moral obligations; he needs to be made aware that what he is doing is wrong.
292. **Very appropriate-** Mark's supervisor would be aware of the guidelines for similar issues so he would be able to advise Mark on what to do and to support him.
293. **Appropriate but not ideal-** It is good to speak to the doctor directly, however, confrontation can make the situation worse, it is best to approach the doctor and clarify the situation; it may have been something innocuous such as a computer virus.
294. **Very inappropriate-** Mark has not clarified the situation with the doctor; this may anger the doctor and may lead to patients losing trust in doctors.
295. **Appropriate but not ideal-** Contacting the hospital IT services to make them aware that these website are accessible so they can firewall these sites would be good, however it does not lead to immediately solving the situation of the doctor watching pornography in a public place.

Scenario 60

296. **Appropriate but not ideal-** She is offering her apologies, however is involving another student and this is not the appropriate step to take.
297. **Inappropriate but not awful-** The change in seminar times was very short notice, so other students may be off sick however Alice would have to justify her absence at a later date.
298. **Very appropriate-** Discussing the issue with the seminar leader, the person who knows best, is proactive and shows that Alice is taking initiative and she has not involved a third party.
299. **Appropriate but not ideal-** Alice has realised that she has to attend the teaching session, it is good to have a work and social life balance so cancelling the dinner plans is not ideal.
300. **Very inappropriate-** The change in seminar times is short notice however; there are ways that Alice could approach the issue without being rude.

UCAT Practice Papers

The Basics

The UCAT consortium do not release past papers…

Well hopefully that is where this book comes in. It contains six unique mock papers written by expert Oxbridge medical tutors at *UniAdmissions*. Having successfully gained places at Oxbridge and other competitive medical schools, our tutors are intimately familiar with the UCAT and its associated admission procedures. So, the novel questions presented to you here are of the correct style and difficulty to continue your revision and stretch you to meet the demands of the UCAT.

Mock Paper A

Section A: Verbal Reasoning

Passage 1

Atomic Structure

Although the existence of atoms has been suggested since ancient Greece, the modern understanding of atomic structure is the product of the hard work of many dedicated scientists. In the early 1800s, John Dalton's experiments with chemical reactions led him to theorise that matter is composed of tiny individual units. These individual units of matter were later understood to be what we call atoms. In 1897, the English Physicist J. J. Thomson discovered that atoms contain both positive and negative electrical charges by performing experiments with cathode ray tubes. Thomson visualised the negative charges as immersed within positively charged material. Although his model of atomic structure is now considered incorrect, it was the most accurate picture of an atom at that time.

In 1909, Ernest Rutherford, a physicist at the University of Manchester, performed his famous alpha particle experiment and concluded that atoms have a positively charged nucleus at their centre. Danish physicist Niels Bohr theorized in 1912 that negatively charged electrons orbit the positively charged nucleus in fixed paths, not unlike planets around the sun. In the 1920s, several scientists modified Bohr's ideas of the orbital paths of electrons by demonstrating that electrons do not behave like other particles and that their location as they orbit the nucleus is difficult to predict.

The rest of the 20th Century saw the discovery of neutrons, which carry a neutral charge, and quarks, which make up all protons, neutrons and electrons. By the 1990s, no less than six different types of quarks had been identified. New discoveries in atomic structure will surely be made in the future.

1. The existence of atoms:

A. is a recent idea.
B. is an old idea.
C. is an early 19th century idea.
D. is a late 19th century idea.

2. Which of the following statements is true according to the above passage:

A. John Dalton proved that matter is composed of tiny individual units.
B. J.J. Thomson proved atoms were made up of negative charges immersed within positively charged material.
C. Niels Bohr discovered that electrons orbit in fixed paths around the nucleus.
D. That atoms do not contain a negatively charged nucleus was discovered in the 20th century.

3. Which of the following statements about quarks is true:

A. There are over six types of quarks.
B. Quarks are made up of neutrons, electrons and protons.
C. The discovery of quarks has settled discussions on atomic structure.
D. Quarks are even smaller than atoms.

4. Which of the following statements is INCORRECT:

A. Electrons' behaviour is dissimilar to other particles' behaviour.
B. Electrons' behaviour is predictable.
C. Electrons contain quarks.
D. Electrons go around a nucleus.

Passage 2

The Space Race

After the Second World War, Western Europe and the United States found themselves at odds with the Soviet Union. Although they never went to war directly, the two sides were in a constant race to develop advanced weapons and other technology.

In 1957, the Soviets launched the first man-made satellite, Sputnik 1, into space. The successful launch and orbit of Sputnik 1 caused the United States to attempt a satellite launch two months later. The rocket carrying the American satellite failed to launch and exploded on the launch pad. Two months after that, the U.S. did successfully launch a satellite into earth's orbit, and the rivalry between the Soviet and American space programs began.

The next goal was to successfully launch a human into outer space, which the Soviets did first in April 1961 when Yuri Gagarin completed almost two hours orbiting the earth. A month later, an American astronaut was successfully launched into space, although not into orbit. U.S. President Kennedy then began campaigning for a space program aimed at reaching the moon faster than the Soviets.

The mid-1960s were spent with both the Americans and Soviets achieving multiple-day manned space flights, the manual manoeuvring of spacecraft, and spacewalks. In 1967, both sides began a series of manned space flights whose ultimate goal was to land on the moon.

The first humans to orbit the moon were American astronauts in December, 1968. The Soviets never achieved manned lunar orbit, as their space program was plagued with difficulties. In June of 1969 American astronaut Neil Armstrong became the first human to set foot on the moon, effectively defeating the rival Soviet lunar program.

After the race to the moon was over, both sides began to focus on developing space stations, as they would be less expensive than lunar programs and would provide valuable opportunities for research. The Soviets launched the first space station, Salyut 1, into orbit in 1971, followed by the American space station Skylab in 1973. In 1975, a joint space mission involving Soviet and American crews in cooperation was the symbolic end of the rivalry.

5. Which of the following statements is correct:
A. Rivalry throughout WWII between the US and the Soviet Union continued after the war's end.
B. The aftermath of WWII caused tensions between the Soviet Union and Western forces including the US and Western Europe.
C. The developments in each other's technology sparked fear and tension between the US and the Soviet Union.
D. The passage does not state the reasons for the US and the Soviet Union being at odds.

6. According to the passage:
A. The US's space programme was inferior to the Soviet Union's.
B. Developments in space technology fuels developments in weapons technology.
C. The Soviet Union was initially more successful in the Space Race.
D. The US won the Space Race.

7. Which of the following statements is supported by the above passage?
A. The Soviet Union's poverty crippled their attempts to achieve the landing of the first man on the moon.
B. The Soviet Union's civil unrest crippled their attempts to achieve the landing of the first man on the moon.
C. Neil Armstrong was the first man to achieve a spacewalk.
D. The moon-landing had political elements to it.

8. According to the above passage, the 1975 space mission was preceded by:
A. Multiple humans orbiting the moon.
B. Political truce between the Soviet Union and the US.
C. Multiple men on the moon.
D. Much valuable research had been achieved by the 1973 space mission.

Passage 3

Childcare

Childcare is a very important service for most families, whether it be day care, preschool, primary school, secondary school, or simply babysitting. Parents generally cherish their children above all other things, so they do not normally hand their children over to just anyone. Parents need to trust that their children will be physically and emotionally safe while they are apart. Furthermore, if the childcare situation is at a school, parents need to trust that their children are receiving an appropriate education, or they may make other arrangements.

Childcare professionals, babysitters, teachers and school staff should make every effort to ensure a safe setting for the children in their care. This normally includes meeting the physical needs of children by providing clean nappies, bathrooms, food, water, shelter, and sleep if necessary. Children also have emotional and intellectual needs that should be met by adults speaking with them, allowing them to make decisions, helping them overcome challenges, giving them advice, allowing them to make friends, and making them feel respected.

People that care for children should also monitor them for signs of emotional and physical abuse. If a teacher, babysitter, or childcare professional were to observe bruises on a child or to notice the child acting unusually aggressive or depressed, he or she should consider that the child may be having serious problems at home. If a teacher, babysitter, or childcare professional confirms that a child is likely experiencing physical or emotional abuse, he or she should contact an appropriate authority to investigate the situation.

9. Parents:
A. All hold childcare as a very important service.
B. All cherish their children above most things, at all times.
C. May be discerning when it comes to childcare providers.
D. Above all, need to trust that their kids will be emotionally safe when apart from them.

10. Which of these is NOT stated as something to consider when caring for someone else's child:
A. Nutrition.
B. The child's feelings.
C. A tidy appearance.
D. The child's feeling respected.

11. People who care for children should know:
A. Bruises mean the child is experiencing serious problems at home.
B. Unusual aggression means the child is being abused.
C. Unusual depressions means the child is being abused.
D. There is a procedure to follow if they suspect child abuse.

12. Which of the following statements is NOT supported by the above passage:
A. People involved in child care include educators.
B. Childcare services include educational establishments, holiday camps and babysitting.
C. People who care for children should make sure the children in their care are getting water.
D. People who care for children should watch out for signs of abuse.

Passage 4

Australia

The first European contact with Australia was apparently with Dutch explorers in the 17th Century, but the English were the first to explore and colonize the enormous island. English settlers arrived in Australia in 1770 and soon English became the dominant language, as opposed to the roughly 250 language groups found in the country before this immigration, and Christianity the dominant religion. Initial settling was through penal transportation, the moving of criminals to the Oceanian land. This practice was also used in the Victorian era, and the fictional character of Sweeney Todd is said to have been sent to this land 'on a trumped up charge'.

The 19th Century saw the development of the territory into a modern economic and political force, making it an important part of the British Empire. During the 20th Century, Australia gained independence from Great Britain and became a major world power.

Most Australians now have European ancestry and Native Australians, also known as Aboriginal Australians, currently make up just a small fraction of the Australian population. Australian society saw little variation for millennia, as the Aborigines inhabited it for at least 40,000 years, but in the last 250 years it has undergone sweeping changes.

13. Australians of European descent may well be able to trace their ancestry back to an 18th century criminal.
A. True.
B. False.
C. Can't tell.

14. Dutch is *not* the dominant language in Australia, because:
A. The English stole the land from them.
B. English is easier to learn than Dutch.
C. The Dutch had the first European contact with Australia, but did not settle there.
D. The natives hated the Dutch.

15. According to the above passage, Australian independence:
A. Improved the conditions of Aboriginal Australians.
B. Decreased the wealth of Great Britain.
C. Embarrassed the English.
D. Resulted in the creation of a new major world power.

16. Which of the following is true according to the passage:
A. Many were sent to Australia on trumped-up charges.
B. Natives have reproduced less since the advent of English immigration to Australia.
C. Immigrants to Australia have all reproduced to a great extent.
D. A quarter of a millennium can be enough time to change a country's demographic situation.

Passage 5

Louis Pasteur

Louis Pasteur, a French scientist, is known as the father of microbiology. Pasteur's work demonstrated once and for all that microorganisms such as mould and bacteria, along with insect larvae, were not the product of spontaneous generation. Spontaneous generation was the ancient and medieval idea that certain types of life could appear on their own, without coming from a parental source, such as mould growing in standing water or maggots growing in uneaten food. Pasteur theorized that microorganisms were responsible for the appearance of these phenomena and proved himself correct in one of his most famous experiments. In 1859, he sterilized several containers and filled them with beef broth. In containers with long, curved necks, the beef broth remained uncontaminated because microbes could not reach the broth within. If a container were opened or turned so that microbes and other particles could reach the broth, its contents became contaminated with bacteria in a matter of hours.

The work of Pasteur and other biologists led to modern food preservation techniques. Canned food was a new development in Pasteur's day and his advancements in microbiology helped perfect and promote the process. Pasteur developed the practice of heating wine and beer to a temperature of 50 – 60 degrees Celsius to prevent spoilage. The practice was later expanded to include milk and other beverages. Boiled wine, beer or milk would be ruined, but if they were heated to this lower temperature, many of the microbes died and the structure of the beverage remained intact. This process was later termed "Pasteurization" after Louis Pasteur.

17. The idea of spontaneous generation:
A. Stated organisms could come into being from nothing.
B. Stated organisms could be utterly different from their parents, like maggots being born from uneaten parents.
C. Started in the middle ages.
D. Ended with the middle ages.

18. Which of the following is Pasteur NOT stated to be in the above passage:
A. European.
B. Male.
C. A genius.
D. A biologist

19. Pasteur's discoveries are stated to have helped modern food production because:
A. It made food more palatable, as micro-organisms are known to be foul-tasting.
B. It made food more attractive, as micro-organisms like mould are unsightly.
C. It stopped food from smelling unpleasant.
D. It helped to keep food from going off.

20. According to the passage, when treating milk, beer and wine through pasteurisation:
A. The fluid becomes ruined by heat.
B. The fluid becomes completely free of microbes.
C. The fluid maintains its structure.
D. The fluid is 100% guaranteed not to cause any sickness through consumption.

Passage 6

Agricultural Reform

The 18th Century saw many advances in agriculture, which spurred Europe into the Industrial Revolution and spawned the modern societies now known by most of the world. Farming had been common in Europe for thousands of years, but few innovations had taken hold. When crops grow in a field, they remove the nutrients and fertilisers from the land. Ancient and Medieval farmers knew to leave fields fallow for a growing season or two to allow the soil to regain its fertility, and this practice remained largely unchanged. In the 1700s, however, British farmers found that if they grew other crops on their unused fields, nutrients returned to the soil faster than if the fields were left fallow.

Clover restores fields well; after growing clover in a field for a season, farmers could replant and grow on that field the next season with success. We now know that this is because clover absorbs nitrogen from the atmosphere and returns it to the soil as a natural fertilizer. Turnips were commonly planted in hitherto unused fields because they would also return fields to fertility. We now know that this is because the deep roots of turnips collect nutrients and bring them to the topsoil where they can be reached by the roots of other crops when the fields are replanted.

21. For thousands of years, farming in Europe was done in roughly the same way.
A. True.
B. False.
C. Can't tell.

22. There was a link between agriculture and industry in 1700s Europe.
A. True.
B. False.
C. Can't tell.

23. What did 18th Century British farmers know that Medieval ones did not:
A. That crops sap nutrients from the land.
B. That crops sap fertilisers from the land.
C. Certain plants replenish nutrients.
D. Leaving fields fallow allows them to recover.

24. According to the passage, turnips and clovers
A. Improve topsoil.
B. Collect nutrients from the atmosphere.
C. Collect nutrients from the earth.
D. Provide an alternative to leaving land fallow.

Passage 7

The Industrial Revolution

The increased production of food in the 18th Century allowed Europe to support a higher population than ever before. Advances in agricultural technology also allowed farms to be operated by fewer labourers than ever before, creating a surplus of labour. Many of these labourers found work in mills, mines and eventually factories, and their manpower helped drive the Industrial Revolution. The excess population in Europe also helped fuel European colonial empires, as a ready supply of colonists appeared to fill the New World.

The cities of Europe soon experienced overpopulation, which brought the problems of disease, poverty and crime. Orphanages and workhouses were common in the 19th Century, as many of the poor lived in squalor. Factories and mills were generally unsafe places to work and workplace accidents were common. The steady supply of labour meant that employers could overwork and underpay their workers. Churches and charities began caring for the poor and campaigning for better living and working conditions. Eventually, laws were enacted across the western world that limited work hours and child labour, promoted workplace safety and public health, and established the minimum wage.

25. Increased food production meant:
A. There were fewer jobs for farm labourers.
B. More people could be fed.
C. More people moved to the colonies.
D. Mills improved.

26. The Industrial revolution was predominately responsible for colonisation.
A. True.
B. False.
C. Can't tell.

27. The passage states:
A. The Industrial revolution was a positive event.
B. The Industrial revolution is an event to be regretted.
C. Things became a lot simpler with the advent of the Industrial Revolution.
D. Higher populations can come with problems.

28. Employers in the above passage are described as possibly:
A. Benevolent.
B. Anxious.
C. Exploitative.
D. Sadistic.

Passage 8

The Ice Age

For much of the last 100,000 years, Earth's climate was colder than it is now and enormous ice sheets covered large parts of North America, Europe and Asia. The Scandinavian Ice Sheet covered what is now Scotland and northern England, as well as what are now Scandinavia and northern Russia. What are now Canada and the northern United States were covered by the Laurentide Ice Sheet. Humans inhabited many of these areas before the ice sheets formed, but were forced out by the cooling climate. By around 12,000 years ago, much of this ice had melted and sea levels had risen to their present state.

As the Earth warmed, the ice sheets slowly receded, creating many of the landforms now present in North America, Europe and Asia. Sand, gravel and rocks of various sizes were all carried northward with the receding ice, and were re-deposited as melting ice formed new rivers and lakes. When melting ice flowed heavily from an ice sheet, a new river could be formed as the flowing water dug a trench through the earth. When a large piece of ice broke off from an ice sheet and was left behind to melt, a lake or pond could be formed. This is how many of the lakes in northern Europe and Canada were created, such as

Osterseen in Germany, Loch Fergus in Scotland, and Wilcox Lake in Canada.

As the ice sheets shrank, humans moved back into the newly inhabitable areas of the arctic. Asians crossed into the Americas, and sea levels rose to separate Siberia from Alaska and the British Isles from Europe.

29. For 100,000 years Earth's climate was colder than it is now.

A. True.

B. False.

C. Can't tell.

30. Which of the following is NOT true:

A. Scotland is covered by the Scandinavian Ice Sheet.

B. The same ice sheet covered what were northern Russia and Scotland.

C. Multiple ice sheets existed.

D. Ice sheets were very large.

31. Loch Fergus was created:

A. By heavy-flowing melting ice.

B. By sand, gravel and rocks being deposited by melting ice.

C. By non-flowing melting ice.

D. By medium-flowing melting ice.

32. The British Isles was once part of mainland Europe:

A. True.

B. False.

C. Can't tell.

Passage 9

Germany

The Federal Republic of Germany (or the *Bundesrepublik Deutschland)* is the most populous country in the European Union and has Europe's largest economy. It also has the fourth largest economy in the world, giving it an influential role in geopolitics. The German language, also widely spoken in Switzerland and Austria, has over 100 million native speakers and some 80 million speakers who learned it as a foreign language. Many Europeans have migrated to Germany to take advantage of job opportunities that are available in its strong economy.

The European Union's Freedom of Movement for Workers principle (described in Treaty on European Union Article 39) means that anyone from an EU country (a state that is a member of the European Union) can seek and gain work in any other EU country, without experiencing discrimination due to their citizenship, excepting the people of Croatia. Accordingly, in 2014 many immigrants from Poland, Romania and Bulgaria came to Germany looking for employment. Croatian citizens also attempted to find paid work in the country, despite their exclusion from the above treaty. There were also those from the Middle East, who were refugees from ongoing conflicts in the region, who sought asylum within Germany's boarders.

33. Germany is a monarchy.
A. True.
B. False.
C. Can't tell.

34. According to the passage, the German language:
A. Is spoken as a mother tongue by over 100 million people.
B. Is spoken as a mother tongue by over 180 million people.
C. Is the dominant language in Austria and Switzerland.
D. Is the second most important language in geopolitics.

35. The German economy:
A. Is strong because of the influx of immigrant workers.
B. Ensures everyone in Germany is well-off.
C. Is in the top ten biggest global economies.
D. Ensures jobs for migrant workers.

36. According to the above passage, Croatians have more right to German jobs than Middle Eastern migrants.
A. True.
B. False.
C. Can't tell.

Passage 10

Thomas Hobbes

Born in 1588 in Malmesbury, Wiltshire, with a clergyman father, Thomas Hobbes was an English political philosopher and political scientist. His birth was linked to acts of war: he was born prematurely, when his mother heard of the approaching Spanish Armada invasion. This instance led to him pithily saying his parent 'gave birth to twins: myself and fear.'

In 1651, he published the book *Leviathan*. The following is an excerpt from this text, which he wrote in France, and is in reference to the English Civil War and its effects on society:

"In such condition, there is no place for industry; because the fruit thereof is uncertain; and consequently no culture of the earth; no navigation, nor use of the commodities that may be imported by sea; no commodious building; no instruments of moving and removing such things as require much force; no knowledge of the face of the earth; no account of time; no arts; no letters
; no society; and which is worst of all, continual fear, and danger of violent death; and the life of man, solitary, poor, nasty, brutish, and short."

37. *Leviathan* considers biblical stances.
A. True.
B. False.
C. Can't tell.

38. Hobbes:
A. Hated the Spanish.
B. Hated war from birth.
C. Was born in a condition of stress.
D. Was born to be a clergyman.

39. The passage states that the seventeenth century:
A. Saw the birth of this great political mind.
B. Saw the birth of a great philosophical mind.
C. Saw the product of a political-philosophical mind.
D. Saw the depression of Thomas Hobbes.

40. Hobbes' speaks on:
A. The necessity of war.
B. The destruction of the enemy through war.
C. The shutting down of society.
D. The problems with the predominate illiteracy of the poor of his time.

Passage 11

Emily Davison

The first-wave feminism movement saw many passionate women fighting for their cause, and sacrificing much in pursuit of equal rights for both sexes. An example of a feminist who paid much for her beliefs in Emily Davison, who campaigned in Britain and had experienced multiple run-ins with the law before her death.

On nine separate occasions she was arrested and thrown into jail. She continued protesting even from a cell, by refusing to eat. Feminist hunger strikes often ended in force-feeding, a horrible process where a tube is passed through the mouth (or, occasionally, the nose) into the stomach so food can be poured directly into the prisoner's body. The inmate would be held down whilst this happened. Davison endured this invasive treatment 49 times.

In 1913, at the Epsom Derby, she ran in front of King George's horse and ended up trampled. It has been debated what exactly her intentions were, with many arguing it was not a suicidal act. Some believe that analysis of the newsreel supports the notion that Davison was trying to attach a scarf to the King's horse's bridle, and that her behaviour was more a publicity stunt than a conscious sacrifice of her life. If this is so, then she paid the ultimate price for her beliefs and died the way she lived: campaigning for male and female equality.

41. Equal rights did not exist at all in the 20th century.
A. True.
B. False.
C. Can't tell.

42. According to the passage, feminists fought for:
A. Superior rights for women.
B. Equal rights for different sexualities.
C. The vote.
D. Men to have the same rights as women.

43. Hunger strikes:
A. Discredited the feminist cause.
B. Were a waste of time.
C. Were countered with awful treatment.
D. Eventually died out.

44. Emily Davison was:
A. Suicidal.
B. Willing to sacrifice personal comfort.
C. A genius.
D. A pre-eminent figure in first wave feminism.

END OF SECTION

Section B: Decision Making

1. Chocolates come in boxes of 6, 9 and 20. What is the largest number of chocolates you CANNOT buy using the above combinations?

A. 19   B. 27   C. 35   D. 43   E. 52

2. "It is best to start medical school aged 18."

Which statement gives the best supporting reason for this statement?

A. Medical schools are unlikely to admit people under 18 years old.
B. At 18, students have reached the right level of maturity to enter medical school.
C. Students cannot live away from their parents before they are 18.
D. You must be an adult before starting medical school.

3. Dr Smith is only able to prescribe drugs. All antidepressants are drugs. Carbamazepine is not an antidepressant. Most home remedies are drugs. Place true and false next to the statements below.

A. Dr Smith can prescribe antidepressants.
B. Dr Smith can prescribe carbamazepine.
C. Carbamazepine is not a drug.
D. Dr Smith can prescribe all home remedies.
E. Most home remedies are antidepressants.

4. The probability Lucas misses the bus to school on a sunny day is 0.3 and on a rainy day is 0.2. The probability he carries an umbrella on any day is 0.4. If he misses the bus, Lucas walks to school. Last week, it rained on the last three days of the school week. Lucas thinks that last week, he was more likely to walk to school in the rain without an umbrella than to walk in the sun with an umbrella. Is he correct?

A. Yes
B. No, there is an equal chance of both occurrences in the last week
C. No because the probability of getting the bus when it is raining is greater than catching the bus when it is sunny
D. No, because the probability that he carries an umbrella on any given day is 0.4

5. All musicians play instruments. All oboe players are musicians. Oboes and pianos are instruments. Karen is a musician. Which statement is true?

A. Karen plays two instruments.
B. All musicians are oboe players.
C. All instruments are pianos or oboes.
D. Karen is an oboe player.
E. None of the above

6. All of James's sons have brown eyes and all of his daughters have blue eyes. His wife has just become pregnant with a boy. Which statement is most likely to be correct?

A. The baby will have brown eyes.
B. James' wife has blue eyes.
C. Brown eyes are more likely than blue eyes.
D. Blue eyes are equally as likely as brown eyes.
E. None of the above.

7. Millie and Ben play a game. There is a stack of pennies and each player takes it in turn to remove one, two or three pennies each turn. The person who takes the last penny wins. If Millie starts the games, how many pennies will she need to start the game with to guarantee a win?

A. 4 pennies.   B. 8 pennies   C. 13 pennies.   D. 16 pennies.

8. "Obesity is a growing problem, therefore there should be a tax on high calorie foods." Which option is the best argument against the above statement?

A. Those from low income backgrounds will be hit hardest from this tax.
B. Cost does not affect choice of food.
C. You are more likely to be overweight if you are rich.
D. Many high calorie foods are healthy

9. B is right of A. C is left of B. D is in front of C. E is in front of B. Where is D is relation to E?

A. D is behind E.
B. E is behind D.
C. D is to the right of E.
D. D is to the left of E.
E. E is to the left of D.

10. Arnold, Carrie and Eric are arguing about the number of cars their father owns. Arnold says "Dad owns at least four cars", Carrie says "No, he owns less than four cars", and Eric says "he owns at least one car". If only one of them is tell the truth, how many cars does their father own?

A. 0 B. 1 C. 3 D. 4 E. 5

11. "Increased traffic is bad for your health." Which statement provides the best evidence for this conclusion?

A. Traffic congested increases carbon monoxide in the environment to harmful levels.
B. Sitting in traffic reduces the amount of time for people to exercise.
C. Towns with higher road tax have healthier people.
D. Pollution from cars causes acid rain.
E. Some traffic congestion is not hazardous to health

12. Fred has a drawer full of socks. There are 1 red, 2 green, 4 blue and 10 orange. In the dark, he cannot distinguish colours. What is the least number of socks he has to pick to ensure he has three matching pairs?

A. 10 B. 8 C. 3 D. 9 E. 11

13. Gabby is older than Maria. Maria's older sister Olivia is older than Gabby. Gabby wins more often than Olivia. Olivia's boyfriend Tom loses the most often. All four play cards. Which statement is true?

A. Maria is the youngest.
B. Olivia wins more than Maria.
C. Gabby hates playing cards.
D. Maria wins more than Tom.
E. Tom is the oldest.

14. Three rats are placed in a maize that is in the shape of an equilateral triangle. They pick a direction at random and walk along the side of a triangle. Sophie thinks they are less likely to collide than not. Is she correct?

A. Yes, mice naturally keep away from each other.
B. No. They are more likely to collide than not.
C. No. they are equally likely to collide than not collide.
D. Yes, the probability they collide is 0.25

15. Jane says, "Plums are not sweets. Some plums are sweet. All sweets are tasty." Which of the below statements is most in keeping with Jane's thoughts?

A. Some sweets are plums
B. Some plums are not tasty.
C. Some plums are tasty
D. No plum is tasty
E. Some plums are not sweet

16. In Leeds, a survey is done on a school. Strawberry ice cream is liked by 8 children, chocolate ice cream is liked by 5 children and vanilla ice cream is liked by 4 children. Three children like all flavours and no children like chocolate and strawberry, or vanilla and strawberry. Only one child likes chocolate and vanilla. Two children in the survey don't like ice cream. How many children took the survey?

A. 15 B. 12 C. 10 D. 19

17. In Newcastle, a survey is done on a school. 4 children like all types of ice cream. 4 children like only strawberry and vanilla, and 12 like chocolate. However, 4 like vanilla ice cream only. Only one child likes everything but strawberry. Which Venn diagram represents this information?

A.

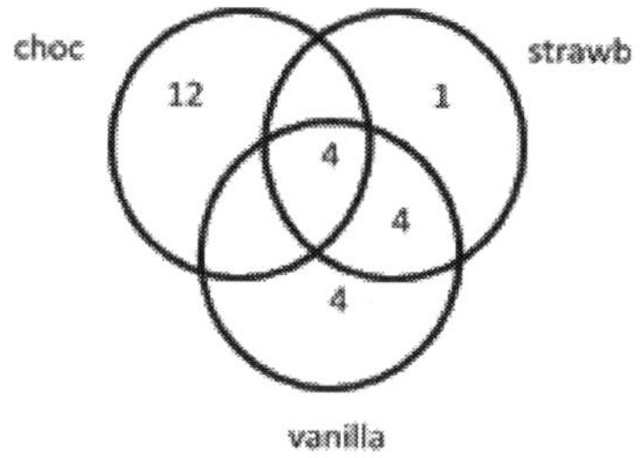

B.

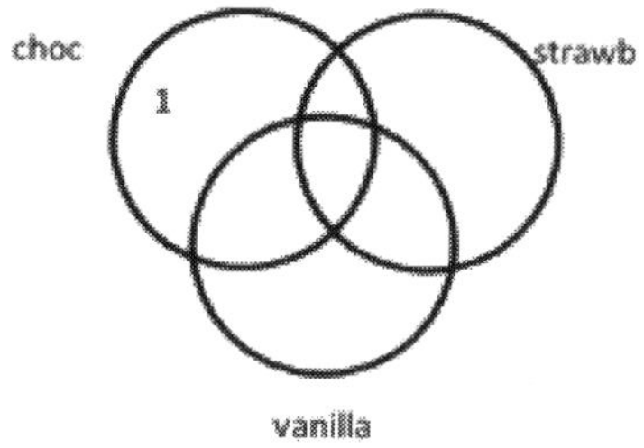

C.

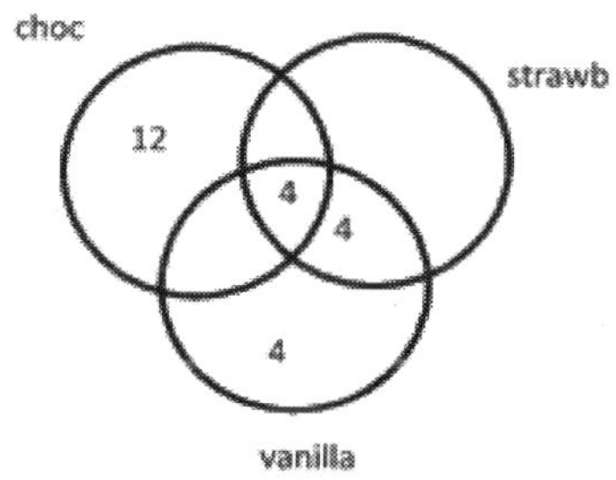

D.

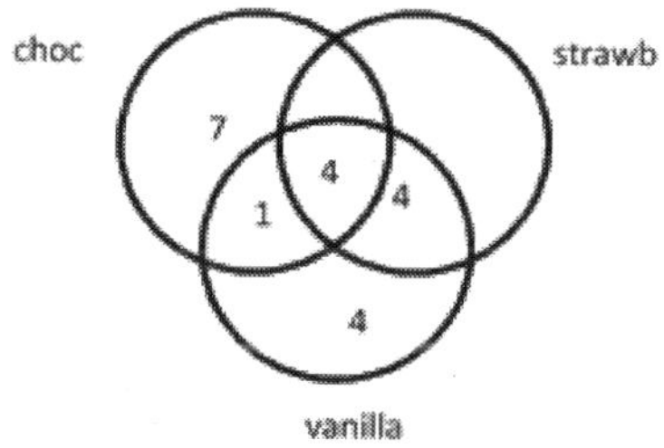

18. Tasha went shopping. She says that every dress she bought was blue and she bought every blue dress she saw. Which statement is true?

A. Blue dresses were the only dresses Tasha saw while shopping.
B. While Tasha was shopping, she bought only blue dresses.
C. In the area that Tasha shopped, there were only blue dresses being sold.
D. All of the dresses that Tasha saw she bought.
E. Tasha did not see any other dress while she was shopping.

19. In a game of kissing catch, everyone put their names in a hat. Each player takes turns to draw a name. If they pick their own name, it is placed back and they draw another. If the last person to pick draws their own name, everyone starts again. John, Kelly and Lisa play and pick in alphabetical order. Which statement is true?

A. Jon has a one in three chance of picking and kissing Lisa
B. Kelly is more likely to pick John than picking Lisa
C. John has an equal chance of kissing Lisa or Kelly
D. Lisa should reverse the order is she wants to increase her chances of kissing John

20. Mary is showing photos to her daughter. She points to a woman and says "her brother's father is the only son of my grandfather." How is the woman in the photo related to Mary's daughter?

A. Cousin B. Mother C. Sister D. Daughter E. Aunt

21. "If vaccinations are now compulsory because society has decided that they should be forced, then society should pay for them." Which of the following statements would weaken the argument?

A. Many people disagree that vaccinations should be compulsory.
B. The cost of vaccinations is too high to be funded locally.
C. Vaccinations are supported by many local communities and GPs.
D. Healthcare workers do not want vaccinations.

22. Tim is going to the doctor for a blood test today. He says that he knows he will be in pain today. What assumption has Tim made?

A. Using a needle will cause pain
B. The doctor will have a hard time finding Tim's vein.
C. He has had pain when he visited the doctor before so it must always happen
D. Tim will have a bruise after his blood is taken
E. The doctor will need repeated attempts to get blood

23. William, Xavier and Yolanda race in a 100m race. All of them run at a constant speed during the race. William beats Xavier by 20m. Xavier beats Yolanda by 20m. How many metres does William beat Yolanda?

A. 30m B. 36m C. 40m D. 60m E. 64m

24. Chris is shorter than Ellen. Jane is shorter than Mark who is shorter than Ellen. Ellen and Jane are shorter than Naomi. Who is the tallest?

A. Chris B. Ellen C. Jane D. Mark E. Naomi

25. Diane, Erica and Harry have Ferraris. Michael and Harry have Fords. Chris just bought an Audi. All the girls have Mercedes, except Lily who has a Volkswagen. Michael, Erica and Chris have BMWs. Who has the most cars?

A. Erica B. Chris C. Harry D. Lily E. Michael

26. Watermelon is 99% water. Penny has 100 grams of watermelon. After drying in the sun, the shrivelled watermelon is 98% water. What is the weight of the watermelon now?

A. 98g B. 75g C. 68g D. 50g E. 49g

27. Jon, Emmanuel and Saigeet are in a Rubik's cube solving competition. They need to solve the cube in less than 30 seconds to qualify. Jon and Saigeet solve faster than Emmanuel. Emmanuel's best time is 32.1 seconds. Which statement must be correct?

A. Only Saigeet qualifies
B. No one qualifies
C. Emmanuel doesn't qualify
D. Only Jon Qualifies
E. Jon and Saigeet qualify

28. All doctors are handsome. Some doctors are popular. Francis is handsome, and Oscar is popular. Choose a correct statement.

A. A doctor can be popular and handsome
B. Oscar is handsome
C. Some popular people are handsome
D. Francis is a doctor
E. Oscar is popular with doctors.

29. There are four houses on a street. Lucy, Vicky and Shannon live in adjacent houses. Shannon has a black dog named Chrissie, Lucy has a white Persian cat and Vicky has a red parrot that shouts obscenities. The owner of a four legged pet has a blue door. Vicky has a neighbour with a red door. Either a cat or bird owner has a white door. Lucy lives opposite a green door. Vicky and Shannon are not neighbours. What colour is Lucy's door?

A. Green
B. Red
C. White
D. Blue
E. Cannot tell

END OF SECTION

Section C: Quantitative Reasoning

Data Set 1

The following graph describes the travel of a car and bike along a road. Study the graph, then answer the following six questions.

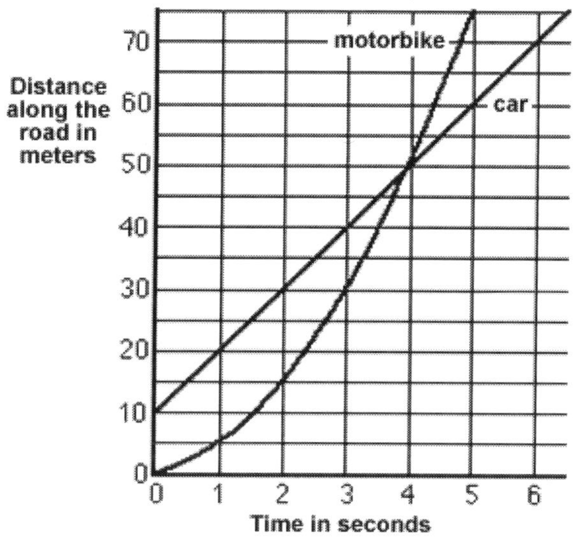

1. After 1 second, what is the speed of the car, in metres per second?

A. 5 m/s
B. 10 m/s
C. 12 m/s
D. 20 m/s
E. 30 m/s

2. Approximately, what is the highest speed the motorcycle reaches?

A. 20 m/s
B. 25 m/s
C. 30 m/s
D. 50 m/s
E. 100 m/s

3. What is the peak acceleration of the car, in m/s^2?

A. 0 m/s^2
B. 1 m/s^2
C. 2 m/s^2
D. m/s^2
E. 10 m/s^2

4. The motorbike accelerates more quickly than the car

A. True
B. False
C. True – but not initially
D. True – but only initially
E. Can't tell

Data Set 2

The following tables describe the cost of making international telephone calls. The cost of any given telephone call is calculated by adding together the connection charge, the duration charge plus a surcharge if applicable. The connection charge is only paid if the call is answered.

Connection charge between two countries (in UK pence):

	UK	France	USA	China	Australia
UK	-	25	47	52	68
France	25	-	51	54	78
USA	47	51	-	43	56
China	52	54	43	-	45
Australia	68	78	56	45	-

Cost per minute for international calls (in UK pence). All calls are rounded up to the nearest minute for calculation purposes. Increasing the duration of the call does not make previous minutes cheaper – only those minutes above any threshold are subject to the lower rate.

	1 – 10 mins	11 – 20 mins	21 – 60 mins	Over 60mins
Peak	42	37	34	28
Off-peak	25	18	16	15

Peak time is recorded as between 0800 and 1800 in the country making the call.

A surcharge of 88 pence is payable on calls over an hour, off peak only. A different surcharge of 10 pence is placed on international calls from Europe to Australia if the phone isn't answered.

5. What is the total cost of a seven-minute peak time call from the UK to France?

A. £ 0.67 B. £ 2.94 C. £ 3.19 D. £ 3.29 E. £ 3.77

6. What is the cost of a call at 0930 local time from France to Australia, that rings for 63 seconds but is unanswered?

A. £ 0.00 B. £ 0.10 C. £ 0.58 D. £ 0.84 E. £ 1.62

7. What percentage of the overall cost of a call (of duration 463 seconds made at 1543 hours local time from USA to China) is represented by fixed (i.e. non-duration dependent) charges?

A. 0% B. 8% C. 11% D. 13% E. 15%

8. What is the total cost of a 75-minute call, from China to France at 1935 local time?

A. £ 11.79 B. £ 12.67 C. £ 13.49 D. £ 14.37 E. £ 21.45

9. What is the total cost of a 763 second call, from France to Australia at 1215 local time?

A. £ 5.31 B. £ 5.59 C. £ 6.09 D. £ 6.19 E. £ 7.19

Data Set 3

The following graph describes the price of gold. The next two questions refer to this graph.

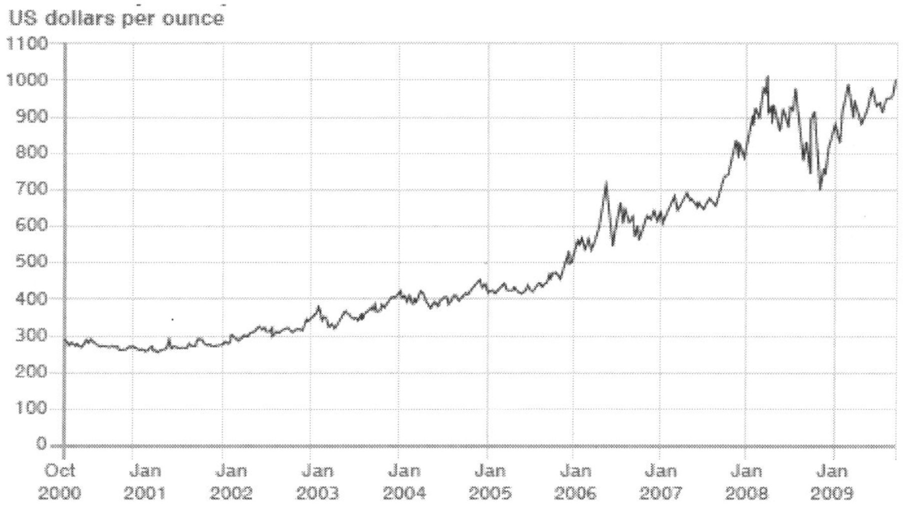

Assume where required that the current conversion rate is 1 USD = 0.68 GBP
One ounce is the equivalent of 28g

10. What is the approximate percentage change in gold value between January 2004 and January 2007?

A. 63% B. 145% C. 155% D. 165% E. 195%

11. What was the approximate total cost (in GBP) of 50g of gold in January 2004?

A. £ 456 B. £ 486 C. £ 714 D. £ 767 E. £ 20,000

Data Set 4

The following table shows the nutritional composition of three different single-portion pre-prepared meals. Read it, and then answer the following questions.

Meal	Energy content / Kcal	Sugar content / g	Total mass / g
Lasagne	427	19	450
Chicken curry	783	24	600
Beef noodles	722	35	475
Ratatouille	359	14	320

12. How much more sugar per unit mass does the Beef Noodle dish contain relative to the Lasagne?

A. 16.0 g/kg
B. 21.5 g/kg
C. 31.5 g/kg
D. 34.3 g/kg
E. 37.1 g/kg

13. Which dish has the least proportion of its energy content provided by sugar?

A. Lasagne
B. Chicken Curry
C. Beef Noodles
D. Ratatouille
E. More information required

Data Set 5

Five respondents were asked to estimate the value of three bottles of wine, in pounds sterling.

Respondent	Wine 1	Wine 2	Wine 3
1	13	16	25
2	17	16	23
3	11	17	21
4	13	15	14
5	15	19	29
Actual retail value	**8**	**25**	**23**

14. What is the mean error margin in the guessing of the value of wine 1?

A. £4.80 B. £5.60 C. £5.80 D. £6.20 E. £6.40

15. Which respondent guessed most accurately on average?

A. Respondent 1
B. Respondent 2
C. Respondent 3
D. Respondent 4
E. Respondent 5

Data Set 6

A sweet shop stocks a range of different products. A new popular product is released, which the shopkeeper is keen to stock. However in order to do this, he must discontinue one of his current lines to create shelf space. The amount of shelf space required for this is 0.2m. The data below show sales figures for four different products currently stocked.

Product	Gobstopper	Bubblegum	Everton mints	Jelly beans
Cost per unit	22p	35p	45p	50p
Sale price	40p	50p	90p	65p
Number sold per week	150	180	300	420
Shelf space taken	0.2m	0.1m	0.2m	0.2m

16. What is the total weekly profit from these four items?

A. £ 189.00
B. £ 225.00
C. £ 252.00
D. £ 295.50
E. £ 472.50

17. What is the total value of sales for Gobstoppers and Everton mints combined, minus the total purchase price of one week's supply of Bubblegum?

A. £ 99.00
B. £ 162.00
C. £ 267.00
D. £ 290.00
E. £ 330.00

18. Based on the information available to you, which of these items would you recommend the shopkeeper replace with the new product?

A. Gobstopper
B. Bubblegum
C. Everton mints
D. Jelly beans
E. Gobstopper and Bubblegum

Data Set 7

The population of Country A is 40% greater than the population of Country B.
The population of Country C is 30% less than the population of Country D (which is has a population 20% greater than Country B).

19. Given that the population of Country A is 45 million, what is the population of country D?

A. 32.1 million people
B. 35.8 million people
C. 36.6 million people
D. 38.6 million people
E. 39.0 million people

20. The population of Country A is still 45 million. If Country B introduced a new health initiative costing $ 45 per capita, what would be the total cost?

A. $ 1.35 bn
B. $ 1.45 bn
C. $ 1.50 bn
D. $ 1.55 bn
E. $ 1.65 bn

21. The population of Country C now changes to 25 million. The ratios are still preserved. Assuming that 52% of the population are female and 28% of the population are aged under 18, how many adult men are there in Country D?

A. 8.6 million
B. 10.3 million
C. 12.3 million
D. 17.1 million
E. 25.7 million

Data Set 8

The table below displays the costs associated with recruiting skilled workers in different industries in euros.

Training sector	**Trade and industry**	**Civil service**	**Liberal professions**	**Crafts and skilled trades**	**Agri-culture**
Application process	1,525	1,168	1,157	664	536
This includes:					
Advertising costs	576	502	337	231	183
Application process (personnel costs)	568	640	562	395	352
External consultants	381	26	258	38	0
Continuing training during the familiarisation period	1,048	1,029	183	329	376
This includes:					
Lost working hours during continuing training	447	431	75	139	168
Cost of continuing training courses	600	598	107	190	208
Difference in productivity during the familiarisation period	2,798	2,183	1,660	1,902	1,399
Total personnel recruitment costs	**5,370**	**4,380**	**3,001**	**2,895**	**2,311**

22. What is the difference in advertising costs per position between the most expensive and least expensive?
What is the difference between the most expensive and the least expensive advertising cost?

A. €271 B. €288 C. €319 D. €363 E. €393

23. In which industry is there the greatest cost due to lost working hours relative to the total overall recruitment cost?

A. Trade and industry
B. Civil service
C. Liberal professions
D. Crafts and skilled trades
E. Agriculture

Data Set 9

The table below shows crime data for some types of crime from the town of Westwich over a three-year period.

Crime code	2011	2012	2013
X632	2,350	2,453	2,670
X652	3,821	3,663	3,231
Y321	230	210	?
Y632	456	490	432
Y115	321	?	431
Y230	763	754	714

24. Data for offence Y321 is missing for 2013, however you are told that the rate is 10% lower than in 2011. What is the rate of crime for Y321 in 2013?

A. 189 B. 195 C. 199 D. 207 E. 210

25. Data for offence Y115 is missing for 2012. You are informed that of the four "Y code" crimes recorded here, there were less than 1,837 in 2012. How many Y115 offences were committed?

A. 373 B. 383 C. 388 D. 393 E. 399

26. Which crime experienced the biggest percentage reduction from 2012 to 2013?

A. X632 B. X652 C. Y321 D. Y632 E. Y230

Data Set 10

This is a bus timetable taken from a route in Southern England. Use the data in the table to answer the following questions.

	Mondays to Fridays	Sch						Sch		Saturdays			
Petersfield Tesco	—	—	0825	1025	1225	1425	1525	1620	1810	—	1025	1325	1625
Petersfield Square	0700	0735	0830	1030	1230	1430	1530	1625	1815	0730	1030	1330	1630
Petersfield Station	0702	0737	0832	1032	1232	1432	1532	1627	1817	0732	1032	1332	1632
Stroud The Seven Stars	0707	0742	0837	1037	1237	1437	1537	1632	1822	0737	1037	1337	1637
East Meon All Saints Church	0717	0752	0847	1047	1247	1447	1547	1642	1832	0747	1047	1347	1647
West Meon The Thomas Lord	0723	0758	0853	1053	1253	1453	1553	1648	1838	0753	1053	1353	1653
Bramdean The Fox Inn	0730	0805	0900	1100	1300	1500	1600	—	1845	0800	1100	1400	1700
Cheriton Cheriton Hall	0736	0811	0906	1106	1306	1506	1606	—	1851	0806	1106	1406	1706
New Alresford Perins School	0744	0819	0914	1114	1314	1514	1614	—	1859	0814	1114	1414	1714
Itchen Abbas Trout Inn	0755	—	0925	1125	1325	—	1625	—	—	0825	1125	1425	1725
Kings Worthy Cart and Horses	0802	—	0932	1132	1332	—	1632	—	—	0832	1132	1432	1732
Winchester City Road	0808	—	0938	1138	1338	—	1638	—	—	0838	1138	1438	1738
Winchester Bus Station	0811	—	0941	1141	1341	—	1641	—	—	0841	1141	1441	1741

No service on Sundays or Public Holidays

	Mondays to Fridays Sch	SH					Sch			Saturdays			
Winchester Bus Station	—	—	0900	1100	1300	1400	—	1650	1750	0900	1200	1500	1750
Winchester City Road	—	—	0904	1104	1304	1404	—	1654	1754	0904	1204	1504	1754
Kings Worthy Cart and Horses	—	—	0911	1111	1311	1411	—	1701	1801	0911	1211	1511	1801
Itchen Abbas Trout Inn	—	—	0918	1118	1318	1418	—	1708	1808	0918	1218	1518	1808
New Alresford Perins School	0727	0729	0929	1129	1329	1429	1529	1719	1819	0929	1229	1529	1819
Cheriton Cheriton Hall	0735	0737	0937	1137	1337	1437	1537	1727	1827	0937	1237	1537	1837
Bramdean The Fox Inn	0741	0743	0943	1143	1343	1443	1543	1733	1833	0943	1243	1543	1833
West Meon The Thomas Lord	0748	0750	0950	1150	1350	1450	1550	1740	1840	0950	1250	1550	1840
East Meon All Saints Church	0755	0757	0957	1157	1357	1457	1557	1747	1847	0957	1257	1557	1847
East Meon Primary School	0757	—	—	—	—	—	—	—	—	—	—	—	—
Stroud The Seven Stars	0807	0807	1007	1207	1407	1507	1607	1757	1857	1007	1307	1607	1857
Petersfield Station	0812	0812	1012	1212	1412	1512	1612	1802	1902	1012	1312	1612	1902
Petersfield Square	0814	0814	1014	1214	1414	1514	1614	1804	1904	1014	1314	1614	1904
Petersfield Tesco	0817	0817	1017	1217	1417	1517	1617	1807	—	1017	1317	1617	—

Liable to change from 11 June 2012

27. On a Monday, how long does the 1225 to Winchester Bus Station take to travel between East Moon All Saints Church and Itchen Abbas Trout Inn?

A. 13 minutes
B. 25 minutes
C. 38 minutes
D. 47 minutes
E. 60 minutes

28. If you were at Cheriton, Cheriton Hall at 1321 on a Tuesday, how long would you have to wait until the next bus to Winchester City Road?

A. 45 minutes
B. 65 minutes
C. 105 minutes
D. 145 minutes
E. 165 minutes

Data Set 11

Tables 1 and **3** show data relating to the cultivation of corn grain. Interpret the tables and answer the subsequent questions. (A hectare is the equivalent of $10000m^2$).

Table 1. Monthly precipitation during the growing season, 1985-1989.

	Precipitatiion (mm)					
	1985	*1986*	*1987*	*1988*	*1989*	*Long-Term Average*
May	69	89	38	15	124	66
June	56	119	64	5	84	89
July	51	71	66	61	46	71
August	104	99	127	97	175	76
September	89	203	102	94	150	64
Total	369	581	397	272	579	366

Table 3. Corn grain yield, seed moisture content, and stand count at harvest for three erosion classes of Marlette soils.

Degree of Erosion	*1985*	*1986*	*1987*	*1988*	*1989*	*Mean*
			Yield (kg/ha)			
Slight	6,770a	8,150a	8,400a	3,510a	9,910a	7,340a
Moderate	5,580ab	7,340a	8,590a	3,820a	9,910a	7,090a
Severe	5,080b	5,960b	6,840b	1,820b	9,280a	5,830b
			Seed moisture content (%)			
Slight	22.6a	22.7a	26.5ab	26.0a	31.6a	25.9a
Moderate	24.8b	26.0a	25.9a	25.1a	30.4a	26.4ab
Severe	24.7b	25.9a	27.2b	31.3b	31.6a	28.2b
			Stand count (plants/ha)			
Slight	43,600a	59,400a	52,000ab	53,600a	57,500a	53,200a
Moderate	33,900a	48,800b	54,500a	46,800ab	57,700a	48,400ab
Severe	33,700a	32,800c	49,000b	34,700b	56,500a	41,300b

29. What is the percentage difference between the July 1987 precipitation levels and the long-term average for the month?

A. 5% B. 6% C. 7% D. 8% E. 9%

30. In what year was the overall mean seed moisture content the lowest?

A. 1985 B. 1986 C. 1987 D. 1988 E. 198

31. What was the difference in corn grain yield between slightly eroded Marlette soil in 1986 and moderately eroded Marlette soil in 1989, expressed in kg/hectare?

A.
B. 0 C. 1330 D. 1640 E. 1760 F. 1920

32. In what month was there the highest average precipitation, taking the years 1985 – 1987 inclusive?

A. May B. June C. July D. August E. September

33. What sized area of ground did each plant occupy, in lightly eroded Marlette soil in 1986?

A. $1262\ cm^2$
B. $1384\ cm^2$
C. $1684\ cm^2$
D. $1836\ cm^2$
E. $2012\ cm^2$

Data Set 12

The following graph plots a child's length and weight up to the age of 36 months.

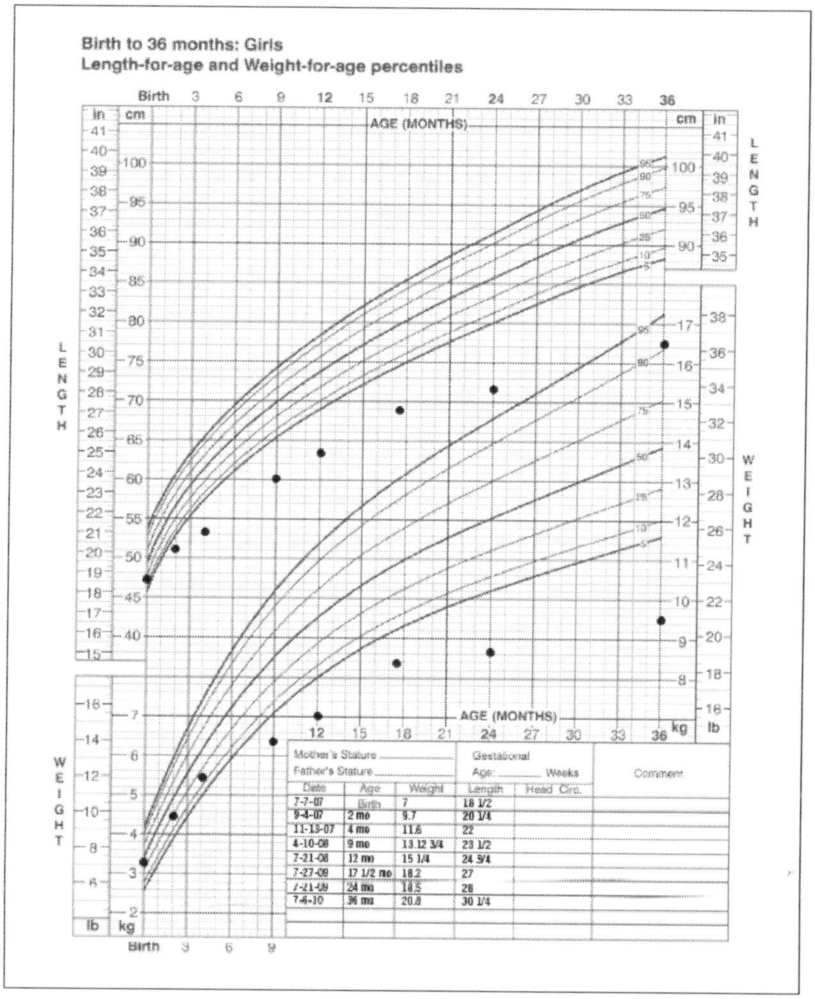

Figure 1 – The patient's weight and length from birth to age 36 months are shown. A deceleration of growth is apparent at age 9 months.

34. After two months, on which centile did the child's weight fall?

A. 75th B. 5th C. 10th D. 25th E. 50th

35. At the 24 month check, what was the child's actual length, in cm?

A. 38.5 B. 70.5 C. 71.5 D. 72.5 E. 73.5

36. What is the mean weight, in pounds (lbs.), of the final three measurements recorded on the chart?

A. 8.5 lbs B. 9.5 lbs C. 18.6 lbs D. 19.2 lbs E. 21.2 lbs

END OF SECTION

Section D: Abstract Reasoning

For each question, decide whether each test shape fits best with Set A, Set B or with neither.

For each question, work through the test shapes from left to right as you see them on the page. Make your decision and fill it into the answer sheet.

Answer as follows:
A = Set A
B = Set B
C = Neither

Set 1: **Set A** **Set B**

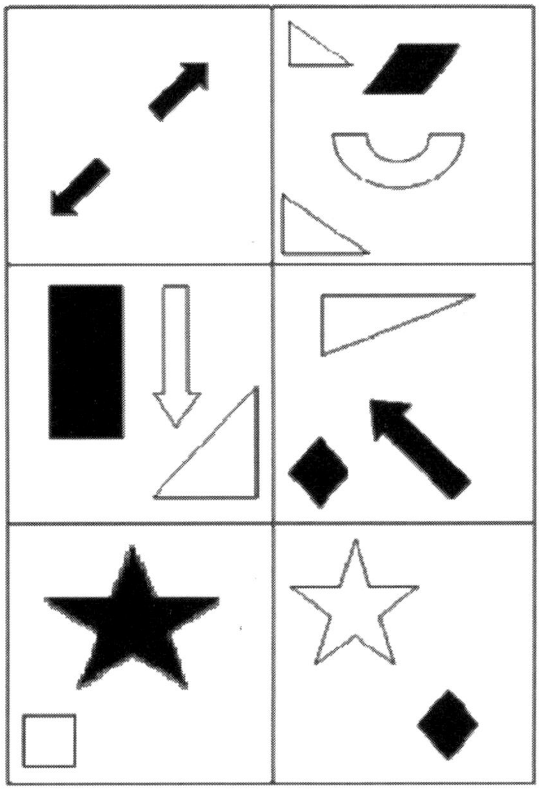

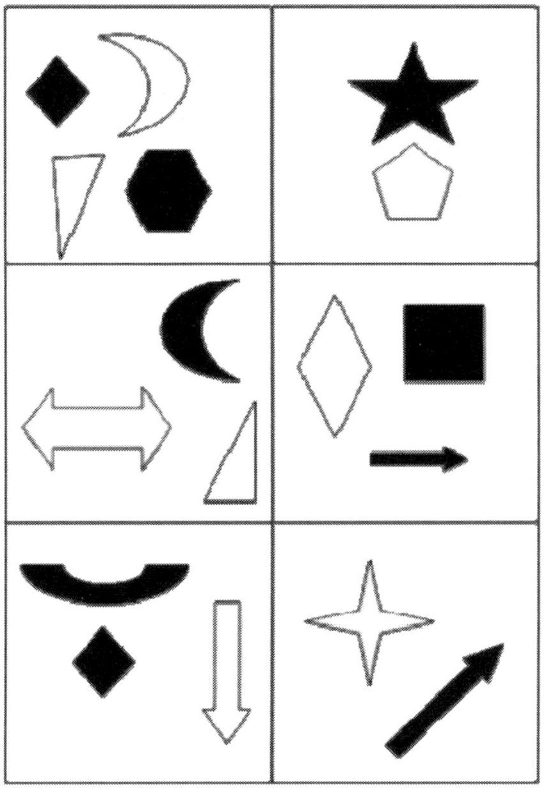

Questions 1-5:

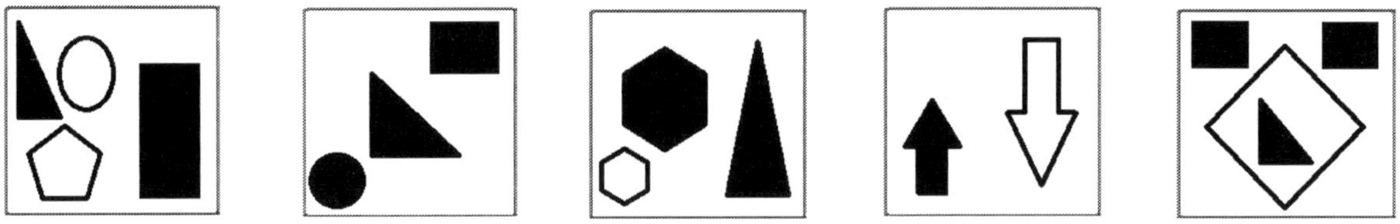

Set 2:

Set A

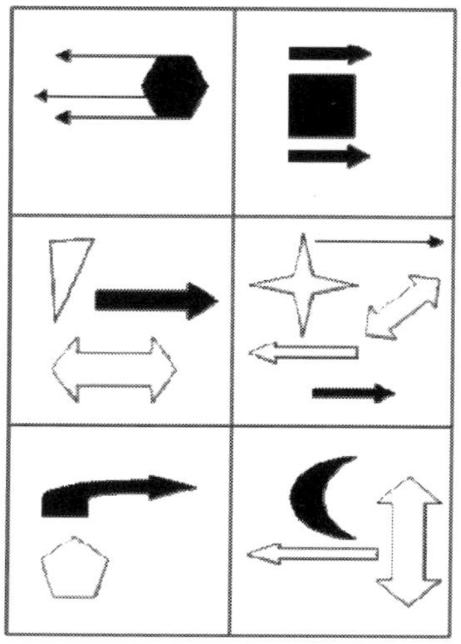

Set B

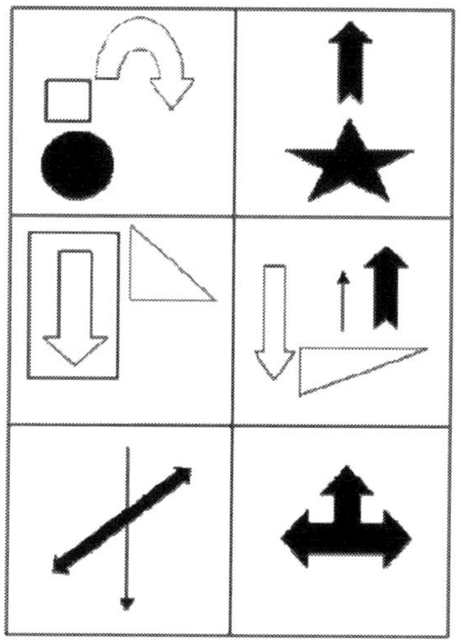

Questions 6-10:

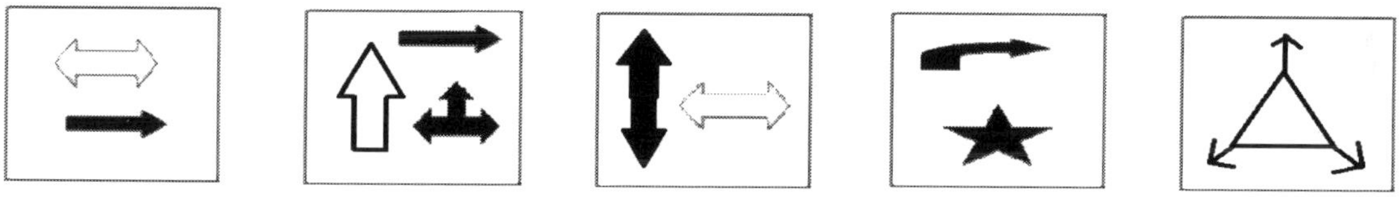

Set 3:

Set A

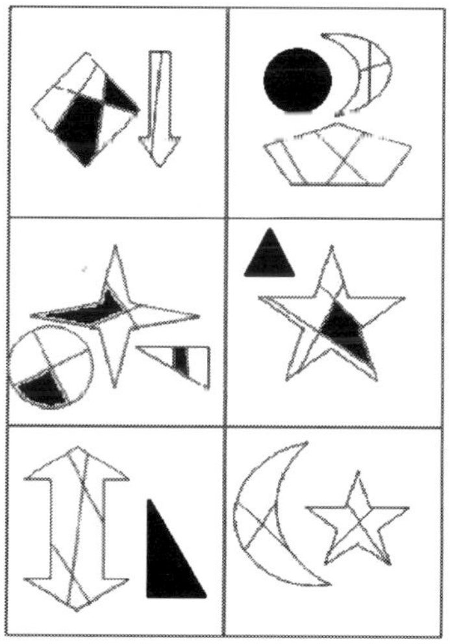

Set B

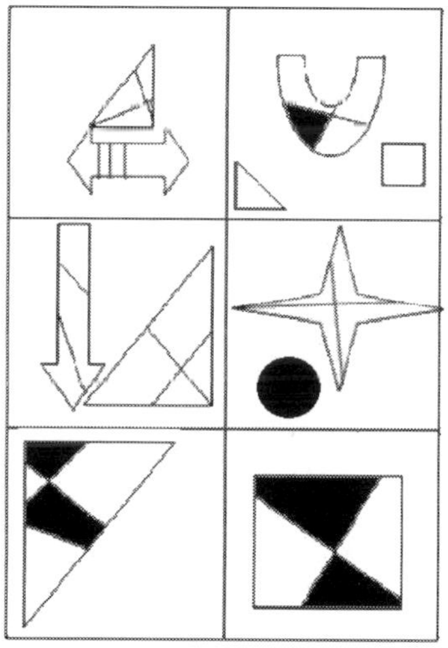

Questions 11-15:

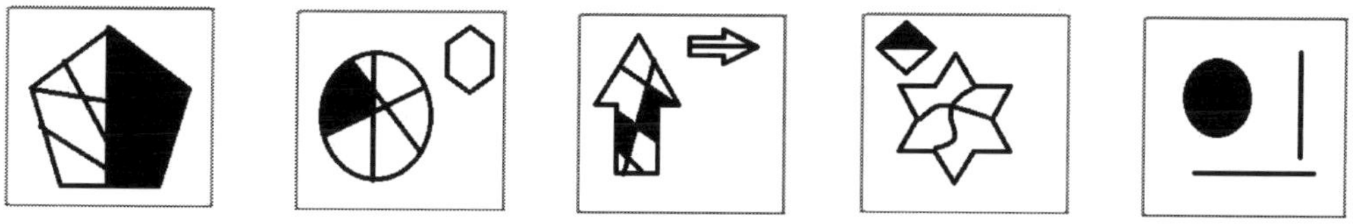

Set 4: **Set A** **Set B**

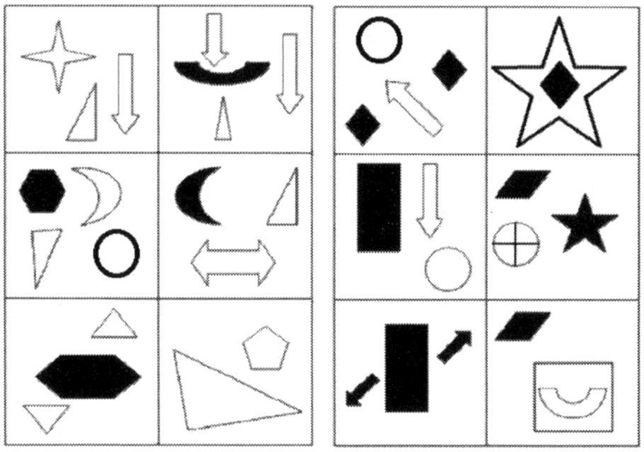

Questions 16-20:

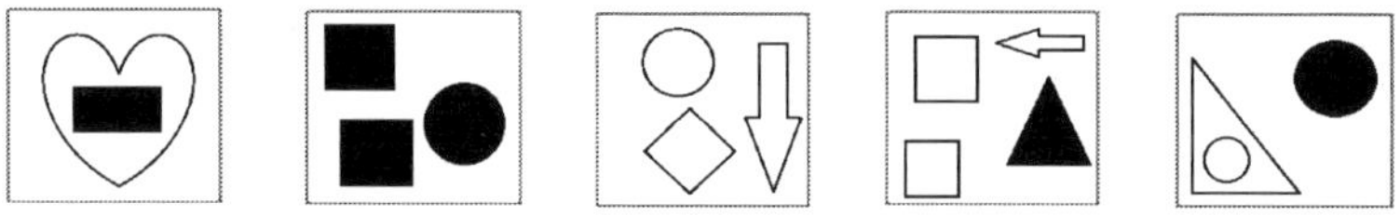

Set 5: **Set A** **Set B**

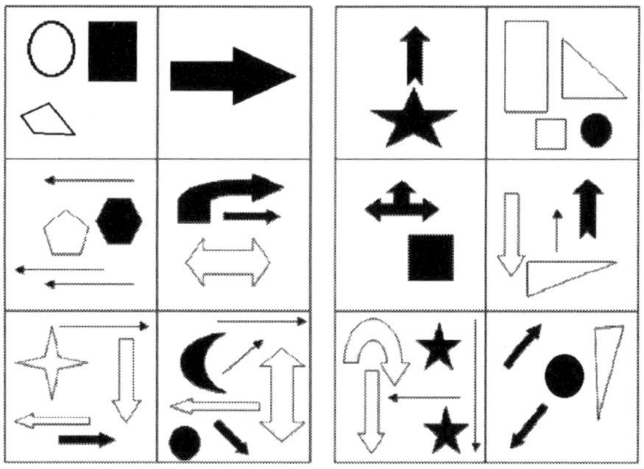

Questions 21-25:

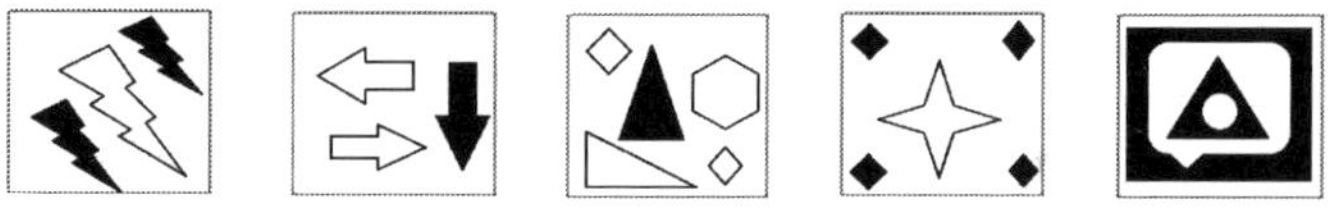

Set 6:

Set A **Set B**

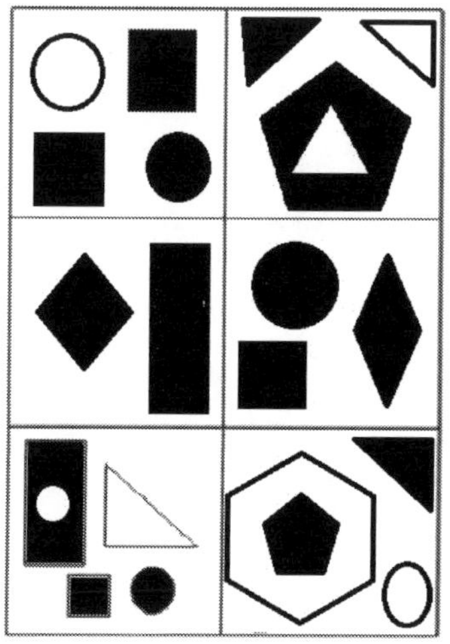

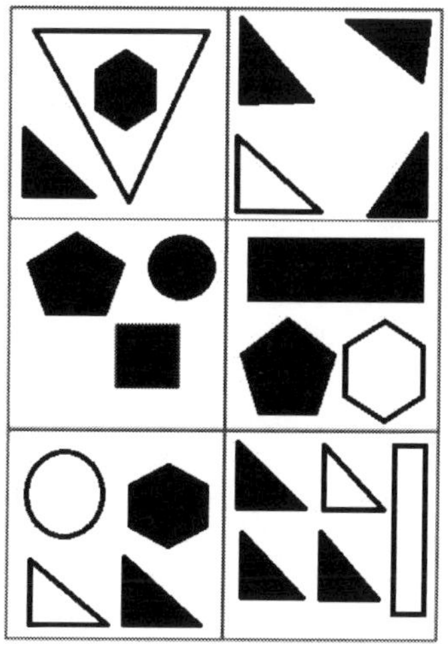

Questions 26-30:

Set 7:

Set A **Set B**

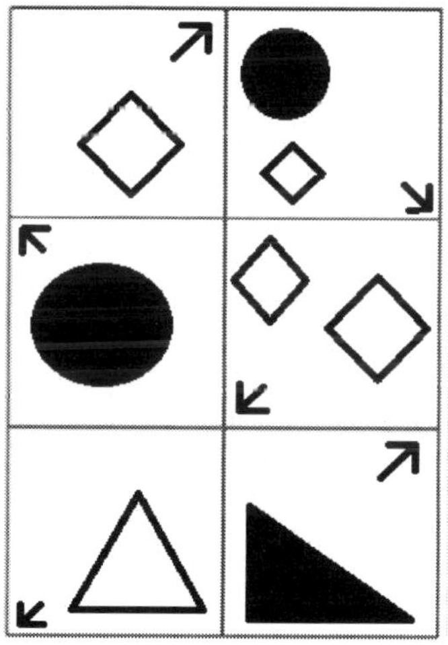

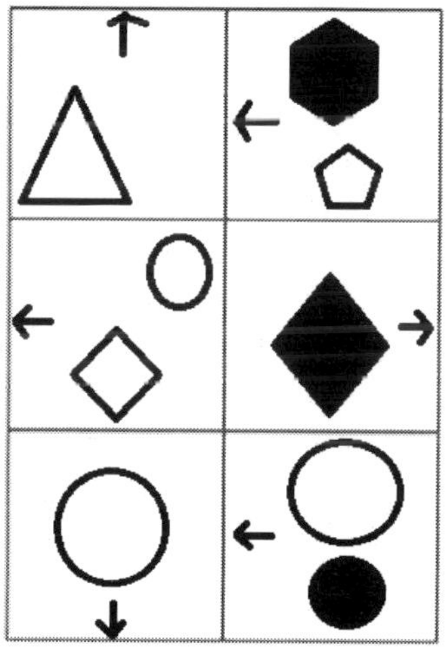

Questions 31-35:

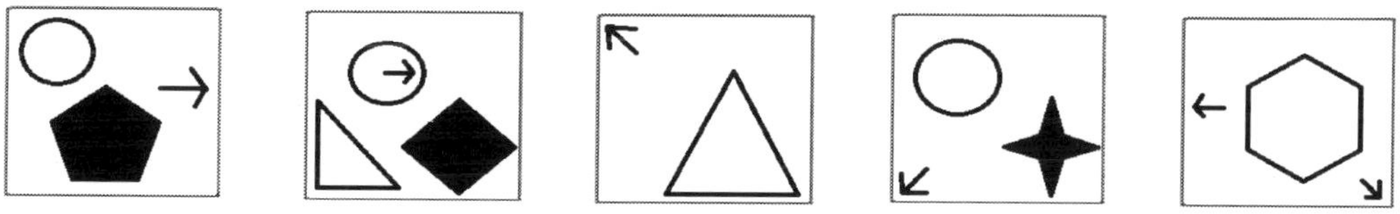

Set 8: **Set A** **Set B**

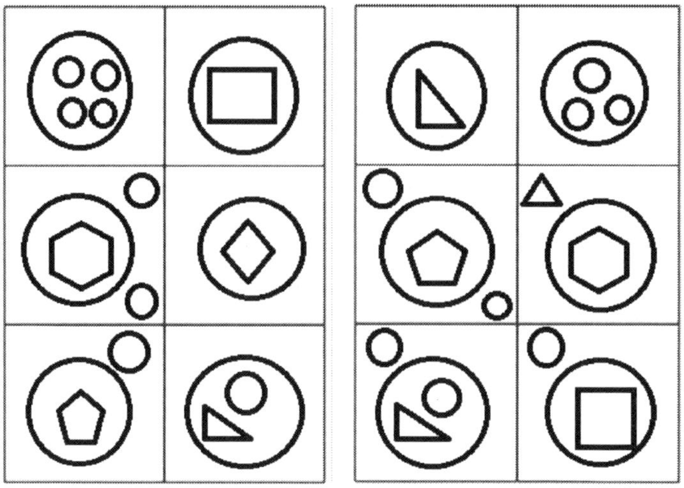

Questions 36-40:

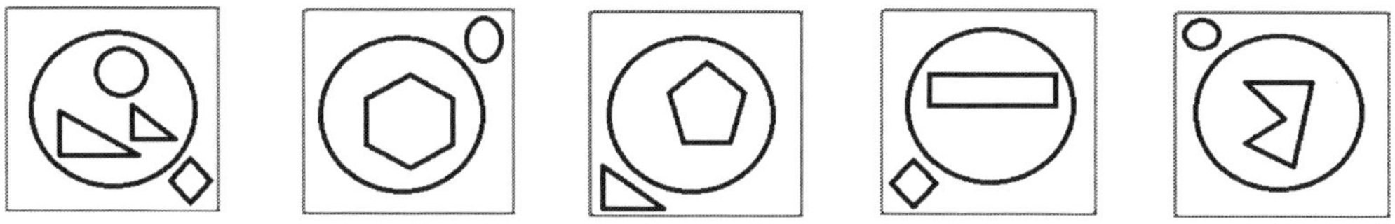

Set 9:

Which answer completes the series?

Question 41:

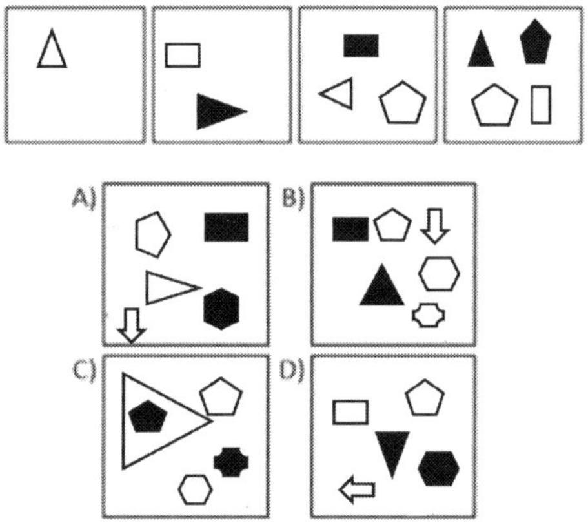

Question 42:

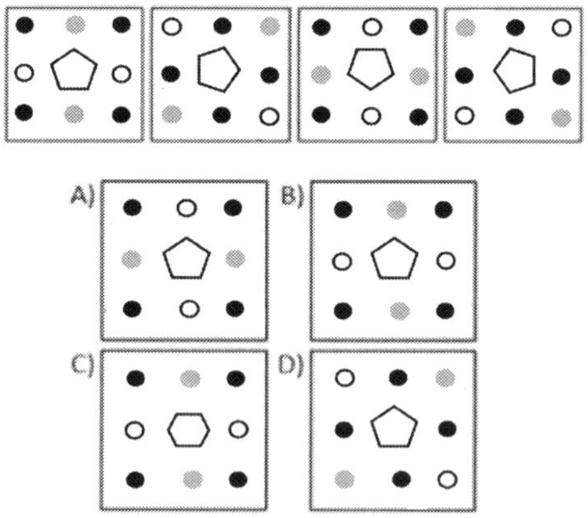

Question 43:

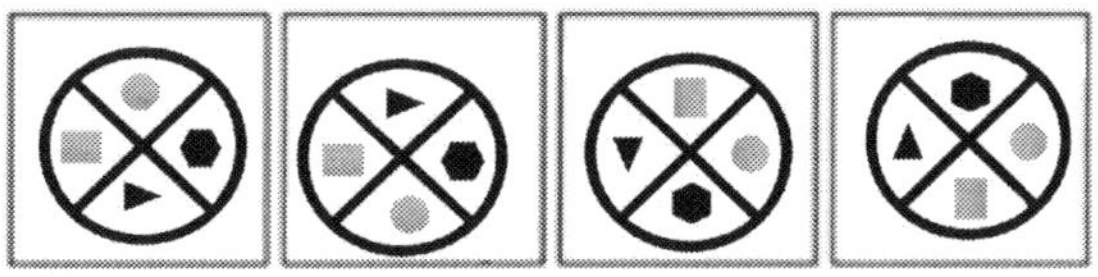

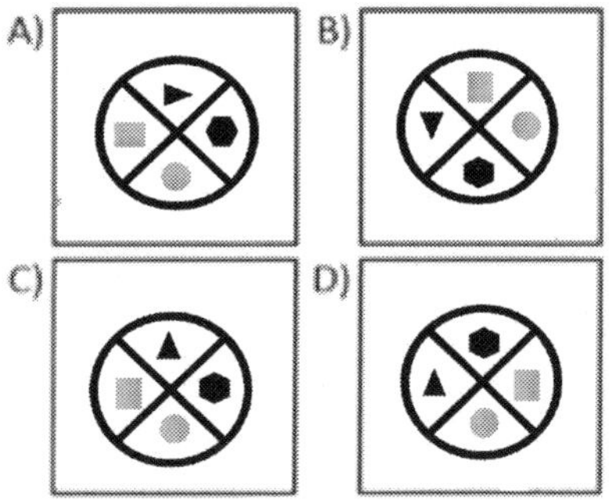

Question 44:

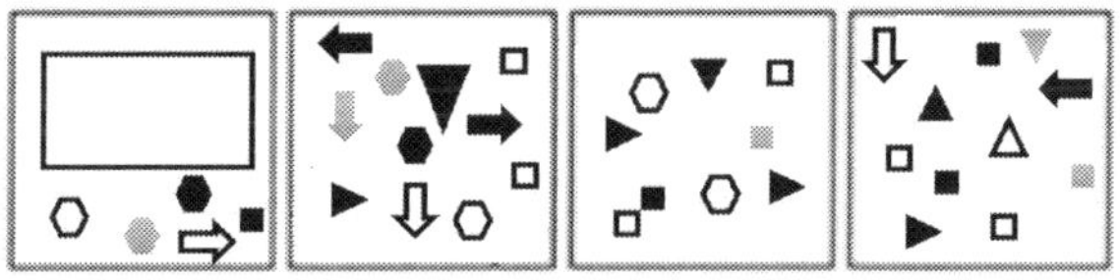

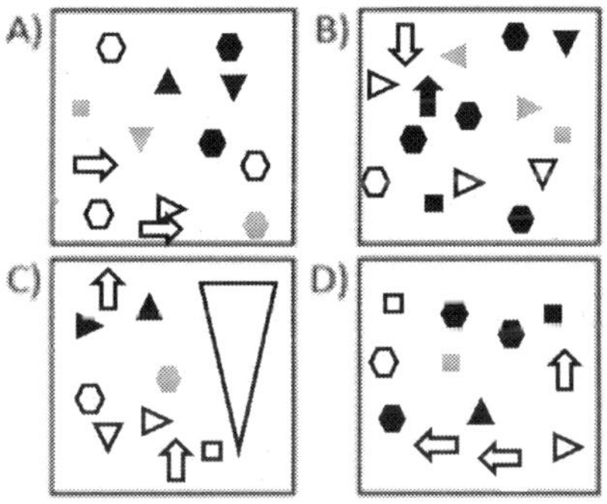

Question 45:

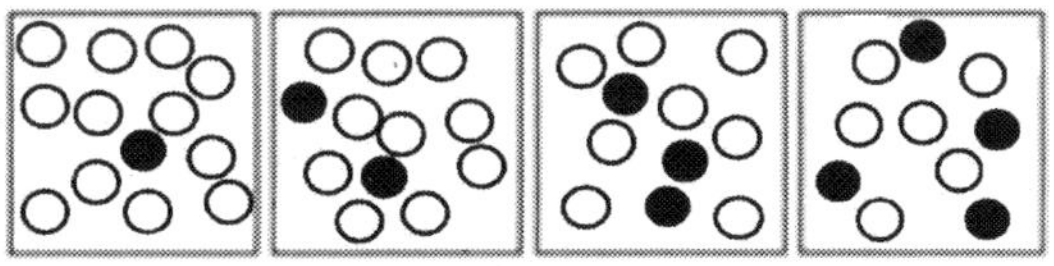

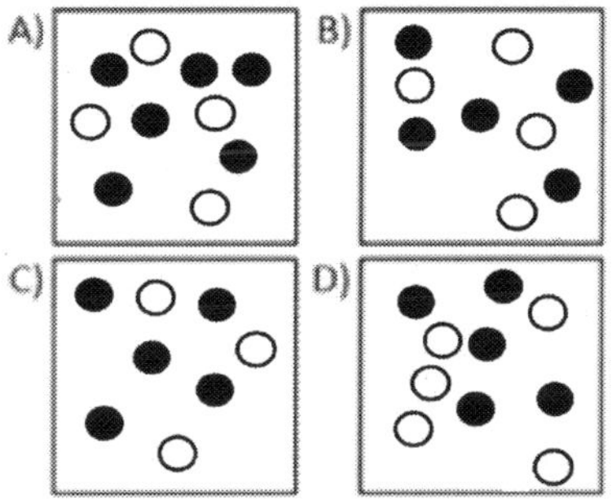

Set 10:
Which answer completes the statement?

Question 46:

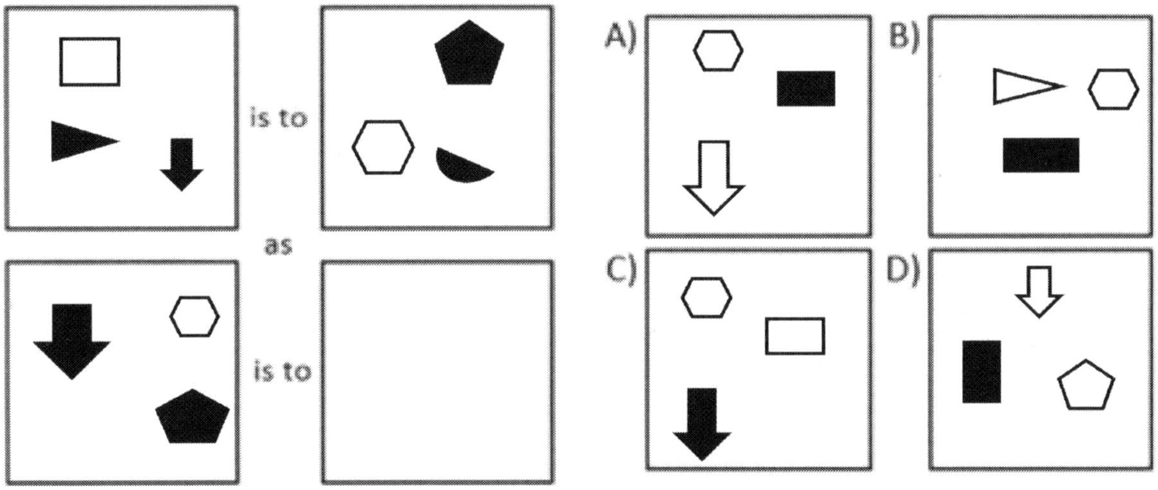

Question 47:

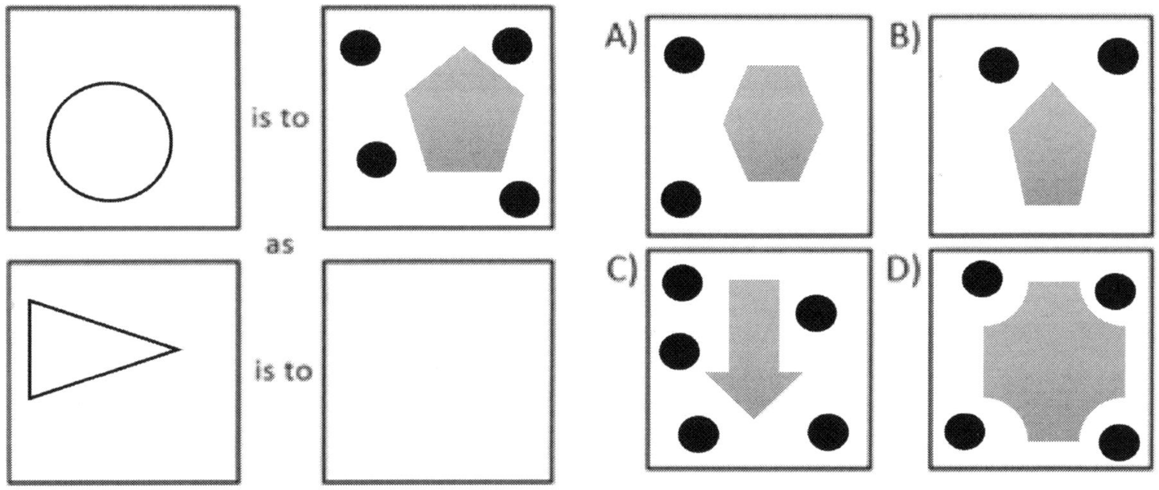

Question 48:

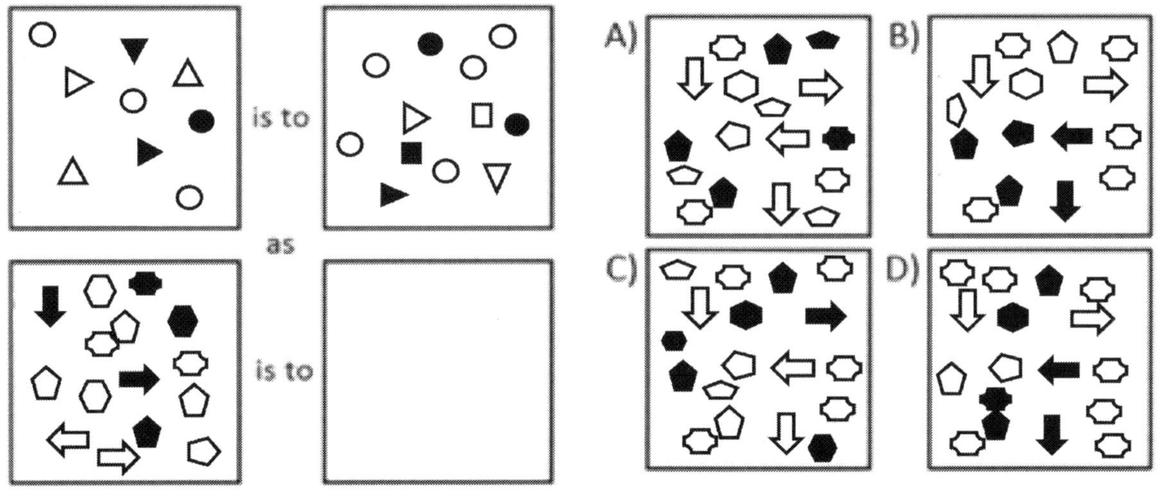

Question 49:

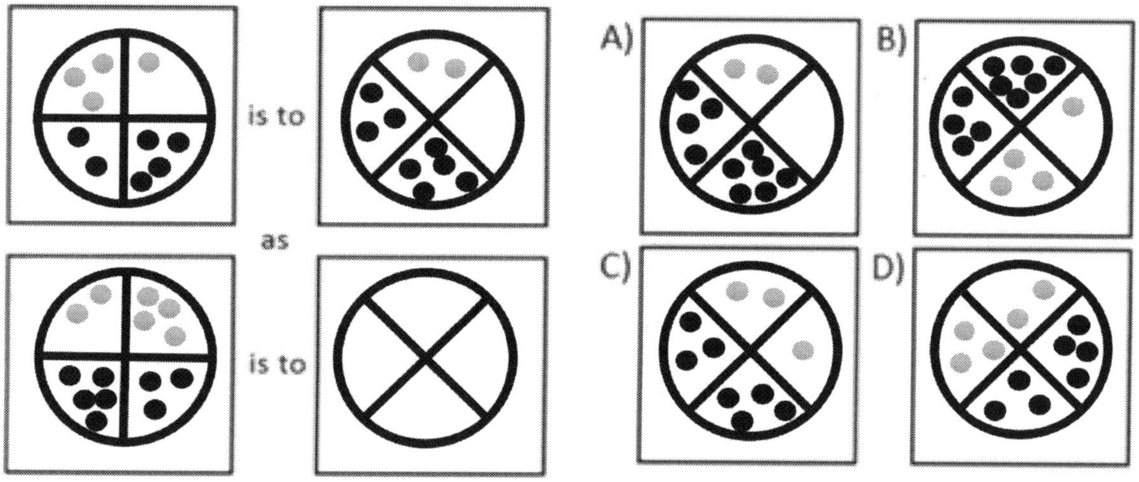

Question 50:

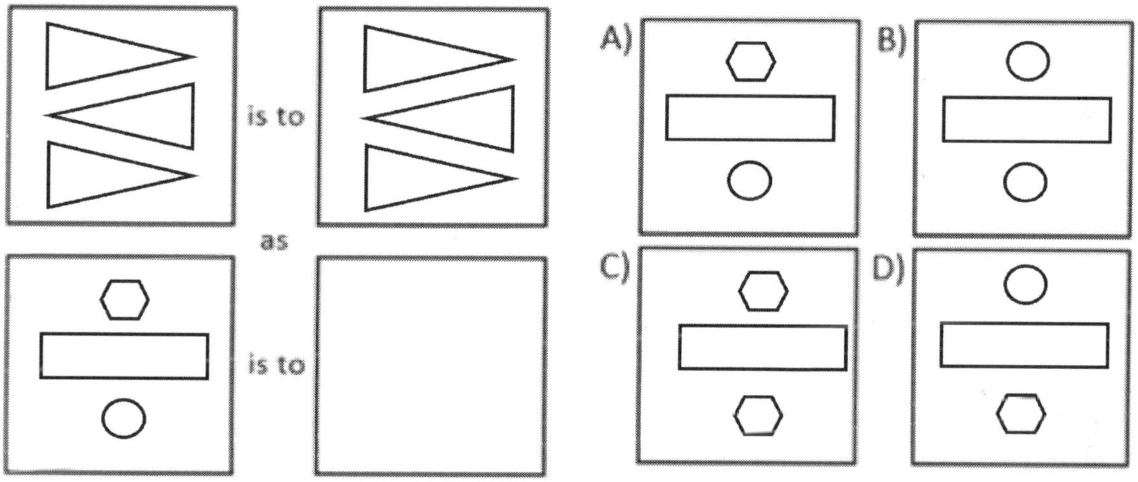

Set 11:

Which of the four response options belongs to either set A or set B?

Set A

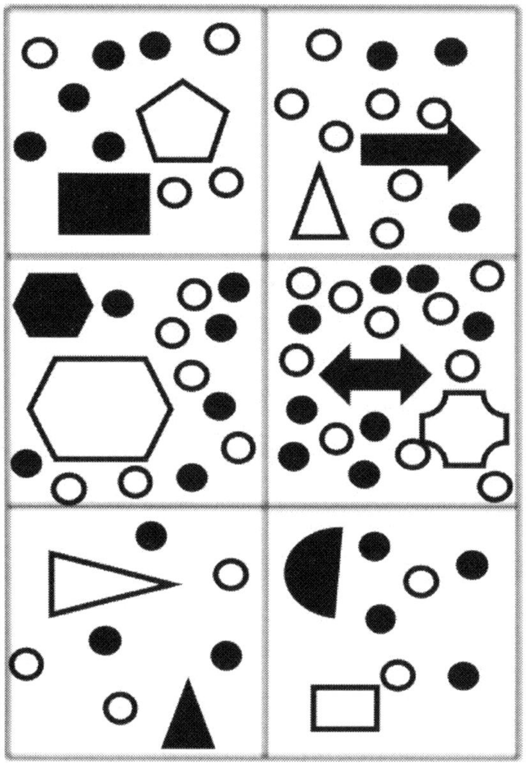

Set B

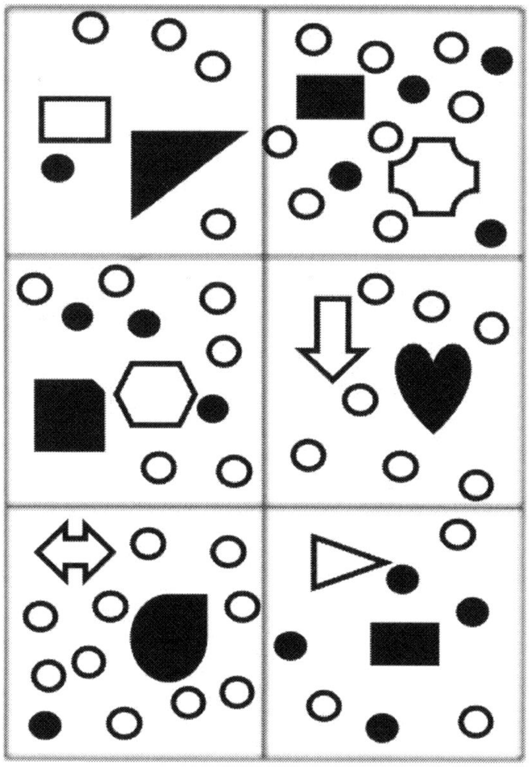

Question 51:

Set A?

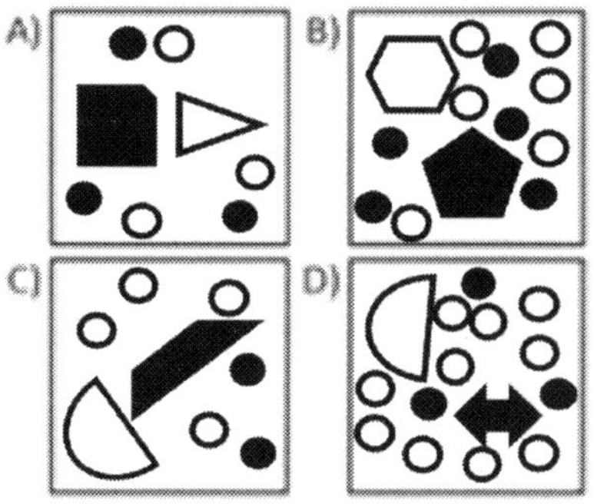

Question 52:

Set B?

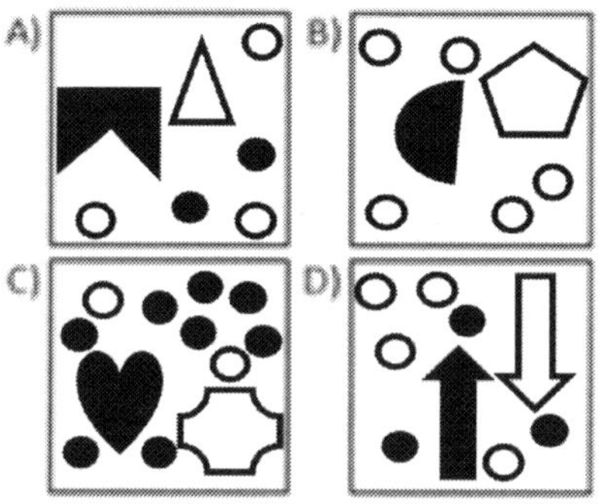

Question 53:

Set A?

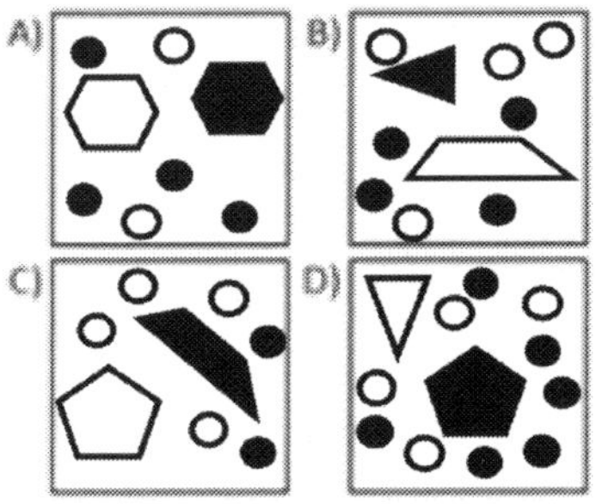

Question 54:

Set B?

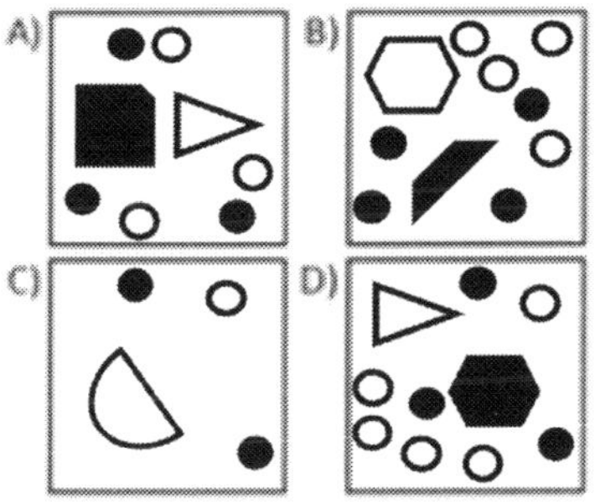

Question 55:

Set B?

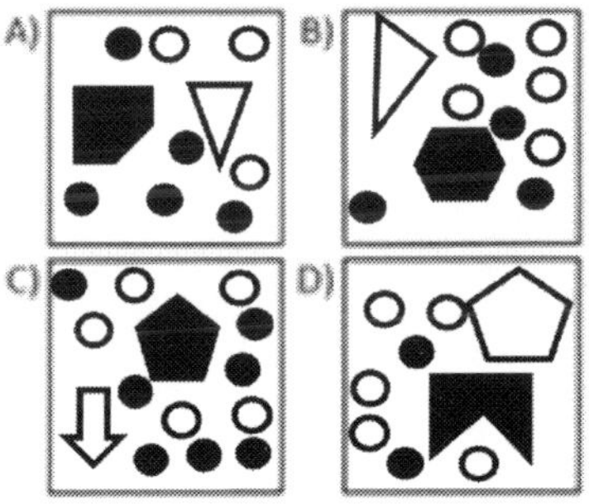

END OF SECTION

Section E: Situational Judgement Test

Read each scenario. Each question refers to the scenario directly above. For each question, select one of these four options. Select whichever you feel is the option that best represents your view on each suggested action.

For questions 1 – 30, choose one of the following options:

A **A highly appropriate action**
B **Appropriate, but not ideal**
C **Inappropriate, but not awful**
D **A highly inappropriate action**

Scenario 1

Emily is a third year medical student. She has been looking forward to the summer holidays for a long time because she has booked a once-in-a-lifetime trip to Tanzania with a group of her best friends from her course. She extended her overdraft to be able to pay for this trip, and has spent a lot of time planning it. Unfortunately, the end-of-year exam results have just come out, and she has only passed 2 out of 3 exams. She only failed by 2%, but must re-sit this final exam in order to continue with her studies. The re-sit is scheduled to be only two days after her return from Tanzania.

How appropriate are the following responses to Emily's dilemma?

1. Go on her trip and cram her revision into the two days before the exam – she only just failed anyway.
2. Cancel the entire trip and let her friends go without her.
3. Ask her friends if they can all reschedule for the following year.
4. Take revision with her to Tanzania – it'll be an active holiday but maybe she can study in her free time.
5. Go for part of the trip but return early to ensure sufficient time for revision.

Scenario 2

Sanjay is a first year medical student who has recently joined the university football team. The word has just got out that this year's sports tour will be abroad. Sanjay is desperate to go as he has heard this is the best week of the academic year, and he wants to have a more active role within the football club. Regrettably, tour will be especially expensive this year and Sanjay is short on funds, having already spent most of his student loan and increased his overdraft.

How appropriate are the following actions to Steve's problem?

6. Ask his other football friends to chip in as they all want him to be there too.
7. Further increase his overdraft to the limit (this would be difficult to pay back).
8. Ask his parents to contribute, despite their own financial hardships.
9. Forget about tour this year – there is always next year when it is likely to be cheaper.
10. Get a part-time job to pay for the tour, even though this will mean sacrificing some of his medical studies.

Scenario 3

Ade is heading into his second year at university. He lived at home with his parents throughout his first year, as the proximity of his home to the university meant that he was not eligible for student accommodation. He struggled to make close friends in his first year and often felt isolated from the other students who all lived together. He has recently seen an advertisement on the year group Facebook page, where several members of his year are looking for another flatmate. He is keen to apply, but is unsure whether his parents would be able to provide financial aid.

How appropriate are the following responses by Ade?

11. Apply to the advertisement without telling his parents.
12. Continue living at home but find other ways to enjoy the student experience – e.g. joining a society.
13. Carry on exactly as he is.
14. Demand his parents pay for him to move out as they are denying him the real student experience.
15. Discuss his concerns with his parents and come up with a financial solution together – e.g. getting a part-time job.

Scenario 4

Gillian has recently been attending communication classes, and has learnt about the importance of having a good manner when talking to patients. That afternoon, she attends a clinic and is shocked to observe the doctor's rude and indifferent manner towards several patients. These patients leave feeling ignored and upset.

How appropriate are the following actions from Gillian?

16. Tell the doctor what she thinks of his rude manner.
17. Inform her supervisor and get their advice on what to do.
18. Do nothing.
19. Talk to the patients and direct them on how to make a complaint.
20. Report the doctor to the dean of education.

Scenario 5

Ethel is a 3rd year medical student observing a prostate cancer clinic. She witnesses her consultant break the bad news of a terminal prognosis to a patient, who clearly struggles to comprehend his situation. Suddenly, the consultant receives a phone call and leaves the room, leaving Ethel alone with the upset patient.

How appropriate are each of the following responses by Ethel in this situation?
21. Say nothing. Leave the patient to his thoughts.
22. Offer words of consolation and support.
23. Leave the room and the patient alone in order to look for the consultant.
24. Share what little information about prostate cancer she knows.
25. Tell the patient everything will be Okay.
26. Ask the patient if he has any questions or concerns.

Scenario 6

Larissa is a third year medical student in her second term of clinical training. Whilst observing in A&E, she is asked by a nurse to perform an ABG (Arterial blood gas). Although she has learnt many of the clinical skills expected at her stage of training, an ABG is a fourth year skill and she has never attempted one before. However, the patient needs the procedure done as soon as possible and no other members of staff are immediately available. She is keen to learn and help out.

How appropriate are the following actions by Larissa in this situation?
27. Refuse to carry out the procedure. It is not worth putting the patient at risk.
28. Wait until a member of staff is available to assist.
29. Go ahead and do the procedure. She has learnt similar skills such as taking blood – how different can it really be?
30. Inform the patient that this would be her first time doing an ABG, and only proceed if they consent.
31. Avoid the embarrassment of telling the nurse she can't do it, and rush off pretending to go to a lecture.

For questions 31 – 69, decide how important each statement is when deciding how to respond to the situation?

A **Very important**
B **important**
C **Of minor importance**
D **Not important at all**

Scenario 7

Romario is a final year medical student. He and his friends have carefully planned a trip to the Caribbean – their last hurrah before graduation. However, his consultant has just offered him a chance to participate in a study that is very likely to be published. Romario has been concerned as he is yet to have any publications to his name, but all of his friends have several. Unfortunately, the study will be carried out at the same time as the Caribbean trip.

How important are the following factors for Romario's decision?
32. The likelihood of the study resulting in a publication – there is no guarantee.
33. This is his last year as a student and a publication will help him when it comes to job applications.
34. This is his last year as a student and the last chance to go away with his university friends.
35. Rejecting the offer may look bad to his consultant.
36. Cancelling the holiday may be letting his friends down.

Scenario 8

Mahood has been offered a one-off teaching session with a senior consultant on the High Dependency Unit (HDU) for respiratory patients. He is very keen to attend as this is a great opportunity to see lots of interesting cases. However, in the preceding days, Mahood comes down with the flu. Whilst he feels able to continue with his day, he is unsure whether to attend the teaching as it could put the patients at risk. He has been told to stay at home if he is unwell, but he is very eager to attend this prestigious teaching.

How important are the following factors for Mahood in deciding what to do?

37. He only has the flu and it seems quite mild to him.
38. This is a one-off teaching session with a top doctor.
39. He has been told to stay at home if he is unwell.
40. This is his only chance to see the interesting cases on HDU.
41. This unit is clearly for very sick patients.

Scenario 9

Theodore is a third year medical student who is captain of his university rugby team. It is his first term on a clinical placement and he is keen to impress his consultant, who will be responsible for his final grade for the year. However, Theodore has noticed that his consultant teaching sessions will always be on a Wednesday afternoon, which clashes with his rugby matches.

How important are the following factors for Theodore in deciding on what to do?

42. He is the team captain – they need him to be present at the matches.
43. His consultant will determine his final grade.
44. His final grade will determine whether he can progress to fourth year.
45. Wednesday afternoons are the only time the consultant can make teaching.
46. His rugby team have the chance to win the championships this year.

Scenario 10

Malaika, a fourth year medical student, has been invited to attend an extra clinic with a senior doctor in a field she is interested in pursuing as a career. Unfortunately, she has not yet finished an important essay that is due in the next day.

How important are the following factors for Malaika to consider in deciding on what to do?

47. How long it will take her to finish the essay.
48. The importance of the essay towards her final mark.
49. She might not learn that much in the clinic.
50. Her reputation with the doctor.
51. Whether or not Malaika will be able to attend another clinic with the doctor.

Scenario 11

Jean and Franklin are medical students and clinical partners. Jean notices that Franklin frequently arrives looking very untidy, and some of their doctors have started to comment on his unprofessional appearance. However, Jean is worried that Franklin would take it personally and get offended if she mentioned something to him.

How important are the following factors for Jean in deciding on what to do?

52. Their reputation with the doctors.
53. Jean's friendship with Franklin.
54. Mentioning his appearance may hurt Franklin's feelings.
55. Their daily contact with patients.
56. Franklin's appearance may reflect badly on Jean as they are clinical partners.

Scenario 12

Rory and Priya have been working on a project together based on an interesting patient they have seen. They divided the work between them so each is responsible for different sections. Rory has been going into the hospital early every day in order to look at the patient's notes and construct his part of the project. However, he notices that Priya has been secretly taking sections of the patient's notes home with her each evening and bringing them back the next morning.

How important are the following factors to Rory's situation?

57. The project must be completed on time.

58. It risks breaking confidentiality for Priya to take identifiable patient notes home.

59. The overnight staff may not be able to access the patient's notes if Priya has taken them home.

60. A member of staff might find out.

61. Rory and Priya will receive a joint mark for their project.

62. Rory has no responsibility towards how Priya works on her part of the project.

Scenario 13

Horatio and Nelson are medical students on a surgical placement. They have been invited to observe an interesting operation, but have been advised to stand back and not to touch any of the sterile equipment. Horatio sees Nelson accidently touch the sterile trolley out of the corner of his eye. Nelson does not say anything, and the procedure is about to begin.

How important are the following factors for Horatio in deciding what he should do?

63. Nelson would be very embarrassed if Horatio told on him.

64. The risk to the patient being operated on with unsterile equipment

65. Nelson only very briefly touched the trolley.

66. The inconvenience for all of the surgical staff if they have to bring out a new sterile trolley.

67. They may be asked to leave the theatre.

68. The procedure may not be able to be carried out if the equipment is contaminated.

69. Nelson is scrubbed in a sterile surgical gown.

END OF PAPER

Mock Paper B

Section A: Verbal Reasoning

Passage 1

Rosa Parks

American Rosa Parks, born Rosa Louise McCauley, met her husband at protests fighting for justice for the Scottsboro boys, a group of young men who were falsely accused and convicted of rape because they were African-Americans. Her vested interest in civil rights had led to her marriage, and would lead to her becoming one of the most recognised names in black history. Montgomery, Alabama, USA had passed a city ordinance in 1900 concerning racial segregation on busses. Conductors were vested in the power to assign seats to their passengers, in order to achieve the sectioning off of black people from white people on the vehicle. Though the law stated no-one should have to give up a seat or move when a bus was crowded, in practice the custom evolved that conductors would get African-Americans to vacate their seat when there were no white-only ones left.

On the 1st of December, 1955, Parks got on a bus after a full day of work. She sat at the front of the 'coloured section' on the bus, a section whose size was determined by a movable sign. At one point during the journey, the driver noticed several white people were standing, and moved the sign back a row, telling the seated black passengers to get up. Three others stood from their seats, but Rosa did not: she instead slid along to a seat next to the window. She refused to give up, and was arrested for this refusal. She said that, contrary to popular belief, she did not remain seated because she was physically tired, but 'tired of giving in'. By not giving in, she made history.

1. Bus segregation was not the only concern for a black person in Rosa Parks' lifetime.

A. True.
B. False.
C. Can't tell.

2. Parks's actions were preceded by:

A. Over half a century of racist law demanding black people vacate seats for white people.
B. Conductors treating African-Americans as inferiors.
C. Her previous arrest for her involvement in the Scottsboro boy protests.
D. Years of tiring hard work being answered by unpleasant bus journeys.

3. A movable sign on a Montgomery bus could NOT:

A. Determine how many seats were for white people.
B. Determine how many black people were allowed to sit.
C. Determine how many African-Americans would be made to stand.
D. Distinguish between the ages, genders and circumstances of black or white customers.

4. Rosa Parks was arrested:

A. For refusing to move.
B. For being black.
C. Wrongly.
D. For not conforming to the behaviours of other black passengers.

Passage 2

Urania Cottage

19th Century social reformers like the author Charles Dickens often desired to help prostitutes leave behind their lives of sex work. Angela Burdett-Coutts, a philanthropist of considerable financial means, approached the novelist in 1846 to talk to him about a project to help save sex workers from their profession. The novelist at first tried to dissuade her from this idea, but ended up persuaded himself, and set up a refuge in Urania Cottage, a building in Shepherd's Bush, London. Unlike other establishments for 'fallen women', which were harsher in their treatments of ex-prostitutes, Dickens and Coutts planned a kind approach to the women who sought help from them.

Dickens sent out an advert to gain the attention of sex workers:

"If you have ever wished (I know you must have done so, sometimes) for a chance of rising out of your sad life, and having friends, a quiet home, means of being useful to yourself and others, peace of mind, self-respect, everything you have lost, pray read... attentively... I am going to offer you, not the chance but the certainty of all these blessings, if you will exert yourself to deserve them. And do not think that I write to you as if I felt myself very much above you, or wished to hurt your feelings by reminding you of the situation in which you are placed. God forbid! I mean nothing but kindness to you, and I write as if you were my sister."

5. Charles Dickens:

A. Wrote on the condition of prostitutes.
B. Used prostitutes.
C. Was romantically engaged with Angela Burdett-Coutts.
D. Wanted to improve working conditions for prostitutes.

6. Dickens:

A. Supported Coutts's idea from the start.
B. Initially opposed Coutts's idea.
C. Greatly admired Coutts.
D. Patronised Coutts.

7. The new refuge was to be:

A. Punishing.
B. Neutral.
C. Heavily religious.
D. Sympathetic.

8. According to the advert, Dickens saw sex workers as:

A. Women who have suffered irredeemable loss.
B. Women who had purposely chosen the way of the devil.
C. Women immensely inferior to himself.
D. Women who could achieve lovely things.

Passage 3

Moral Relativism

Despite the good intentions of those who would reform policies, such people must always be aware of their audience and ask if those they would help actually wish to receive this 'help'. Though it is tempting to project personal ideas of happiness and value onto another, it is not always correct. Human beings do not all hold the same desires or ideals, and what is misery for one person could be contentment for another. The phrase 'one man's trash is another man's treasure' may spring to mind.

A good example of this can be found in an 1858 British incident involving a letter in the newspaper, *The Times*. An unnamed 'Unfortunate' had written two columns on being a prostitute that had gained the attention of Angela Burdett-Coutts. Coutts then asked Charles Dickens to find out the writer, so that she may reach out and help this 'unfortunate' herself.

Unfortunately, neither of the well-meaning people had read the two columns in full. By the end of her letter, the prostitute stated she was happy doing what she did, and rather angered by those who would actively try to get rid of her means of earning. She scorned the type of person who would seek to redeem her:

"You the pious, the moral, the respectable, as you call yourselves ... why stand you on your eminence shouting that we should be ashamed of ourselves? What have we to be ashamed of, we who do not know what shame is?"

9. The above passage states:

A. We should all mind our own business.
B. A good deed is its own punishment.
C. Good deeds are not necessarily considered 'good' by all.
D. Other people's views on morality are wrong.

10. When the above passage states 'one man's trash is another man's treasure', they specifically refer to the fact that:

A. Poor people will enjoy things rich people do not.
B. Prostitutes love their profession, whereas non-prostitutes would not.
C. Dickens demands has higher expectations of happiness than sex workers do.
D. There is no universal route to happiness for all humans.

11. According to the passage, the letter accused do-gooders like Coutts of:

A. Prudishness.
B. Making working conditions worse.
C. Depriving people of work.
D. Conservatism.

12. The excerpt from the letter:

A. Personally attacks Coutts and Dickens.
B. Is from the 18th century.
C. Questions reformers' definition of piety.
D. States do-gooders should be ashamed of *their* actions.

Passage 4

Dystopias in Fiction

Literature and popular culture have seen a great range of dystopias. George Orwell's *1984* depicts a surveillance state where every individual is being constantly watched and assessed, where the 'truth' may be destroyed and rewritten by those in the Ministry of Truth and where those who don't toe the line may be subject to horrendous torture. The novel sees children informing on their parents and love being sacrificed to fear. Considering the severity of all of this, it may seem odd that the reality TV show 'Big Brother' took both its name and concept from such a frightening piece of fiction, replicating a house where one can never find privacy. One wonders what Orwell would have made of his work being used in this populist way. Another oddity is the fact that the awful torture chamber of the book, Room 101, has been used as the title of a BBC comedy programme where people discuss their pet hates - not, as in the novel, their greatest fear.

Other dystopian works include the graphic novel *V for Vendetta* written by Alan Moore, *A Clockwork Orange* written by Anthony Burgess and episodes of Charlie Brooker's *Black Mirror* TV series. The literal translation of dystopia is 'not-good-place' and many audiences are very much drawn to nightmarish imaginings of awful places and societies.

13. *V for Vendetta* and *A Clockwork Orange* both describe horrible future realities.

A. True.
B. False.
C. Can't tell.

14. George Orwell would be pleased with the way *1984* has inspired TV.

A. True.
B. False.
C. Can't tell.

15. Which of the following is NOT described as occurring within *1984*:

A. Constant camera surveillance.
B. Honesty being undermined.
C. Children turned against parents.
D. Love being destroyed.

16. Which of the following is true according to the passage:

A. *Black Mirror* voices the same concerns previously brought up in *A Clockwork Orange* and *1984.*
B. Audiences universally love dystopias.
C. Dystopias help us feel good about things as they are.
D. Horrible fictional realities do not necessarily repel people.

Passage 5

Oscar Wilde on Art
Oscar Wilde wrote the following as a preface to the only novel he wrote, *The Picture of Dorian Grey:*

'The artist is the creator of beautiful things. To reveal art and conceal the artist is art's aim. The critic is he who can translate into another manner or a new material his impression of beautiful things.

The highest as the lowest form of criticism is a mode of autobiography. Those who find ugly meanings in beautiful things are corrupt without being charming. This is a fault.

Those who find beautiful meanings in beautiful things are the cultivated. For these there is hope. They are the elect to whom beautiful things mean only beauty.

There is no such thing as a moral or an immoral book. Books are well written, or badly written. That is all.

The nineteenth century dislike of realism is the rage of Caliban seeing his own face in a glass.

The nineteenth century dislike of romanticism is the rage of Caliban not seeing his own face in a glass...No artist desires to prove anything. Even things that are true can be proved. No artist has ethical sympathies. An ethical sympathy in an artist is an unpardonable mannerism of style....

All art is quite useless.'

17. The above excerpt is cited as being written by:

A. A playwright.
B. A writer of fiction.
C. A Victorian-era man.
D. A comedian.

18. According to Wilde, the critic:

A. Is a beast.
B. Should find beautiful meanings in ugly things.
C. Should avoid all things that are not beautiful.
D. Can be corrupt or cultivated.

19. Beautifully written books:

A. Are immoral.
B. Are moral.
C. Are the highest form of art.
D. Are simply beautifully written.

20. The book to follow this preface, according to the writer himself:

A. Is well written.
B. Has no purpose.
C. Will have no impression of the creator.
D. Will be translated into further beauty by critics.

Passage 6

G.K. Chesterton on Eugenics

The following is from G.K. Chesterton's 1922 'Eugenics and Other Evils':

'It is not really difficult to sum up the essence of Eugenics: though some of the Eugenists seem to be rather vague about it. The movement consists of two parts: a moral basis, which is common to all, and a scheme of social application which varies a good deal. For the moral basis, it is obvious that man's ethical responsibility varies with his knowledge of consequences. If I were in charge of a baby (like Dr. Johnson in that tower of vision), and if the baby was ill through having eaten the soap, I might possibly send for a doctor. I might be calling him away from much more serious cases, from the bedsides of babies whose diet had been far more deadly; but I should be justified. I could not be expected to know enough about his other patients to be obliged (or even entitled) to sacrifice to them the baby for whom I was primarily and directly responsible. Now the Eugenic moral basis is this; that the baby for whom we are primarily and directly responsible is the babe unborn. That is, that we know (or may come to know) enough of certain inevitable tendencies in biology to consider the fruit of some contemplated union in that direct and clear light of conscience which we can now only fix on the other partner in that union. The one duty can conceivably be as definite as or more definite than the other. The baby that does not exist can be considered even before the wife who does. Now it is essential to grasp that this is a comparatively new note in morality.'

21. G.K. Chesterton accuses Eugenicists of being:

A. Too blunt.
B. Too pithy.
C. Imprecise in their definition of their belief.
D. Crude in their definition of anti-Eugenicists.

22. Chesterton acknowledges one might criticise the guardian of the soap-eating baby for:

A. Allowing the baby to consume soap.
B. Not treating the baby himself.
C. Having a baby with no self-preservation instincts.
D. Taking up a doctor's valuable time for a case that may not be as serious as others.

23. 'The babe unborn' can be contemplated because:

A. Of the inherent value of human life.
B. Our ability to predict the products of a union through science.
C. Babies are essentially just like their mothers.
D. Babies are all the same.

24. The 'new note in morality' described in the passage is:

A. A belief that the living babies of others are more important than yours.
B. A belief that we should use biology to stop births of undesirable babies.
C. That non-existent babies can be more important than existing women.
D. People should have as many babies as possible.

Passage 7

Asylums in the 19th Century

The following is an extract from a column from Fanny Fern, describing a visit to an American insane asylum in the 19th century:

'It is a very curious sight, these lunatics – men and women, preparing food in the perfectly-arranged kitchen. One's first thought, to be sure, is some possibly noxious ingredient that might be cunningly mixed in the viands; but further observation showed the impossibility of this under the rigid surveillance exercised. As to the pies, and meats, and vegetables, in process of preparation, they looked sufficiently tempting to those who had earned a good appetite like ourselves, by a walk across the fields. Some lunatic-women who were employed in the laundry, eyed me as I stood watching them, and, glancing at the embroidery on the hem of my skirt, a little the worse for the wet and dust of the road, exclaimed, "Oh, fie! A soiled skirt!" In fact, I almost began to doubt whether our guide was not humbugging us as to the real state of these people's intellects; particularly as some of them employed in the grounds, as we went out, took off their hats, and smiled and bowed to us in the most approved manner.'

25. It is curious for the author to see men in a kitchen.

A. True.
B. False.
C. Can't tell.

26. The writer wonders whether the inmates of the asylum:

A. May burn themselves working in a kitchen.
B. Should be kept away from sharp objects like knives.
C. Would be distressed by food preparation.
D. May poison the asylum's food.

27. The laundry-women demonstrate they are women of their trade through:

A. Busily washing the sheets.
B. Cleaning the writer's skirt.
C. Commenting on the dirtiness of clothing.
D. The fine state of everyone's apparel in the asylum.

28. The writer doubts that the inmates are insane, specifically as:

A. They all demonstrate good intelligence.
B. Some demonstrate good courtesy.
C. They are not violent.
D. They speak good English.

Passage 8

Self-immolation

The following is an excerpt from a Victorian era newspaper column:

I RECENTLY witnessed one of the most extraordinary and horrid scenes ever performed by a human being – namely, the self-immolation of a woman on the funeral pile of her husband. The dreadful sacrifice has made an impression on my mind, that years will not efface...

Yesterday morning, at seven o'clock, this woman was brought in a palanquin to the place of sacrifice. It is on the banks of the Ganges, only two miles from Calcutta. Her husband had been previously brought to the river to expire. His disorder was hydrophobia – think of the agony this must have occasioned him. He had been dead for twenty-four hours, and no person could prevail on the wife to save herself. She had three children, whom she committed to the care of her mother. A woman, called to be undertaker, was preparing the pile. It was composed of bamboo, firewood, oils, resin, and a kind of flax, altogether very combustible. It was elevated above the ground, I should say twenty inches, and supported by strong stakes. The dead body was lying on a rude couch, very near, covered with a white cloth. The eldest child, a boy of seven years, who was to light the pile, was standing near the corpse. The woman sat perfectly unmoved during all the preparation, apparently at prayer, and counting a string of beads which she held in her hand. She was just thirty years old; her husband twenty-seven years older.

29. Which of the following terms could NOT be used to correctly describe the Indian wife in the passage:

A. A daughter.
B. A mother.
C. A wife.
D. Alive.

30. The agony of the husband is due to:

A. The painfulness of his condition.
B. The knowledge of his imminent death.
C. The fear he held of water.
D. The knowledge of his wife's imminent sacrifice.

31. Which of the following is the seven year old boy NOT described to do:

A. Enable his mother's suicide.
B. Burn his father's body.
C. Become an orphan.
D. Become the support of his younger siblings.

32. Which of the following is definitely true:

A. The wife was in prayer during the preparation of the pile.
B. The wife was immobilised during the preparation of the pile.
C. The wife was three decades the junior of her husband.
D. The wife chose to leave her children.

Passage 9

Advice for Boys

The following is an excerpt from a Victorian era newspaper:

A WORD TO BOYS. – Who is respected? It is the boy who conducts himself well, who is honest, diligent, and obedient in all things. It is the boy who is making an effort continually to respect his father, and obey him in whatever he may direct to be done. It is the boy who is kind to other little boys, who respects age, and who never gets into difficulties and quarrels with his companions. It is the boy who leaves no effort untried to improve himself in knowledge and wisdom every day – who is busy and attentive in trying to do good acts towards others. Show us a boy who obeys his parents, who is diligent, who has respect for age, who always has a friendly disposition, and who applies himself diligently to get wisdom and to do good towards others, and if he is not respected and beloved by everybody, then there is no such thing as truth in this world. Remember this, boys, and you will be respected by others, and will grow up and become useful men.

33. A boy must be and do several things before he can be 'respected'.

A. True.
B. False.
C. Can't tell.

34. Girls, unlike boys, cannot hope to be 'respected' for qualities like honesty, diligence and obedience.

A. True.
B. False.
C. Can't tell.

35. A boy should avoid unnecessary confrontation.

A. True.
B. False.
C. Can't tell.

36. Respected boys will one day be valuable men.

A. True.
B. False.
C. Can't tell.

Passage 10

Renaissance Revenge Tragedy

Renaissance Revenge tragedies were very popular dramas, often filled with sexuality and murder. Shakespeare himself wrote two revenge tragedies, *Titus Andronicus* (set in ancient Roman times) and *Hamlet*, and though he is often considered the greatest English playwright (if not, writer) that ever lived, he has a sense of wickedness that thrilled through his dark plays. For example, Titus Adronicus involves an act of familial cannibalism, as Tamora's two sons (who had raped and mutilated Titus' daughter) are killed and baked into a pie, to be served to their mother (who had committed a series of deeds to destroy the family and happiness of Titus). Other such tragedies involve unusual scenes, like a Duke being killed by a poisoned skull he believes to be a living woman (*The Revenger's Tragedy*) or a man biting off his own tongue so that he will not reveal secrets when he is tortured (*The Spanish Tragedy*).

The avengers in revenge tragedies often die themselves: having killed a wrong-doer, they become murderers themselves, and often have lost their previous moral high-ground. Morality dictates that they must be served with a bloody end. Though the plays do not protect innocents, who may be raped or murdered, the genre does not allow its killers to go unpunished - even when the killers are also the protagonists.

37. Shakespeare was not above writing in a populist genre.

A. True.
B. False.
C. Can't tell.

38. Only Shakespeare named his revenge tragedies after characters in the play.

A. True.
B. False.
C. Can't tell.

39. Revenge tragedies are NOT described as involving:

A. A sexually abused woman.
B. Deadly bones.
C. Self-mutilation.
D. Suicide.

40. Revenge tragedies are described as:

A. All set in European places like Italy and Spain.
B. Poems and plays involving tales of avengers.
C. Following an ethical code.
D. Obsessed with cannibals.

Passage 11

Cats have been domesticated for thousands and thousands of years, but as yet there has been no conclusive explanation for what started off this trend of making felines pets.

One theory for the origins of cat domestication lies in the animal's ability to kill rodents. Washington University's Wesley Warren suggests that originally people would welcome the predators, as they would destroy pests that would otherwise eat up grain harvests. The human may then have offered, as a reward, food, to make sure the cat would stay.

One can see in this a possible beginning in human's affectionate relationship with felines: having done such a good job in controlling rodents, an owner would be pleased with their pet and perhaps even grateful. It may well be this very practical use of the creature that led to our modern culture of keeping the animal as a pampered pet.

To this day, domestic cats, with their simple gut suited for raw meat, are mostly carnivorous. Their bodies have another feature suited to this diet of flesh: a rough tongue. The tongue's textured surface helps the cat take every last morsel of meat from the bone of some other animal.

Of course, even if the cat's owner attempts to limit their intake of meat, a wily feline can still hunt for their own prey, perhaps outside the home, even if they are 'domesticated'.

41. There is no longer such a thing as a wild cat.

A. True
B. False
C. Can't tell

42. Which of the following statements is NOT supported by the passage:

A. Cats may have been traditionally used as hunters.
B. Cats are currently used for their killing ability.
C. Cats are anatomically suited for a diet of meat.
D. Cats may not exclusively rely on their owners for food.

43. Which of the following statements is supported by the passage:

A. Wesley Warren is a student of Washington University.
B. Wesley Warren is an acclaimed professor of Washington University.
C. Wesley Warren is affiliated with an academic institution.
D. Wesley Warren is a man.

44. According to the passage, humans:

A. All love cats.
B. Love only those that do something for them in return.
C. Have as a race conducted relationships with another species for millennia.
D. All hate rats.

END OF SECTION

Section B: Decision Making

1. "All chemistry exams are written. All written exams are flammable. Some written exams are double sided." If the above is true which of the below statements are also true?

I. Some chemistry papers are double sided.
II. All flammable exams are chemistry exams
III. All double sided exams are flammable

A. I only
B. II only
C. III only
D. II and III
E. All of the above

2. The Government is starting a new health initiative to sponsor athletic shoes, in the hopes of improving the fitness of the public by encouraging more walking. Outdoor activities are cheaper than gym memberships. What can be concluded from this?

A. Athletics is the best form of exercise
B. Outdoor training is better than indoor training
C. Gym memberships are a poor investment
D. New shoes will mean fewer people go to the gym
E. Walking is a good form of exercise

3. There are 30 medical students in a classroom, discussing their subjects. Everyone states a preference for at least one subject. 6 medical students like anatomy only. 14 medical students like pharmacology, and 19 like biochemistry. 5 like all three. 3 hate pharmacology but like the others. No one enjoys pharmacology and anatomy. How many medical students like pharmacology and biochemistry.

A. 7
B. 4
C. 0
D. 6
E. 3

4. "Medical knowledge and supplies are urgently needed around the world. People in developing countries need better medical care." Which statement supports these?

A. The majority of people in the world have never seen a doctor
B. People in developing countries are not getting minimum medical aid
C. Doctors are selfish and only care about money
D. Insurance companies have increased their prices
E. Developed countries have a lot of medical supplies

5. Which diagrams shows the relationship between women, mothers and doctors?

A.
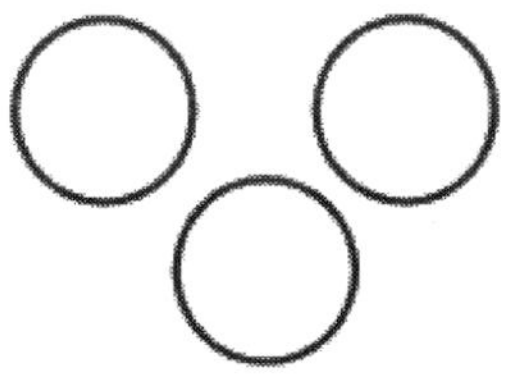

C.
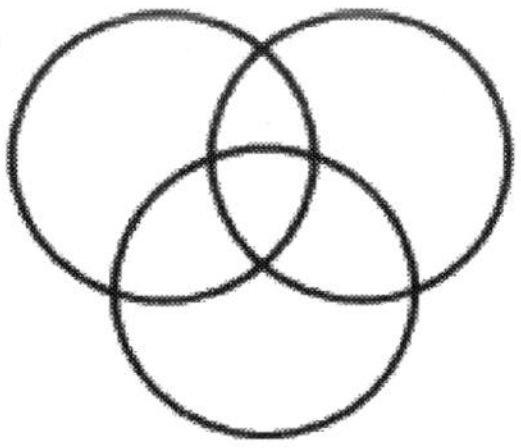

E.
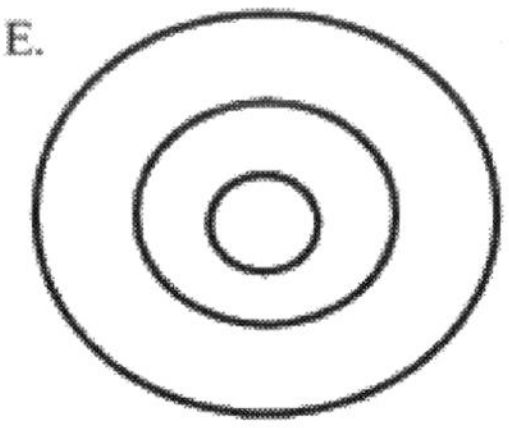

B.
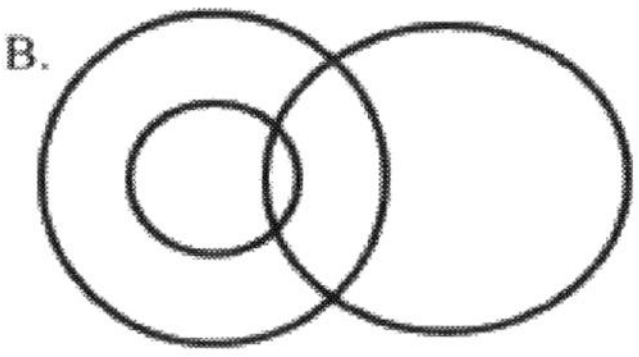

D.
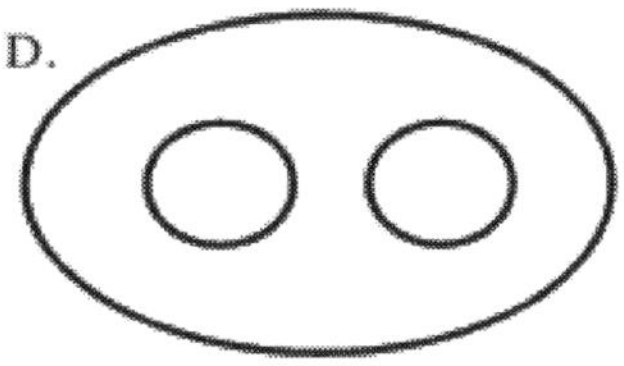

6. A survey is down on pets owned in a town.

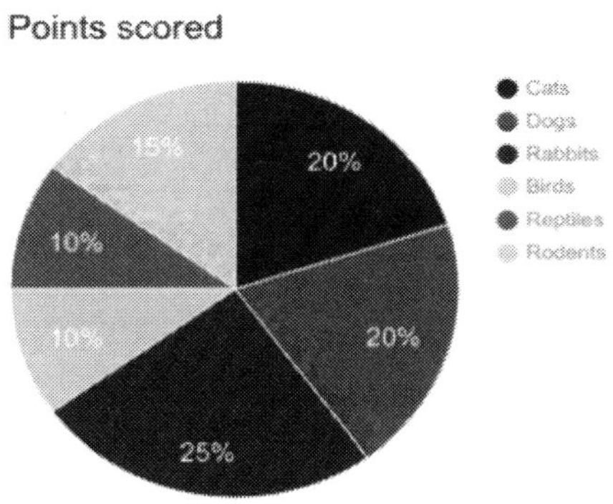

Which statement is correct?

A. There are 25% fewer rodents than cats.
B. It is more expensive to feed dogs than birds.
C. Only 65% of pets have four legs
D. Reptiles and rodents must be sold together
E. Rabbits are less popular than dogs.

7. The chart shows the profits between three competing shops: Jake's, Lauren's and Nathan's, over the course of 5 years.

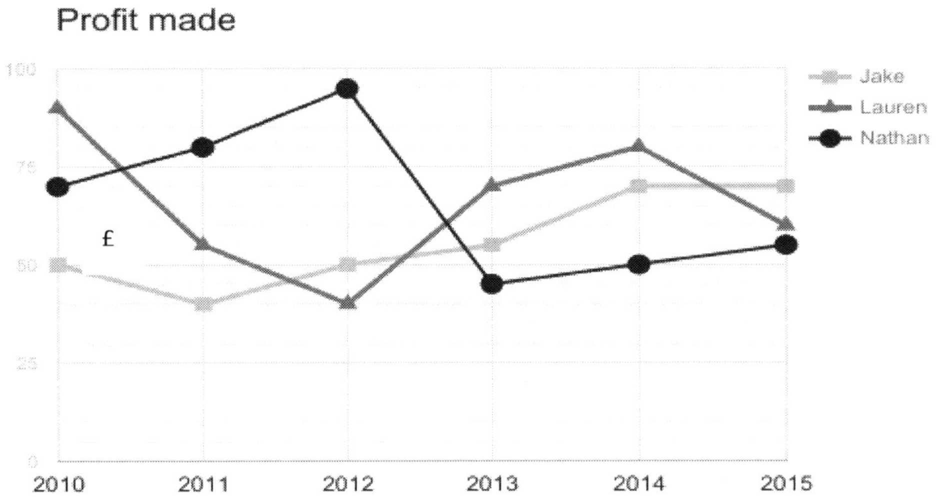

Which statement is correct?

A. The greatest overall loss of profits was 2012 to 2013.
B. Jake has the greatest percentage change in profit at the end of 5 years.
C. Lauren made more than Nathan for 2 years.
D. Everyone made the same amount of money from 2010 to 2012

8. Scores are taken from a recent exam period.

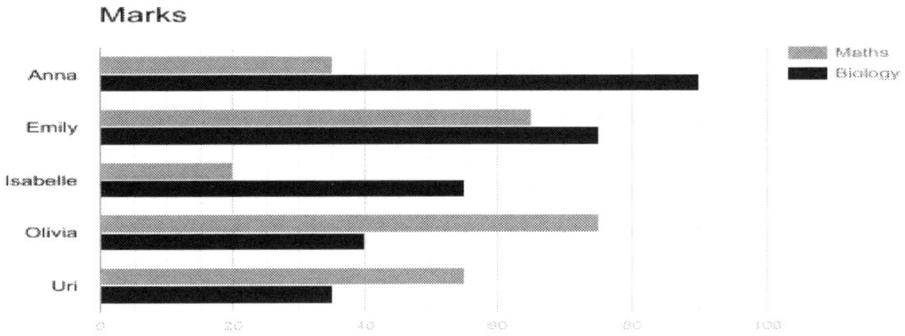

Which statement is correct?

A. Anna beats Olivia in biology by double the number of marks that Oliva beat Anna in Maths
B. Maths was a harder exam than Biology
C. Emily has the highest average score
D. Isabelle and Uri combined have the highest Biology score
E. It is an all girls' school.

9. Millie's Marvellous Cars is reviewing their yearly sales and profit.

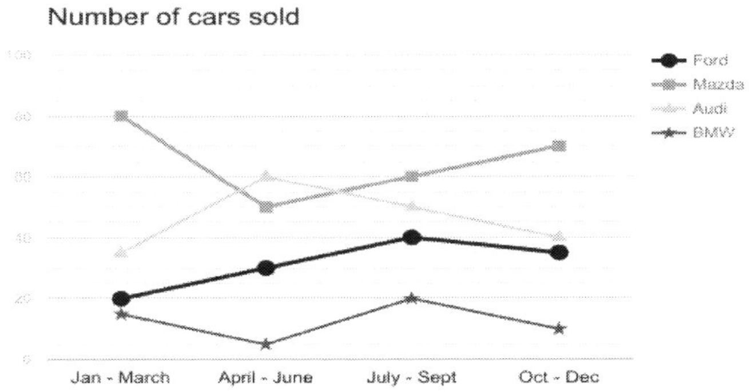

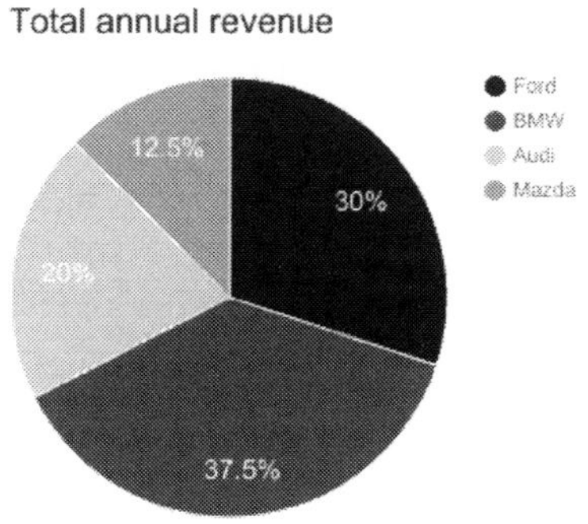

Which statement is true?

A. Millie did not make money selling Audi cars
B. All the cars increased in value throughout the year
C. BMW and Ford sold fewer cars in the second half of the year than Audi did in the first half
D. Mazda cars are cheaper than BMWs

10. The table shows the proportion of female students and swimmers in a school. There are 200 students in Y10, Y11 and Sixth Form. 80% of students are in Sixth form and there are an equal number of Y10 and Y11 students.

	Female	Swimmers
Year 10	0.3	0.65
Year 11	0.7	0.5
Sixth form	0.45	0.3
Total	0.46	0.355

Which statement is true?

A. The percentage of swimmers in the school that are in Y11 is 65%
B. The total number of swimmers in the school is 82
C. There are the same number of male students in the Sixth Form as there are in Y11.
D. You are more likely to be a male swimmer than a female non swimmer.
E. There are twelve times as many girls in Sixth form as in Y10.

11. Queenie, Rose, and Susanna are playing a game where the loser gives half her money to the other players, who share it equally. They play three games and each loses a game, in alphabetical order. At the end of last game, each girl has 32p. If Queenie started with the least money, who had the most money?

A. They all started with the same amount
B. Rose
C. Susanna
D. Rose and Susana started with the same amount

12. Communism is the only truly just social system where everybody is equal.

Which of the following statements **most strongly** argues against this point?

A. Communism must fail because humans inherently strive for personal gain.
B. Communism has so far always failed to produce functioning state systems.
C. Communist societies always fail economically.
D. Capitalism is better than Communism.

13. In a shooting competition, an individual is awarded 5 points for hitting a target. Missing a target results in no points being added, but there is no penalty for missing. Each shooter fires 5 shots at the target. 5 Shooters take part in the competition.

Pat achieves 15 points.
Lauren misses 4 targets, but does not finish last.
Peter hits 4 targets.
Dave achieves 5 more points than Lauren.

Which of the following statements is correct?

A. Joe finishes last.
B. Dave finishes second
C. Pat is a poor shot.
D. Dave shoots better than Pat.

14. Mr Smith is a surgeon. One day, Mr Smith and his wife decide to sort through his wardrobe. He has a total of 20 shirts, of which ¼ striped. Mrs Smith doesn't like Mr Smith's pink shirt. Mr Smith has 3 blue shirts. He only wears his white shirts with black trousers.
Select if the following statements are true or false from the information provided.

A. Mrs Smith is a surgeon.
B. Mr Smith has black shirts.
C. Mr Smith only wears black trousers with white shirts
D. Mr Smith owns white shirts.

15. Explorers in the US in the 18th Century had to contend with a great variety of obstacles ranging from natural to man-made. Natural obstacles included the very nature and set up of the land, presenting explorers with the sheer size of the land mass, the lack of reliable mapping as well as the lack of paths and bridges. On a human level, challenges included the threat from outlaws and other hostile groups. Due to the nature of the settling situation, availability of medical assistance was sketchy and there was a constant threat of diseases and fatal results of injuries.

Which of the following statements is correct with regards to the above text?

A. Medical supply was good in the US in the 18th Century.
B. The land was easy to navigate.
C. There were few outlaws threatening the individual.
D. Crossing rivers could be difficult.

16. People who practice extreme sports should have to buy private health insurance.

Which of the following statements most strongly supports this argument?

A. Exercise is healthy and private insurance offers better reward schemes.
B. Extreme spots have a higher likelihood of injury.
C. Healthcare should be free for all.
D. People that practice extreme sports are more likely to be wealthy.

17. A group of scientists investigates the role of different nutrients after exercise. They set up two groups of averagely fit individuals consisting of the same number of both males and females aged 20 – 25 and weighing between 70 and 85 kilos. Each group will conduct the same 1hr exercise routine of resistance training, consisting of various weighted movements. After the workout they will receive a shake with vanilla flavour that has identical consistency and colour in all cases. Group A will receive a shake containing 50 g of protein and 50 g of carbohydrates. Group B will receive a shake containing 100 g of protein and 50 g of carbohydrates. All participants have their lean body mass measured before starting the experiment.

Which of the following statements is correct?

A. The experiment compares the response of men and women to endurance training.
B. The experiment is flawed as it does not take into consideration that men and women respond differently to exercise.
C. The experiment does not consider age.
D. The experiment mainly looks at the role of protein after exercise.

18. When considering the reproductive behaviour of animals, different factors have to be considered. On one hand, there are social structures within the local animal population that play a role. In herd animals for example, it is common for only the lead male or female to reproduce in order to ensure that offspring have optimal genetic material. In addition to that, different animals reproduce during different times of the year in order to optimise survival chances for their offspring based on different gestation periods. Animals with longer periods of gestation, for example, are more likely to reproduce in the spring so that the young are born in late summer, allowing them to grow during the fall months in order to prepare for the winter months. In areas where there are less marked differences between winter and summer months, this behaviour is less relevant.

Which of the following statements is correct?

A. In herd animals lead animals are always the only individuals reproducing.
B. Animal reproductive behaviour is complex.
C. Animals with longer gestation periods are more likely to deliver in spring in colder climates.
D. All of the above.

19. A restaurant re-prints their menus and decides to display their range of beers according to alcohol content.

The Monk's Brew is brewed in Germany and has an alcohol content of 4.5%.
Fisher's Ale has the least alcohol content at 3.8% and is brewed using triple filtered spring water.
Knight's Brew has more alcohol than Fisher's, but less than Monk's.
Ferrier Ale has 5% alcohol, but is not the strongest beer.

Which of the following is true?

A. Brewer's Choice is the strongest beer.
B. German beer is the weakest.
C. Spring water makes for particularly strong beers.
D. Fischer's Ale is not the weakest beer.

20. Jack sets up a vegetable garden. He starts out with 10 potato plants. For every potato plant, he plants twice as many carrots. He also plants twice as many tomatoes as he plants carrots. In the end, he also plants 10 heads of salad.

Which of the following is true?

A. There are a total of 70 plants
B. He plants more potatoes than heads of salad.
C. There must be 20 tomato plants.
D. There are four times as many tomatoes than heads of salad.

21. A group of scientists investigate the prevalence of allergies in the population. In order to do that, they use medical files of those treated for allergies or diagnosed with allergies. They find that over the last 30 years the overall prevalence of allergies has increased. This is particularly the case for food intolerances and allergies to inhaled substances such as dust and pollen, which represent the majority of all allergies documented. The scientists also find that there is a proportionally larger increase in younger individuals being diagnosed with allergies than there was 30 years ago. The scientists find that 30% of diagnoses are being made within the first 5 years of live, 20% of diagnoses are being made in the second 5 years of life and the remaining 50% are being made between age 10 and 50.

Which of the following statements is true?

A. Contact allergies are very common.
B. The majority of diagnoses are being made between 6 and 10 years.
C. The scientists used unreliable data.
D. Allergy prevalence in the young has increased over the past 3 decades.

22. Rowing is a complex sport that requires a variety of different skills in order to perform well. On one hand, a good rower must possess physical strength in order to move the heavy boats as well as his own body effectively through the water. The more power a rower can exert on the oars, the more his boat will accelerate. Due to the length of rowing races of 2000m, rowers also need a high degree of cardiovascular fitness and muscular endurance in order to be able to perform well for the duration of their race. The final aspect of rowing is not a physical one but a mental one, requiring the individual to perform complex motor patterns with technical perfection in order to reduce opposing forces on the motion of his boat and in order to maintain constant and even acceleration.

Which of the following is true?

A. Rowing has little technical skill involved.
B. Physics plays no role in rowing.
C. Rowing requires a combination of physical and mental abilities.
D. Being strong is the most important aspect of rowing.

23. A group of scientists conduct a study into the density of fast food restaurants in different income neighbourhoods and relate this to the incidence of obesity. After collecting their data they find that the density of fast food restaurants in low-income neighbourhoods is higher than in high-income neighbourhoods. They also find that there are comparatively more fast food restaurants in the vicinity of schools than there is in the vicinity of housing areas. With regards to obesity, the study finds that with increasing density of fast food restaurants, the incidence of obesity increases.

Which of the following statements is true?

A. The incidence of obesity is higher in low-income neighbourhoods.
B. The most fast food restaurants exist around housing areas.
C. Places that serve fast food can hardly be called restaurants.
D. In order to tackle the obesity crisis, fast food needs to be more expensive.

24. Jason is unsure of what to get his little sister for her birthday, so he conducts a poll amongst his friends.

5 friends think that new ear rings are a good idea.
Out those that think earrings are a good idea, 3 also support a necklace and 2 also support shoes.
2 other friends also think that shoes are a good idea, but one of those also thinks a handbag is a good idea.
3 friends only support the idea of a dress.

Which of the following most accurately describes the distribution of opinion?

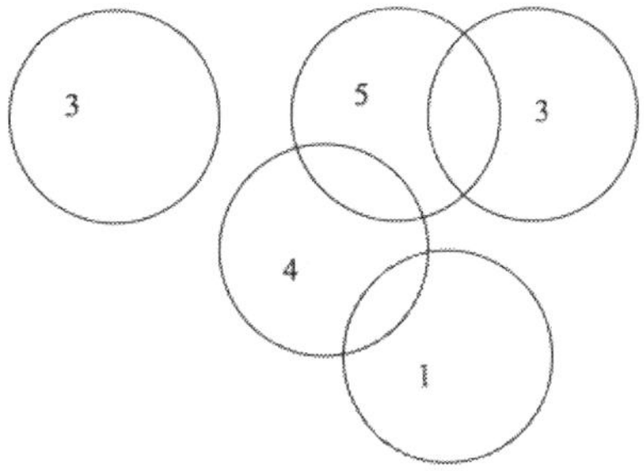

A.

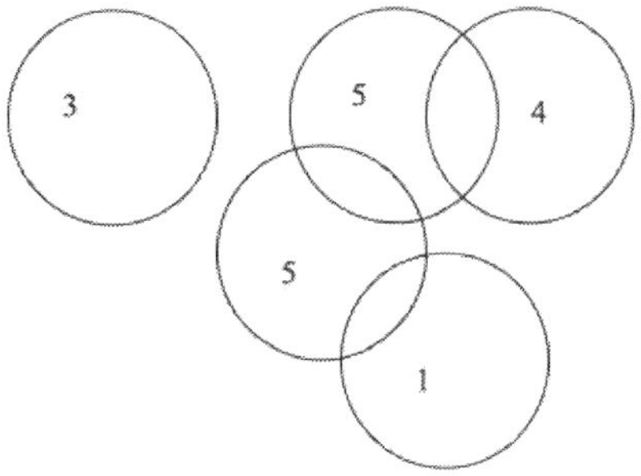

C.

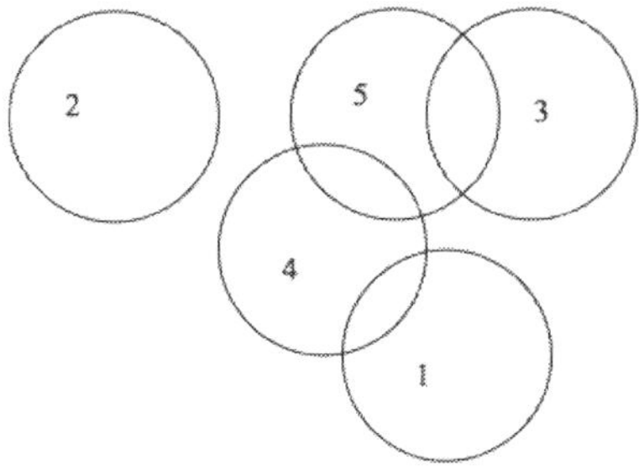

B.

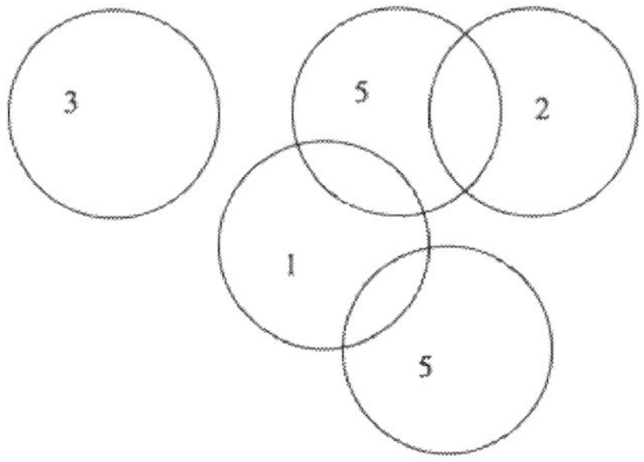

D.

25. Parents with high incomes should pay more school fees so the extra money can be used to subsidise the fees of poorer children.

Which of the following arguments supports this statement the most?

A. By law, everybody has to go to school.
B. Children from poorer backgrounds are more likely to undergo poorer education due to financial constraints.
C. Wealthy families have a social responsibility to support others.
D. It is not justifiable to charge wealthier families for being more successful.

26. Antibiotic resistance is an increasingly important problem for modern medicine. There are several key mechanisms with which bacteria aim to evade the action of antibiotics including the mutation of target structures or the production of lytic enzymes that destroy antibiotic molecules before they can act on the bacteria. This represents an important resistance mechanism. It is also common for bacteria to develop mutations in important transporter molecules that reduce the entry of antibiotic molecules into the cell or increase their extrusion from the cell. The worst case scenario is that one lineage of bacteria has developed multiple mechanisms of resistance that allow it to counteract the action of many different types of antibiotics.

Which of the following is correct?

A. Antibiotic resistance is of little relevance today.
B. Bacteria rarely develop lytic enzymes that destroy antibiotic molecules.
C. Bacteria have no way to reduce uptake of antibiotic molecules.
D. Antibiotic resistance can be caused by more than one mechanism simultaneously.

27. Stan collects stamps. He has stamps from Europe. He also has a half a dozen from Asia, and 3 from Canada. Select whether each statement is true or false.
A. Stan has no stamps from North America.
B. Stan may have stamps from Germany.
C. There are fewer stamps from Asia in Stan's collection than from Canada.
D. Stan may have stamps from France.

28. A survey asks a group of universities are asked for what they consider the most important quality in students applying for medicine.

- Dependability receives 28% of the votes,
- Intelligence receives 10% less of the votes.
- Communication skills receives 5% of the votes.
- Mental flexibility receives 10% more than communication skills.

Communication skills				

Which of the following is correct?

A. Intelligence is less important than mental flexibility.
B. Mental flexibility is the most important.
C. Dependability is not the most important skill in a prospective medical student.
D. Empathy receives less than 30% of votes.

29. Sugar should be taxed like alcohol and cigarettes.

Which of the following arguments most supports this claim?

A. Sugar can cause diabetes.
B. Sugar has a high addictive potential and is associated with various health concerns.
C. High sugar diets increase obesity.
D. People that eat a lot of sugar are more likely to start abusing alcohol.

END OF SECTION

Section C: Quantitative Reasoning

SET 1

Anne is looking to buy food from a takeaway. A sample of the menu is shown:

Item	Cost	Item	Cost
Plain Rice	£1.55	Chicken Satay	£4.30
Egg Fried Rice	£2.00	Kung Po Chicken	£3.40
Special Fried Rice	£5.00	Sichuan Pork	£5.60
Special Curry	£4.30	Roast Pork	£6.00
Chicken Curry	£4.00	Prawn Chow Mein	£5.50

1. Anne wishes to purchase 2 portions of egg fried rice, 1 special fried rice, a special curry, roast pork and a portion of Kung Po Chicken. What proportion of her bill comes from rice (to 2 s.f)?

A. 1:2.3 B. 1:2.5 C. 1:3.2 D. 1:4.2

2. The shop offers a set menu whereby someone can buy 2 portions of rice (either plain or egg fried) and any two different main meals for £10. Suppose Hannah buys the most expensive options. What percentage of the bill does she save?

A. 32% B. 36% C. 40% D. 44%

3. The shop charges £2.50 delivery on orders under £25 and 10% of the cost of the order otherwise. If Anne buys two set menus consisting of Special Curry and Chicken Curry, each with Egg Fried Rice, how much has she saved on delivery relative to if she bought the items separately?

A. £0.00 B. £0.30 C. £0.60 D. £1.00

4. The shop wishes to offer a new deal, when a customer spends more than £40, they get free delivery. Anne is planning to spend £39.40 and wants delivery. What percentage of her bill does she save by purchasing an extra portion of egg fried rice?

A. 2.3% B. 4.5% C. 6.8% D. 9.2%

SET 2

Bob is looking to insure his car. He gets the following three quotes:

Company	Cost
Red Flag	£25 a month, 10% discount for 5+ years with no claims, 2 free months a year for 10+ years with no claims (the final two deals accumulate together).
Chamberlain	£350 a year, 3% discount for each year with no claims.
Meerkat Market	£300 a year, but for every year with no claims £10 is saved.
Munich	£250 a year, no discounts.

5. Bob has 4 years with no claims. Which is the cheapest company for him to go with?

A. Red Flag B. Chamberlain C. Meerkat Market D. Munich

6. What percentage of the Red Flag normal cost is saved by a driver with 11 years without claims?

A. 12.5% B. 25.0% C. 37.5% D. 40.0%

7. Laura is insured with Chamberlain. She has 3 years no claims discount and is thinking about switching to Meerkat Market. How much money would she save by switching?

A. £58.50 B. £62.00 C. £68.50 D. £72.00

8. Munich decides to introduce a system whereby if two people buy a policy from them, they save 10%. Suppose that Delia and Elliot have 3 and 5 year no claims discounts respectively. Delia buys her insurance from Meerkat market and Elliot buys his from Chamberlain. Which of the following proportions gives the total new cost:old cost?

A. 0.79:1 B. 0.88:1 C. 1:1.14 D. 1:1.32

SET 3

The figure gives details of the number of students in a school who play any of the four games – cricket, basketball, football and hockey.

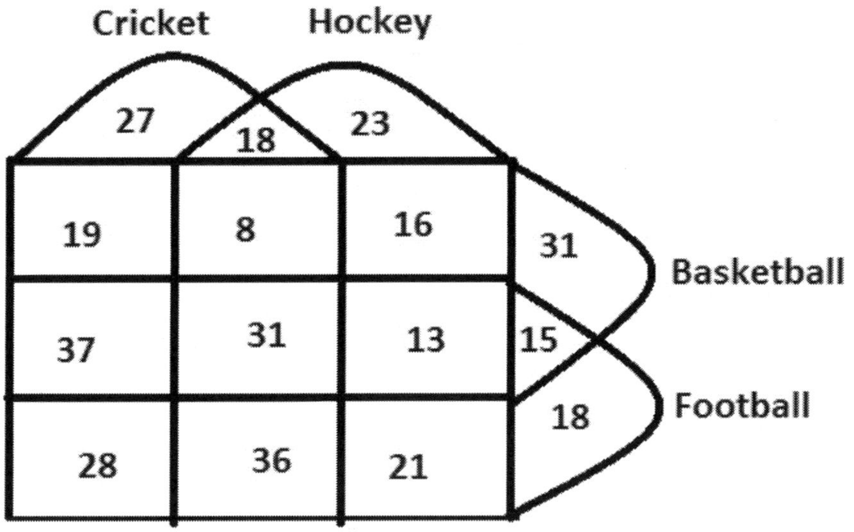

The total number of students in the school is 500.

9. How many of the students play at most one game?

A. 99 B. 159 C. 258 D. 341

10. What is the number of students who play either cricket or basketball, but not football?

A. 92 B. 119 C. 126 D. 138

11. How many students play at least three games?

A. 75 B. 125 C. 175 D. 225

12. The number of students playing at most one game exceeds those playing at least two games by

A. 8 B. 16 C. 18 D. 36

13. How many students do not play cricket, football or hockey?

A. 160 B. 180 C. 190 D. 200

14. By what number did the number of students playing none of the games **outnumber** the number of students playing exactly one game?

A. 20 B. 30 C. 60 D. 90

SET 4

The table below shows the daily number of passengers (in thousands ('000)) using trains as a means of transportation from 1998–2005.

Year	Number (in '000)
1998	200
1999	150
2000	300

For the year 2000, the following table shows the daily break-down of the proportion of passengers using different transportation modes:

Mode of Transport	Percentage
Taxis	8.33
Trains	41.67
Buses	33.33
Private Cars	16.67
Total	**100**

15. In 2000, how many people used a private car as a daily means of transportation?

A. 120,000 B. 180,000 C. 280,000 D. 320,000

16. If the same proportional break-down in 2000 is also applicable for 1999, the number of persons using taxis as a daily means of transport in 1999 is closest to:

A. 20,000 B. 30,000 C. 40,000 D. 50,000

17. If in 1998, one quarter of the total passengers travelled by train, what is the percentage change in the total number of daily passengers from 1998 to 2000?

A. 10% increase B. 10% decrease C. 20% increase D. 20% decrease

18. From 1998 to 2000, the number of passengers using taxis as a means of transportation increased by 50%. What is the percentage of passengers using daily taxis in 1998, given that the total population using public transport was 0.8 million in that year?

A. 5% B. 10% C. 15% D. 20%

19. If the ratio of number of people using buses as a means of transport in 1998, 1999 and 2000 is 8:5:6 and the bus fares in these three years are in the ratio of 2:3:4, then find the total amount collected in 1998 and 1999 together, given that fare in 2000 was £2 per person and the buses operate for 358 days a year.

A. £22,196,000 B. £211,360,000 C. £221,960,000 D. £235,020,000

20. If the same break-down as for 2000 is also applicable for 1999, then the number of persons using buses and private cars combined as a means of transport in 1999 is closest to:

A. 140,000 B. 160,000 C. 180,000 D. 200,000

SET 5

The following are the details of different steps involved in opening a fully functional computer centre.

S. No.	Work	Work Code	Duration (Weeks)	Other works that should be completed before the work
1.	Planning by architect	A	2	-
2.	First painting of roof	B	1	-
3.	First painting of walls	C	1	B
4.	Partitioning the workspace	D	2	A, B
5.	Networking	E	4	A
6.	Air-conditioning	F	6	D
7.	Electrical work	G	3	B
8.	False ceiling	H	4	E, F, J
9.	False flooring	I	1	L
10.	Fire safety systems	J	1	G
11.	Final painting of ceiling	K	2	H
12.	Final painting of walls	L	2	K, C

Note: In any week one or more activities are in progress.

21. The earliest time by which the false ceiling work can start is:

A. 8th week B. 9th week C. 10th week D. 11th week

22. If the work is to be done at the earliest, then the latest by which the fire safety systems work can start is:

A. 8th week B. 9th week C. 10th week D. 11th week

23. If not more than one activity can be undertaken at any given time, then what is the minimum possible time in which all of the above-mentioned works can be completed?

A. 25 weeks B. 29 weeks C. 31 weeks D. 33 weeks

24. What can be the maximum time gap between the start of the air-conditioning work and the start of the final painting of walls, if no time is wasted in between?

A. 17 weeks B. 19 weeks C. 21 weeks D. 23 weeks

25. If the work is to be done at the earliest, then the latest the air-conditioning work can start is:

A. 5th week B. 6th week C. 7th week D. 8th week

SET 6

The production of 5 food grains is listed in the following table:

Food Grain	Year 1989–90	Year 1999–2000
A (Rice)	75	90
B (Wheat)	50	70
C (Coarse Cereals)	35	30
D (Total Cereals)	160	190
E (Pulses)	15	13

Note:
Food Grains = Total Cereals + Pulses
Total Cereals= Total of A, B and C

26. The production target for food grains from 1999-2000 was 20% more than that of 1989-90, but this target was missed. What was the percentage deficit of production in 1999-2000 relative to the target production?

A. 1.3% B. 2.3% C. 3.3% D. 4.3%

27. The percentage decrease in the production of pulses from 1989-90 to 1999-2000 is equal to the percentage increase in the price of the pulses during the same period. If the average price of pulses is £1.80 per kg in 1989-90, what is the price in 1999-2000?

A. £2.00 B. £3.00 C. £4.00 D. £5.00

28. What is the percentage of total cereal production in 1999-2000 relative to total cereal production in 1989-90?

A. 112.5% B. 118.75% C. 143.95% D. 145.25%

SET 7

Four countries (USA, Kenya, Russia and Australia) participated in a 4 × 400 metre relay race. This is a race around a 400m athletic track with each team comprising four runners, each of whom completes 1 complete lap of 400 metres before handing a baton over to the next runner, who starts at the moment the previous runner finishes their lap. The winning team is the team whose final runner finishes their lap first.

The following bar graph gives the average speeds at which runners from the four teams ran to complete their laps.

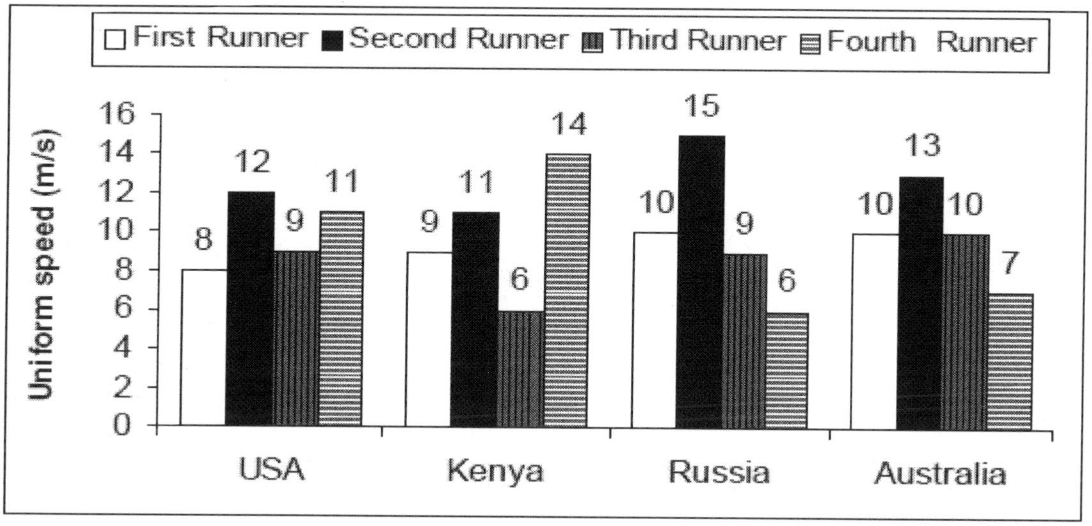

29. Which country won the event?

A. USA B. Australia C. Russia D. Kenya

30. Which country finished last in the event?

A. USA B. Australia C. Russia D. Kenya

31. Which of the following statements is <u>definitely</u> true?

A. A runner from Australia was never behind the corresponding numbered runner from USA.
B. The third runners from Russia and Kenya never met during the course of the event.
C. The second runner from Kenya and Russia definitely met once during the event.
D. A runner from Kenya was always behind the corresponding numbered runner from Russia.

32. Taking all four countries into account, which runners were the slowest on average?

A. First Runners B. Second Runners C. Third Runners D. Fourth Runners

SET 8

The table below shows data for export and import for Simuland, a hypothetical country.

Year	Exports (Million USD)	Imports (Million USD)
1996	100	90
1997	120	130
1998	130	110
1999	140	180
2000	190	220
2001	160	150

Trade Surplus = Exports – Imports

Trade Deficit = Imports – Exports

33. During the year 1999, the average cost of exports was USD 7000 per tonne and that of imports was USD 6000 per tonne. By what percentage is the total weight of exports less than the total weight of imports in 1999?

A. 30.33%
B. 31.33%
C. 32.33%
D. 33.33%

34. The percentage decrease in trade surplus from 2001 to 2002 is the same as during the period 1998 to 2001 overall. Given that imports in 2002 increased by 20%, what is the value of exports in 2002 in Million USD?

A. 175
B. 180
C. 185
D. 190

35. If imports grow at a rate of 10% per year from 2001 onwards, what is the approximate total import value in 2004?

A. 100 Million USD
B. 150 Million USD
C. 200 Million USD
D. 250 Million USD

36. What is the approximate compound annual growth rate (CAGR) for exports during 1996 to 2001?

A. 5%
B. 10%
C. 15%
D. 60%

END OF SECTION

Section D: Abstract Reasoning

For each question, decide whether each test shape fits best with Set A, Set B or with neither.

For each question, work through the test shapes from left to right as you see them on the page. Make your decision and fill it into the answer sheet.

Answer as follows:
A = Set A
B = Set B
C = **N**either

Set 1:

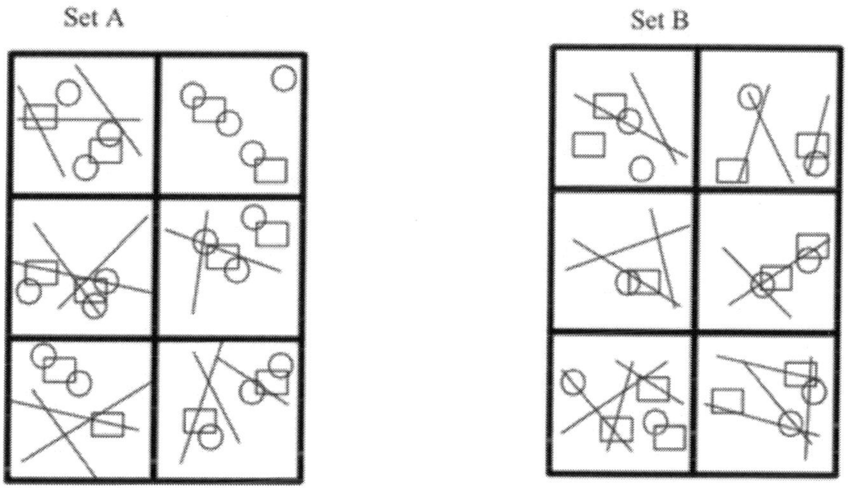

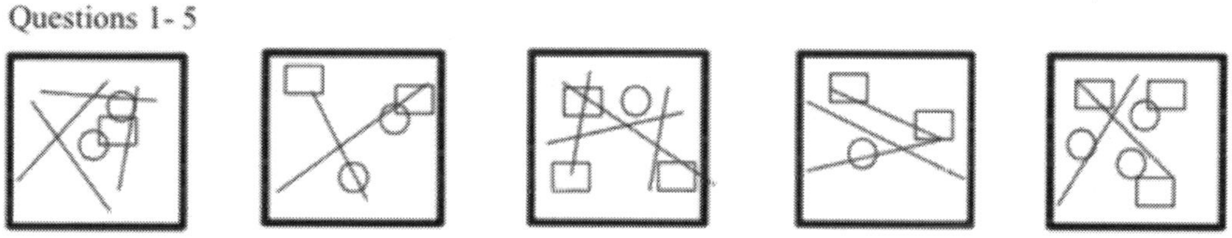

Set 2:

Set A

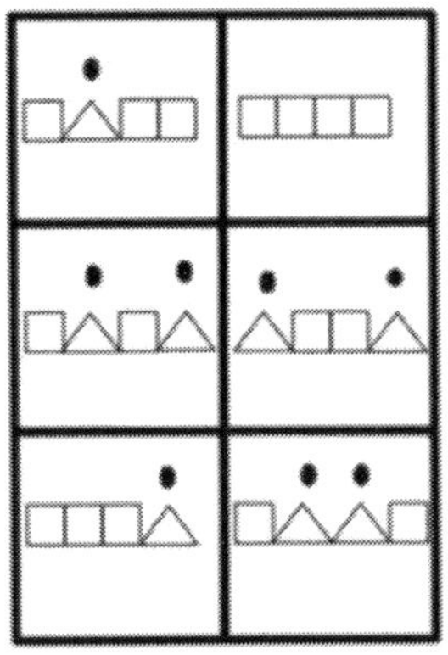

Set B

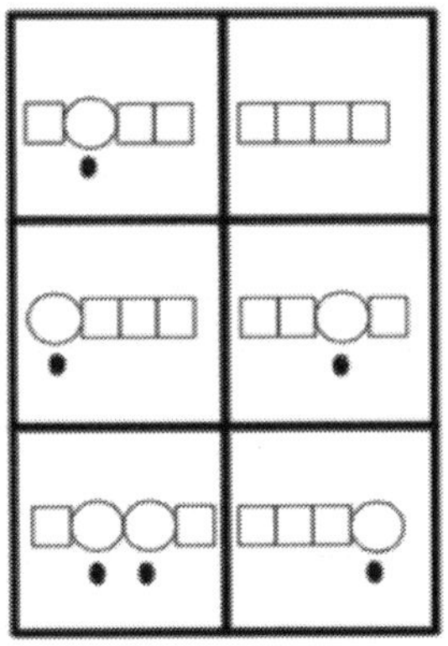

Questions 6 - 10

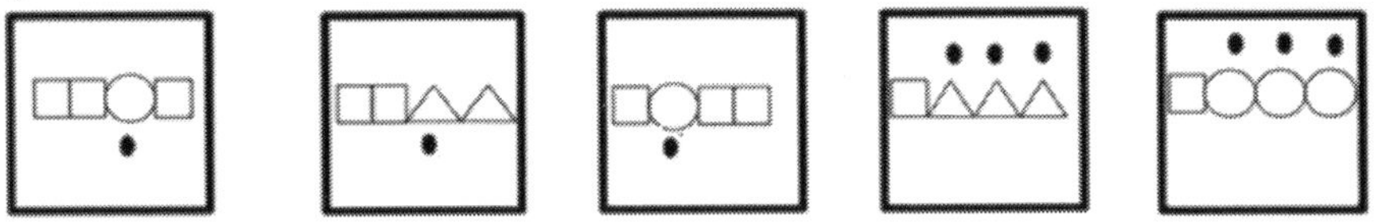

Set 3:

Set A

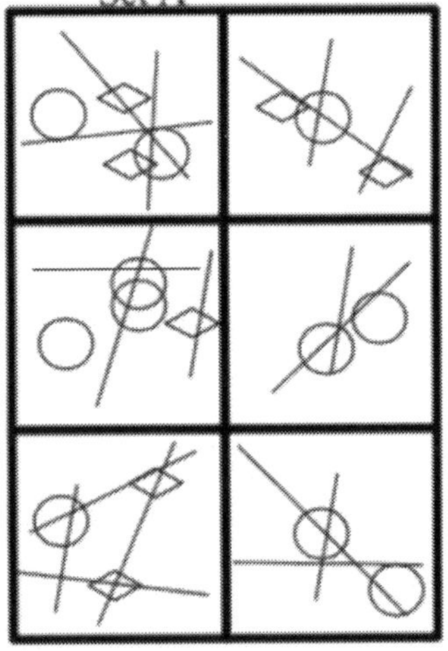

Set B

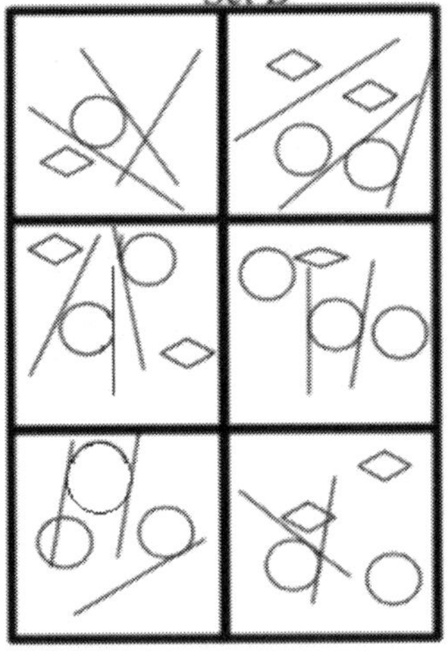

Questions 11 - 15

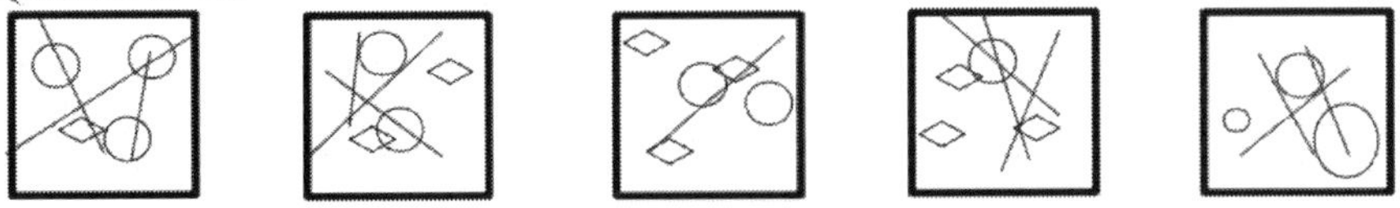

Set 4

Set A

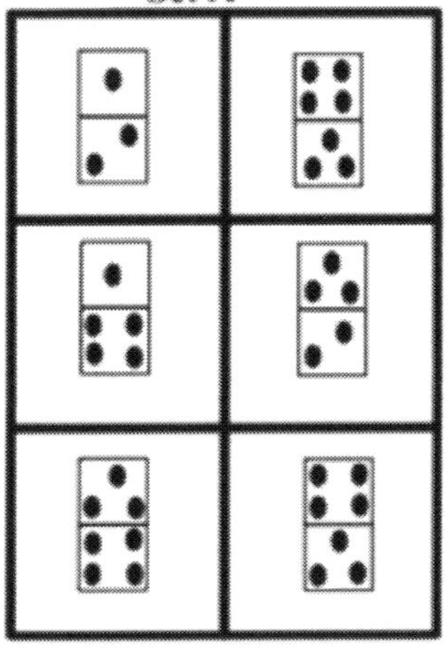

Set B

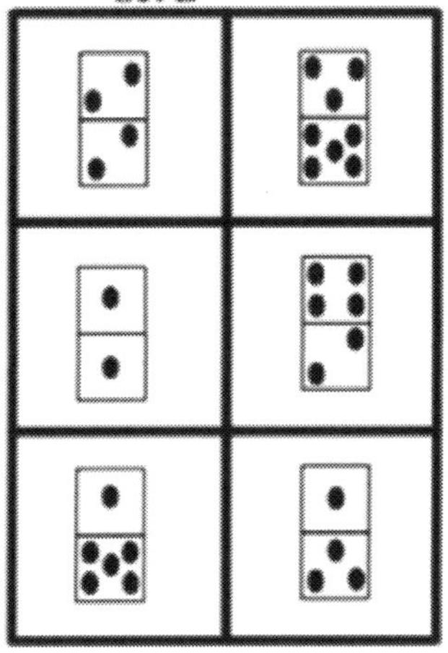

Questions 16 - 20

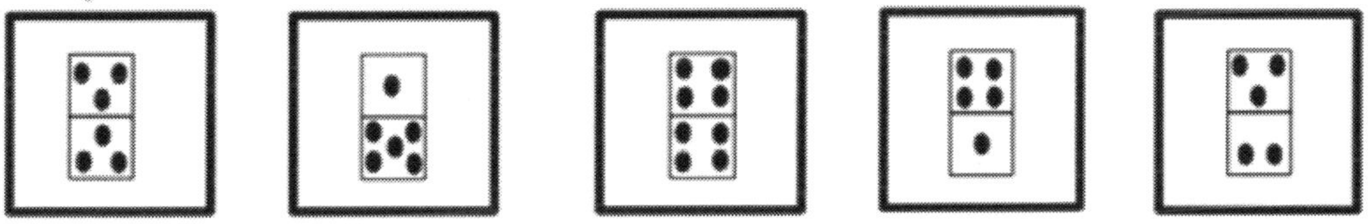

Set 5

Set A

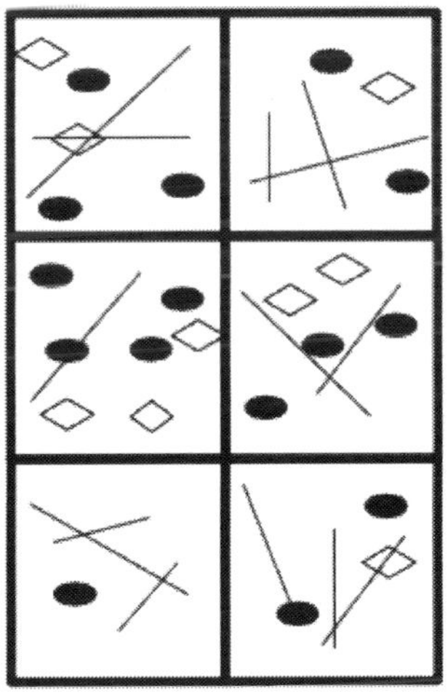

Set B

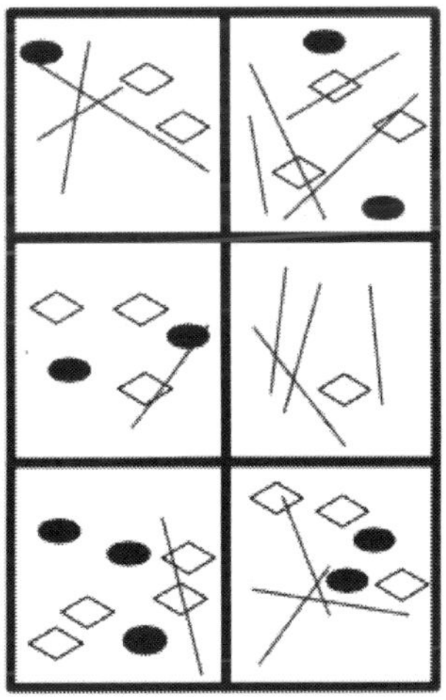

Questions 21 - 25

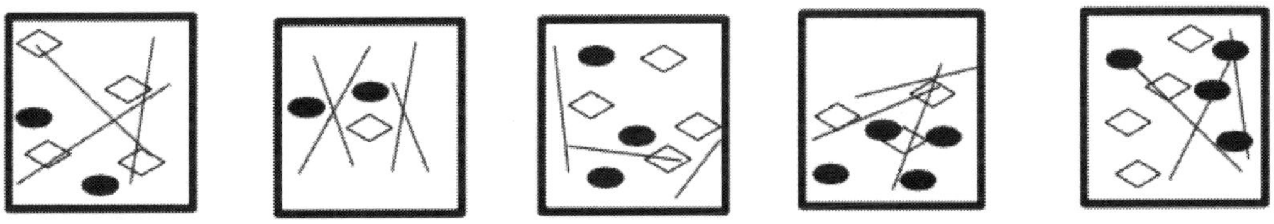

Set 6

Set A

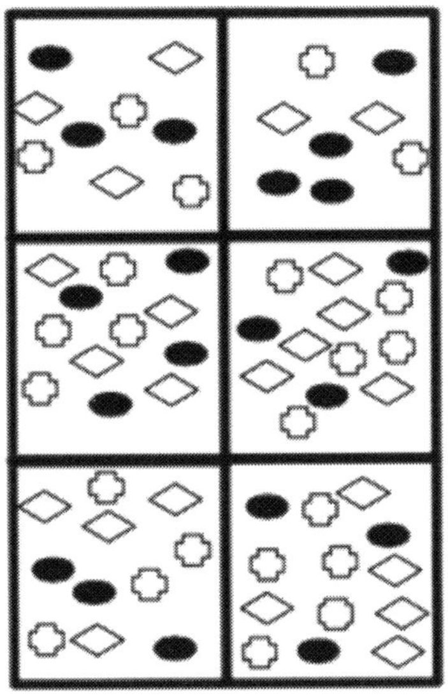

Set B

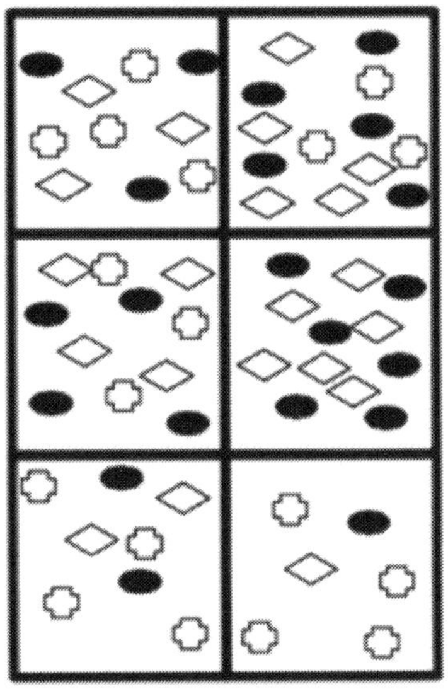

Questions 26 - 30

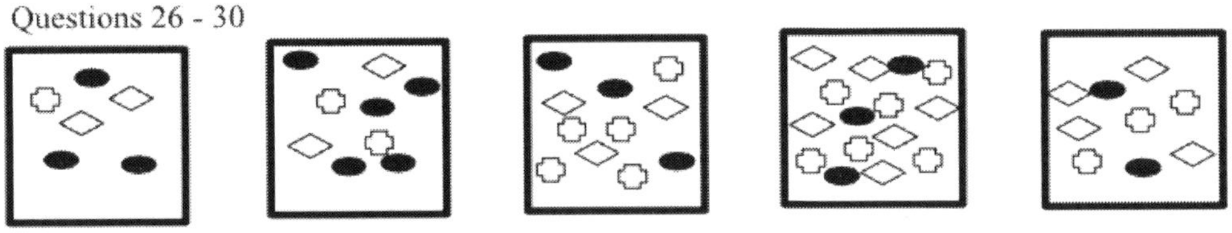

Set 7

Set A

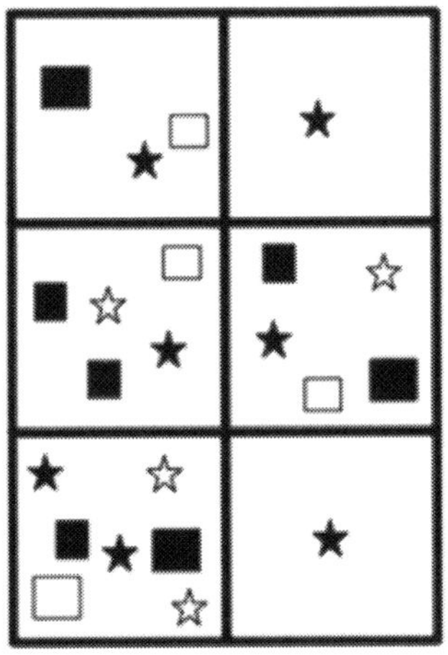

Set B

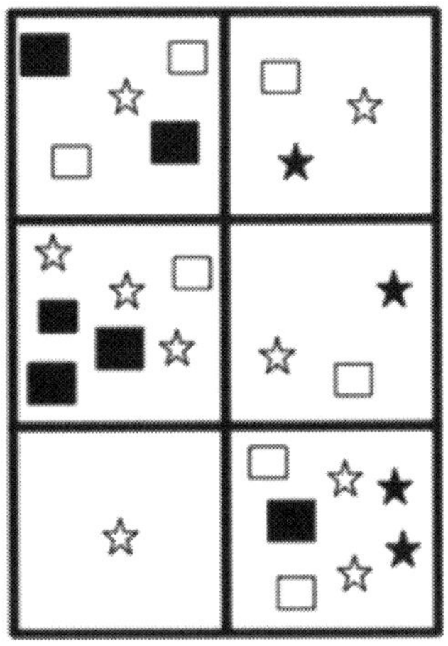

Questions 31 - 35

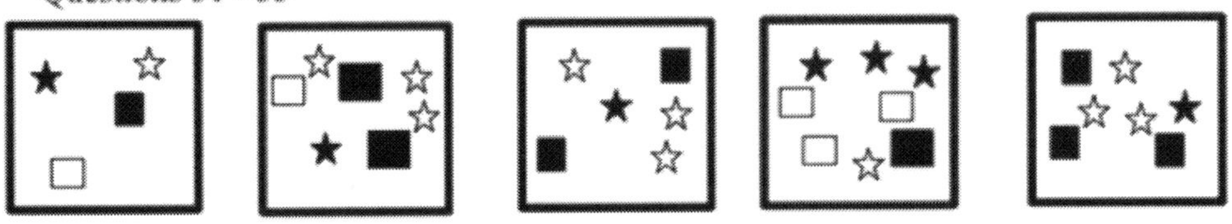

Set 8

Set A

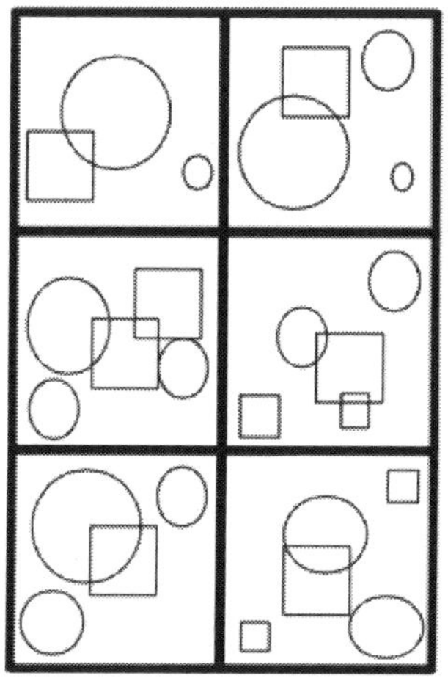

Set B

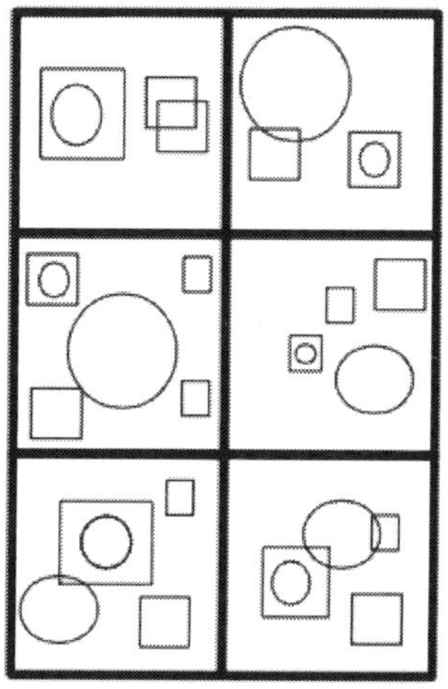

Questions 36 – 40

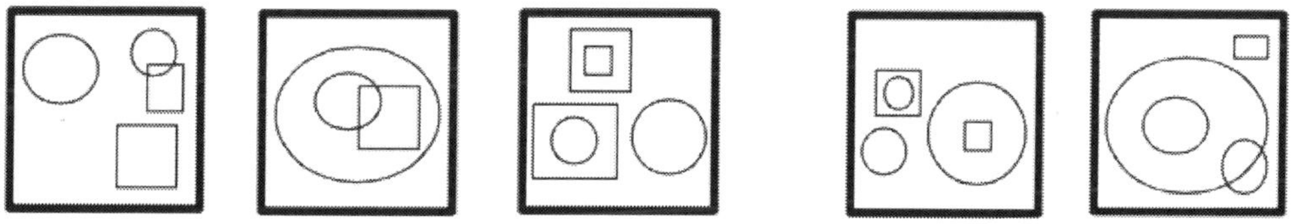

Set 9

Which answer completes the series?

Question 41:

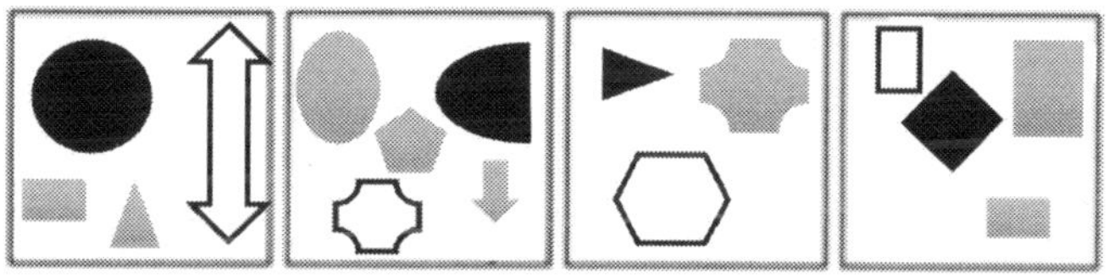

A)

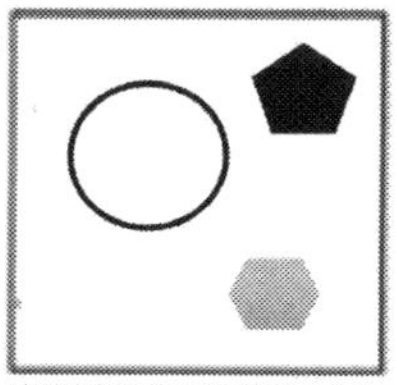

B)

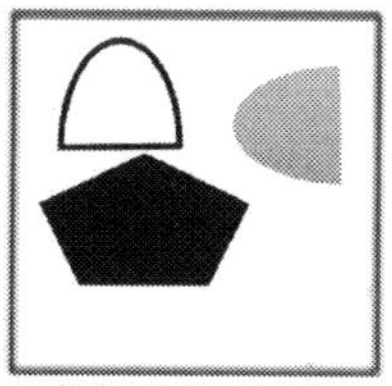

C)

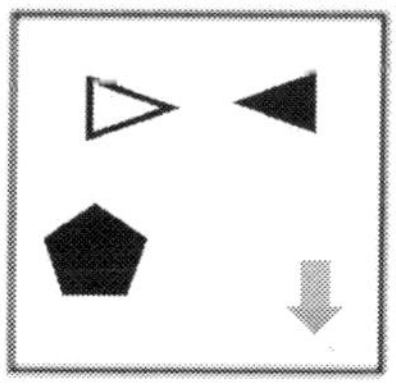

D)

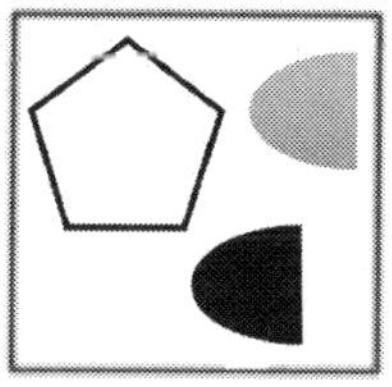

Question 42:

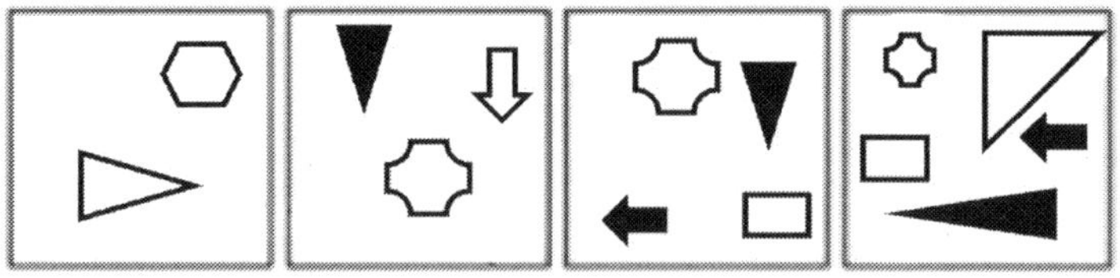

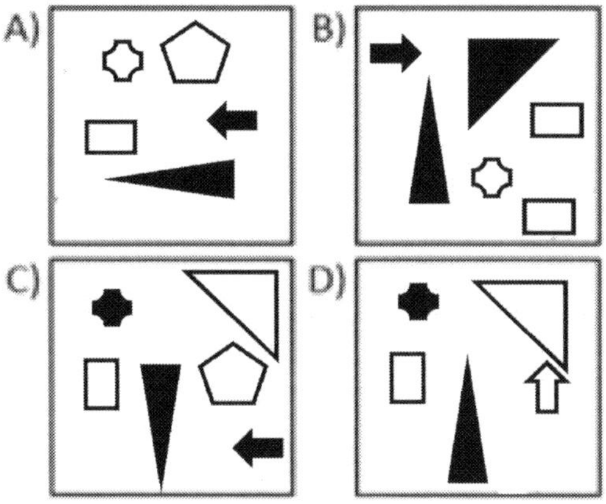

Question 43:

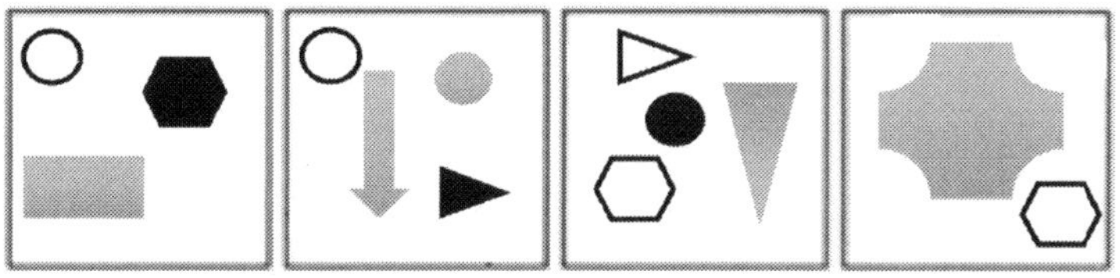

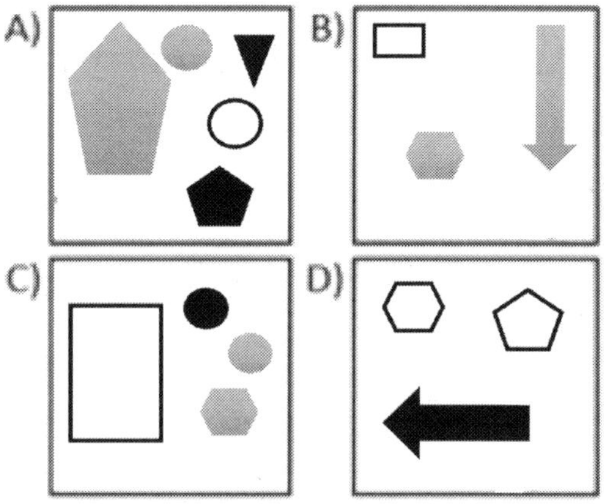

Question 44:

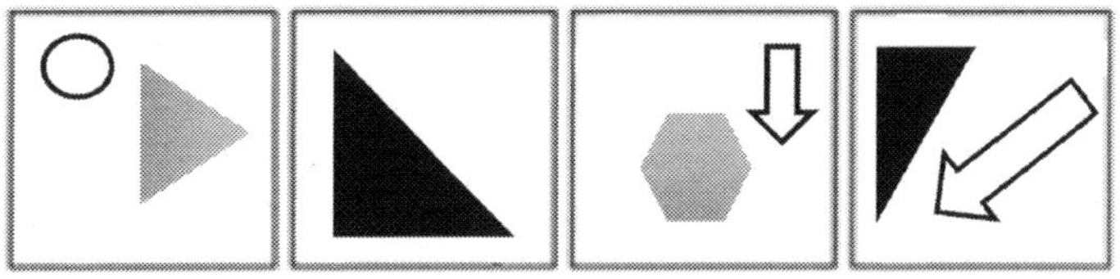

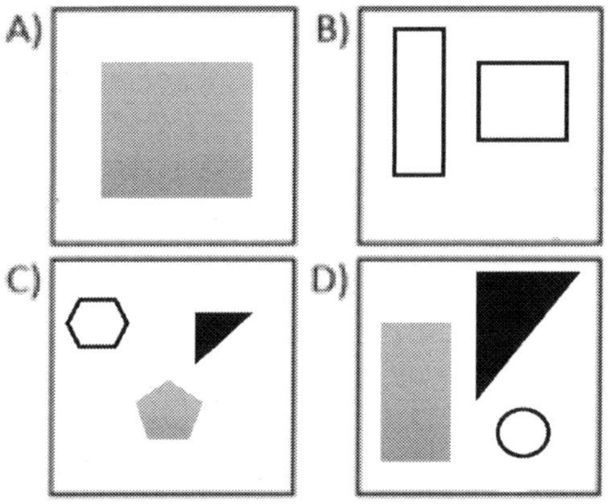

Question 45:

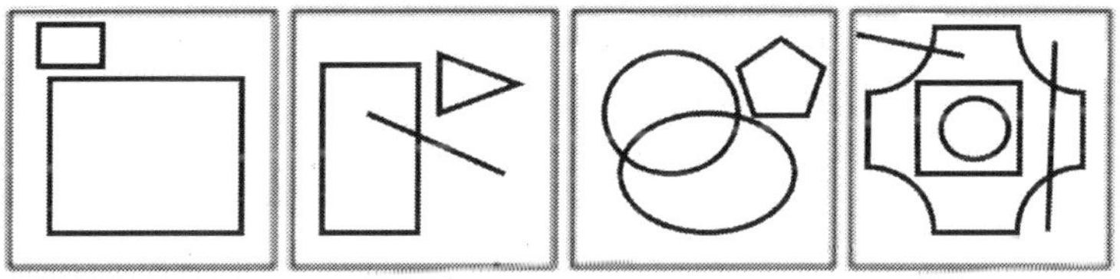

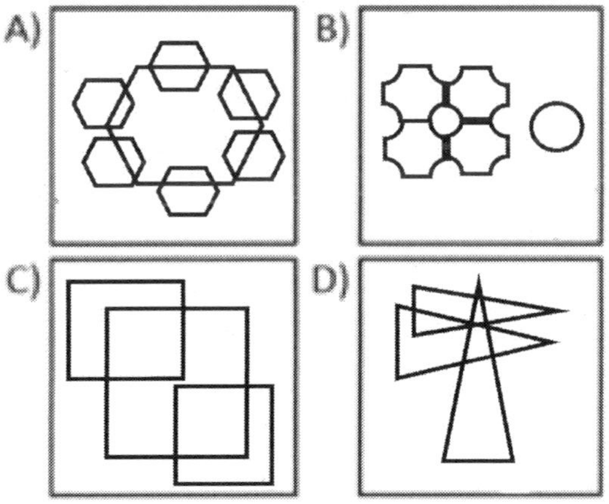

Set 10

Which answer completes the statement?

Question 46:

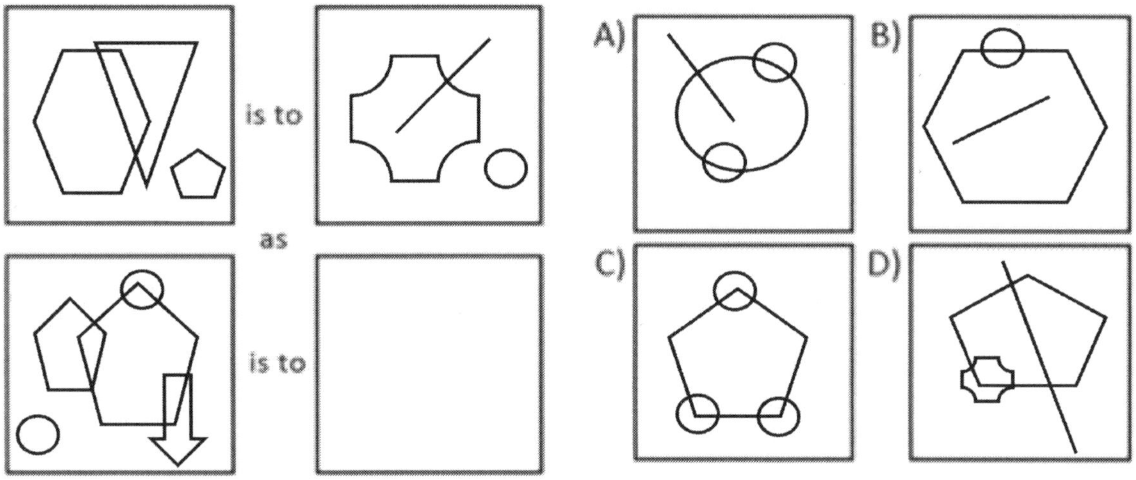

Question 47:

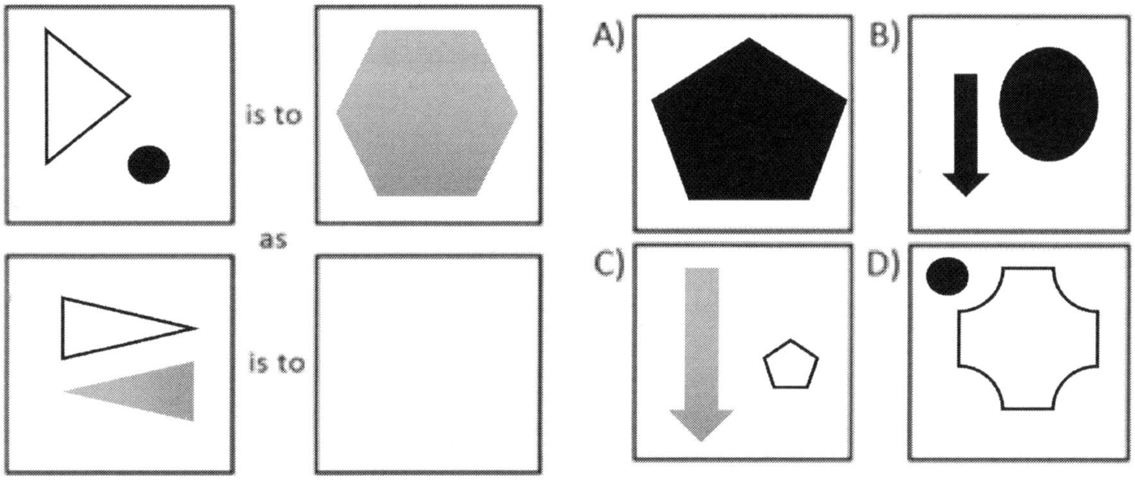

Question 48:

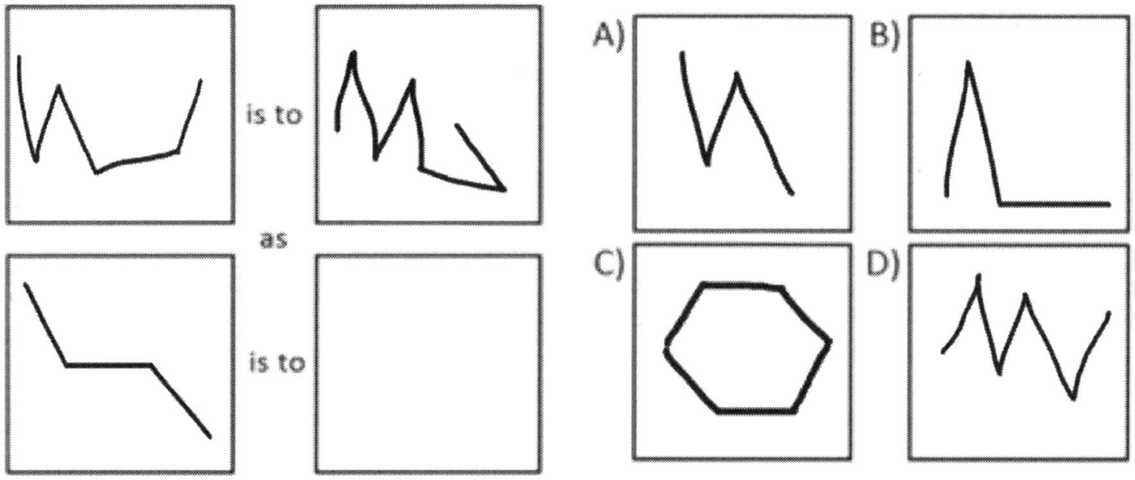

Question 49:

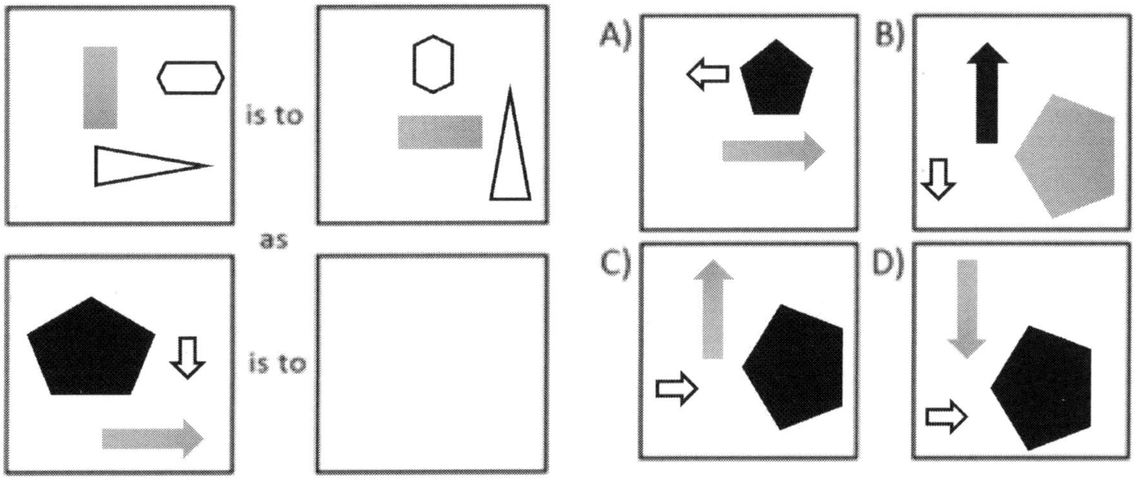

Question 50:

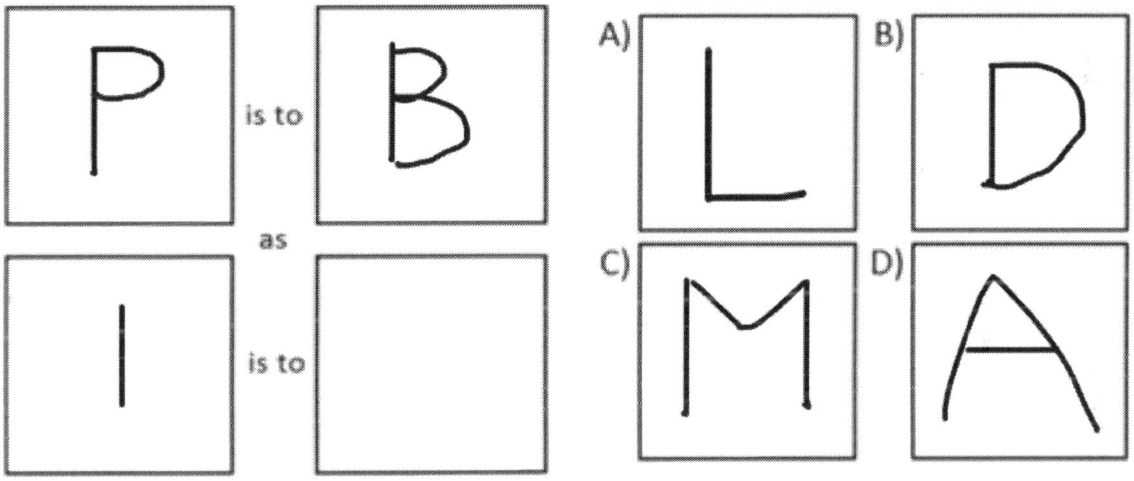

Set 11

Which of the four response options belongs to either set A or set B?

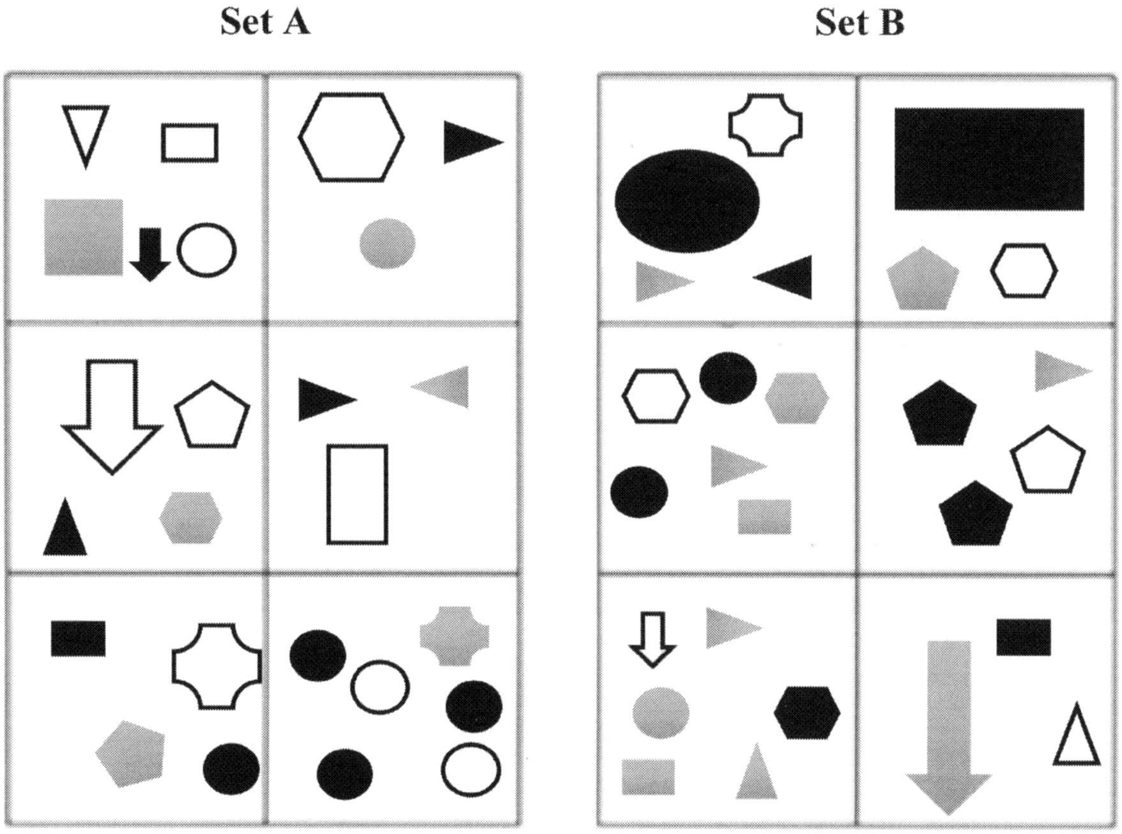

Question 51:

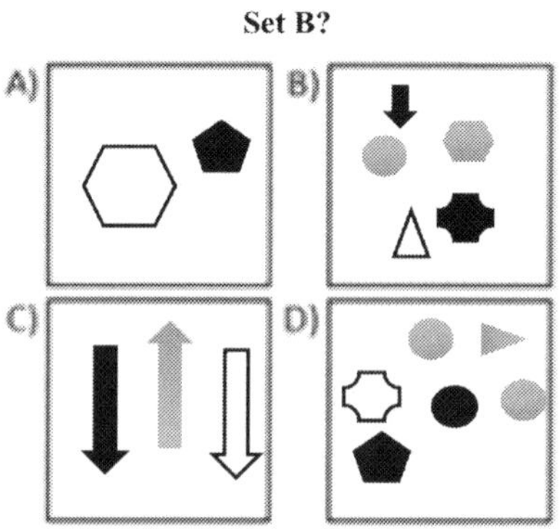

Question 52:

Set A?

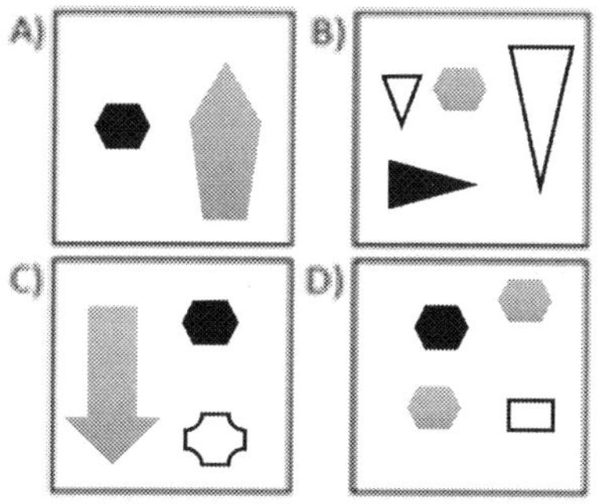

Question 53:

Set A?

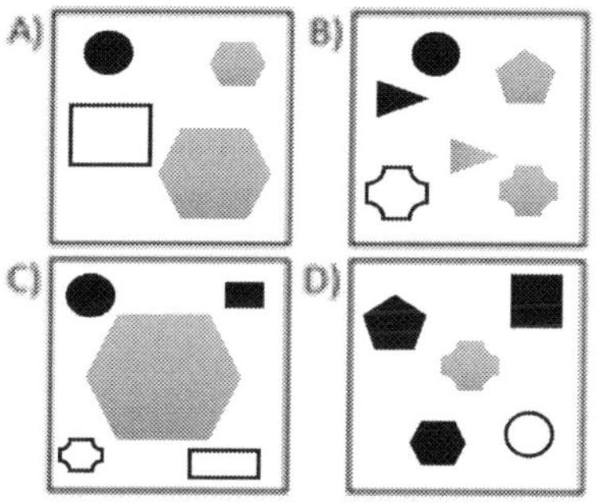

Question 54:

Set B?

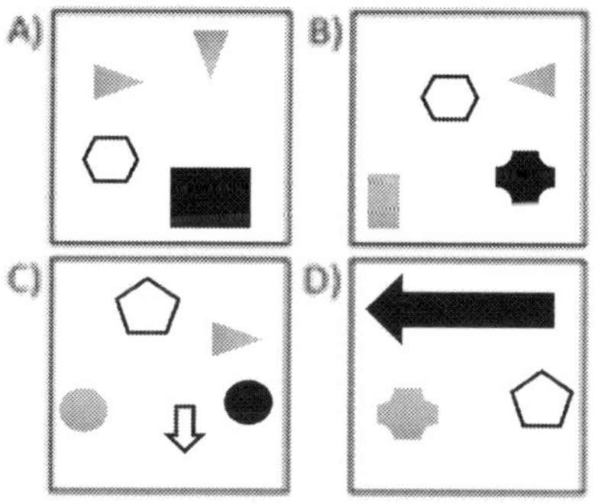

Question 55:

Set B?

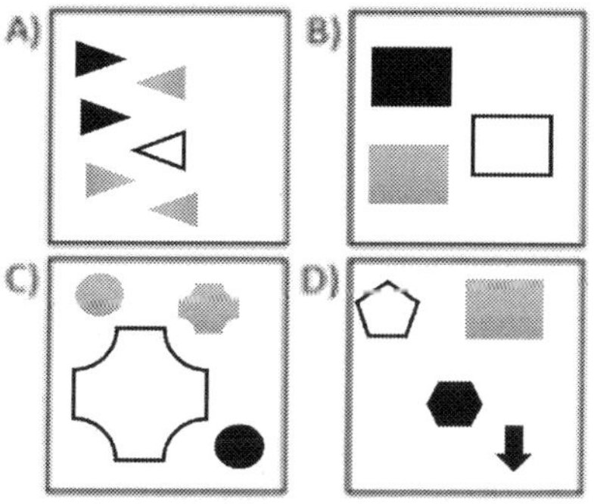

END OF SECTION

Section E: Situational Judgement Test

Read each scenario. Each question refers to the scenario directly above. For each question, select one of these four options. Select whichever you feel is the option that best represents your view on each suggested action.

For questions 1 – 40, choose one of the following options:

A Very appropriate
B Appropriate, but not ideal
C Inappropriate, but not awful
D Very inappropriate

Scenario 1
Arthur is a final year medical student on his GP placement. Having just observed the doctor take a history from a new patient, the doctor quickly steps outside to discuss something with a colleague. In her absence, the patient reveals to Arthur that he has been having suicidal thoughts. These feelings had not been shared with the doctor. The patient pleads with Arthur to not share this information.

How appropriate are the following responses to Arthur's dilemma?

1. Encourage the patient to share his feelings with the doctor on her return.
2. When the doctor returns, Arthur should reveal what the patient shared whilst the patient is still present – ignoring the patient's request.
3. After the patient has left, take the doctor aside and tell her his concerns over the patient. It is worth breaking confidentiality to potentially save a life.
4. Say nothing.
5. Don't explicitly inform the doctor, but hint to her that there might be more than meets the eye with this patient.

Scenario 2
Nico is studying for his first year medical exams. He is feeling very unprepared and starting to panic about how much he last left to do. The prospect of failing is very embarrassing to him, and he would rather tell his friends and family that he is too ill to take the exams, rather than face the truth. It is the rules of the medical school that an exam can only not be taken for a valid medical reason with a certified doctor's letter.

How appropriate are the following actions for Nico to take?

6. Speak to his personal tutor about his concerns.
7. Refuse to attend the exam.
8. Make an efficient revision timetable for the few remaining days and do the best he can.
9. Feign an illness and obtain a sick note.
10. Bury his head in the sand and ignore how much he has left to do – what will be will be.

Scenario 3
Alan is a fourth year medical student. On his way home from the hospital one afternoon, he notices Mrs Hamilton, a patient whose case he was previously involved in, on the bus.

How appropriate are the following actions for Alan to take?

11. Politely acknowledge Mrs Hamilton and ask her how she is.
12. Pretend not to see her and look the other way.
13. Discuss her medical history openly on the bus.
14. Get off the bus early without acknowledging her, even though she has clearly spotted him.
15. Not go out of his way to talk to her.

Scenario 4
Sabrina is a final year medical student. On her way home from hospital one evening, she spots two girls from the year below her. She overhears their conversation, and realises they are openly discussing a patient in detail, including mentioning the patient's name.

How appropriate are the following responses to Sabrina's situation?

16. Ignore the girls and hope no one else recognises the patient's name.
17. Report the girls for breaking patient confidentiality.
18. Inform the girls that they should not be talking about patients publically.
19. Advise the girls to speak more quietly.
20. Pretend she does not recognise the girls.

Scenario 5
Maxine is a second year medical student visiting the hospital for the first time since she started at medical school. The doctor supervising her and her group had previously emailed saying they should prepare for a small assessment. Unfortunately, Maxine is the only one who did not receive the email and is therefore unprepared.

How appropriate are the following responses to Maxine's dilemma?

21. Ask the doctor not to hold the test as she was not informed.
22. Tell the doctor that she did not receive the email.
23. Decide not to turn up to the session.
24. Quickly ask the other students what they have learnt and attempt to understand it before the assessment.
25. Copy one of the other students' work.

Scenario 6
Marcus is a third year medical student attending a clinic with his consultant. He observes the consultant inform a patient that their condition is terminal. However, he does not believe that the patient has fully understood this as he thinks the consultant gave the patient false hope.

How appropriate are the following responses to Marcus' situation?

26. Follow the patient and bluntly inform them of their prognosis.
27. Tell the consultant he believes he gave the patient false hope.
28. Ask the consultant why they chose to deliver the information in this way.
29. Say nothing.
30. Inform the patient's family of the reality of the patient's condition.

Scenario 7
Tunde is a third year medical student on a clinical placement. His consultant informed him a week in advance that their group of students would be having a test. However, Tunde completely forgets to inform the other students in his group, and only remembers the night before the test. The results of the test will contribute towards the final placement mark.

How appropriate are the following responses to Tunde's problem?

31. Pretend to the consultant that he had told all of the students and that they are lying.
32. Inform the consultant the night before of his mistake, and ask to reschedule.
33. Inform the other students and apologise profusely.
34. Deny the consultant told him anything about a test.
35. Decide not to come in to avoid the situation.

Scenario 8
Delilah is a third year medical student on a sexual health rotation. Whilst she is taking the history of a young male patient, she feels like he is being rather inappropriate towards her. At the end of the consultation, the patient asks if she would like to go for a drink with him.

How appropriate are the following responses to Delilah's situation?

36. Go for a drink with him, he is a nice young man after all.
37. Thank the patient politely, but inform him that she is unable to do so.
38. Report the patient for inappropriate behaviour.
39. Become very offended by the patient and storm out of the room.
40. Ask another student to take over from her.

For questions 40 – 69, decide how important each statement is when deciding how to respond to the situation?

- **A Very important**
- **B Important**
- **C Of minor importance**
- **D Not important at all**

Scenario 9

Chad is a second year medical student approaching his end-of-year exams. He also plays football for the medical school, and joins the team in the national inter-university tournament. After they bring home the cup, Chad is approached by a scout for a professional football team, and asked if he would like to trial for them.

How important are the following factors for Chad in deciding what he should do?

41. His end-of-year exams may be compromised if he focuses on football rather than studying.
42. He has only been offered a trial; this may not be worth compromising his exams for.
43. He has been offered a trial, which may lead to bigger things.
44. There are still a few weeks remaining before the exams.
45. His parents don't think being a footballer is an appropriate profession.

Scenario 10

Troy is a medical student at a busy GP surgery. The doctor has been delayed and there is a long queue in the waiting room. Troy enters the waiting room to inform the patients that the waiting time will be two hours. One of the patients becomes very aggressive and starts to verbally abuse Troy.

How important are the following factors for Troy in determining what he should do?

46. The patient may be feeling very unwell or might be in pain.
47. The patient may have something important to go to after his appointment.
48. There are many other patients in the waiting room who have not become aggressive.
49. The doctor was delayed due to an emergency.
50. Troy needs to look professional to patients.
51. Troy is just a student, there are plenty of other staff around.
52. The patient has dementia.

Scenario 11

Leroy and Byrony are fourth year medical students who are in a relationship. Byrony has recently won an award for a poster she submitted, and has been asked to present it at a conference. One evening, Byrony tells Leroy in confidence that some of the work on the poster is not her own, and was copied from elsewhere.

How important are the following factors in determining what Leroy should do?

53. Leroy and Byrony are in a relationship.
54. Byrony only told Leroy her secret because she thought he would keep it to himself.
55. Byrony has plagiarised and could get into serious trouble.
56. The award Byrony has won is very prestigious.
57. If Byrony is caught presenting plagiarised work at the conference, the reputation of the medical school could be damaged.

Scenario 12

Benson is a first year medical student. He has become concerned about how many books he will need to help him in his studies, as he does not think he will be able to afford them. He thinks he may need to extend his overdraft in order to pay for these books, or else get a part-time job.

How important are the following factors in determining what Benson should do?

58. These books will greatly help Benson in his studies.
59. The library is likely to have many of the books he needs.
60. An overdraft can be difficult to pay back.
61. A part-time job may compromise his studies.
62. His parents may be able to contribute towards these books.
63. If he spends all of his money on books, he will not have any left for a sports tour later in the year.

Scenario 13

Albert-Clifford, a medical student, has been keen to do a particular project for a long time. He has even spoken to the project supervisor and begun to outline it. However, he knows that this project is a very popular one and lots of other people want to do it too. Despite putting it down as his first choice, Albert-Clifford is randomly allocated to a different project instead. Bitterly disappointed, he discovers that his friend, Anna-Theresa, has been allocated his chosen project, despite putting it down as her last choice. Albert-Clifford would like to make an official appeal.

How important are the following factors for Albert-Clifford in deciding whether or not to appeal?

64. Anna-Theresa did not put the project down as her first choice.

65. Albert-Clifford was not allocated his first choice of project.

66. Many other people wanted to do this project too.

67. Albert-Clifford already started planning the project.

68. Albert-Clifford has no interest in the project he has been allocated.

69. Albert-Clifford has spoken to the project supervisor.

END OF PAPER

Mock Paper C

Section A: Verbal Reasoning

Passage 1

Modern Considerations in Pigeon Pest Control
For much of the 20th century, controlling intra-city pigeon populations primarily meant killing them. To this day culling remains a common fallback position (the United States Department of Agriculture kills 60,000 pigeons a year in response to complaints). However the trade journal "Pest Control" cautions local authorities that with "millions of bird lovers out there," one must consider "the publicity you would receive if your local paper runs photos of hundreds of poisoned pigeons flopping around on Main Street." In an apparent paradoxical situation whilst we have become less tolerant of the birds, we have also, somehow, grown more concerned for their welfare.

Studies have allowed for the calculation of estimates that a single pigeon dispenses over 11 kilograms of excrement each year. Often this muck must be blasted off hard-to-reach places by climbing teams using steam hoses. Pigeon-related damage in America alone has been estimated to cost $1.1 billion a year. But the full scope of our disdain and prejudice for the birds is impossible to quantify. Marketing circulated by the bird-control industry (a profitable offshoot of the $6.7-billion-a-year pest-control business) describes how pigeons and their faeces can spread more than 60 diseases communicable between humans. However one must consider that whilst this is true, it is not necessarily panic-inducing given the vanishingly small incidences of respiratory infections like cryptococcosis.

1. The bird-control industry profits around $6.7 billion a year by controlling the pigeon population.

A. True

B. False

C. Can't tell

2. Millions of bird lovers out there:

A. Are responsible for an increasing risk of cryptococcosis

B. Must feel partly to blame for the $1.1 billion of pigeon related damage every year in America

C. Outnumber those who are intolerant of pigeons

D. Have made it difficult to use traditional pigeon-control methods

3. The necessity of pigeon control is to reduce the number disease vectors.

A. True

B. False

C. Can't tell

4. In light of our growing concern for pigeon well-being there has seen a significant move away from traditional killing practices.

A. True

B. False

C. Can't tell

Passage 2

Little Wars *H G Wells*

"LITTLE WARS" is the game of kings—for players in an inferior social position. It can be played by boys of every age from twelve to one hundred and fifty—and even later if the limbs remain sufficiently supple—by girls of the better sort, and by a few rare and gifted women. This is to be a full History of Little Wars from its recorded and authenticated beginning until the present time, an account of how to make little warfare, and hints of the most priceless sort for the recumbent strategist....

The beginning of the game of Little War, as we know it, became possible with the invention of the spring breechloader gun. This priceless gift to boyhood appeared some when towards the end of the last century, a gun capable of hitting a toy soldier nine times out of ten at a distance of nine yards. It has completely superseded all the spiral-spring and other makes of gun hitherto used in playroom warfare. These spring breechloaders are made in various sizes and patterns, but the one used in our game is that known in England as the four-point-seven gun. It fires a wooden cylinder about an inch long, and has a screw adjustment for elevation and depression. It is an altogether elegant weapon and it was with one of these guns that the beginning of our war game was made. It was at Sandgate—in England.

5. The author created the game of little wars.

A. True B. False C. Can't tell

6. The spring breechloader gun has a 90% toy soldier hit rate at 10 yards.

A. True B. False C. Can't tell

7. The four-point-seven gun used by the author adopts the use of a spiral spring mechanism.

A. True B. False C. Can't tell

8. The game of little wars:

A. Was invented at Sandgate
B. Requires a spiral spring breechloader
C. Uses wooden ammunition
D. Is an expensive hobby

Passage 3

A New German Shipping Canal

The gates which admit the water into the new canal which is to connect the Baltic with the North Sea have been recently opened by the Emperor William. This canal is being constructed by the German government principally for the purpose of strengthening the naval resources of Germany, by giving safer and more direct communication for the ships of the navy to the North German ports. The depth of water will be sufficient for the largest ships of the German navy. The canal will also prove of very great advantage to the numerous timber and other vessels trading between St. Petersburg, Stockholm, Dantzic, Riga, and all the North German ports in the Baltic and this country. The passage by the Kattegat and Skager Rack is exceedingly intricate and very dangerous, the yearly loss of shipping being estimated at half a million of money. In addition to the avoidance of this dangerous course, the saving in distance will be very considerable. Thus, for vessels trading to the Thames the saving will be 250 miles, for those going to Lynn or Boston 220, to Hull 200, to Newcastle or Leith 100. This means a saving of three days for a sailing vessel going to Boston docks, the port lying in the most direct line from the timber ports of the Baltic to all the centre of England. Considering that between 30,000 and 40,000 ships now pass through the Sound annually, the advantage to the Baltic trade is very apparent.

9. The new German shipping canal was constructed to reduce the distance trading ships had to travel when making port.

A. True B. False C. Can't tell

10. It could be hoped that the new German shipping canal will save £500,000 by reducing the chance of ships running aground in Kattegat and Skager Rack.

A. True B. False C. Can't tell

11. The main aim of this article is demonstrating that the opening of the new German shipping canal is an example of

A. How military developments often benefit many aspects of society
B. A human engineering solution to reduce the costs of transport
C. A human engineering solution to reduce the loss of life at sea
D. Germany's booming trade across the Baltic Sea

12. The opening of the German shipping canal has benefited the shipping trade more than the navy.

A. True B. False C. Can't tell

Passage 4

Darwin's Geological Observations of South America

Of the remarkable "trilogy" constituted by Darwin's writings which deal with the adventures of the "Beagle," the member which has perhaps attracted least attention up to the present time is that which describes of the geology of South America. The actual writing of this book appears to have occupied Darwin a shorter period than either of the other volumes of the series; his diary records that the work was accomplished within ten months, namely, between July 1844 and April 1845; but the book was not actually issued till late in the year following, the preface bearing the date "September 1846." Altogether, as Darwin informs us in his "Autobiography," the geological books "consumed four and a half years' steady work," most of the remainder of the ten years that elapsed between the return of the "Beagle," and the completion of his geological books being, it is sad to relate, "lost through illness!"

Concerning the "Geological Observations on South America," Darwin wrote to his friend Lyell, as follows: "My volume will be about 240 pages, dreadfully dull, yet much condensed. I think whenever you have time to look through it, you will think the collection of facts on the elevation of the land and on the formation of terraces pretty good."

13. The author is discussing one of Darwin's books out of a trilogy that he wrote on the geology of South America

A. True B. False C. Can't tell

14. The author believes Darwin's work is boring.

A. True B. False C. Can't tell

15. Darwin was delayed 12 months in publishing his Geological Observations on South America due to ill health.

A. True B. False C. Can't tell

16. Darwin's first draft of his Geological Observations of South America was greater than 200 pages.

A. True B. False C. Can't tell

Passage 5

Cattle

The wealth-producing possibilities of cattle-raising are written into the history, literature and art of every race; and with every nationality riches have always been counted in cattle and corn. We find cattle mentioned in the earliest known records of the Hebrews, Chaldeans and Hindus, and carved on the monuments of Egypt, thousands of years before the Christian era.

Among the primitive peoples wealth was, and still is, measured by the size of the cattle herds, whether it be the reindeer of the frigid North, the camel of the Great Sahara, or herds of whatsoever kind that are found in every land and in every climate. The earliest known money, in Ancient Greece, was the image of the ox stamped on metal; and the Latin word *pecunia* and our own English "pecuniary" are derived from *pecus*—cattle.

Although known to the Eastern Hemisphere since the dawn of history, cattle are not native to the Western Hemisphere, but were introduced into America during the sixteenth century. Cortez, Ponce de Leon, De Soto and the other *conquistadores* from Old Madrid, who sailed the seas in quest of gold, brought with them to the New World the monarchs of the bull ring, and introduced the national sport of Spain into the colonies founded in Peru, Mexico, Florida and Louisiana.

17. The rearing of cattle had a major influence on the development of economy in the Eastern Hemisphere.

A. True B. False C. Can't tell

18. The Spanish are the reason that cattle exist in America.

A. True B. False C. Can't tell

19. The main conclusion to draw from the second paragraph is that

A. Cattle are valuable

B. Cattle does not necessarily refer to cows

C. Cattle are a historical symbol of attaching wealth to goods

D. Cattle are an integral part of modern economy

20. The Conquistadores landed in Peru, Mexico, Florida and Louisiana.

A. True B. False C. Can't tell

Passage 6

Succession of Forest Growths

It is the prevailing and almost universal belief that when native forests are destroyed they will be replaced by other kinds, for the simple reason that the soil has been impoverished of the constituents required for the growth of that particular tree or trees. This I believe to be one of the fallacies handed down from past ages, taken for granted, and never questioned. Nowhere does the English oak grow better than where it grew when William the Conqueror found it at the time he invaded Britain. Where do you find white pines growing better than in parts of New England where this tree has grown from time immemorial?

The question why the original growth is not reproduced can best be answered by some illustrations. When a pine forest is burned over, both trees and seeds are destroyed, and as the burned trees cannot sprout from the stump like oaks and many other trees, the land is left in a condition well suited for the germination of tree seeds, but there are no seeds to germinate. It is an open field for pioneers to enter, and the seeds which arrive there first have the right of possession.

21. The author agrees with the prevailing belief of forest growth succession and the influence of impoverished soil.

A. True
B. False
C. Can't tell

22. White pine grows best in New England.

A. True
B. False
C. Can't tell

23. In conclusion

A. Soil nutrient depletion is not an issue for forest growth unless the population is entirely destroyed
B. The most pioneering species of trees succeed in colonising the remains of forest fires
C. When native forests are destroyed they are replaced by a different species of tree
D. The English oak grows best in England

24. The author believes that the species of seed which arrives first holds possession of the land.

A. True
B. False
C. Can't tell

Passage 7

The Neutral Use of Cables

Eleven submarine cables traverse the Atlantic between 60 and 40 degrees north latitude. Nine of these connect the Canadian provinces and the United States with the territory of Great Britain; two (one American, the other Anglo-American) connect France. Of these, seven are largely owned, operated or controlled by American capital, while all the others are under English control and management. There is but one direct submarine cable connecting the territory of the United States with the continent of Europe, and that is the cable owned and operated by the Compagnie Francais Cables Telegraphiques, whose termini are Brest, France, and Cape Cod, on the coast of Massachusetts.

All these cables between 60 and 40 degrees north latitude, which unite the United States with Europe, except the French cable, are under American or English control, and have their termini in the territory of Great Britain or the United States. In the event of war between these countries, unless restrained by conventional act, all these cables might be cut or subjected to exclusive censorship on the part of each of the belligerent states.

25. In the event of War, America would take control of all submarine cables.
A. True B. False C. Can't tell

26. America owns all nine of the submarine cables connecting the United States with Great Britain.
A. True B. False C. Can't tell

27. The neutral use of cables
A. Adopts the use of 11 underwater telecommunication cables crossing the Pacific
B. Occurs less than 60 degrees north
C. Presents a significant benefit to belligerent states during times of war
D. Is integral in maintaining peace between Great Britain, America and France.

28. France receives least use of the submarine cables
A. True B. False C. Can't tell

Passage 8

Tombs of the First Egyptian Dynasty

For many years various European collections of Egyptian antiquities have contained a certain series of objects which gave archæologists great difficulty. There were vases of a peculiar form and colour, greenish plates of slate, many of them in curious animal forms, and other similar things. It was known, positively, that these objects had been found in Egypt, but it was impossible to assign them a place in the known periods of Egyptian art. The puzzle was increased in difficulty by certain plates of slate with hunting and battle scenes and other representations in relief in a style so strange that many investigators considered them products of the art of Western Asia.

The first light was thrown on the question in the winter of 1894-95 by the excavations of Flinders Petrie in Ballas and Neggadeh, two places on the west bank of the Nile, a little below ancient Thebes. This persevering English investigator discovered here a very large necropolis in which he examined about three thousand graves. They all contained the same kinds of pottery and the same slate tablets mentioned above, and many other objects which did not seem to be Egyptian. It was plain that the newly found necropolis and the puzzling objects already in the museums belonged to the same period. Petrie assumed that they represented the art of a foreign people—perhaps the Libyans—who had temporarily resided in Egypt in the time between the old and the middle kingdoms.

29. The peculiar vases referred to in the text originated from Western Asia.
A. True B. False C. Can't tell

30. Flinders Petrie undertook is excavation of Ballas and Neggadeh in December 1895.
A. True B. False C. Can't tell

31. For a period after the middle kingdoms Libyans may have resided in Egypt.
A. True B. False C. Can't tell

32. Flinders Petrie examined 3,000 bodies during his excavation along the west bank of the Nile
A. True B. False C. Can't tell

Passage 9

How to Raise Turkeys

The best feed for young turkeys and ducks is the yolks of hard-boiled eggs, and after they are several days old the white may be added. Continue this for two or three weeks, occasionally chopping onions fine and sometimes sprinkling the boiled eggs with black pepper; then give rice, a teacupful with enough milk to just cover it, and boil slowly until the milk is evaporated. Put in enough more to cover the rice again, so that when boiled down the second time it will be soft if pressed between the fingers. Milk must not be used too freely, as it will get too soft and the grains will adhere together. Stir frequently when boiling. Do not use water with the rice, as it forms a paste and the chicks cannot swallow it. In cold, damp weather, a half teaspoonful of Cayenne pepper in a pint of flour, with lard enough to make it stick together, will protect them from diarrhea. This amount of food is sufficient for two meals for seventy-five chicks. Give all food in shallow tin pans. Water and boiled milk, with a little lime water in each occasionally, is the best drink until the chicks are two or three months old. When loppered, buttermilk may take the place of the boiled milk. Turkeys like best to roost on trees, and in their place artificial roots may be made by planting long forked locust poles and laying others across the forks.

33. Turkeys are best raised on a vegetarian diet.

A. True B. False C. Can't tell

34. In conclusion turkeys

A. Are best reared on the ground with dairy and grains
B. Should eat a varied diet dependent upon the time of year
C. Are difficult to raise
D. Require separate items of food and drink to sustain them despite the water and milk in the food paste

35. A mixture of rice and water will cause turkey chicks to choke.

A. True B. False C. Can't tell

36. For the first month of their life turkey chicks should primarily eat whole eggs.

A. True B. False C. Can't tell

Passage 10

Pneumatic Malting

According to K. Lintner, the worst features of the present system of malting are the inequalities of water and temperature in the heaps and the irregular supplies of oxygen to, and removal of carbonic acid from, the germinating grain. The importance of the last two points is demonstrated by the facts that, when oxygen is cut off, alcoholic fermentation - giving rise to the well-known odour of apples - sets in the cells, and that in an atmosphere with 20 percent of carbonic acid, germination ceases. The open pneumatic system, which consists of drawing in warm air through the heaps spread on a perforated floor, should yield better results. All the processes are thoroughly controlled by the eye and by the thermometer, great cleanliness is possible, and the space requisite is only one-third of that required on the old plan. Since May, 1882, this method has been successfully worked at Puntigam, where plant has been established sufficient for an annual output of 7,000 qrs. of malt. The closed pneumatic system labours under the disadvantages from the form of the apparatus; germination cannot be thoroughly controlled, and cleanliness is very difficult to maintain, while the supply of oxygen is, as a rule, more irregular than with the open floors.

37. The author believes that the present system of malting is flawed due to inefficient removal of carbonic acid from the germinating grain.

A. True B. False C. Can't tell

38. The open pneumatic system is more hygienic than the closed.

A. True B. False C. Can't tell

39. Germination would not be possible in an atmosphere of 30% carbonic acid.

A. True B. False C. Can't tell

40. Pneumatic malting

A. Is the first step in the process of alcoholic fermentation.
B. Is a general method of malting with several subtypes.
C. Has only been adopted in Puntigam
D. Was invented in 1882.

Passage 11

The Anglesea Bridge in Cork

The river Lee flows through the city of Cork in two branches, which diverge just above the city, and are reunited at the Custom House. The central portion of the city is situated upon an island between the two arms of the river, both of which are navigable for a short distance above the Custom House, and are lined with quays on each side for the accommodation of the shipping of the port.

The Anglesea bridge crosses the south arm of the river about a quarter of a mile above its junction with the northern branch, and forms the chief line of communication from the northern and central portions of the city to the railway termini and deep-water quays on the southern side of the river.

The new swing bridge occupies the site of an older structure which had been found inadequate to the requirements of the heavy and increasing traffic, and the foundations of the old piers having fallen into an insecure condition, the construction of a new opening bridge was taken in hand jointly by the Corporation and Harbour Commissioners of Cork.

The new bridge, which has recently been completed, is of a somewhat novel design, and the arrangement of the swing-span in particular presents some original and interesting features, which appear to have been dictated by a careful consideration of the existing local conditions and requirements.

41. The river Lee flows north of Cork

A. True
B. False
C. Can't tell

42. Local conditions make it difficult to engineer river structures in Cork

A. True
B. False
C. Can't tell

43. The Anglesea bridge has always been a swing bridge

A. True
B. False
C. Can't tell

44. Cork train station is south of the northern branch of the river Lee

A. True
B. False
C. Can't tell

END OF SECTION

Section B: Decision Making

1. Magazine Zleda provides biased opinions praising President Trump. Thus nobody should read magazine Zleda. What is the assumption in this statement?

A. Readers do not want to read magazines with bias
B. President Trump has done nothing worth praising
C. Magazines should publish balanced opinions
D. Magazine Zleda is not a good magazine

2. A survey by a university Students' union found that 2 students liked beer, wine and spirits, 13 students liked wine, 4 students liked beer and spirits, 4 liked only spirits and nobody liked only beer and wine. How many students liked beer alone from the 25 who took part in the survey?

A. 11 B. 10 C. 8 D. 6

3. "Humans can live off 3 hours of sleep a night". Which statement would allow us to refute this conclusion?

A. Most people sleep between 6-8 hours a day
B. Scientists recommend more than 5 hours of sleep for a functional immune system
C. Sleeping less than 6 hours a night increases mortality
D. The need for sleep increases as animals reach the top of the food chain

4. "Australia was the latest country to approve gay marriage. Next thing we know, Australians will be marrying monkeys and dogs". Which statement would weaken this argument?

A. Gay marriage is not equivalent to marrying animals
B. Australians are not known to be animal lovers
C. Every individual has a right to decide who they love, no matter their gender
D. Animals and gays are not equal

5. In an accident at a coal factory, 18 people were reported injured or dead. The factory claimed that 28% of the casualties had been mishandling ignition that caused the accident. Which statement is correct?

A. The factory was trying to get out of paying compensations to all the casualties
B. There is not enough information to draw any conclusions
C. 5 individuals were the cause of the accident
D. 72% of the individuals did not deserve to die at the coal factory

6. The probability of a professor turning up to their lecture is 0.92. The probability of at least half the cohort of students attending a lecture is 0.8. The probability that more than half of the students turn up to the lecture, but not all is 0.7. What is the probability a professor not turning up to the lecture, and all the students attending it?

A. 0.129
B. 0.011
C. 0.045
D. Not enough information known

7. Marbles can be bought in bags of 7, 16 and 28 from Master Maena. Pervill claimed that he bought a certain number of marbles from Master Maena, but everybody knew he was lying. How many marbles had he bought?

A. 55 B. 51 C. 63 D. 67

8. During admissions interviews at Lewisons Medical School, 60% of the candidates interviewed are have a chance to get in. 8% of the candidates are considered "gifted" but will not get in. About 17% are "gifted international students" who will get in. Which Venn diagram represents the given data?

A.

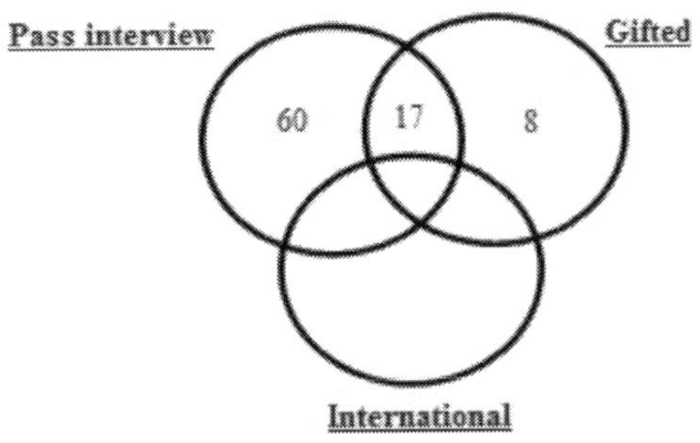

C.

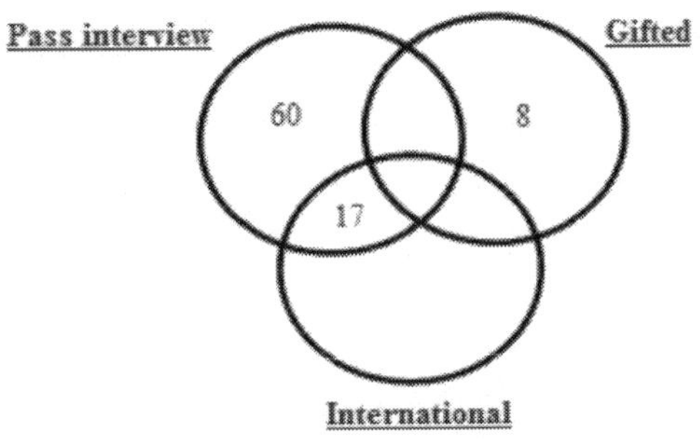

B.

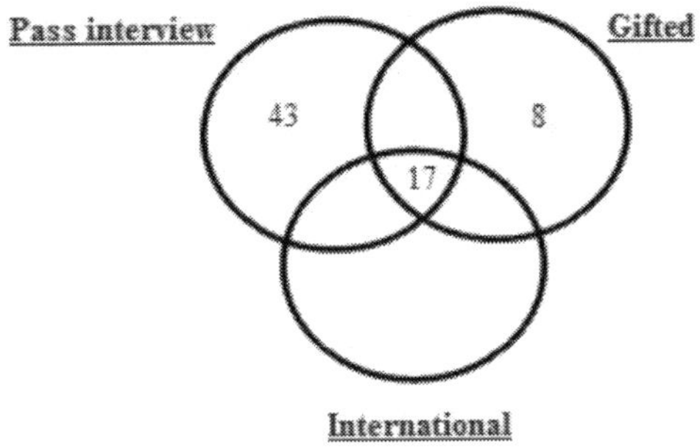

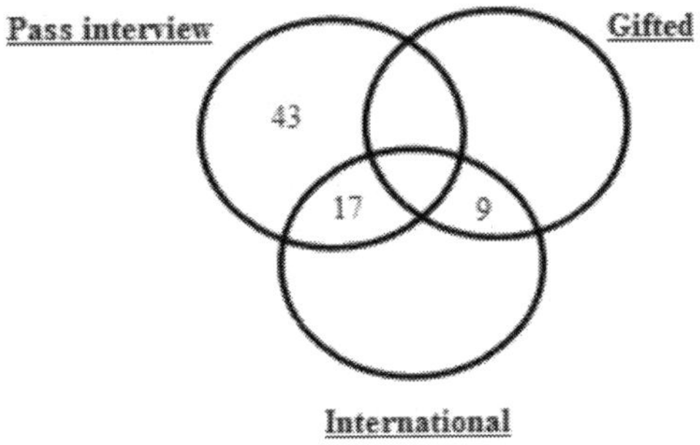

9. In a dance formation, 5 dancers have to make a diamond with the lead dancer in the middle. Jake stands to the left of Macy and Hans, and Amelia stands behind him. Hans stands at the tip of the diamond, with everybody else behind him. Lola stands in front of Amelia and next to Jake. Who is the person in the middle?

A. Amelia B. Jake C. Lola D. Macy

10. Dora has taken up a job as a warehouse assistant. She was sorting through Adidas shoes when the lights went off. There were 4 pairs of Adidas Stan Smiths, 7 pairs of Adidas originals and 3 pairs of Adidas BAIT. What is that probability that she will pick 1 pair of Stan Smiths and 1 pair of BAIT.

A. $\frac{6}{49}$ B. $\frac{3}{49}$ C. $\frac{1}{12}$ D. $\frac{7}{12}$

11. Smoking is the leading cause of lung cancer. The NHS is in debt and cannot afford to treat everyone for free. The NHS should charge smokers for lung cancer treatment. Which statement would support this argument?

A. Children have the most potential and should get preference in free treatment
B. Non-smokers should get free treatment preference
C. Smokers have brought the disease upon themselves
D. All of the above

12. At a conference about reducing anxiety, all the participants were asked to hug one another to relieve stress. 28 hugs were counted in total. How many participants attended the conference?

A. 4 B. 7 C. 8 D. 11

13. A Russian president has never agreed with a British prime minister on trade borders. The American president has always managed to make trade deals with the Russian president, but sometimes fails with the British Prime minister. Which of the following statements are true?

A. Putin and Theresa May will not agree on a trade borders
B. It is likely that Trump will make trade deals with both Putin and Theresa May
C. Trump is the best negotiator amongst the three
D. None of the above

14. Medical students are known to party hard. Most medical students get good grades. Janet gets good grades. Felix is the life of every party

A. Janet is a medical student
B. People can party hard and get good grades
C. Felix gets good grades
D. All medical students party hard and work hard

15. In a 200M medley swimming competition, Jon, Alex and Holly swim at constant speeds. Jon beats Alex by 15m and Holly loses by 15m. At what distance was Holly at when Jon touched the finish line?

A. 156 B. 170 C. 171 D. 185

16. "It is better to do something imperfectly than to do nothing flawlessly". Which of the below options supports this statement?

A. It is impossible to do "nothing" flawlessly
B. We cannot improve by doing nothing
C. Imperfections build the path to success
D. None of the above

17. Doctors are likely to be sued by their patients. Thus, they should hire medicolegal services. Which statement can be an argument against this?

A. If a doctor works towards the greater good, they will not be sued
B. It is expensive to pay for medicolegal services every year
C. Hospitals lawyers can protect doctors
D. Not all doctors are sued by their patients

18. Cybersecurity is a big problem in this day and age. Thus, pornography sites should be banned. What assumption does this conclusion make?

A. Cybersecurity hacks lead to the loss of valuable personal data
B. Pornography sites are a risk to cyber security
C. Pornography sites increase the probability of viewing child pornography
D. The cybersecurity of pornography videos is low

19. Of 130 seafood restaurants in Bali, 63 served shark fin, 28 served lobster, 45 served oysters. 9 restaurants served shark fin and lobster, 9 served lobster and oyster and 12 served shark fin and oyster. How many served all three assuming all restaurant served one of the above?

A. 0 B. 18 C. 24 D. 27

20. Douglas struggles with understanding Venn Diagrams. He was asked to draw one with the following information:
At a swimming pool, children and men above the age of twenty are not allowed to share changing rooms.
Women are allowed to use the same rooms as men above twenty, children or some swim instructors.
Swim instructors are allowed to use any room but some men above twenty have exclusive access and can deny the instructors room use.

Douglas produced the image below.

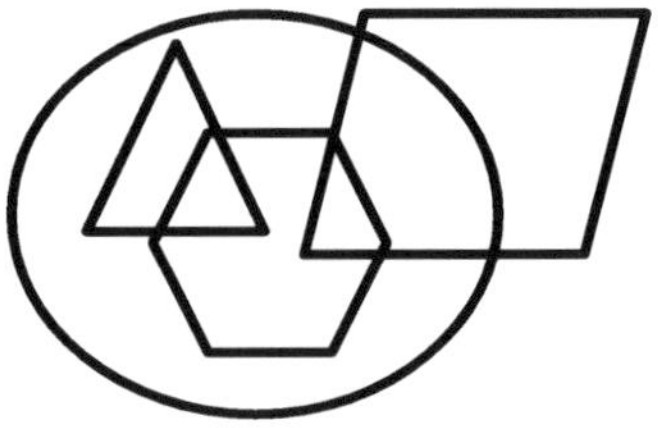

What does the hexagon represent?

A. Children
B. Men above twenty
C. Swim instructors
D. Women

21. Halep can choose to either dissect the cerebellar cortex, or the brain stem. The probability of completing 85% of her assignment before the class ends is 0.7 if she chooses the cortex. The probability choosing the brain stem and completing 85% of the assignment is 0.3. There is a 0.1 likelihood of her finishing all of her assignment if she chooses the cortex. If she chooses the brain stem, there is a probability of 0.1 that she will finish between 85% and all of the assignment. Which is the better brain region to dissect and why?

A. Brain stem because she is more likely to complete her assignment
B. Brain stem because she is more likely to do 85% of her assignment
C. Cerebellar cortex because she is more likely to complete her assignment
D. Cerebellar cortex because she is more likely to do 85% of her assignment

22. This Dalmatian barks loudly. All dogs that bark loudly are wild. Which conclusion can be drawn?

A. All Dalmatians are wild
B. All dogs are wild
C. Some Dalmatians bark loudly
D. This Dalmatian is wild

23. The cheapest flights from Tokyo to Seoul are provided by Airlines B, F and N. Airline F is the cheapest of the three except on Thursday. Airline B provides extremely low fares for a single flight every Thursday and Saturday. Airline N is the most popular for its good customer service. Which of the following statements is false.

A. Airline B is the cheapest on Thursday
B. Airline F is the cheapest on Saturday, but customer service is not the best
C. Airline N is the cheapest on Saturday
D. Travel with Airline N on Wednesday if you want a cheap flight with good service

24. 83 students indicated their interest to watch the Lion King musical in theatre on Saturday. The probability that any given student will get to watch the play is 0.6. Students are chosen by a random number generator and then informed that there is a 25% chance of them wining a drinks voucher. How many students will watch the play but NOT win the voucher.

A. 50 B. 38 C. 12 D. 63

25. Methane is flammable. Methane is a pollutant. Methane is a greenhouse gas. Greenhouse gases are released in cow faeces.

A. All greenhouse gases are flammable
B. Greenhouse gases are pollutants
C. Methane may increase pollution by causing car fires
D. Methane is released in cow faeces

26. In a game of marbles, Jess and Tim scatter several marbles on the floor. Each can pick 1 or 2 marbles in turn. The person who takes the last marble is the loser. Jess badly wants to win. How many marbles will she need to ensure she defeats Tim, if she starts the game?

A. 4 B. 8 C. 13 D. 16

27. When NASA first sent men to the moon, the probability that Neil Armstrong would place the first step on the moon was 0.7. The probability that Buzz Aldrin would not place the American flag on the moon surface was 0.4. The probability that Armstrong would make the first step, place the flag and then communicate with NASA was 0.14. Either of the two had to do each action. What was the probability that Buzz Aldrin would communicate with NASA

A. 0.2 B. 0.3 C. 0.4 D. 0.5

28. Aspirin is an NSAID (pain reliever). Aspirin causes peptic ulcers. Doctors are recommended not to prescribe Aspirin to patients with gastrointestinal issues. Which of the statements is correct?

A. NSAIDs will always cause peptic ulcers
B. Doctors can prescribe herbal drugs to patients with gastrointestinal pain
C. Patients in pain can be prescribed aspirin
D. None of the above

29. Mike, James, Carrie and Leia decided amongst themselves to cook lunch for the group on one of the four days of the week, Monday, Tuesday Wednesday and Thursday. Each day had a different dish; chicken, fish, lentils and noodles.

James made food on Wednesday. Leia did not food on Thursday. Leia cooked fish on Tuesday. On Monday, chicken was cooked but not by Carrie. Mike did not make noodles and lentils were not cooked on Thursday. Which statement is true about noodles?

A. It was made on Thursday by Carrie
B. It was made on Thursday by Mike
C. It was made on Wednesday by James
D. It was made on Monday by Carrie

END OF SECTION

Section C: Quantitative Reasoning

SET 1

Chris is cooking paella for 10 of his friends from the recipe seen below:

CHRIS' SUPER SECRET PAELLA RECIPE

170g/6oz chorizo, cut into thin slices
110g/4oz pancetta, cut into small dice
2 cloves garlic finely chopped
570ml/1pint calasparra (Spanish short-grain) rice
8 chicken thighs, each chopped in half and browned
110g/4oz fresh or frozen peas
12 jumbo raw prawns, in shells
450g/1lb squid, cleaned and chopped into bite-sized pieces

- Chris' recipe makes 6 portions
- Each portion contains 575kcal which is 25% of Chris' recommended daily kcal intake
- It takes Chris 7 minutes per portion to cook the meal
- The cost per portion is £1.80
- Chris is not eating

1. What quantity of squid does Chris need?

A. 0.45kg B. 0.6kg C. 0.75kg D. 0.9kg E. 1.35k

2. Chris' friends are due to arrive at 8.30pm. He wants the food to be ready 10 minutes before. What time does Chris need to start preparing the meal?

A. 19:00 B. 19:10 C. 19:15 D. 19:20 E. 19:25

3. If Chris were to eat all 10 portions himself, by how many kcal would he be exceeding his recommended daily intake?

A. 2300 B. 2875 C. 3450 D. 4600 E. 5750

4. Two of Chris' friends are unable to attend. So as not to leave Chris out of pocket his remaining friends agree to split the difference in cost. What is the new cost per portion?

A. £1.95 B. £2.05 C. £2.15 D. £2.25 E. £2.35

5. If Chris had decided to eat with his 10 friends, how many jumbo prawns would he have needed altogether?

A. 2 B. 4 C. 18 D. 20 E. 22

SET 2

The table of admission prices for a cinema is shown below:

	Peak	Off-peak
Adult	£11	£9.50
Child	£7	£5.50
Concession	£7	£5.50
Student	£5	£5

- Peak times include weekends and Friday's from 5pm
- A £2 surcharge is added to any ticket for a film premiere
- A £1 surcharge is added per ticket for the use of 3D glasses
- On Tuesday a special offer means all tickets are charged at the student price

6. How much will it cost for a family of 2 adults, 2 children and 1 concession to watch a premiere 3D film on Saturday evening?

A. £35.50
B. £43
C. £48
D. £53
E. £5

7. How much change would 3 adults receive from a £50 note when viewing a 3D film on a Tuesday?

A. £15
B. £18.50
C. £21.50
D. £32
E. £35

8. Joe buys 4 student tickets for a standard Wednesday afternoon film on his credit card which charges 30% interest. How much does he actually pay?

A. £20
B. £22
C. £24
D. £26
E. £28

9. What is the maximum number of children that could attend an off-peak premiere with £100?

A. 12
B. 13
C. 14
D. 15
E. 16

10. How much money would 1 adult, 2 children and 2 students save by watching a premiere 3D film on a Tuesday instead of a Saturday?

A. £2.50
B. £5
C. £7.50
D. £10
E. £12.50

SET 3

Shown below is a table of figures outlining average energy consumption per property type per year.

	Electricity usage (kWh)	Gas usage (kWh)	Total cost (£)
1 bedroom flat	2,000	0	300
2 bedroom flat	2,000	8,000	700
3 bedroom house	4,750	18,000	1612.50
4 bedroom house	6,000	22,000	2000
Microbusiness	5,000	4,500	635
Small business	15,000	9,000	1770
Medium Business	30,000	12,000	3360

- Gas and electricity are priced differently
- Business and household rates are different

11. What is the cost per kWh for household gas?

A. £0.04
B. £0.05
C. £0.06
D. £0.07
E. £0.08

12. Given that businesses receive gas at a rate of 3p per kWh, what is the difference in price between household and business electricity per kWh?

A. £0.03
B. £0.04
C. £0.05
D. £0.06
E. £0.1

13. If Kate owns both a small business and a 3 bedroom house, what is her expenditure on gas every two years?

A. £900
B. £1170
C. £1350
D. £2340
E. £2700

14. If Luke owns 50% of a medium business in addition to his 1 bedroom flat, what is his monthly energy expenditure?

A. £165
B. £305
C. £440
D. £1980
E. £3660

15. Installing 1m^2 of photovoltaic cells cuts electricity costs by 1%. Approximately what area of photovoltaic cells would be required to reduce household electricity rates to those of businesses?

A. 0.33m^2
B. £0.5m^2
C. 0.66m^2
D. 33m^2
E. 66m^2

SET 4

A sports retailer offers discounts on item pricing when bulk buying. Their graph of item prices can be seen below:

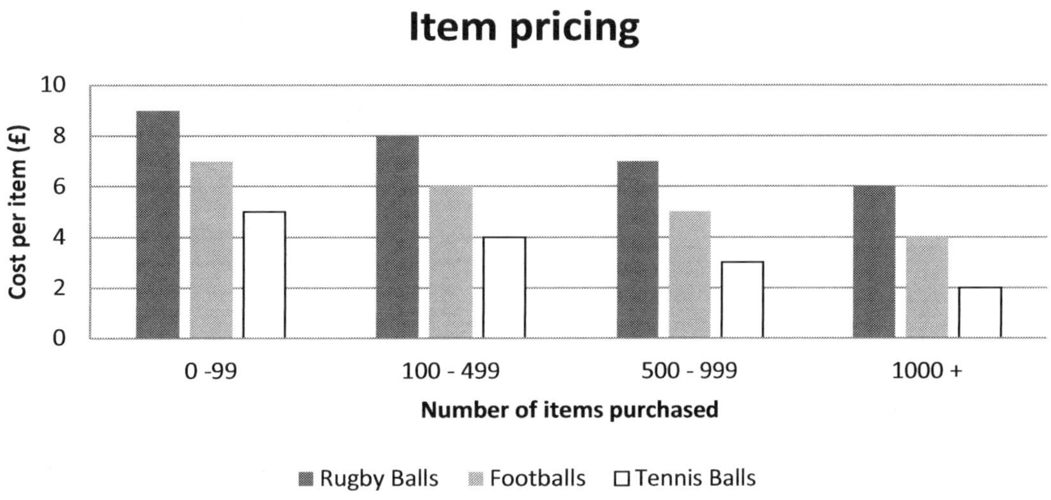

- Rugby balls and footballs are sold separately but tennis balls come in packs of 3. (i.e. 3 tennis balls = 1 item)
- Home delivery is charged at £10 within a 15 mile radius and £20 thereafter
- Home delivery is free on orders exceeding £75

16. How much would it cost to collect 50 rugby balls and 60 tennis balls in store?

A. £550
B. £570
C. £750
D. £770
E. £980

17. Alex plans to buy 8 footballs, how many more should she buy to qualify for free delivery?

A. 1
B. 2
C. 3
D. 4
E. 5

18. What is the maximum number of tennis balls that could be delivered to a home 36 miles away on a budget of £75?

A. 11
B. 33
C. 39
D. 45
E. 58

19. What is the difference in price when the quantity of items in an order of 1000 footballs and 500 rugby balls is halved?

A. £2,750
B. £3,000
C. £3,250
D. £3,500
E. £3,750

20. The following year the retailer revokes their free delivery policy and increases all prices by 20%. Now how much does an order of 6,000 tennis balls cost when delivered to a factory 78 miles away?

A. £4,800
B. £4,820
C. £4,824
D. £14,400
E. £14,420

SET 5

The figure shown below is a plan of 4 cattle fields:

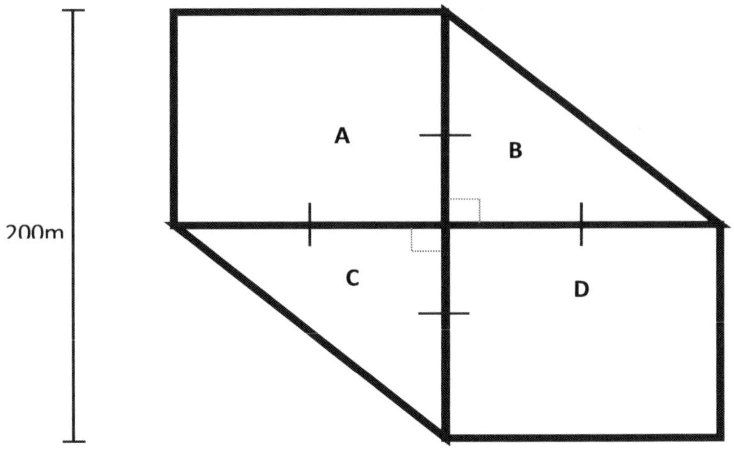

- Each cow legally requires $2m^2$ of space
- A cow drinks 3.5L of water and eats 4kg of pellet food each day
- The farmer's water rate equates to 2p/L and pellet food is purchased at £10 per 20kg
- On average each cow produces 1.5L of milk upon milking
- Milking can only happen every other day

21. What is the total area of all 4 fields?

A. $0.03km^2$
B. $0.3km^2$
C. $3km^2$
D. $300km^2$
E. 30,000km

22. How many cattle could be legally housed within field A alone?

A. 50
B. 500
C. 5,000
D. 10,000
E. 50,000

23. How much money is spent providing the cattle with food and water each day if the maximum legal number of cattle are present?

A. £10,350
B. £31,050
C. £35,000
D. £86,750
E. £135,000

24. Assuming there is a total of 200 cattle in the fields, what is the maximum volume of milk that could be obtained in a week?

A. 300L
B. 600L
C. 900L
D. 1,200L
E. 1,500L

25. If the farmer changed to a higher-grade pellet feed instead costing him £2.93 per day, what is the maximum number of cattle that could be housed on a daily budget of £1,000?

A. 288
B. £315.33
C. 333
D. 333.33
E. 50

SET 6

Shown below is a table of statistics from a race track.

- The statistics shown are for 1 lap of the track
- MPG = miles per gallon
- 1 gallon = 4.5L
- Current fuel prices are 102 pence per litre

CAR	Top Speed (MPH)	Average Speed (MPH)	Fuel consumption (MPG)	Fuel Tank Capacity (L)
A	150	130	54	60
B	180	150	22.5	50
C	165	140	36	60
D	220	180	13.5	40

26. Given that car B completed the lap in 3 minutes exactly, what is the length of the race track?

A. 7.5 miles
B. 9 miles
C. 50 miles
D. 450 miles
E. 540 miles

27. How much does it cost for car C to drive the 10 miles to the race track?

A. 12.75p
B. 87.5p
C. 120p
D. 127.5p
E. 130p

28. How far could car D travel on a full tank of fuel at its average track speed?

A. 105 miles
B. 115 miles
C. 120 miles
D. 125 miles
E. 130 miles

29. If car A was 1.8 miles in front of car B when both cars simultaneously hit top speed; how long would it take for car B to overtake car A–assuming both cars remain travelling at top speed?

A. 0.06 seconds
B. 0.6 seconds
C. 60 seconds
D. 0.06 hours
E. 0.6 hours

30. On a track 8 miles in length, how many whole laps could car A complete on a full tank of petrol assuming that fuel consumption remains constant?

A. 9
B. 90
C. 405
D. 720
E. 3

SET 7

Average annual house prices are shown below.

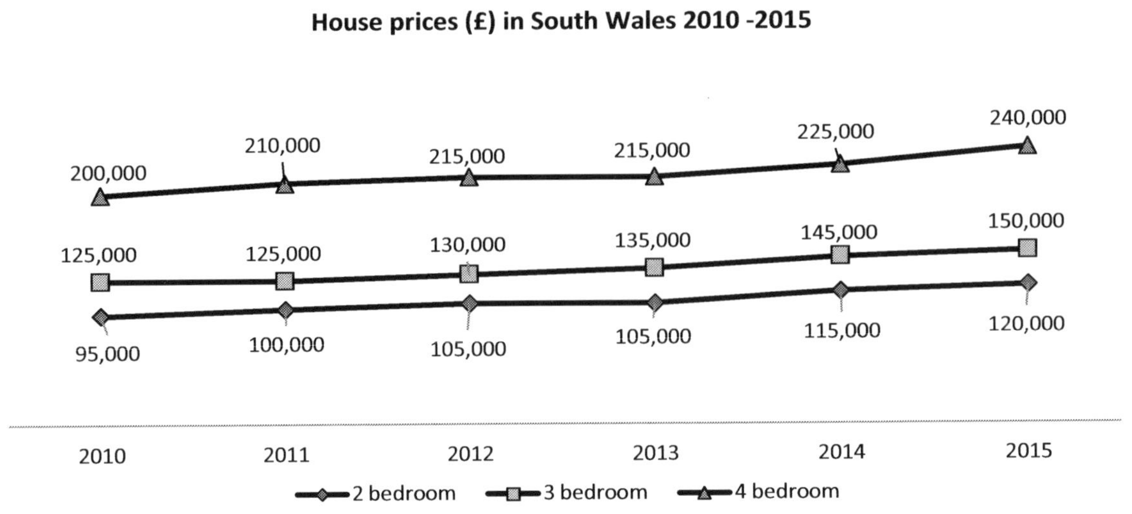

31. What is the percentage rise in 4 bedroom house prices from 2010 to 2015?

A. 17%
B. 20%
C. 23%
D. 26%
E. 29%

32. A couple wants to upgrade from a 2 bedroom to a 4 bedroom house in 2014. They are able to save £5,000 a year for the first 10 years and £10,000 a year thereafter; from what year would they needed to have started saving in order to make their desired move?

A. 1992
B. 1996
C. 1998
D. 2001
E. 2003

33. If house prices rose a staggering 25% between 2009 and 2010, how much would a 4-bedroom house have cost in 2009?

A. £40,000
B. £80,000
C. £120,000
D. £160,000
E. £200,000

34. If an investor buys a 2,3 and 4 bedroom house in 2010, then sells the: 2 bedroom after 2 years, the 3 bedroom after 3 years and the 4 bedroom after 4 years how much profit does he make?

A. £5,000
B. £15,000
C. £25,000
D. £35,000
E. £45,000

35. If a house can only ever be let for 20% of its initial purchase price per annum, for how many years must a 2010, 3 bedroom house be let in order to receive the same profit as if it were sold 4 years later?

A. 0.6
B. 0.8
C. 3.6
D. 5.6
E. 5.8

36. A street has 2, 3, and 3 2 bedroom, 3 bedroom and 4 bedroom houses respectively. What percentage of the streets value do 2 bedroom houses comprise in 2015?

A. 10% B. 14% C. 17% D. 20% E. 25%

END OF SECTION

Section D: Abstract Reasoning

For each question, decide whether each box fits best with Set A, Set B or with neither.
For each question, work through the boxes from left to right as you see them on the page. Make your decision and fill it into the answer sheet.

Answer as follows:
A = Set A
B = Set B
C = neither

Set 1: **Set A** **Set B**

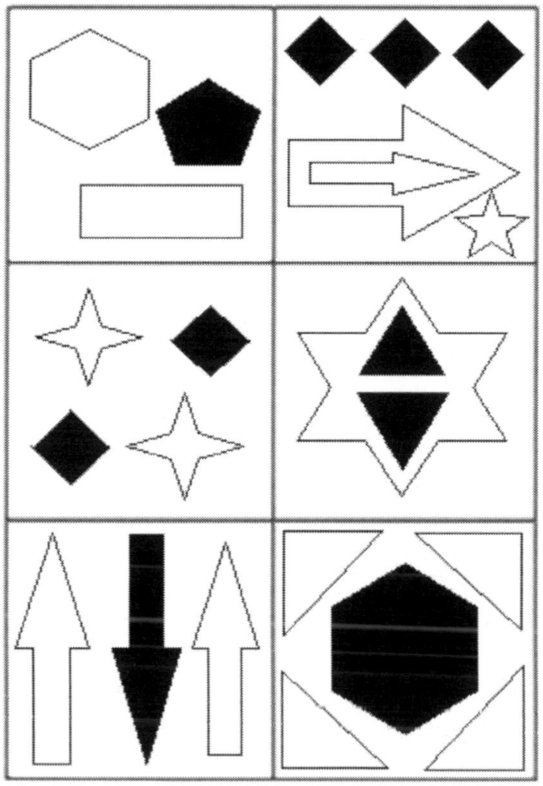

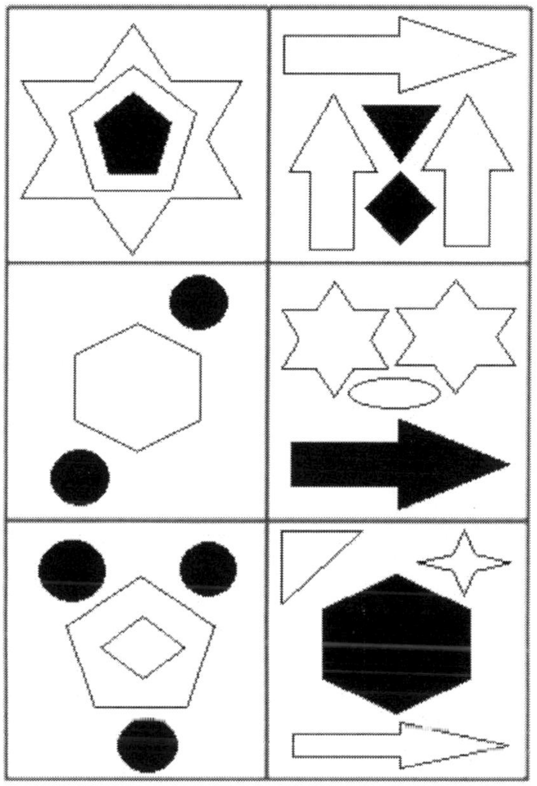

Questions 1-5:

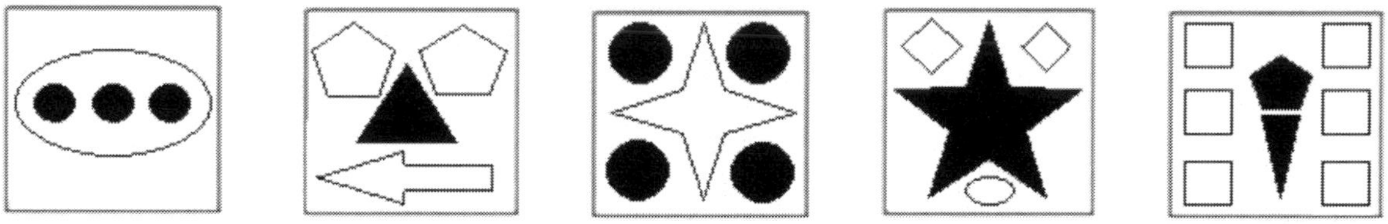

Set 2:

Set A

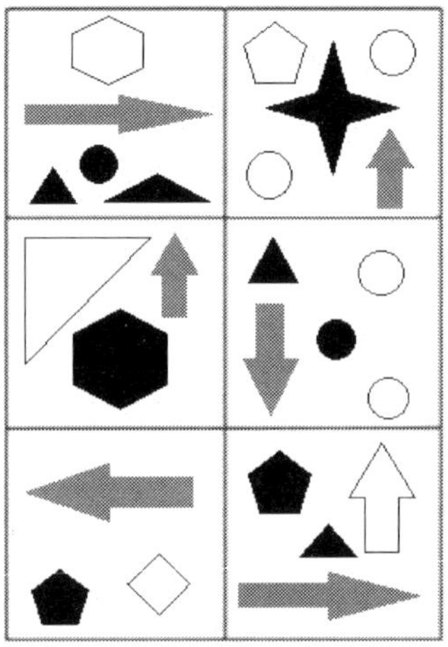

Set B

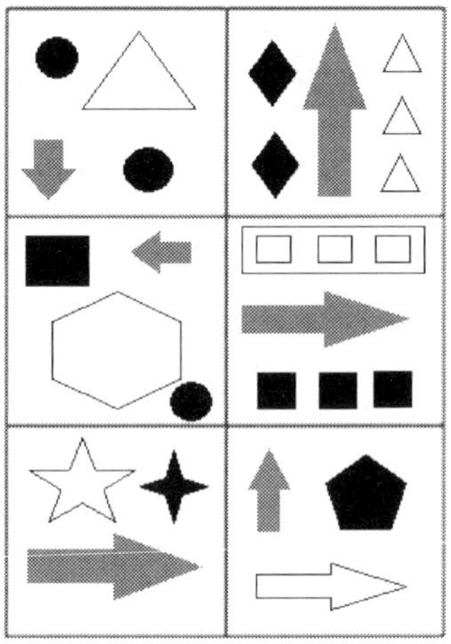

Questions 6-10:

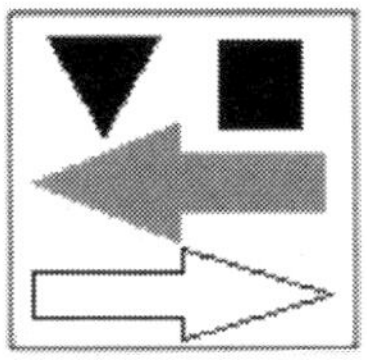
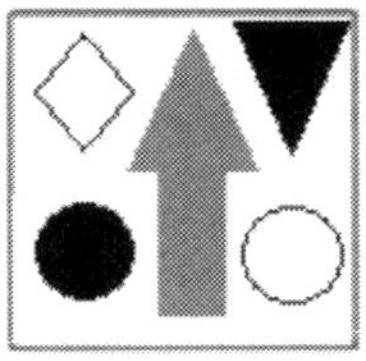
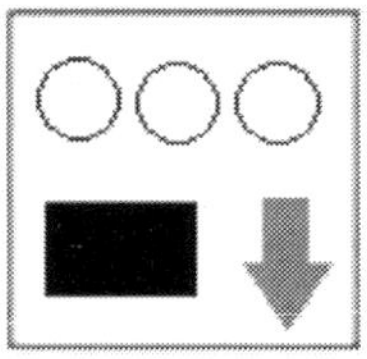

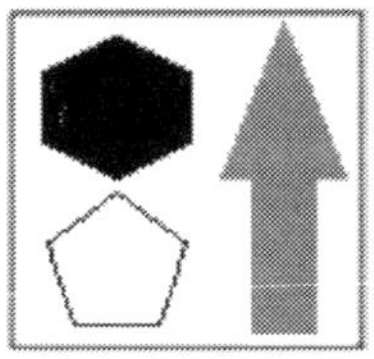

Set 3:

Set A

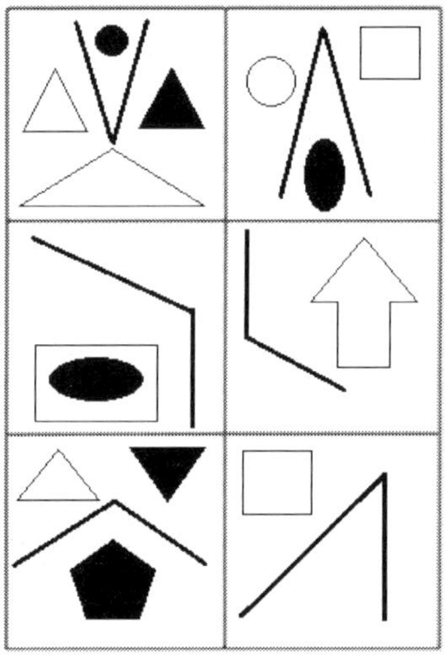

Set B

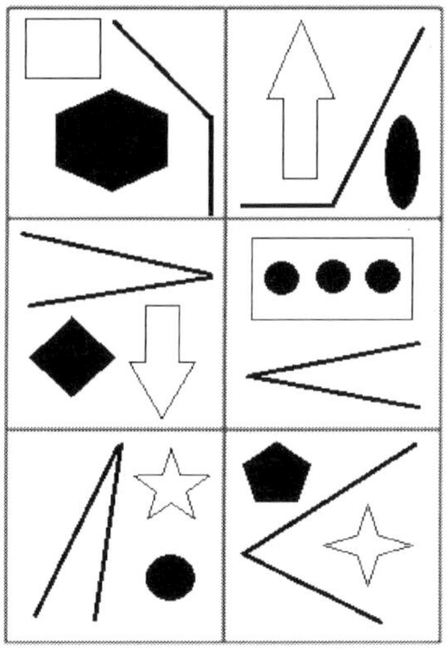

Questions 11-15:

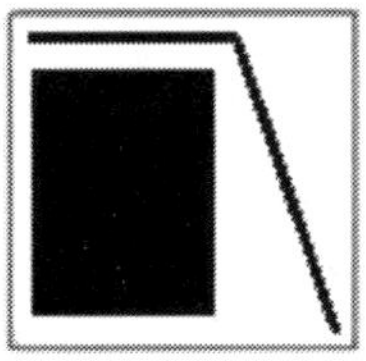
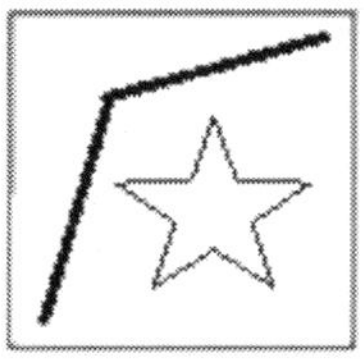
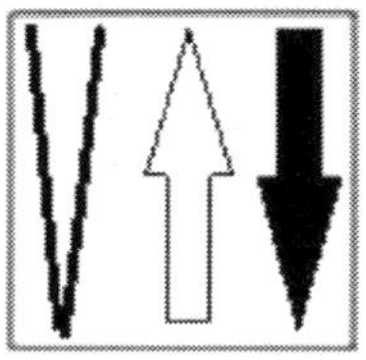

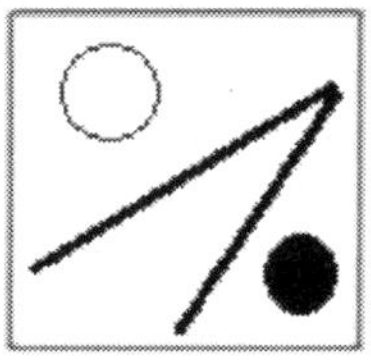

Set 4: **Set A** **Set B**

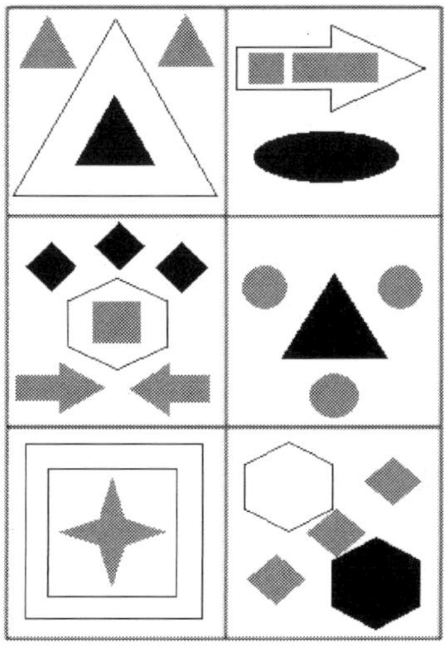

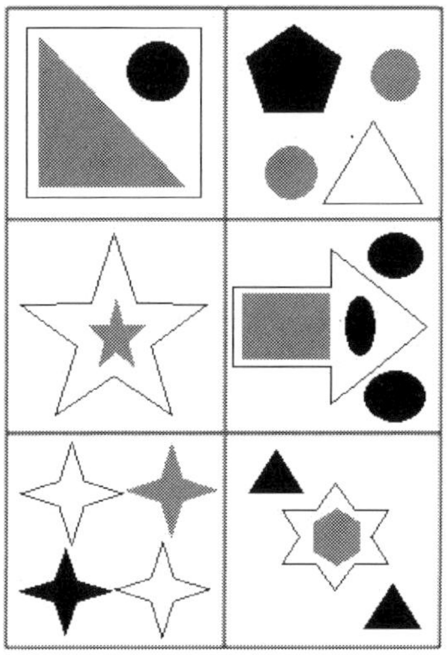

Questions 16-20:

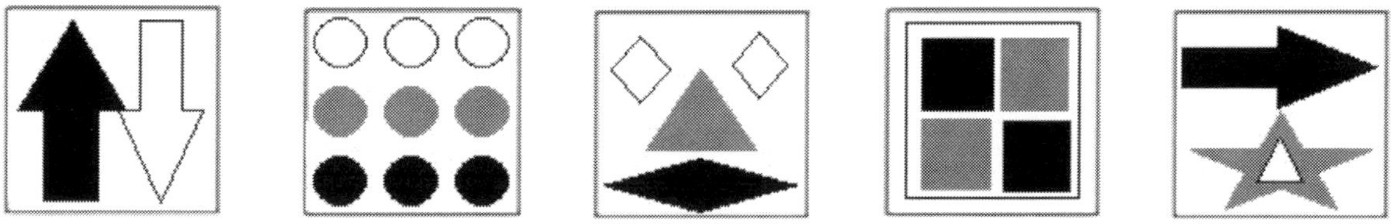

Set 5: **Set A** **Set B**

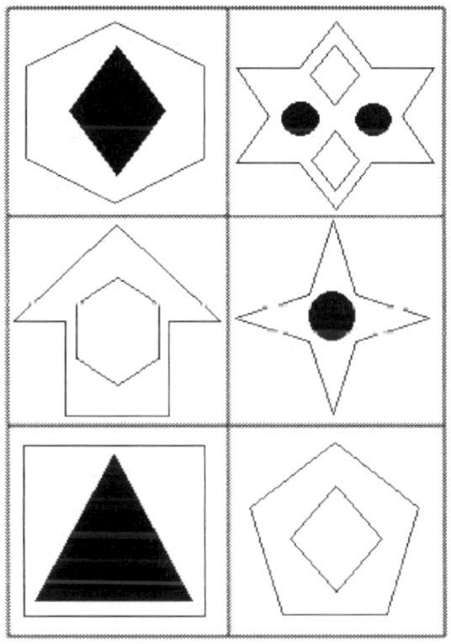

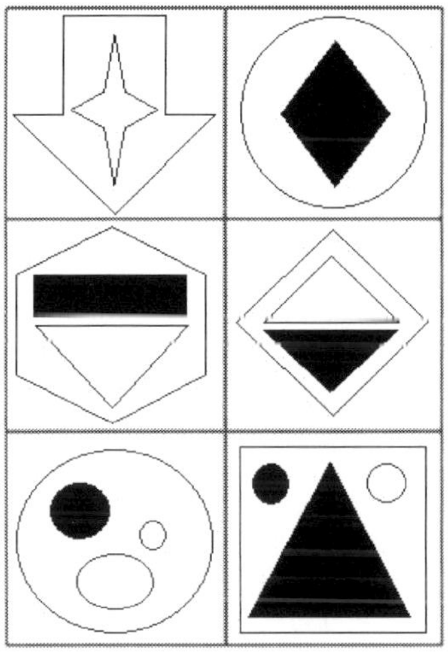

Questions 21-25:

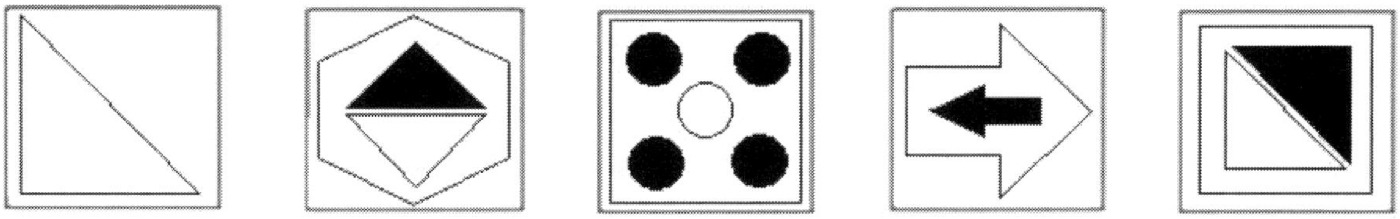

Set 6

Which answer completes the series?

Question 26:

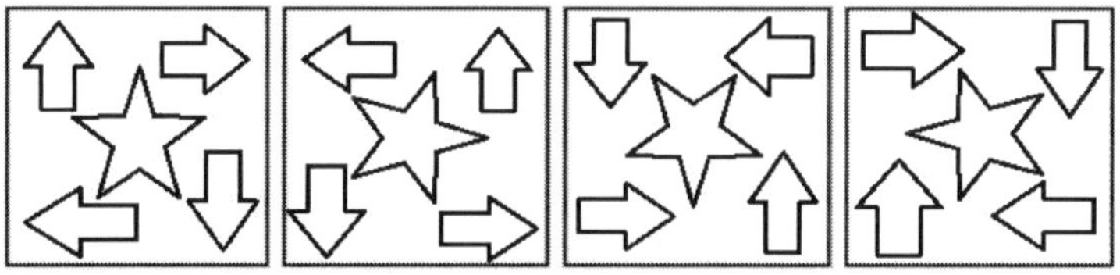

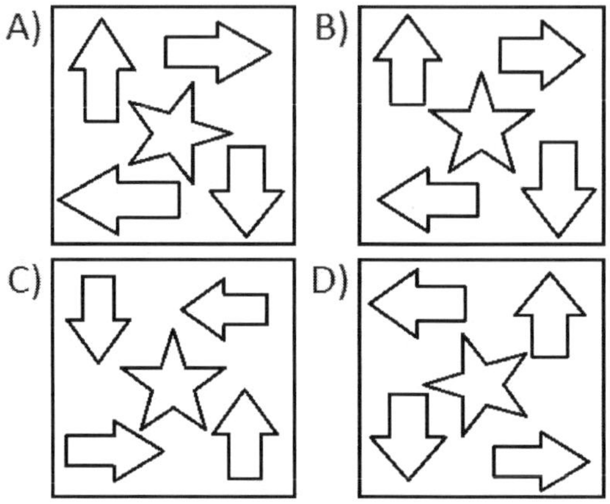

Question 27:

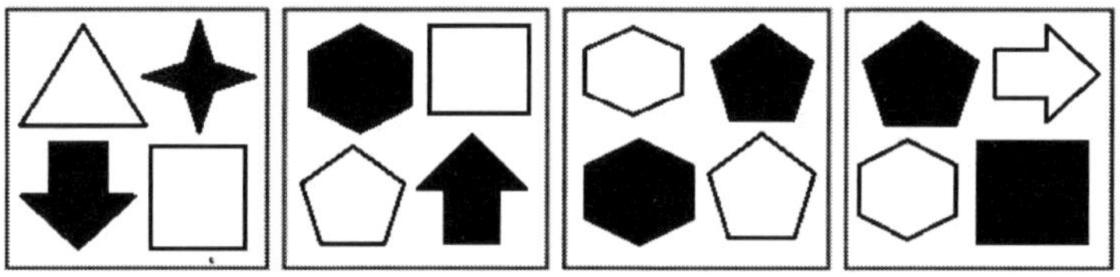

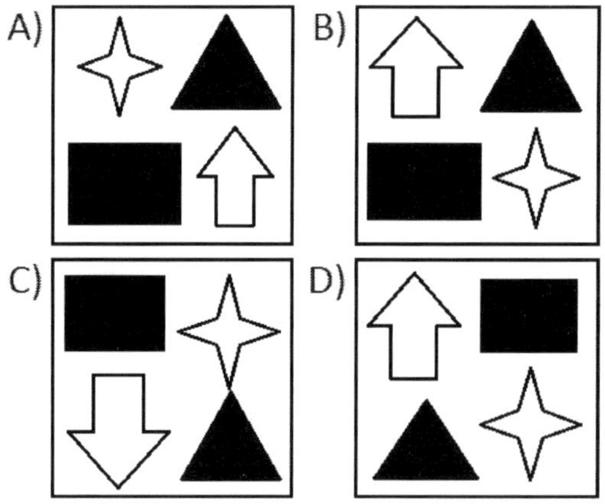

Question 28:

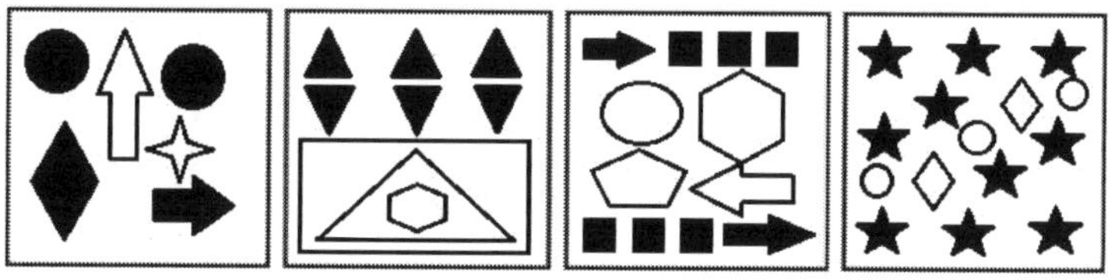

A) 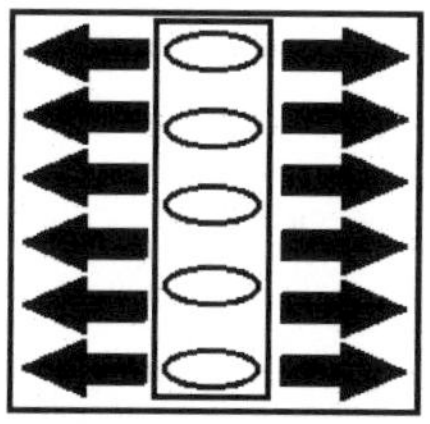 B) 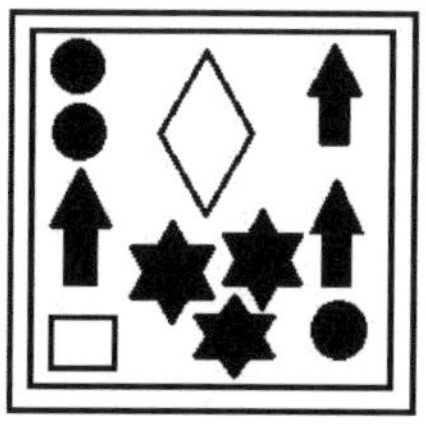

C) 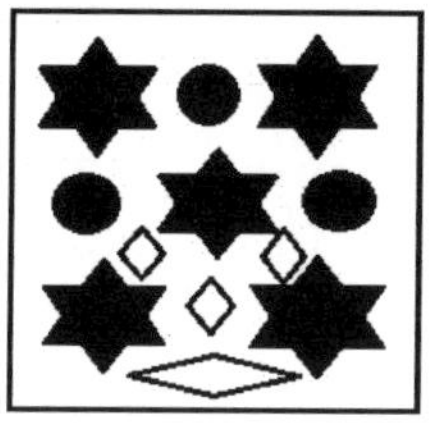 D) 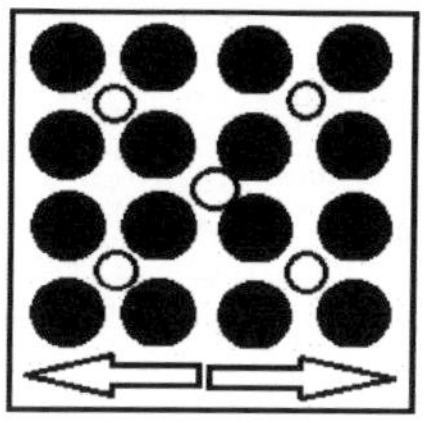

Question 29:

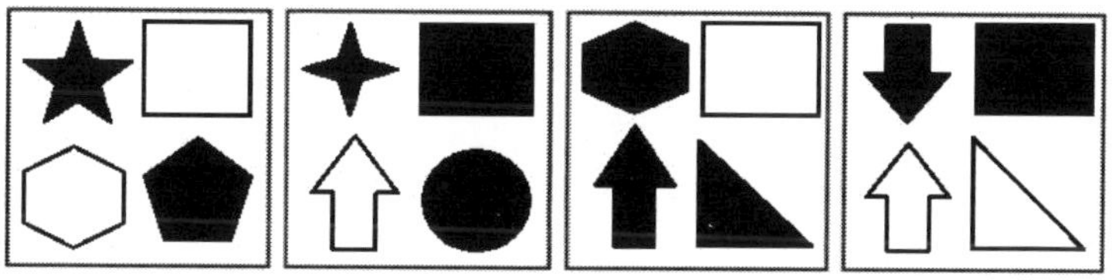

A) 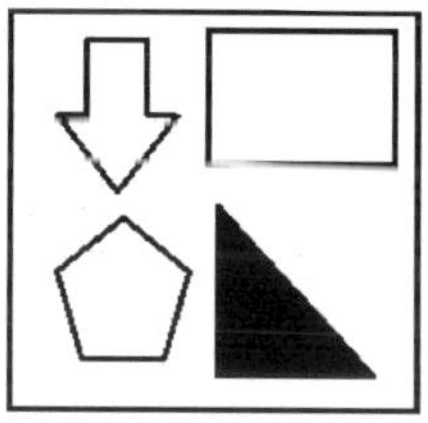 B) 

C)  D) 

Question 30:

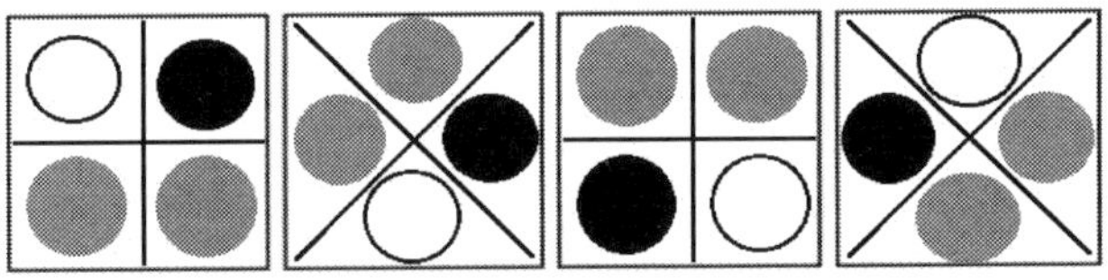

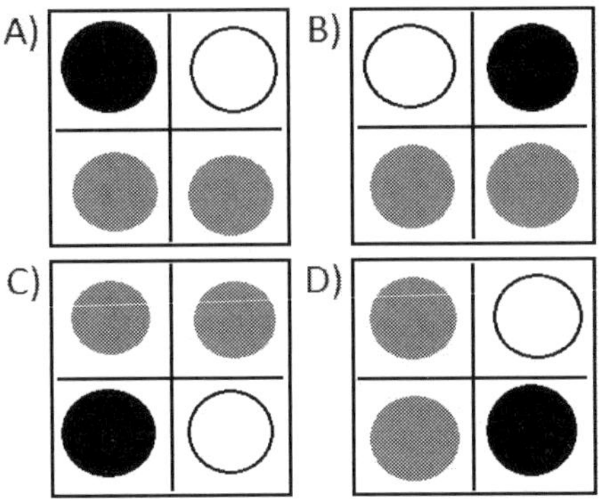

Set 7

Which answer completes the statement?

Question 31:

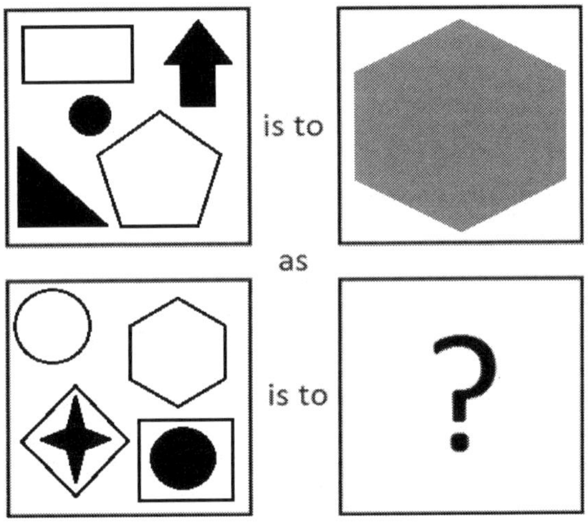

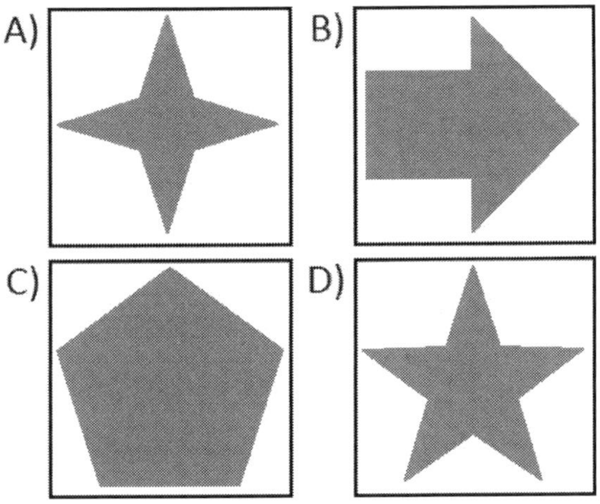

Question 32:

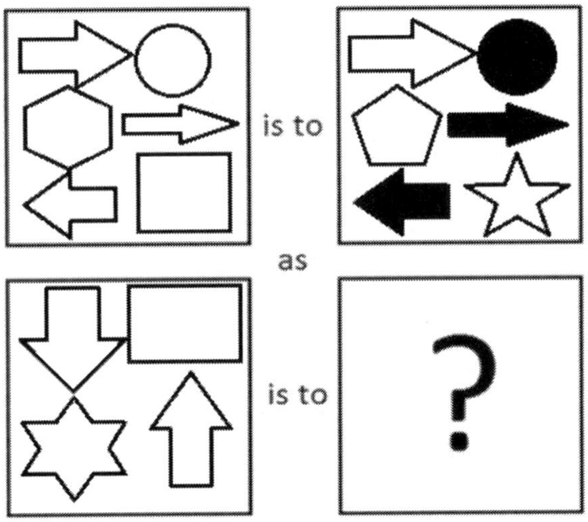

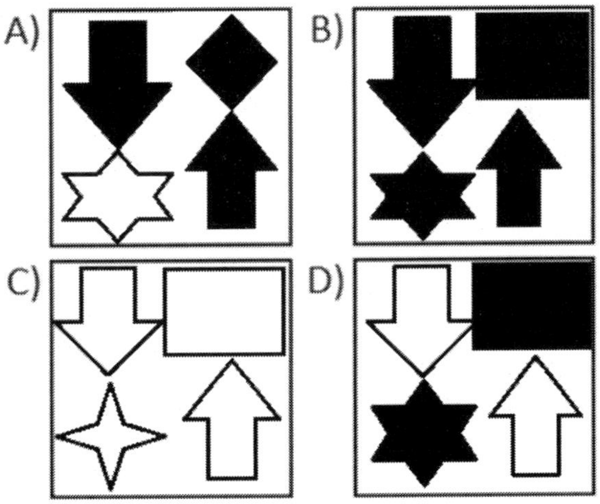

Question 33:

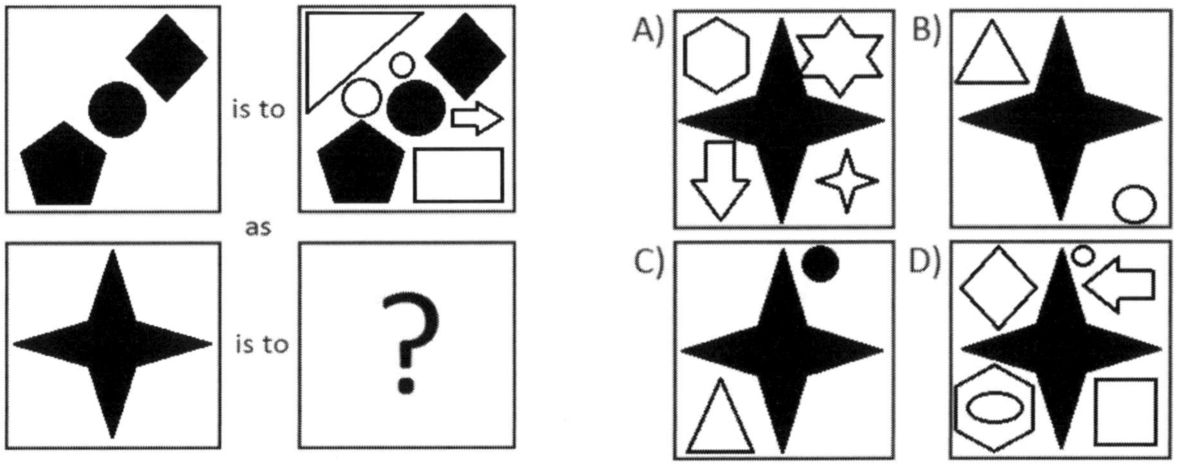

Question 34:

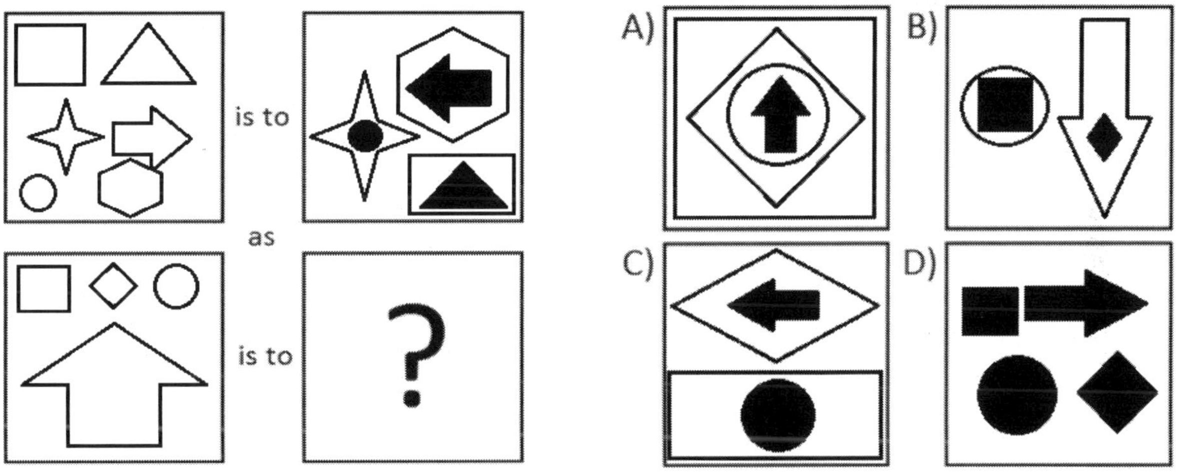

Question 35:

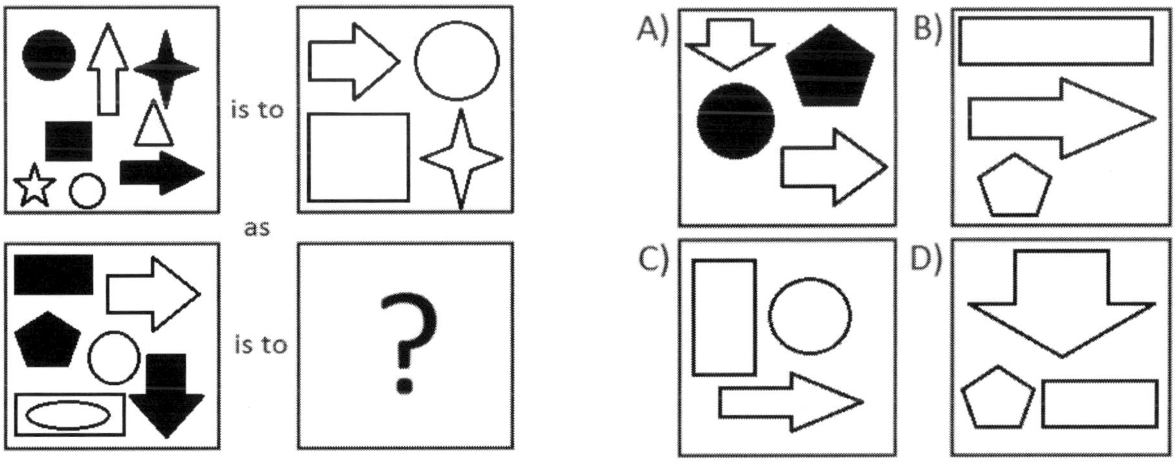

Set 8

Which of the four response options belongs to either set A or set B?

Set A **Set B**

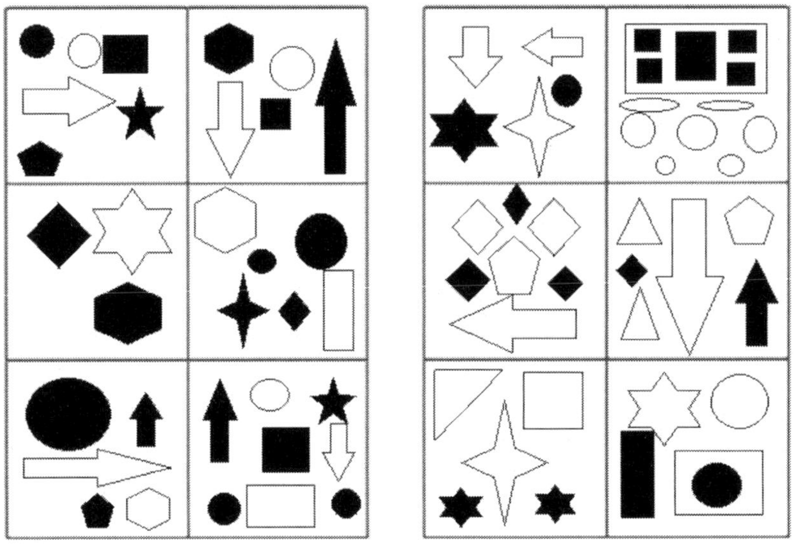

Question 36:

Set A?

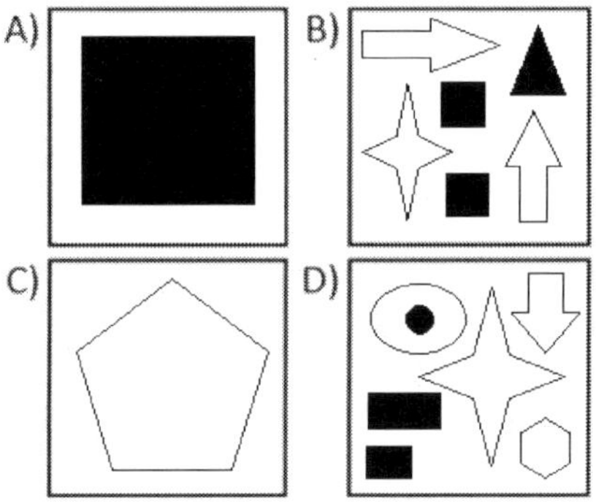

Question 37:

Set B?

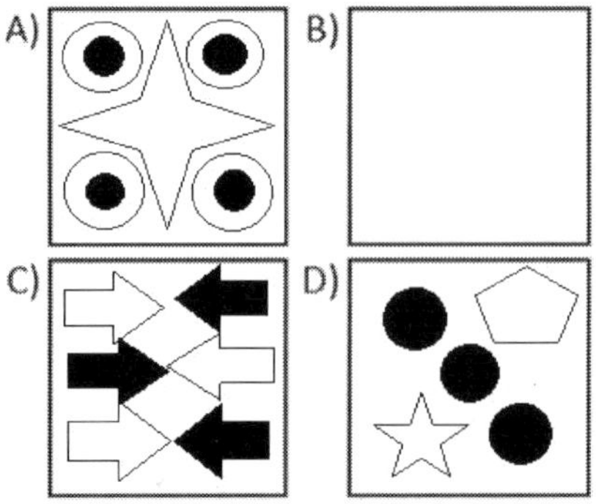

Question 38:

Set A?

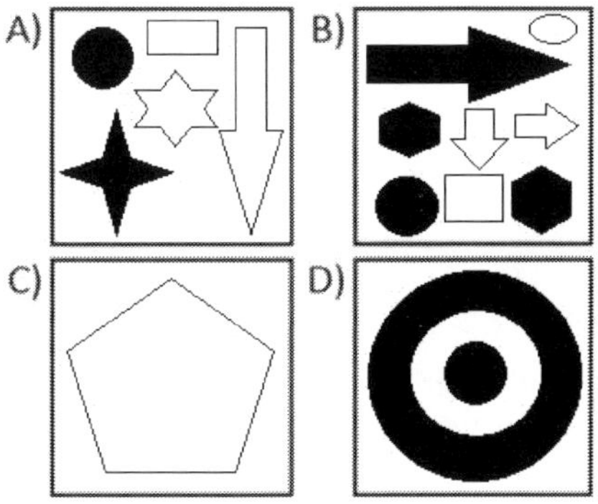

Question 39:

Set A?

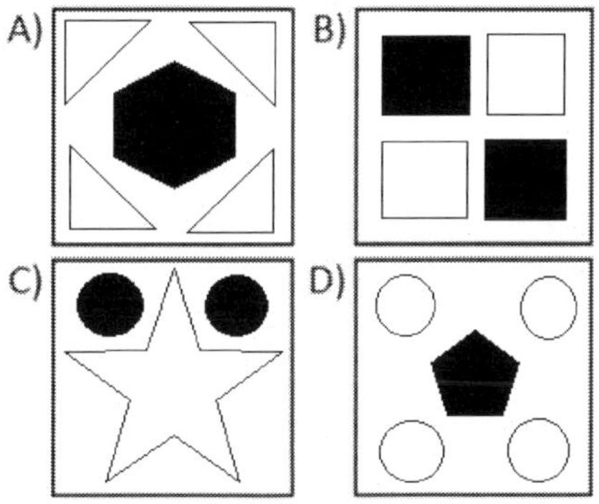

Question 40:

Set B?

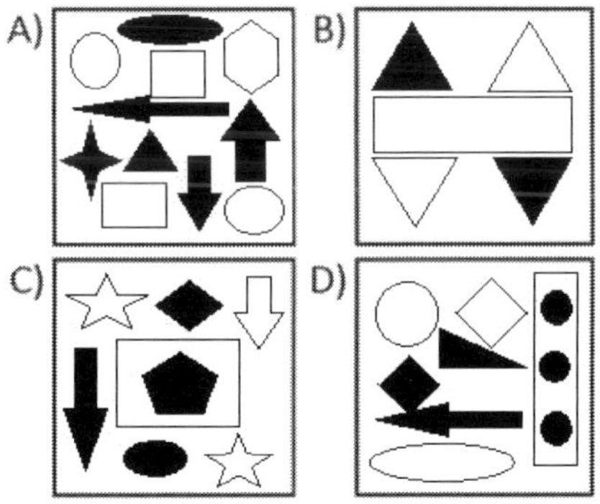

Set 9

Decide whether each box fits best with Set A, Set B or with neither.

Answer as follows:
A = Set A
B = Set B
C = neither

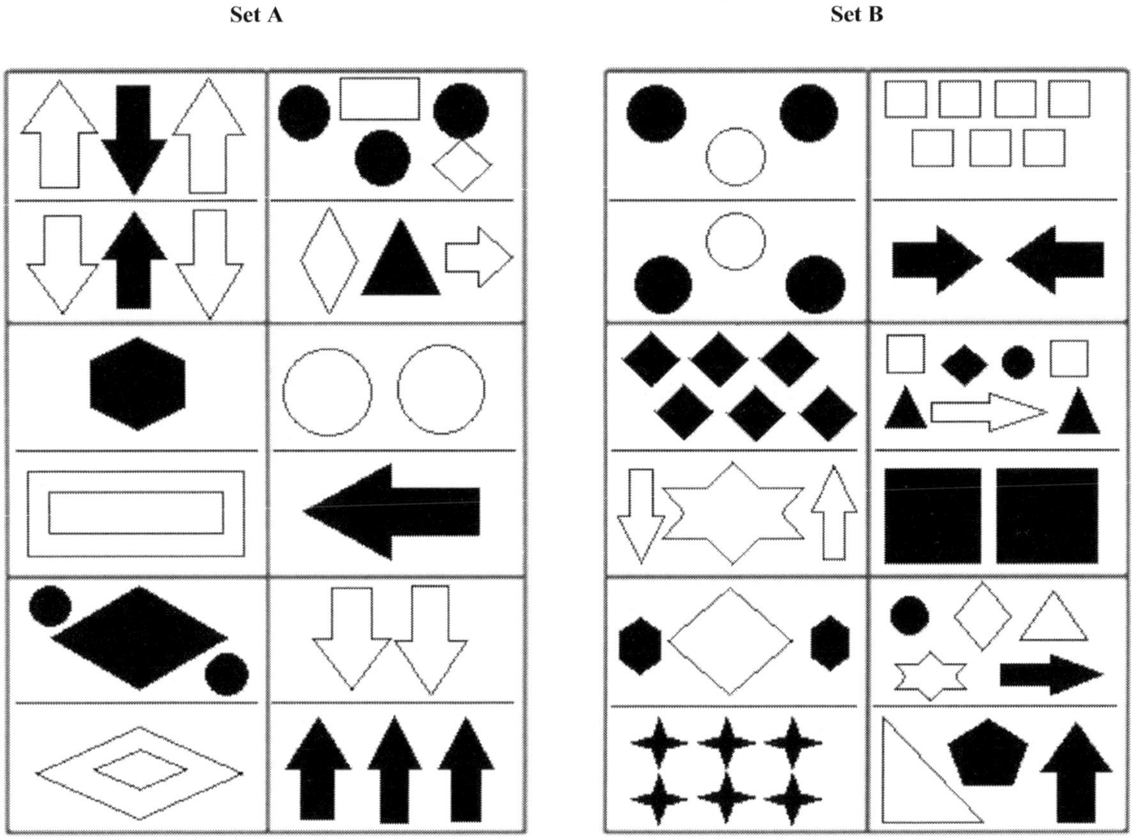

Questions 41-45:

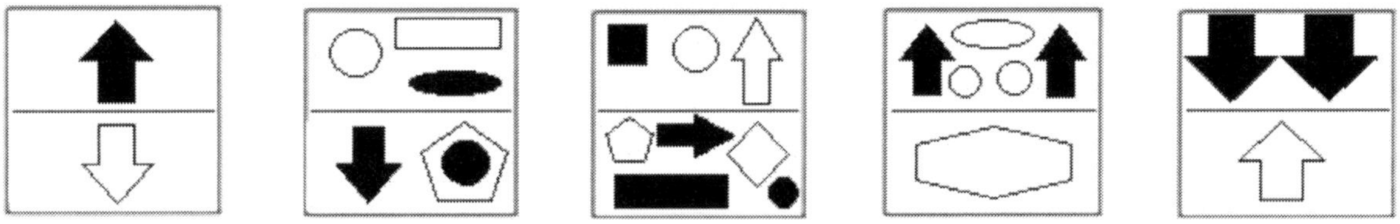

Set 10 **Set A** **Set B**

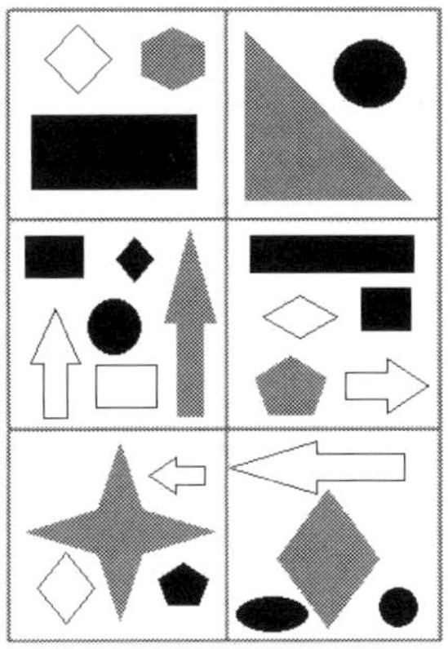

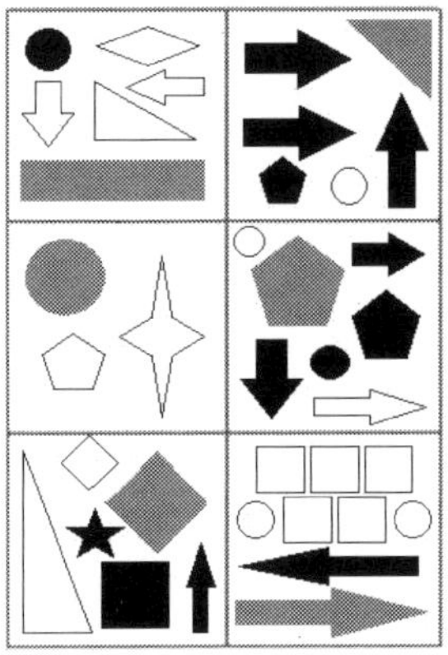

Questions 46-50:

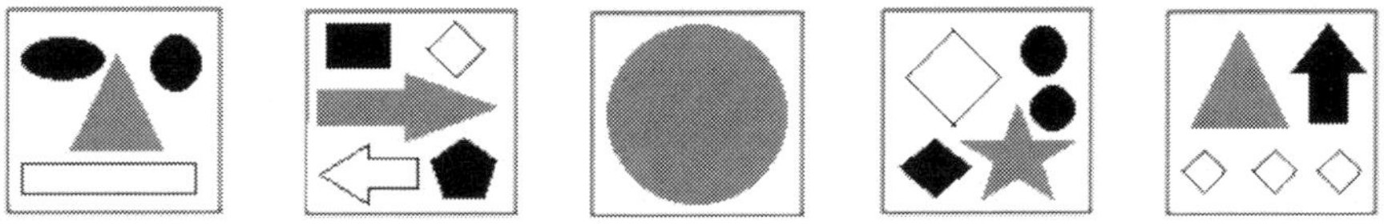

Set 11 **Set A** **Set B**

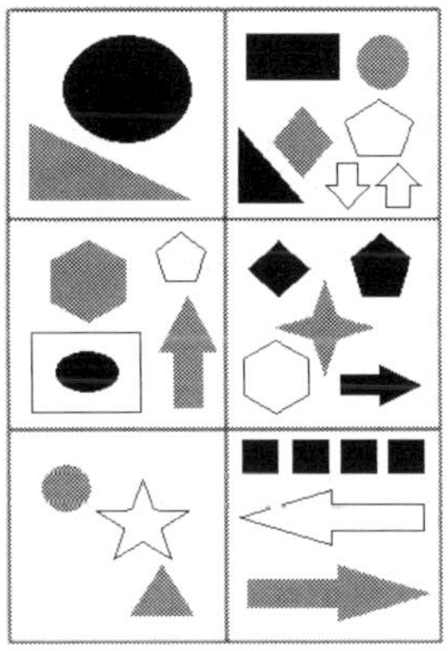

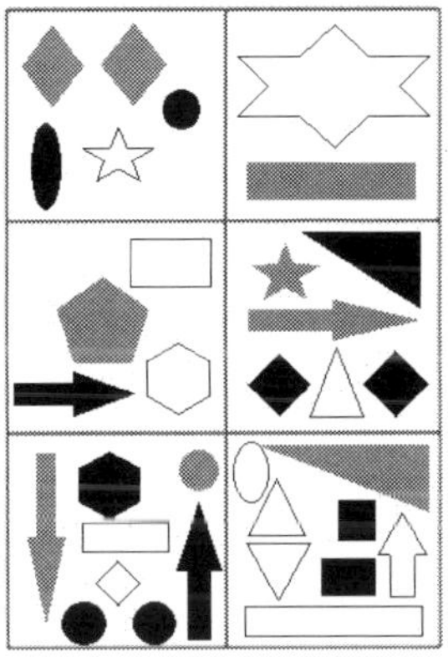

Questions 51-55:

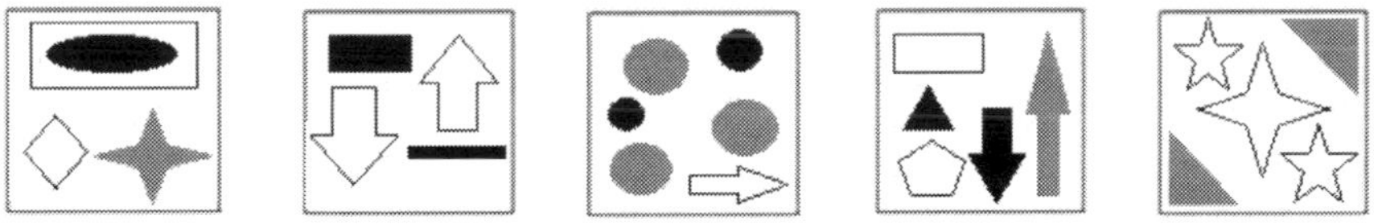

END OF SECTION

Section E: Situational Judgement Test

Read each scenario. Each question refers to the scenario directly above. For each question, select one of these four options. Select whichever you feel is the option that best represents your view on each suggested action.

For questions 1 – 30, choose one of the following options:

A A highly appropriate action
B Appropriate, but not ideal
C Inappropriate, but not awful
D A highly inappropriate action

Scenario 1
Maya is a 2nd year medical student who has clinical placement once a week at the GP. She is asked by the GP to see a patient in clinic and take a full history. When she talks to the patient, she notices bruises down the patient's left arm. The patient is a young mother with children aged two and 4 months, and upon further questioning, Maya learns that the patient is going through domestic abuse at home at the hands of her husband. The patient is insistent that Maya tells no one of this information, as she fears that the situation could escalate at home.

How appropriate are the following responses to Maya dilemma?

1. Reassure the patient that she will tell no one of what is happening at home.
2. Reassure the patient that she will not say anything and then, once the patient has left the room, immediately phone the police and report what she has learnt.
3. Tell the patient that everything she says is confidential but if Maya is worried, she may discuss the situation with the GP and the GP may call the patient in again to talk to her.
4. Discuss the situation with the GP and leave it to her to take further action.
5. Discuss this with her parents and get their opinion on this issue.

Scenario 2
Abdul is a 3rd year medical student. He is on clinical placement for two days a week. He is starting his placement in the paediatric ward today. When he arrives at the hospital for 9am, the consultant he's supposed to see with regards to this placement isn't in and there is no one else on the ward he can refer to.

How appropriate are each of these responses to the situation?

6. Go home.
7. Ask a junior doctor or nurse on the ward, if there is anything of interest to see or any patients he can take a history from.
8. Join his friends on their placement, in a different ward.
9. Email his supervisor and ask them what to do.
10. Go around the ward and take some histories from patients as long as they are willing.

Scenario 3
Mike is a final year medical student working in the hospital. While in the canteen at lunch time, he hears some younger medical students he recognises from the ward round, discussing and joking about the case of a patient very loudly over their lunch. At that moment, a relative of the patient being discussed enters the canteen and overhears the students making a joke at the expense of the patient. They look very upset about what they've heard.

How appropriate are Mike's responses to this situation?

11. Tell the students that they are breaking confidentiality in front of everyone and then, immediately email their supervising consultant to report them.
12. Leave his lunch and seek out the senior consultant supervising them to report their behaviour.
13. Take the students aside and quietly tell them they are breaking confidentiality and ask them to apologise to the relative.
14. Take the relative aside and apologise on the student's behalf.
15. Do nothing.

Scenario 4
Alisha is a 4th year medical student on her way home after clinical placement. She is rushing as she is going on a date tonight and is already late. As she is walking home, she sees an elderly man collapsed and half-conscious on the side of the road. Everyone else is ignoring him and walking past him.

How appropriate are each of these responses to Alisha's situation?

16. Point someone in the direction of the elderly man and continue her journey.
17. Walk past him as well.
18. Stop and help him by performing first aid as best as possible and by calling an ambulance. Then call her date and inform them that she may be a little late.
19. Call an ambulance
20. Call a friend and ask them to call an ambulance.

Scenario 5
George is a 2nd year medical student. He is on the respiratory ward when the senior consultant he is shadowing is bleeped and has to leave him to go and see another patient. A nurse that is passing, mistakes him for a junior doctor and asks him to take some bloods from a patient. George does not know how to do this procedure, but the nurse has already left him to get the equipment.

How appropriate are these responses to the situation?

21. Do the procedure.
22. Tell the nurse that he is only a student when she comes back and that he hasn't been taught how to so this clinical skill and therefore does not want to carry out the procedure. It is not worth putting the patient at risk.
23. Ask an FY1 doctor in passing to do the procedure and slip out quietly.
24. Slip out quietly before the nurse comes back.
25. Tell the nurse he is just a student and offer to find someone else to do the procedure.

Scenario 6
Tracy is a first year medical student and it is her first day on the ward. An FY2 shows her around the ward and as he introduces one particular patient makes a racist joke. When Tracy looks uncomfortable, the FY2 tells her to 'lighten up' and that this patient doesn't understand English.

How appropriate are the responses to this situation?

26. Do nothing and laugh along.
27. Lodge a complaint with her senior as soon as possible.
28. Lodge a complaint with her senior the next week, when she is less busy.
29. Repeat the joke to her friends later as they sit in the canteen for lunch.
30. When she is out of earshot of the other patients on the ward, take the FY2 aside and explain to him how she feels about the joke and that she is going to take this further to her senior.

Scenario 7
Mark is a 3rd year medical student on a very busy ward. While he is looking at the drug charts in one of the patient's records, he realises that the patient has been prescribed a drug that they are allergic to by mistake. The chart hasn't been signed off yet.

How appropriate are these responses to Mark's situation?

31. Say nothing – everyone is busy.
32. Cross the medication off the list himself.
33. Alert the junior doctor he is with so that the chart may be changed immediately.
34. Wait until everyone becomes less busy, then alert them about the chart.
35. Remove the chart from the patient's records.
36. Tell the patient to advise the doctors when they try to give them the medication.

For questions 36 – 69, decide how important each statement is when deciding how to respond to the situation?

A Extremely important
B Fairly important
C Of minor importance
D Of no importance whatsoever

Scenario 8

Meena, a 5th year medical student is working on a project with her clinical partner, Tom. The project involves auditing patient records. Meena has been coming in early and staying late to look at the patient records, but she notices that Tom has been taking pictures of the records on his phone.

How important are the following factor's in Meena's situation?

37. The project is due in a week's time, and they still have a lot of records to get through.
38. Their supervisor could find out.
39. They have a shared mark.
40. Patient confidentiality could be broken if someone finds the pictures.
41. He could delete the pictures later.

Scenario 9

Maria is a 5th year medical student. She is taking an online course on digital professionalism and has learnt about the importance of using social media responsibly. When she goes into placement the next day, she hears some patients talking about how one of her colleagues has tagged the hospital page on a picture of a party she was at last night. They are not impressed. When she checks her own social media, she sees she has been tagged on the same post and it shows some of the other students present at the party, drinking and smoking.

How important are the following factors in Maria's situation?

42. The reputation of the hospital may be damaged because of this post.
43. Future employers may link her back to this post and this could impact her chances of getting a job.
44. Maria is not actually in the picture and so there is a slim chance anyone at the hospital will recognise her.
45. It's not her post, and therefore not her responsibility.
46. She will be leaving the hospital in a few weeks as her rotation will change.

Scenario 10

Muhammed has been invited to a neurology conference taking place in London, where he will have the chance to listen to some talks and interact with some consultants who are specialists in their field. He has an interest in neurology and is hoping to specialise in it in the future. However, the conference is on the same day as his meeting with the educational supervisor at the hospital to sign some forms, which he cannot miss as he may not have a chance to see his supervisor again before the deadline.

How important are the following factors in Muhammed's decision?

47. The conference will be taking place next year as well.
48. If he does not submit the forms in on time, then it may go down against his record as professionalism issues.
49. His educational supervisor has specifically made the time for Muhammed to come and see him.
50. Muhammed wanted to acquire some chances for work experience in a laboratory setting with one of the researchers in the summer.
51. The conference may not be in London next year.

Scenario 11

Melissa is a 2nd year medical student in the neonatal ward. While she is talking to a patient, she notices a nurse has dropped a piece of paper with patient information, as she walked past. The patient Melissa is with has just launched into an interesting story about her condition and Melissa feels it would be rude to stop her.

How important are the following factors in Melissa's decision?

52. The patient is in full flow with her story.
53. It would be rude to stop the patient.
54. Patient details are on full display.
55. Someone else could pick up the piece of paper.
56. It is a drug chart.
57. The patient is receiving palliative care.

Scenario 12

Jeremy is a 3rd year medical student at the GP on placement. His clinical partner, Tariq has been looking increasingly dishevelled every day. Jeremy has started to notice that some of the staff have been commenting about Tariq's appearance and some of the patients have been giving Tariq nasty looks.

How important are the following factors for Jeremy in deciding what to do?

58. Jeremy's friendship with Tariq.
59. Tariq's feelings.
60. Their daily contact with patients.
61. Tariq's reputation with the staff.
62. Issues with professionalism.

Scenario 13

Edgar is a 4th year medical student on surgical placement at the hospital. While he is observing an emergency surgery, he notices that one of the nurses does not use the correct sterile technique while putting on her gloves. He knows that the surgery must be done immediately in order to save the patient's life.

How important are the following factors in Edgar's decision?

63. The patient is losing a lot of blood very quickly.
64. Everyone else is gloved up and would have to wait for the nurse to leave the theatre and get some more gloves.
65. The patient could end up contracting an infection
66. They are on a tight time limit, as there are countless other patients waiting for surgery.
67. He is only a student.
68. Everything else is sterile.
69. The nurse doesn't actually touch the surgical site.

END OF PAPER

Mock Paper D

Section A: Verbal Reasoning

Passage 1

The Teeth of Children

Children have twenty temporary teeth, which begin making their appearance about the sixth or seventh month. The time varies in different children. This is the most dangerous and troublesome period of the child's existence, and every parent will do well to consult a reputable dentist. About the second or third year the temporary teeth are fully developed. They require the same care to preserve them as is exercised toward the permanent set.

About the sixth year, or soon after, four permanent molars, or double teeth, make their appearance. Some parents mistakenly suppose these belong to the first set. It is a serious error. They are permanent teeth, and if lost will be lost forever. No teeth that come after the sixth year are ever shed. Let every parent remember this.

At twelve years the second set is usually complete, with the exception of the wisdom teeth, which appear anywhere from the eighteenth to the twenty-fourth year. When the second set is coming in the beauty and character of the child's countenance is completed or forever spoiled. Everything depends upon proper care at this time to see that the teeth come with regularity and are not crowded together. The teeth cannot have too much room. When a little separated they are less liable to decay.

1. Children's teeth begin to appear:

A. Around June or July.
B. Typically before they have their first birthday.
C. At the same time in all children.
D. Before birth.

2. Which of the following statements are true according to the above passage:

A. Temporary teeth require less care than permanent teeth.
B. Temporary molars appear when the child is around six years of age.
C. All teeth that appear after six years of age are permanent.
D. Usually wisdom teeth are finished growing at twelve years of age.

3. Which of the following statements about permanent teeth are true:

A. Permanent teeth require the same level of care as temporary teeth.
B. Permanent teeth often appear when children are four years old.
C. Permanent teeth if lost are naturally regenerated by the body.
D. All teeth are permanent.

4. Which of the following statements is INCORRECT:

A. Wisdom teeth tend to appear when a person is a young adult.
B. You never naturally shed any teeth that appear after six years of age.
C. When teeth are a little separated, decay can easily develop in between.
D. Some parents mistake molars that appear when children are six as temporary teeth.

Passage 2

The Mysteries of Hypnotism

Animal magnetism is the nerve-force of all human and animal bodies, and is common to every person in a greater or less degree. It may be transmitted from one person to another. The transmitting force is the concentrated effort of will-power, which sends the magnetic current through the nerves of the operator to the different parts of the body of their subject. It may be transmitted through the eyes, or the application of the finger tips or the whole open hands, to different regions of the body of the subject, as well as to the mind. The effect of this force upon the subject will depend very much upon the health, mental capacity and general character of the operator. Its action in general should be soothing and quieting upon the nervous system; stimulating to the circulation of the blood, the brain and other vital organs of the body of the subject. It is the use and application of this power or force that constitutes hypnotism.

Magnetism is a quality that inheres in every human being, and it may be cultivated like any other physical or mental force of which men and women are constituted. From the intelligent operator using it to overcome disease, a patient experiences a soothing influence that causes a relaxation of the muscles, followed by a pleasant, drowsy feeling which soon terminates in refreshing sleep. On waking, the patient feels rested; all their troubles have vanished from consciousness and they are as if they had a new lease of life.

In the true hypnotic condition, when a patient voluntarily submits to the operator, any attempt to make suggestions against the interests of the patient can invariably be frustrated by the patient. Self-preservation is the first law of nature, and some of the best-known operators who have recorded their experiments assert that suggestions not in accord with the best interest of the patient could not be carried out. No one was ever induced to commit any crime under hypnosis, that could not have been induced to do the same thing much easier without hypnosis.

The hypnotic state is a condition of mind that extends from a comparatively wakeful state, with slight drowsiness, to complete somnambulism, no two subjects, as a rule, ever presenting the same characteristics. The operator, to be successful, must have control of their own mind, be in perfect health and have the ability to keep their mind concentrated upon the object they desires to accomplish with his subject.

5. Which of the following statements is correct:
A. Animal magnetism cannot be transmitted from one person to another.
B. Transmission of animal magnetism is limited to transmission through the eyes.
C. The effect of animal magnetism on a person is not at all related to the health of the operator.
D. Animal magnetism can be cultivated by men and women alike.

6. According to the passage:
A. The first law of nature is self-preservation.
B. No one has ever committed a crime whilst in a hypnotic state.
C. Upon waking from a hypnotic state the patient feels very tired and stressed.
D. All hypnotic operators are healthy people.

7. Which of the following statements is supported by the above passage:
A. The initial steps required to enter a hypnotic state involve relaxation of the patient's muscles.
B. The hypnotic state is often a turbulent state of mind and results in disturbed sleep.
C. Hypnotism is a skill that can only be performed by doctors.
D. Hypnotism causes raised blood pressure and increases risk of heart attack.

8. According to the above passage, refreshing sleep during hypnotism is preceded by:
A. A pleasant feeling that is accompanied with drowsiness.
B. Muscle ache and general soreness
C. Watching a metronome for extended periods of time.
D. Disturbed sleep.

Passage 3

Tea and Coffee

Tea is a nerve stimulant, pure and simple, acting like alcohol in this respect, without any value that the latter may possess as a retarder of waste. It has a special influence upon those nerve centres that supply will power, exalting their sensibility beyond normal activity, and may even produce hysterical symptoms, if carried far enough. Its principle active ingredient, theine, is an exceedingly powerful drug, chiefly employed by nerve specialists as a pain destroyer, possessing the singular quality of working toward the surface. That is to say when a dose is administered hypodermically for sciatica, for example, the narcotic influence proceeds outward from the point of injection, instead of inward toward the centres, as does that of morphia, atropia, etc. Tea is totally devoid of nutritive value, and the habit of drinking it to excess, which so many American women indulge in, particularly in the country, is to be deplored as a cause of our American nervousness. Coffee, on the contrary, is a nerve food. Like other concentrated foods of its class, it operates as a stimulant also, but upon a different set of nerves from tea. Taken strong in the morning, it often produces dizziness and that peculiar visual symptom of overstimulus which is called muscae volilantes--dancing flies. But this is an improper way to take it, and rightly used it is perhaps the most valuable liquid addition to the morning meal. Its active principle, caffeine, differs in all physiological respects from theine, while it is chemically very closely allied, and its limited consumption makes it impotent for harm.

9. Coffee:

A. Operates as a depressant.
B. If rightly used is the most important liquid ingested with breakfast.
C. Has an active principle named theine.
D. Acts on the same nerves that tea acts upon.

10. Which of these is NOT stated as an effect of tea:

A. Pain reduction.
B. American nervousness.
C. Nerve stimulation.
D. Hysteria

11. Which of the following statements does the above passage support?

A. Tea and coffee both are drunk habitually by American women.
B. Dizziness and peculiar vision symptoms are an effect of excess caffeine
C. Theine and caffeine are both chemically and physiologically closely allied
D. Theine is a weak drug.

12. Which of the following statements is NOT supported by the above passage:

A. Caffeine when taken in high dosage can cause flies to dance.
B. The active principles in tea and coffee are chemically similar.
C. Hypodermic administration of theine proceeds outward from the point of injection.
D. Tea does not have any nutritional value.

Passage 4

How to Care for a piano

The most important thing in the preservation of a piano is to avoid atmospheric changes and extremes and sudden changes of temperature. Where the summer condition of the atmosphere is damp all precautions possible should be taken to avoid an entirely dry condition in winter, such as that given by steam or furnace heat. In all cases should the air in the home contain moisture enough to permit a heavy frost on the windows in zero weather. The absence of frost under such conditions is positive proof of an entirely dry atmosphere, and this is a piano's most dangerous enemy, causing the sounding board to crack, shrinking up the bridges, and consequently putting the piano seriously out of tune, also causing an undue dryness in all the action parts and often a loosening of the glue joints, thus producing clicks and rattles. To obviate this difficulty is by no means an easy task and will require considerable attention. Permit all the fresh air possible during winter, being careful to keep the piano out of cold drafts, as this will cause a sudden contraction of the varnish and cause it to check or crack. Plants in the room are desirable and vessels of water of any kind will be of assistance. The most potent means of avoiding extreme dryness is .to place a single-loaf bread-pan half full of water in the lower part of the piano, taking out the lower panel and placing it on either side of the pedals inside. This should be refilled about once a month during artificial heat, care being taken to remove the vessel as soon as the heat is discontinued in the spring. In cases where stove heat is used these precautions are not necessary.

13. If the piano is exposed to humidity in summer, it must remain exposed to humidity during the following winter.

A. True.
B. False.
C. Can't tell.

14. Absence of frost indicates a dry atmosphere because:

A. Dryness makes frost melt.
B. Frost causes humidity.
C. Humidity during cold temperatures in winter causes frost.
D. The melting of frost causes dryness.

15. According to the above passage, avoiding dryness:

A. Is a straight forward process.
B. Requires plant life in the same room as the piano.
C. Is essential to maintaining a piano's tuning.
D. In the summer following a humid winter may cause clicks and rattles.

16. Which of the following is true according to the passage:

A. Out of tune keys produce clicks and rattles.
B. Cracking of the sounding board causes clicks.
C. Clicks and rattles are never produced by pianos in a humid environment.
D. Stiffness in action parts and glue joints is less likely to produce clicks and rattles

Passage 5

Theosophy

Much is said nowadays about theosophy, which is really but another name for mysticism. It is not a philosophy, for it will have nothing to do with philosophical methods; it might be called a religion, though it has never had a following large enough to make a very strong impression on the world's religious history. The name is from the Greek word theosophia--divine wisdom--and the object of theosophical study is professedly to understand the nature of divine things. It differs, however, from both philosophy and theology even when these have the same object of investigation. For, in seeking to learn the divine nature and attributes, philosophy employs the methods and principles of natural reasoning; theology uses these, adding to them certain principles derived from revelation.

Theosophy, on the other hand, professes to exclude all reasoning processes as imperfect, and to derive its knowledge from direct communication with God himself. It does not, therefore, accept the truths of recorded revelation as immutable, but as subject to modification by later and personal revelations. The theosophical idea has had followers from the earliest times. Since the Christian era we may class among theosophists such sects as
Neo-Platonists, the Hesychasts of the Greek Church, the Mystics of mediaeval times, and, in later times, the disciples of Paracelsus, Thalhauser, Bohme, Swedenborg and others. Recently a small sect has arisen, which has taken the name of Theosophists. Its leader was an English gentleman who had become fascinated with the doctrine of Buddhism. Taking a few of his followers to India, they have been prosecuting their studies there, certain individuals attracting considerable attention by a claim to miraculous powers. It need hardly be said that the revelations they have claimed to receive have been, thus far, without element of benefit to the human race.

17. The idea of theosophy:

A. Is a combination of philosophy and theology.
B. Is based entirely upon scriptures.
C. Was born from the ancient Greeks.
D. Does not involve any natural reasoning.

18. Which of the following is NOT stated to be a sect of theosophy in the above passage:

A. Mystics from the mediaeval ages.
B. Hesychasts of the Roman Church.
C. Neo-Platonists.
D. Paracelsus' disciples.

19. The leader of the Theosophists:

A. Was a Buddhist monk.
B. Is a British lady that lives in India.
C. No longer practices Theosophy.
D. Was fascinated by Buddhist teachings.

20. According to the passage, the point of theosophy:

A. Is to learn about Buddhism and its teachings.
B. Is to learn how to use natural reasoning to understand religion.
C. Is to understand and learn more about God.
D. Is to spread teachings of God to the rest of the world.

Passage 6

Dreams

The Bible speaks of dreams as being sometimes prophetic, or suggestive of future events. This belief has prevailed in all ages and countries, and there are numerous modern examples, apparently authenticated, which would appear to favour this hypothesis. The interpretation of dreams was a part of the business of the soothsayers at the royal courts of Egypt, Babylon and other ancient nations.

Dreams and visions have attracted the attention of mankind of every age and nation. It has been claimed by all nations, both enlightened and heathen, that dreams are spiritual revelations to men; so much so, that their modes of worship have been founded upon the interpretation of dreams and visions. Why should we discard the interpretation of dreams while our mode of worship, faith and knowledge of Deity are founded upon the interpretation of the dreams and visions of the prophets and seers of old. Dreams vividly impressed upon the mind are sure to be followed by some event.

We read in the Holy Scripture the revelation of the Deity to His chosen people, through the prophet Joel: "And it shall come to pass, afterward, that I will pour out My Spirit on all flesh, and your sons and your daughters shall prophesy, your old men shall dream dreams, your young men shall see visions, and also upon the servants and the handmaids in those days will I pour out My Spirit." (Joel ii, 28.) Both sacred and profane history contain so many examples of the fulfilment of dreams that he who has no faith in them must be very sceptical indeed. Hippocrates says that when the body is asleep the soul is awake, and transports itself everywhere the body would be able to go; knows and sees all that the body could see or know were it awake; that it touches all that the body could touch. In a word, it performs all the actions that the body of a sleeping man could do were he awake. A dream, to have a significance, must occur to the sleeper while in healthy and tranquil sleep. Those dreams of which we have not a vivid conception, or clear remembrance, have no significance. Those of which we have a clear remembrance must have formed in the mind in the latter part of the night, for up to that time the faculties of the body have been employed in digesting the events of the day.

21. Dreams of significance only occur during a peaceful slumber.

A. True.
B. False.
C. Can't tell.

22. It is written in religious texts that dreams are divine interventions.

A. True.
B. False.
C. Can't tell.

23. What did Hippocrates NOT say about dreams:

A. That the body and soul are both alive and awake during the dreaming state.
B. That the soul sees all that the body would during the dreaming state.
C. Whilst dreaming, the soul can travel everywhere that the body would be able to in a waking state.
D. The soul can do everything the body can when we dream.

24. According to the passage, dreams:

A. Were never claimed to be spiritual by heathen nations.
B. Are only considered spiritual by religious people.
C. Have inspired some people in the way they worship deities.
D. That are vivid are less likely to be followed by an event suggested by the dream.

Passage 7

What Different Eyes Indicate

The long, almond-shaped eye with thick eyelids covering nearly half of the pupil, when taken in connection with the full brow, is indicative of genius, and is often found in artists, literary and scientific men. It is the eye of talent, or impressibility. The large, open, transparent eye, of whatever colour, is indicative of elegance, of taste, of refinement, of wit, of intelligence. Weakly marked eyebrows indicate a feeble constitution and a tendency to melancholia, Deep sunken eyes are selfish, while eyes in which the whole iris shows indicate erraticism, if not lunacy. Round eyes are indicative of innocence; strongly protuberant eyes of weakness of both mind and body. Eyes small and close together typify cunning, while those far apart and open indicate frankness. The normal distance between the eyes is the width of one eye; a distance greater or less than this intensifies the character supposed to be symbolized. Sharp angles, turning down at the corners of the eyes, are seen in persons of acute judgment and penetration. Well-opened steady eyes belong to the sincere; wide staring eyes to the impertinent.

25. Deep sunken eyes mean:

A. Lunacy.
B. Erraticism.
C. A lack of selflessness.
D. Melancholic depression.

26. If the distance between the eyes is twice the width of 1 eye means the person is more erratic.

A. True.
B. False.
C. Can't tell.

27. The passage states:

A. A person's entire personality is dependent on their eye shape.
B. A person with very small pupils are always lunatics.
C. That people with eyes that are far apart and open are more honest.
D. Elegant and intelligent people have thick eyelids.

28. Geniuses in the above passage are described as:

A. Having deep sunken eyes.
B. Always being scientists.
C. Artists or writers only.
D. Having long almond-shaped eyes.

Passage 8

Physical Exercise

The principal methods of developing the physique now prescribed by trainers are exercise with dumbbells, the bar bell and the chest weight. The rings and horizontal and parallel bars are also used, but not nearly to the extent that they formerly were. The movement has been all in the direction of the simplification of apparatus; in fact, one well-known teacher of the Boston Gymnasium when asked his opinion said: "Four bare walls and a floor, with a well-posted instructor, is all that is really required for a gymnasium."

Probably the most important as well as the simplest appliance for gymnasium work is the wooden dumbbell, which has displaced the ponderous iron bell of former days. Its weight is from three-quarters of a pound to a pound and a half, and with one in each hand a variety of motions can be gone through, which are of immense benefit in building up or toning down every muscle and all vital parts of the body.

The first object of an instructor in taking a beginner in hand is to increase the circulation. This is done by exercising the extremities, the first movement being one of the hands, after which come the wrists, then the arms, and next the head and feet. As the circulation is increased the necessity for a larger supply of oxygen, technically called "oxygen-hunger," is created, which is only satisfied by breathing exercises, which develop the lungs. After the circulation is in a satisfactory condition, the dumbbell instructor turns his attention to
exercising the great muscles of the body, beginning with those of the back, strengthening which holds the body erect, thus increasing the chest capacity, invigorating the digestive organs, and, in fact, all the vital functions. By the use of very light weights an equal and symmetrical development of all parts of the body is obtained, and then there are no sudden demands on the heart and lungs.

29. The most important appliance for gymnasium work is the wooden dumbbell.

A. True.
B. False.
C. Can't tell.

30. Which of the following is NOT true:

A. The heaviest dumbbells are a pound and a half.
B. Increasing circulation is the first objective an instructor has when teaching a beginner.
C. Increasing circulation involves exercising all the limbs as well as the abdomen.
D. Use of light weights results in symmetrical muscle development.

31. Oxygen-hunger is:

A. Something that causes increased circulation.
B. Resolved by breathing pure oxygen.
C. A consequence of lunge development.
D. Resolved through breathing exercises.

32. The muscles of the back help maintain posture:

A. True.
B. False.
C. Can't tell.

Passage 9

Facts about Sponges

Sponges belong to the animal kingdom, and the principal varieties used commercially are obtained off the coasts of Florida and the West Indies; the higher grades are from the Mediterranean Sea, and are numerous in variety.

A sponge in its natural state is a different-looking object from what we see in commerce, resembling somewhat the appearance of the jelly fish, or a mass of liver, the entire surface being covered with a thin, slimy skin, usually of a dark colour, and perforated to correspond with the apertures of the canals commonly called "holes of the sponge." The sponge of commerce is, in reality, only the skeleton of a sponge. The composition of this skeleton varies in the different kinds of sponges, but in the commercial grades it consists of interwoven horny fibres, among and supporting which are epiculae of silicious matter in greater or less numbers, and having a variety of forms. The fibres consist of a network of fibriles, whose softness and elasticity determine the commercial quality of a given sponge. The horny framework is perforated externally by very minute pores, and by a less number of larger openings. These are parts of an interesting double canal system, an external and an internal, or a centripetal and a centrifugal. At the smaller openings on the sponge's surface channels begin, which lead into dilated spaces. In these, in turn, channels arise, which eventually terminate in the large openings. Through these channels or canals
definite currents are constantly maintained, which are essential to the life of the sponge. The currents enter through the small apertures and emerge through the large ones.

33. Commercial sponges look exactly like what you would find in the wild.

A. True.
B. False.
C. Can't tell.

34. According to the passage, sponges:

A. Are a type of jellyfish.
B. Are typically light coloured.
C. Can be found in many different varieties in the Mediterranean Sea.
D. Typically found of the coast of Mexico.

35. Definite currents:

A. Are critical to sponge life.
B. Enter through small apertures and exit through them as well.
C. Are the name given to waves that carry sponges onto the shore.
D. Fluctuate depending on the tide.

36. According to the above passage, the skeletal organisation of a sponge is uniform in all sponges.

A. True.
B. False.
C. Can't tell.

Passage 10

The Claims of Osteopathy

Strictly construing the claims of osteopathic doctors, it is an anti-medicine system of practice for the cure of every disease to which the human body is liable.

Dr. Andrew T. Still, who claims to have made the discoveries that led to the establishment of the school of Osteopathy, asserts that all diseases and lesions are the result of the luxation, dislocation, or breakage of some bone or bones; this, however, is not now maintained to any great extent by his followers. Osteopathists, though, do generally claim that all diseases arise from some maladjustment of the bones of the human body, and that treatment, therefore, must be to secure the normal adjustment of the bones and ligaments that form the skeleton. They claim that a dislocation is not always necessarily the result of external violence; it may be caused by the ulceration of bones, the elongation of ligaments, or excessive muscular action.

The constriction of an important artery or vein, which may be caused by a very slightly displaced bone, an indurated muscle, or other organ, may produce an excess of blood in one part of the body, thereby causing a deficiency in some other part. A dislocated member will generally show alteration in the form of the joint and axis of the limb; loss of power and proper motion; increased length or shortening of the limb; prominence at one point and depression at another; greatly impaired circulation, and pain due to the obstruction of nerve force in the parts involved.

37. Osteopathy is the study of bones.

A. True.
B. False.
C. Can't tell.

38. Dr Andrew T. Still:

A. Established the school of Osteopathy.
B. Lied in order to gain fame.
C. Imparted teachings to his followers which are not believed by all to be true today.
D. Was the first Osteopathist.

39. The passage states that the constriction of an artery:

A. Can cause a heart attack.
B. Is only fatal if the artery is important.
C. Always causes an excess of blood at the site of constriction.
D. Can be caused by a dislocated bone impinging upon it.

40. Most osteopathists believe:

A. That all medical issues occur due to breakage of bones.
B. The incorrect positioning of bones is involved to an extent in all diseases.
C. That if all bones are in their correct position then all ligaments must be okay as well.
D. The skeleton is the most important component of the human body.

Passage 11

Hints on Bathing

There has been a great deal written about bathing. The surface of the skin is punctured with millions of little holes called pores. The duty of these pores is to carry the waste matter off. For instance, perspiration. Now, if these pores are blocked up they are of no use, and the body has to find some other way to get rid of its impurities. Then the liver has more than it can do. Then we take a liver pill when we ought to clean out the pores instead. The housewife is very particular to keep her sieves in good order; after she has strained a substance through them they are washed out carefully with water, because water is the best thing known. That is the reason water is used to bathe in. But the skin is a little different from a sieve, because it is willing to help along the process itself. All it needs is a little encouragement and it will accomplish wonders. What the skin wants is rubbing. If you should quietly sit down in a tub of water and as quietly get up and dry off without rubbing, your skin wouldn't be much benefited. The water would make it a little soft, especially if it was warm. But rubbing is the great thing. Stand where the sunlight strikes a part of your body, then take a dry brush and rub it, and you will notice that countless little flakes of cuticle fly off. Every time one of these flakes is removed from the skin your body breathes a sigh of relief. An eminent German authority contends that too much bathing is a bad thing. There is much truth in this. Soap and water are good things to soften up the skin, but rubbing is what the skin wants. Every morning or every evening, or when it is most convenient, wash the body all over with water and a little ammonia, or anything which tends to make the water soft; then rub dry with a towel, and after that go over the body from top to toe with a dry brush. Try this for two or three weeks, and your skin will be like velvet.

41. Rubbing of the skin is essential to softening it.

A. True.
B. False.
C. Can't tell.

42. According to the passage, pores:

A. Are large holes found in the skin.
B. Are responsible for exuding waste material from the body.
C. Have the singular function of perspiring.
D. Are the only method employed by the body to exude waste.

43. Bathing without rubbing:

A. Does not clean you at all.
B. Is good for cleaning the skin if hot water is used.
C. Is how to make skin soft.
D. Causes no real harm or benefit to the skin.

44. Ammonia is used when bathing because:

A. It kills bacteria.
B. It dislodges dead skin from your pores.
C. There is no other alternative.
D. It softens the water.

END OF SECTION

Section B: Decision Making

1. Tennis balls come in packs of 5, 8 and 18. Which of the following denotes an exact number of balls that cannot be reached purchasing these packs.

A. 188. B. 44. C. 13 D. 21. E. 27.

2. "It is best for teenagers to start driving when they are 17.". Which statement gives the best supporting reason for this statement?

A. Teenagers are immature and driving a car before 17 is unsafe.
B. It is illegal to drive without a provisional license which can only be obtained at 17 years of age or older.
C. Most teenagers cannot afford to buy a car until they are 17.
D. At 17 years old most teenagers have the cognitive abilities to successfully drive a vehicle.

3. Professor Moriarty is only able to give lectures on physics. All lectures on philosophy are given by physics professors. Identity is a topic in philosophy. Some maths lectures are given by physics professors. Which statement below is TRUE.

A. Professor Moriarty can give lectures on philosophy.
B. Professor Moriarty can lecture on Identity.
C. All professors that give philosophy lectures can also lecture on physics.
D. All philosophers know a lot about physics.
E. Professor Moriarty gives all of the maths lectures.

4. There are 4 different coloured cars parked in a parking lot. The yellow, red and blue cars are parked adjacent to each other. The blue car has green coloured cotton seats, the yellow car has fluffy pink cotton seats and the red car has shiny black leather seats. One of the cars with non-leather seats has white tires. A car next to the red car has orange tires. Either a car with pink or black seats has silver tires. The yellow car is opposite a car with gold tires. The red car is not next to the blue car. What colour are the yellow car's tires?

A. Gold. C. Silver. E. Cannot tell.
B. Orange. D. White.

5. All engineers are intelligent. Some engineers are funny. Jamal is intelligent and Derek is funny. Choose a correct statement.

A. An engineer can be funny as well as intelligent.
B. Derek is both intelligent and funny.
C. All funny people are intelligent as well
D. Jamal is an engineer.
E. None of the above.

6. Prakash, Ryan and Harvey are 100-metre sprinters. In order to qualify for district finals, they need to be able to set a time of less than 12 seconds. Prakash and Harvey are faster sprinters than Ryan. Ryan's best time is 12.2 seconds. Which statement must be correct?

A. Prakash and Harvey qualify.
B. All 3 sprinters qualify.
C. None of the three qualify.
D. Ryan doesn't qualify
E. None of the above.

7. Jennifer is drinking a cup of coffee which contains 95% water and 5% is dissolved coffee granules. The weight of the coffee in the cup is 100g. The cup weighs 10g. She leaves the coffee in the sun for an hour and then returns to it an hour later. Some of the water has evaporated in the sun and now the water content of the cup of coffee is 75%. What is the weight of the cup of coffee now?

A. 75g. B. 110g. C. 30g. D. 20g. E. 50g.

8. Julia, Polly and Fred own sweet shops. James and Fred own bakeries. Harrison recently became the owner of a grocery store. All the women own pharmacies, except for Holly who owns a sports shop. James, Polly and Harrison own shoe shops. Who owns the most shops?

A. Polly. B. Fred. C. James. D. Julia. E. Harrison.

9. Brian weighs less than Archith. Clarissa weighs less than Mike who weighs less than Archith. Archith and Christy weigh less than Billy. Who weighs the most?

A. Billy. B. Christy. C. Archith. D. Mike. E. Clarissa.

10. The odds of Sanjay losing his football match on a hot day is 0.1 and on a cold day is 0.3. The probability that Sanjay goes for ice cream on any day is 0.5. Sanjay has a match every single day of the week. Last week, it was cold for the last 3 days of the week. Sanjay thinks that last week he was more likely to lose his match in the cold and not eat ice cream after than he was to lose his match in the heat and eat ice cream after. Is he correct?

A. Yes.
B. No because the chance of winning the match when it is cold is greater than winning the match when it is hot.
C. No because he eats ice cream most days.
D. No because the chance of losing his match on a hot day is almost certain and the chance he loses his game on a cold day is less than half.

11. All athletes play sports. All footballers are athletes. Football and rugby are sports. Drogba is an athlete. Which statement is true?

A. All athletes play football or rugby
B. Drogba can play rugby.
C. All athletes play football as well as another sport.
D. Drogba plays football.
E. None of the above.

12. Homer has flipped 2 regular 10 pence coins 17 times. 11 times he has flipped the result has been 2 heads and 6 times the result has been 2 tails. Homer flips the 2 coins again and one lands as heads. Which statement is most likely to be correct?

A. The other coin also will land as heads.
B. The other coin will land as tails.
C. Homer is flipping both coins the same way.
D. Flipping heads is just as likely as flipping tails.
E. None of the above.

13. Alaric, David and Alex compete in a 500m cycling race. All of them cycle at a constant speed throughout the race. Alaric beats David by 50m and David beats Alex by 50m. How many metres does Alaric beat Alex by?

A. 100m. B. 95m. C. 90m. D. 80m. E. 150m.

Question 14:
Corrine has an exam today. She says that she knows she will cry later this evening. What assumption has Corrine made?

A. That the exam will have a lot of maths questions.
B. That she will be caught cheating during the exam by invigilators.
C. That the exam is going to cause Corrine stress and sadness.
D. That she will have to resit this exam multiple times.

15. "If the public elections have decided that Jed Arksey is to be the new prime minister, then the public should pay for his inauguration ceremony." Which of the following statements would weaken the argument?

A. The cost of the ceremony is too much to be funded locally.
B. Jed Arksey has the support of most of the MPs.
C. Many people did not vote for Jed Arksey.
D. Many politicians think that inauguration ceremonies are outdated.

16. Whilst discussing their family history, Isabella points to a name on their family tree and says to her son that "her sister's mother is the only daughter of my grandmother." How is the name that Isabella points to related to her?

A. Niece B. Sister C. Cousin D. Aunt E. Mother

17. In Oxford, a survey is done on a primary school. 5 children like all types of cake. 3 children like only chocolate and banana, and 13 like carrot. However, 2 like banana cake only. Only one child likes all flavours of cake but chocolate. Which Venn diagram represents this information?

A.

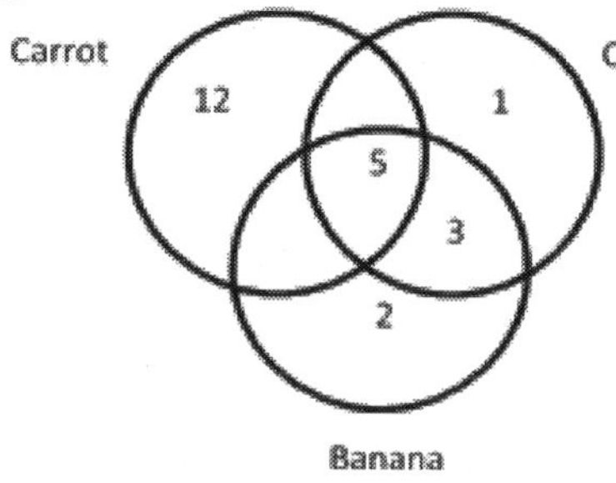

C.

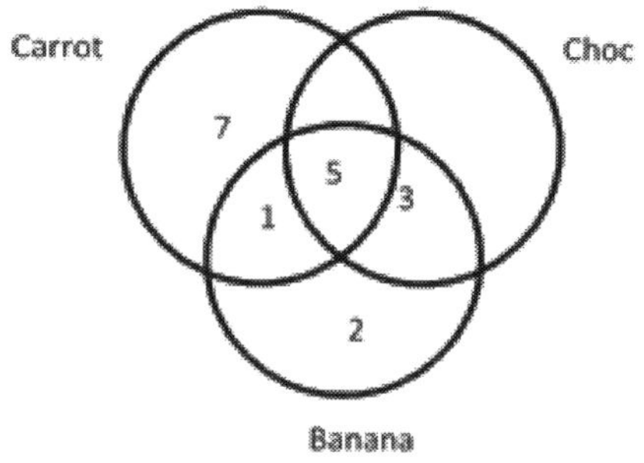

B.

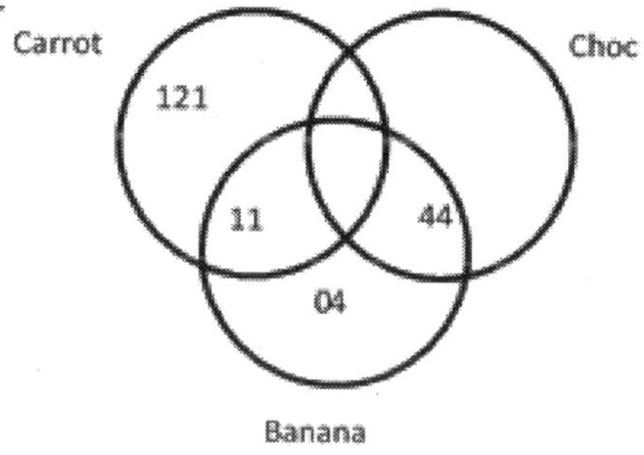

D.

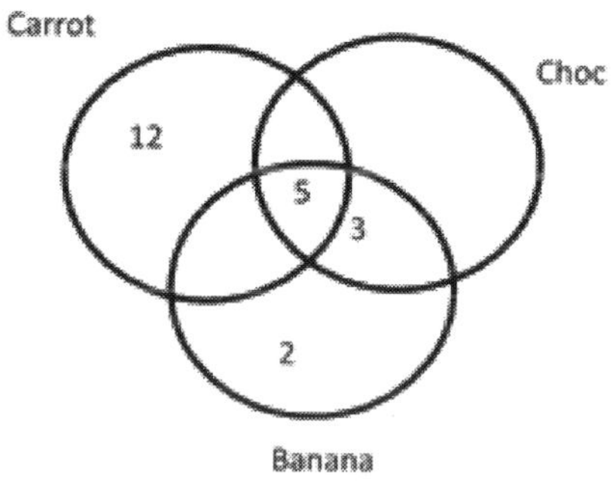

18. Harold and Fletcher play a game of 11. They have to take turns counting numbers up to 11. In a turn, they can say 1, 2 or 3 numbers. The person who says 11 wins the game. If Harold starts the game, how many numbers does he have to say to guarantee a win.

A. 1
B. 2
C. 3
D. It is impossible for Harold to win if he starts the game.

19. In a game of dance off, everyone puts their names in a hat. Each player takes turns to draw a name. If they pick their own name, it is placed back and they draw another. If the last person to pick draws their own name, everyone starts again. Imogen, Lucy and Norden play and pick in alphabetical order. Which statement is true?

A. Imogen has a one in three chance of picking and dancing against Norden.
B. Lucy is more likely to pick Imogen than picking Norden.
C. Imogen has an equal chance of dancing against Norden or Lucy.
D. Norden should reverse the order is he wants to increase his chances of dancing against Imogen.

20. Barry is sat to the right of Andrew. Charlie is sat next to Barry and Andrew. David is in front of Charlie. Eric is sat in front of Andrew. Where is David with respect to Eric?

A. David is behind Eric.
B. Eric is behind David.
C. Eric is to the right of David.
D. David is to the left of Eric.
E. Eric is to the left of David.

21. "The growing population is a growing problem, therefore there should be a tax on having more than one child." Which of the following statements would weaken the argument?

A. Having more than one child is already a high financial cost due to schooling costs.
B. People from low income backgrounds are more likely to have more than one child.
C. Cost has no effect on how many children people have.
D. People who only want 1 child will be unfairly benefited.

22. Three brothers, Peter, Max and Edwin are arguing over how many times they have been to the swimming pool this year. Peter says "We have been at least 5 times", Max says "No we have been less than 5 times", and Edwin says "We have been at least once". If only one of the brothers is telling the truth, how many times have they been to the swimming pool this year?

A. 3
B. 1
C. 0
D. 4
E. 6

23. "Living in cities is injurious to health." Which statement provides the best evidence for this conclusion?

A. People in cities exercise less than people in rural areas.
B. Fast food is cheaper in cities.
C. Cities have harmful levels of carbon monoxide in the air.
D. Increased traffic in cities means increased pollution.
E. Healthy food is more accessible in cities.

24. Will has many shoes in his wardrobe. He has 1 blue, 2 black, 4 orange and 10 red shoes. He is trying to find a pair of shoes but his house has had a power cut so he cannot see anything. How many shoes does Will have to pick to make sure he has 3 matching pairs?

A. 4.
B. 10.
C. 12.
D. 5.
E. 9.

25. Felix is taller than Bob. Bob's friend Gerard is taller than Felix. They all are basketball players. Felix is better at basketball than Gerard. Felix's brother Chris is the worst at basketball. Which statement is true?

A. Bob is better at basketball than Chris.
B. Gerard is better at basketball than Bob.
C. Bob is the shortest.
D. Chris is the tallest.
E. Felix is the worst at basketball.

26. 4 mice are placed in a square shaped maze. They each pick a random direction and walk along the edge of the square. Are the mice less likely to collide than not?

A. No because the likelihood of the mice colliding or not colliding is equal.
B. Yes as the probability they collide is 12.5%.
C. No because they are more likely to collide than they are to not collide.
D. Yes as mice do not like to be near each other.

27. "Lizards are not mammals. Some lizards are poisonous. All mammals produce offspring." Which of the following statements fits best with the given facts?

A. No lizards produce offspring.
B. Some lizards are not poisonous.
C. Some mammals are lizards.
D. Some lizards do not produce offspring.
E. Some lizards produce offspring.

28. Jacob played a game of football. He says every goal he scored was from a free kick and he scored every free kick his captain let him take. Which statement is true?

A. No goals were scored in the match that weren't from free kicks.
B. Jacob scored every goal in the match.
C. Jacob didn't have any other opportunities to score goals apart from free kicks.
D. Free kick goals were the only goals Jacob scored in the match.
E. Jacob didn't see any goals during the match that weren't from free kicks.

29. A survey was conducted in a city to learn about preferences for sport. 80 people said they liked football, 50 people said they liked rugby and 40 people said they liked cricket. 30 people said they liked all 3 sports. 0 people said they liked only football and rugby. 0 people said they only liked football and cricket. 10 people said they liked only rugby and cricket. How many people took the survey?

A. 75 B. 68 C. 110 D. 150 E. 100

END OF SECTION

Section C: Quantitative Reasoning

Data Set 1

Jake decided to take a trip up to Manchester from London. The journey by train took 2 hours 8 minutes over a distance of approximately 210 miles.

1. What was the average speed the train was travelling from London to Manchester?

A. 104.7 mph
B. 98.4 mph
C. 89.6 mph
D. 95.9 mph
E. 100.2 mph

2. If there are 1.6 kilometres in a mile, how many kilometres did Jake travel over his journey?

A. 346 km
B. 340 km
C. 336 km
D. 353 km
E. 338 km

3. Jake's sister Martha decided to drive to Manchester from London instead. It took her 3 hours 32 minutes (over approximately the same distance). How much slower was Martha's journey than Jake's, as a percentage to the nearest whole number?

A. 54%
B. 74%
C. 47%
D. 59%
E. 66%

Data Set 2

Sam is a farmer and owns a field to grow his crops. The characteristics of the field are as follows:

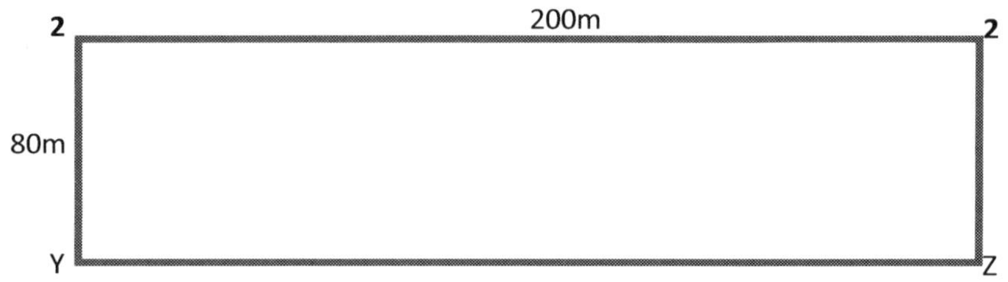

4. What is the area of the field?

A. $8000m^2$
B. $16000m^2$
C. $10000m^2$
D. $18000m^2$
E. 16000m

5. Sam's wife, Helen, jogs along the edge of the field every Saturday morning to exercise. How long does it take her to jog around the field once? Assume that she jogs at a pace of 6km/hr.

A. 5min 27sec
B. 4min 54sec
C. 5min 43sec
D. 5min 36sec
E. 5min 16sec

6. Sam uses the field to grow cabbages in rows parallel to the WX edge of the field. The first and last rows grow on the WX and YZ edges of the field, respectively. There are 50cm between each row. How many rows of cabbages are there on Sam's field?

A. 150
B. 142
C. 161
D. 156
E. 148

Data Set 3

The table shows the population of Town X, divided up into age groups.

Age Group	Population	Age Group	Population
0 - 5	6900	**46 - 50**	9050
6 - 10	6750	**51 - 55**	8400
11 - 15	8200	**56 - 60**	7850
16 - 20	7150	**61 - 65**	8350
21 - 25	6350	**66 - 70**	7500
26 - 30	6400	**71 - 75**	6450
31 - 35	8750	**76 - 80**	6000
36 - 40	7750	**81 - 85**	5700
41 - 45	9950	**86 and over**	3650

7. How many people are older than 65?

A. 25900
B. 30650
C. 29300
D. 28600
E. 23900

8. If everyone in town X retires at 65 years, what percentage of the population is within 14 years of retiring?

A. 18.76%
B. 15.42%
C. 22.87%
D. 19.53%
E. 16.68%

9. Approximately what number of the population is of working age, assuming this starts at 16?

A. 85000
B. 79000
C. 82000
D. 87000
E. 80000

10. Approximately what fraction of the population is under 30 years?

A. 1/4
B. 1/5
C. 1/3
D. 1/6
E. ½

Data Set 4

The pie chart below shows the popularity of different sports offered by a leisure centre.

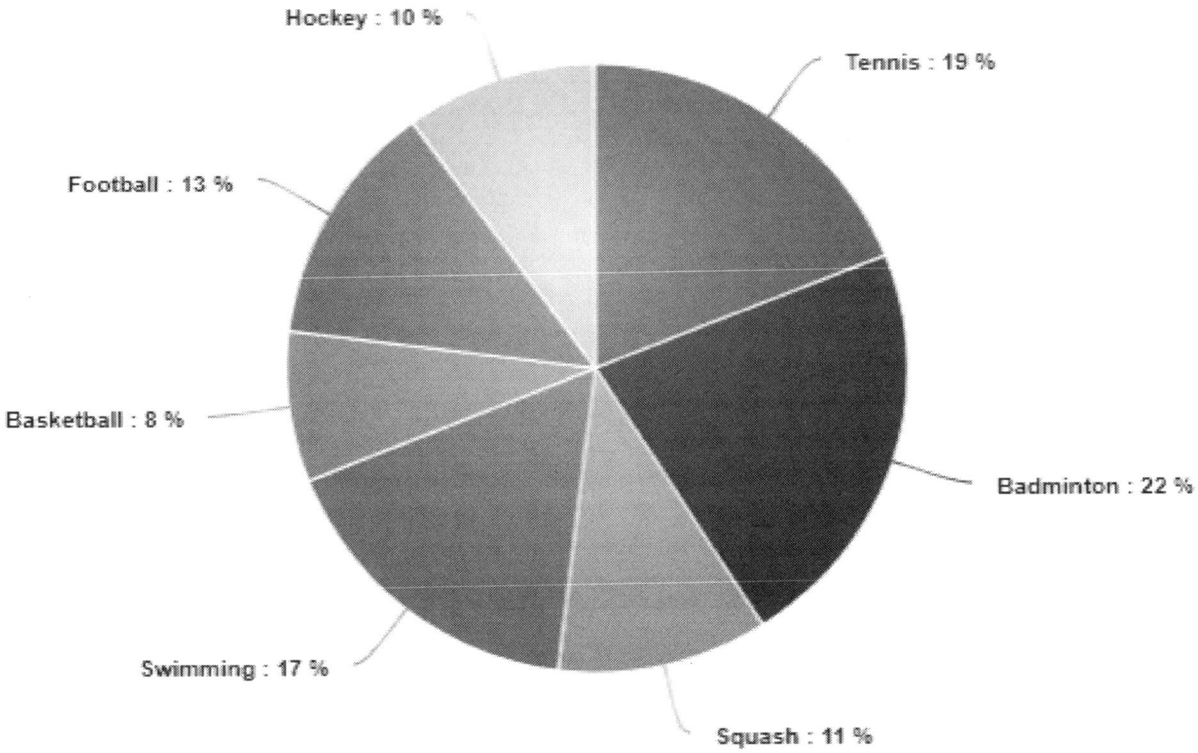

11. What is the ratio of popularity between badminton and basketball?

A. 13:6 B. 11:5 C. 15:8 D. 11:4 E. 9:3

12. By how much is football less popular than tennis, as a fraction?

A. 6/19 B. 7/18 C. 5/16 D. 7/19 E. 2/15

13. On average, approximately 570 people play a sport at the leisure centre each week. How many people play a racquet sport each week?

A. 283 B. 301 C. 294 D. 308 E. 295

Data Set 5

The graph below shows company D's sales of hot chocolate over a year.

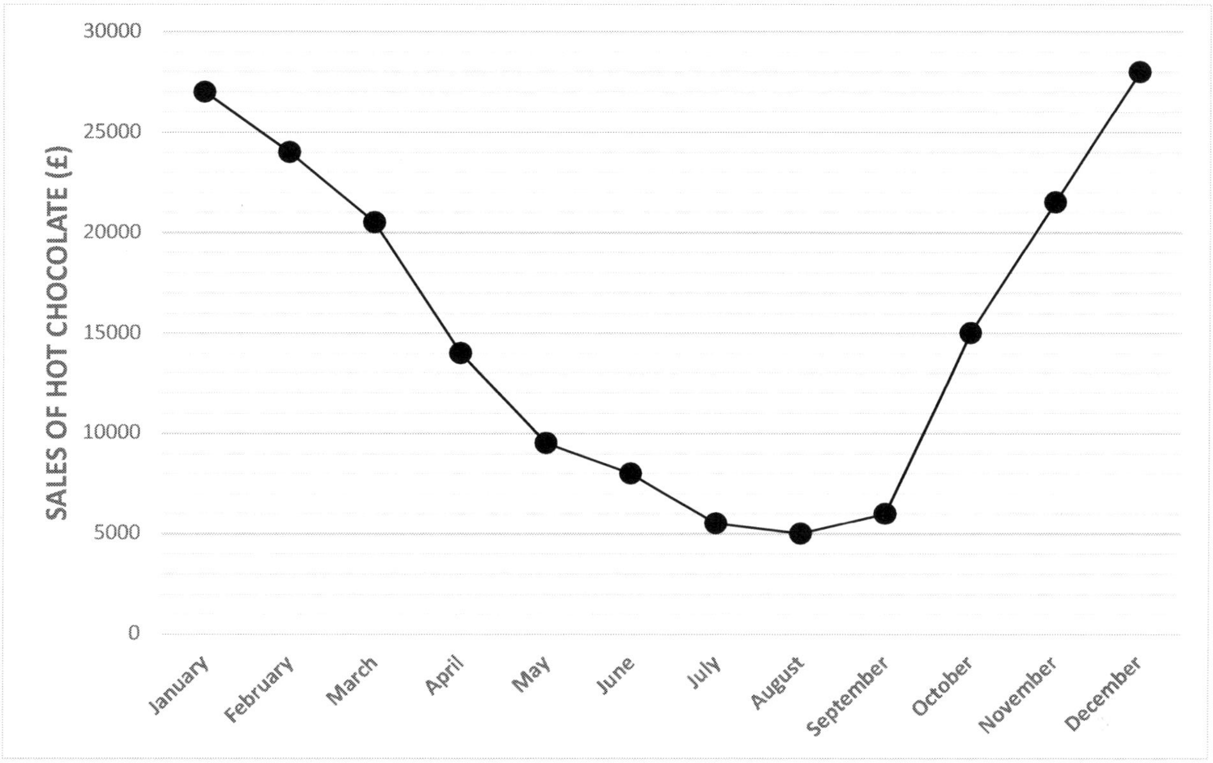

14. By how much do the sales increase from August to December?

A. 21000 B. 21500 C. 22000 D. 22500 E. 23000

15. In October company D falls short of their expected sales by 12%, how much were they expecting to make to the nearest whole number?

A. £16500
B. £17045
C. £18110
D. £17000
E. £15075

16. If each hot chocolate costs £2.50, how many hot chocolates did the company make in January?

A. 11400 B. 10800 C. 13200 D. 9900 E. 10000

Data Set 6

A company produced two variations of mango juice. They meet with two focus groups to decide which variation is preferred.

	Focus Group A	Focus Group B
Mango Juice 1	70%	55%
Mango Juice 2	25%	30%

17. What fraction of focus group B did not have a preference?

A. 3/20 B. 1/8 C. 7/40 D. 1/5 E. 7/25

18. If there are 108 people in focus group A and 110 in focus group B, how many people preferred mango juice 2 in total?

A. 55 B. 62 C. 58 D. 60 E. 63

Data Set 7

The following diagram presents student's percentages scored in the exam 'Methods in Mathematics'.

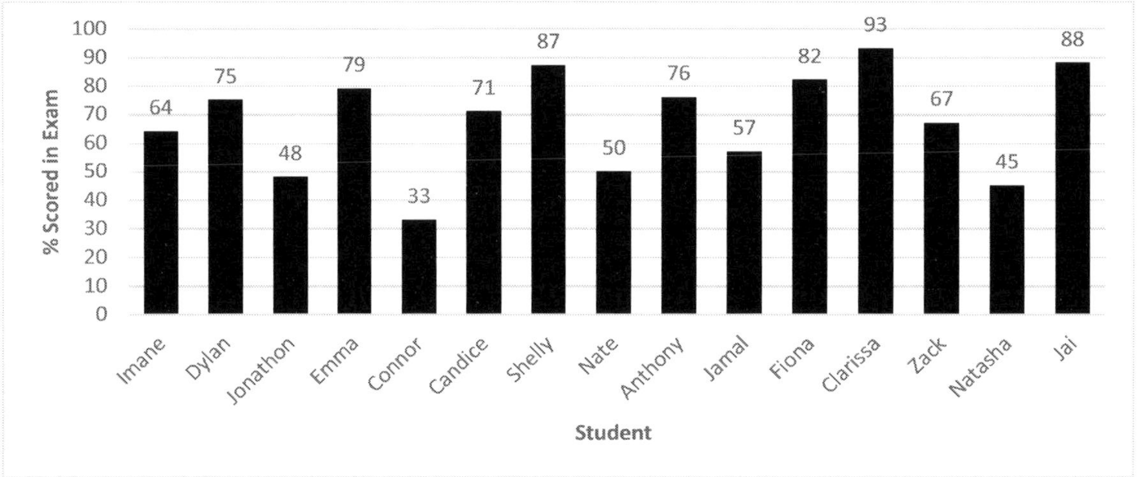

19. What is the average percentage obtained by the students?

A. 60.7%
B. 67.7%
C. 59.8%
D. 70.1%
E. 68.2%

20. If the school exam board decides that only up to 15% of students in the class should receive the maximum grade, what is the minimum threshold mark value for this?

A. 79%
B. 82%
C. 93%
D. 87%
E. 88%

21. If all students attended an extra class and the marks went up by 2% for all students, how many students would score higher than the 2 lowest scores combined?

A. 3 B. 5 C. 4 D. 1 E. 6

Data Set 8

The graph below shows the fluctuations of Company R's share price in 2007.

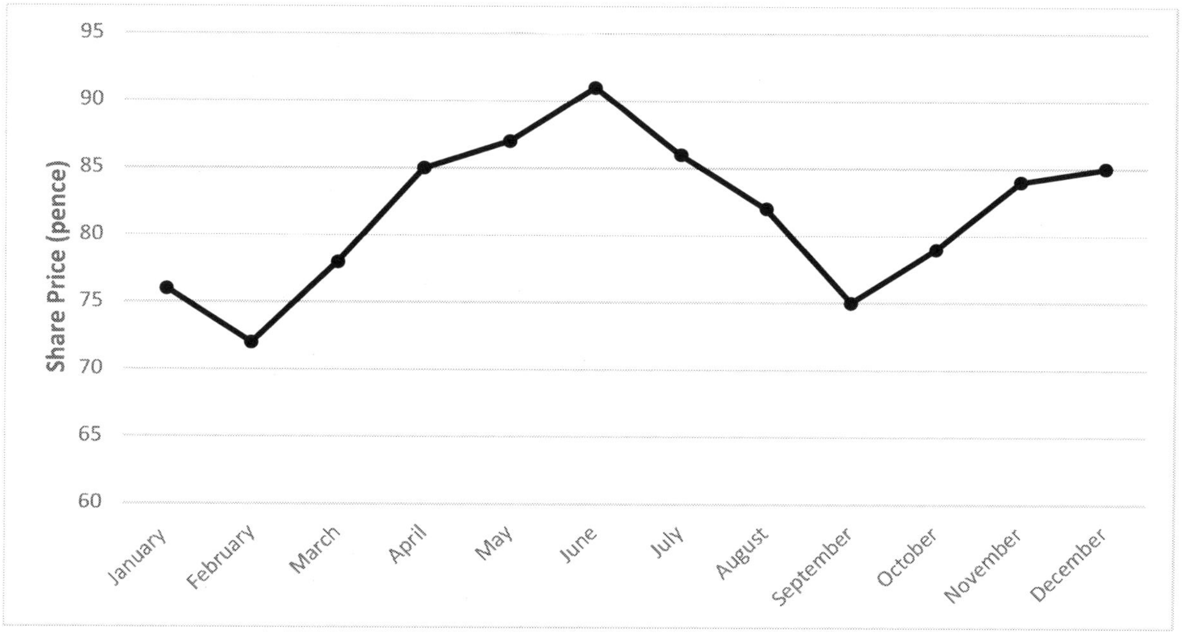

22. What fraction of the April share price is the September price?

A. 15/16 B. 14/21 C. 13/18 D. 15/17 E. 12/15

23. If the company's share price increased by 13% in January 2008, what would be its value?

A. 95.10 p B. 92.04 p C. 96.05 p D. 100.00 p E. 91.80 p

Data Set 9

The table right presents the Body Mass Index (BMI) for a group of people.

- BMI = Weight in kg / (Height in m)^2
- Normal Range: 18.5-24.9
- Overweight: 25.0-29.9
- Obese: 30.0 or more

Person	Weight (kg)	Height (m)
A	72	1.70
B	49	1.55
C	54	1.40
D	68	1.80
E	57	1.60

24. Which person has the lowest BMI?

A. A B. B C. C D. D E. E

25. Person F has a BMI of 17.6 but would like to be within the normal range. If person F currently weighs 45kg, how much weight would they need to gain?

A. 4kg B. 7.5kg C. 2.5kg D. 1kg E. 5kg

26. Person G is 1.7m and has a BMI of 28.0. Approximately what fraction of their weight would they have to lose to be within the normal BMI range?

A. 1/8 B. 1/10 C. 1/15 D. 1/6 E. 1/12

Data Set 10

The next set of questions concerns the cost of chicken and chips at a fast food restaurant.

27. If 3 portions of chicken and 4 portions of chips cost a total of £20.95, and 4 portions of chicken and 5 portions of chips cost £27.10, what equations would be used to determine the price of each item?

A. $3x + 4y = 20.95$; $4x + 5y = 27.10$
B. $6c + 8g = 2095$; $2c + y = 2600$
C. $h + t =$ £6.10 ; $2h + 3t =$ £14
D. $f =$ £4.20 ; $e =$ £2.65
E. $2x + 6y = 20.95$; $5x + 4y = 27.10$

28. If the price of chicken increases by 10% and the price of chips increase by 5%, what would be the cost of a portion of chicken and chips, to the nearest penny?

A. £7.54 B. £8.88 C. £6.00 D. £10.02 E. £6.65

29. The restaurant also accepts payment in other currencies. If a tourist purchases 2 portions of chicken and 5 portions of chips in dollars ($) at the original prices, how much would they pay? Assume that £1 = $1.39.

A. $29.55 B. $32.46 C. $25.98 D. $27.52 E. $30.72

Data Set 11

A weightlifting team were required to check the weights of their entrants before a competition.

Team Member	Alex	Jay	Thomas	Kyran	James
Weight	78kg	13 stone 7lb	11 stone 11lb	82kg	97kg

1kg = 2.2 lb

1stone = 14 lb

30. How much does Kyran weigh in lb?

A. 176.3 lb B. 184.0 lb C. 180.4 lb D. 192.5 lb E. 169.8 lb

31. How much does Alex weigh in stones and lb?

A. 10 stone 4 lb
B. 12 stone 0 lb
C. 12 stone 4 lb
D. 11 stone 9 lb
E. 13 stone 2 lb

32. What is the total weight of the boys in kg?

A. 398.4kg B. 417.9kg C. 476.3kg D. 502.8kg E. 454.7kg

33. Approximately how much lighter is Alex than James, as a fraction?

A. 1/5 B. 1/8 C. 1/4 D. 1/6 E. 1/10

Data Set 12

The graph shows the production of weed killer by a company in 10,000 litres between the years 1998-2005.

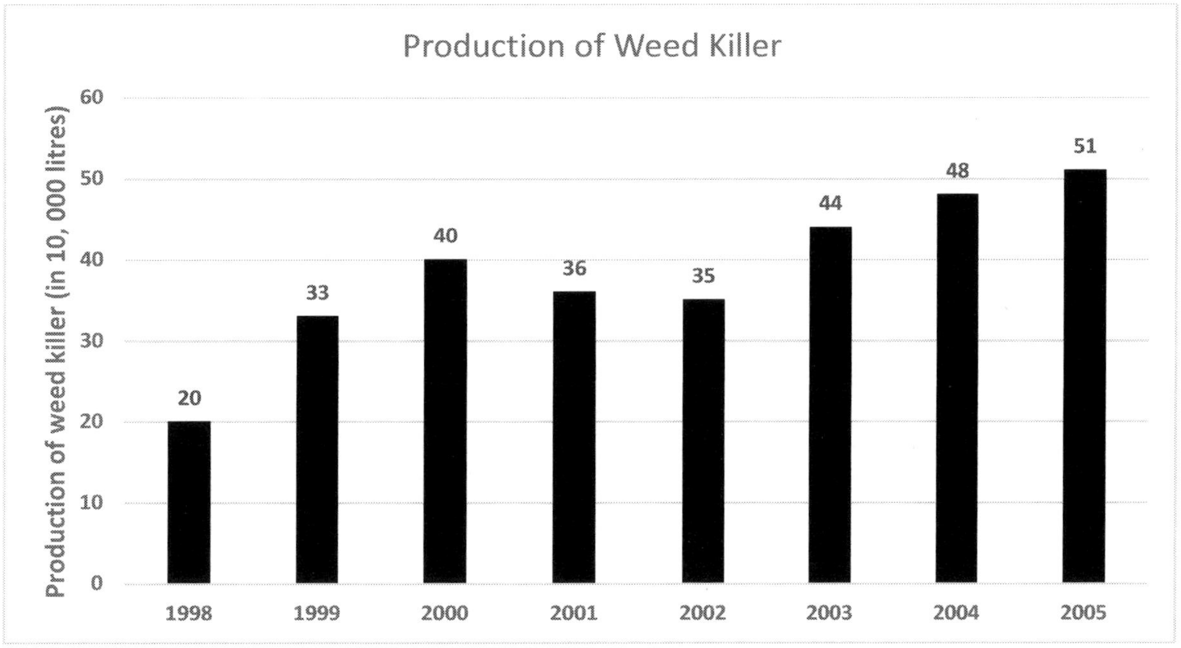

34. What was the percentage increase in the production of weed killer from 1998 to 1999?

A. 54% B. 72% C. 65% D. 49% E. 73%

35. In how many of the years was the production of weed killer more than the average production in the period shown above?

A. 1 B. 2 C. 3 D. 4 E. 5

36. In 2006 the company shut down one of the factories producing the weed killer, reducing the amount produced to 350,000 litres for that year. What was the decrease in production of weed killer from 2005 to 2006 as a decimal?

A. 0.431 B. 0.517 C. 0.298 D. 0.314 E. 0.277

END OF SECTION

Section D: Abstract Reasoning

For each question, decide whether each box fits best with Set A, Set B or with neither.

For each question, work through the boxes from left to right as you see them on the page. Make your decision and fill it into the answer sheet.

Answer as follows:
A = Set A
B = Set B
C = neither

Set 1:

Set A

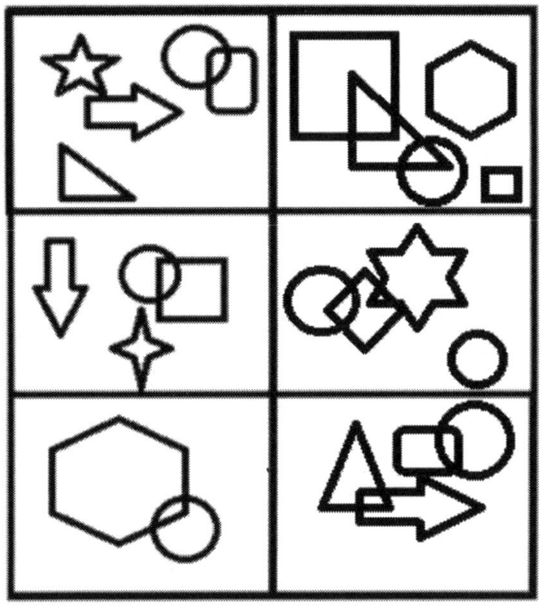

Set B

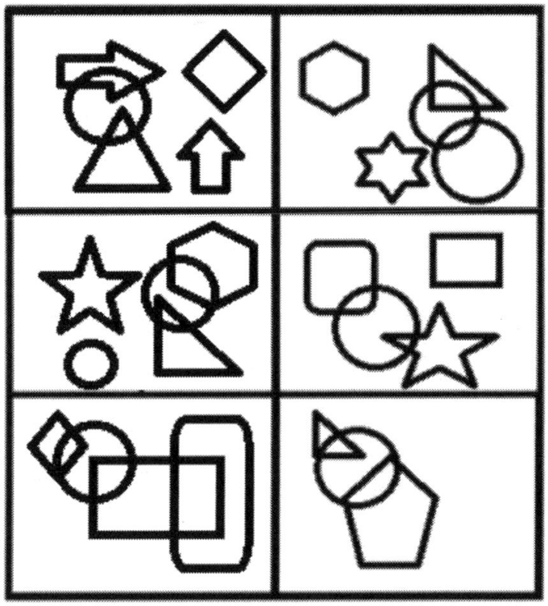

Questions 1-5

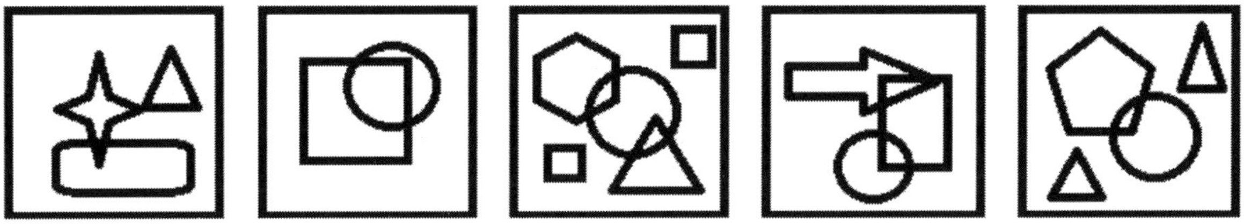

Set 2: **Set A** **Set B**

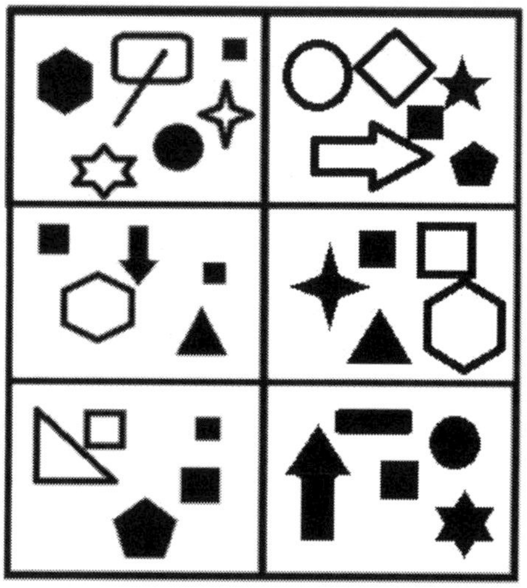

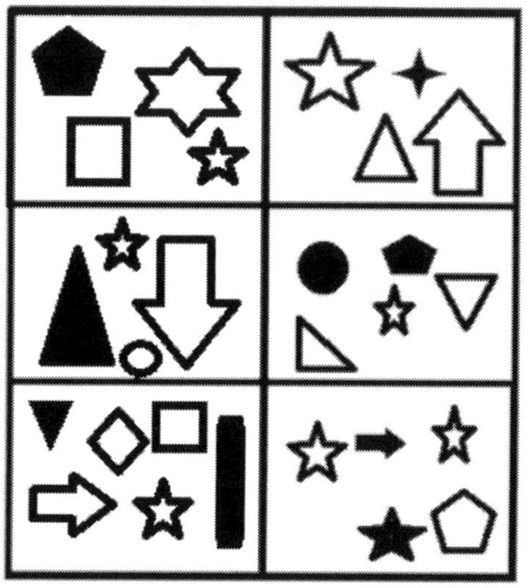

Question 6-10

Set 3: **Set A** **Set B**

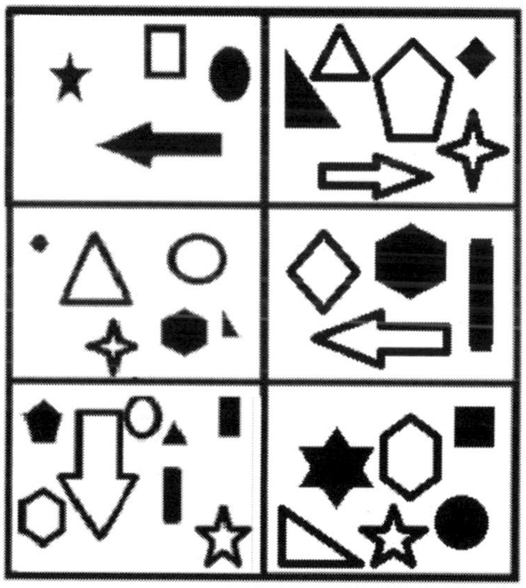

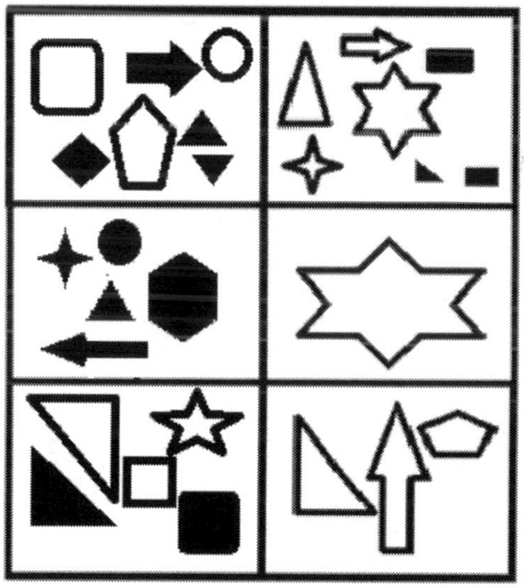

Questions 11-15:

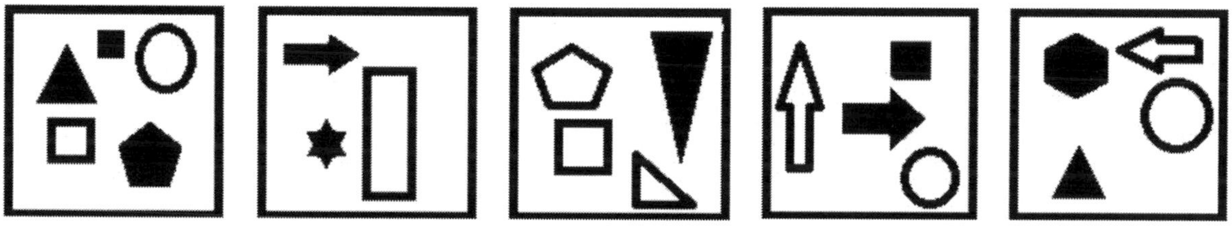

Set 4: **Set A** **Set B**

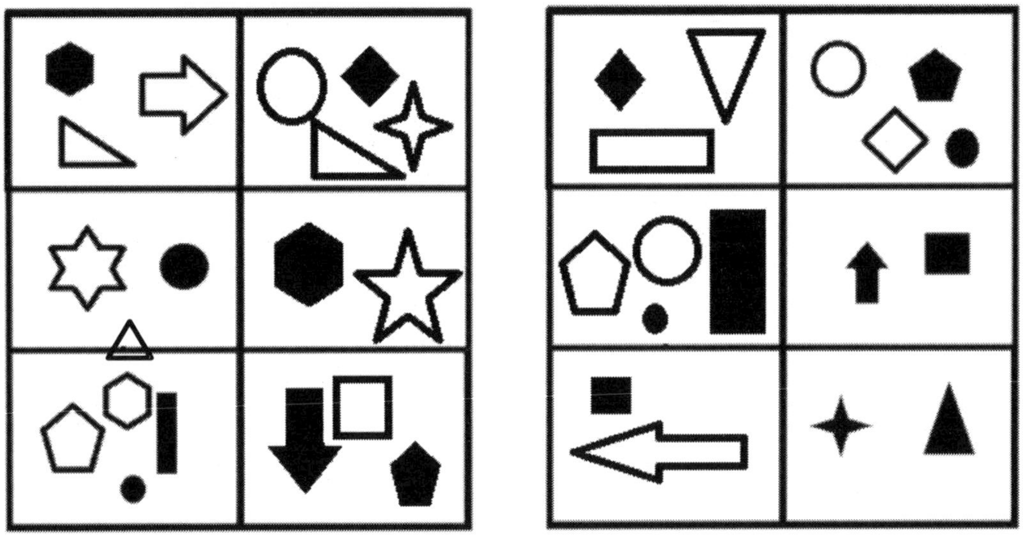

Question 16-20

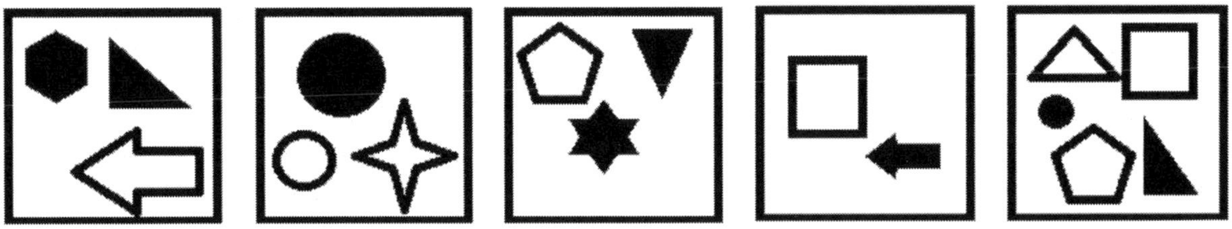

Set 5: **Set A** **Set B**

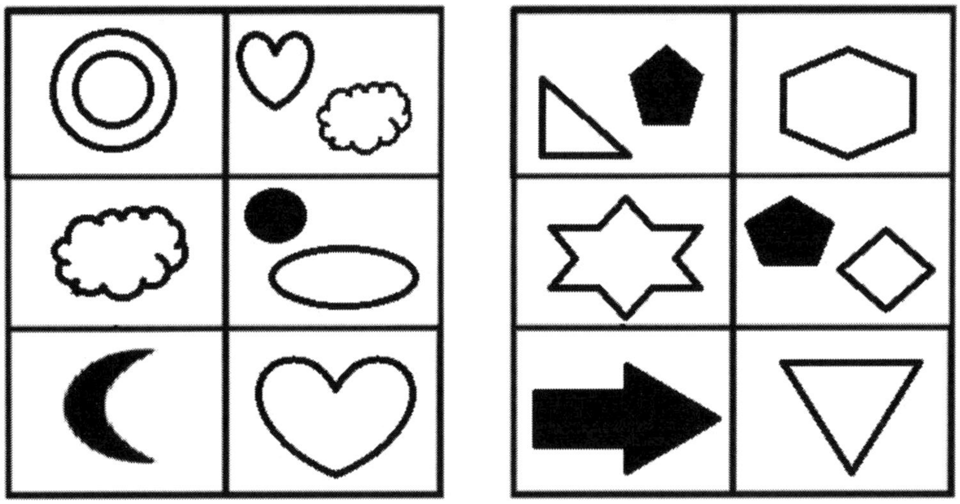

Questions 21-25

For the next set of questions, decide which figure completes the series.

Set 6:

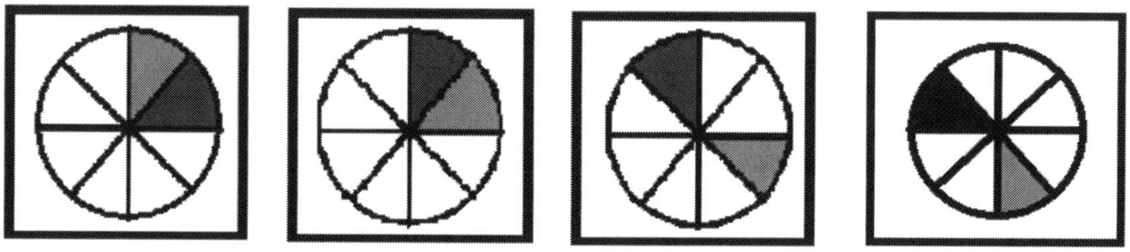

Question 26

A B C D

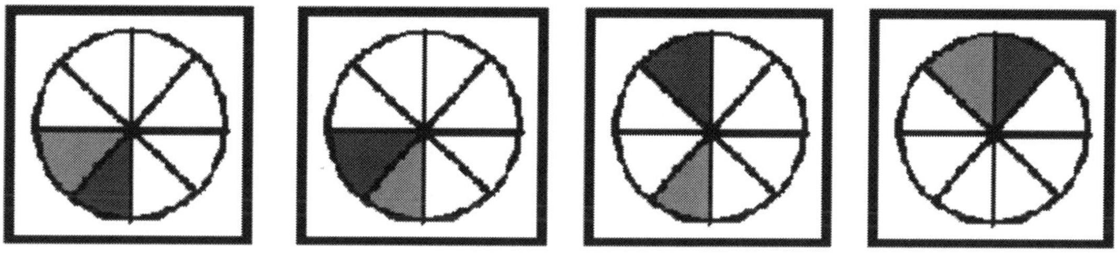

Set 7:

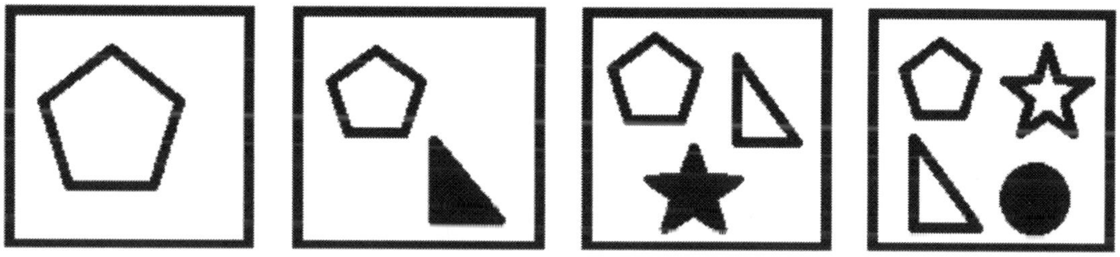

Question 27

A B C D

For the next set of questions, decide which figure completes the statement

Set 8:

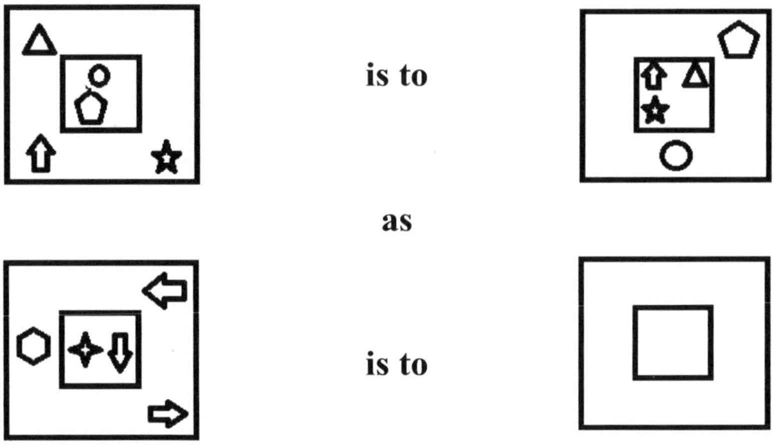

Question 28

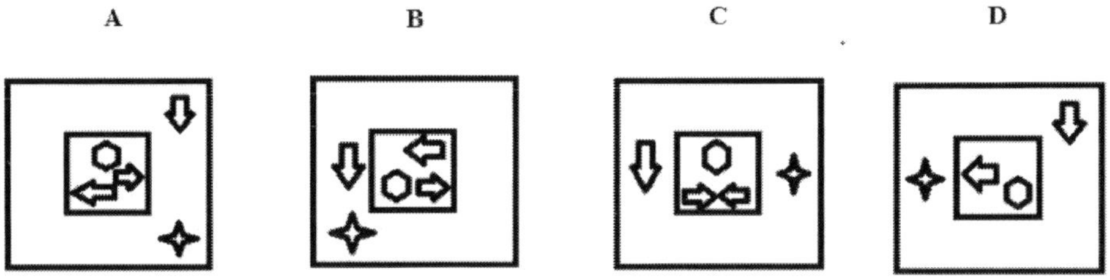

Set 9:

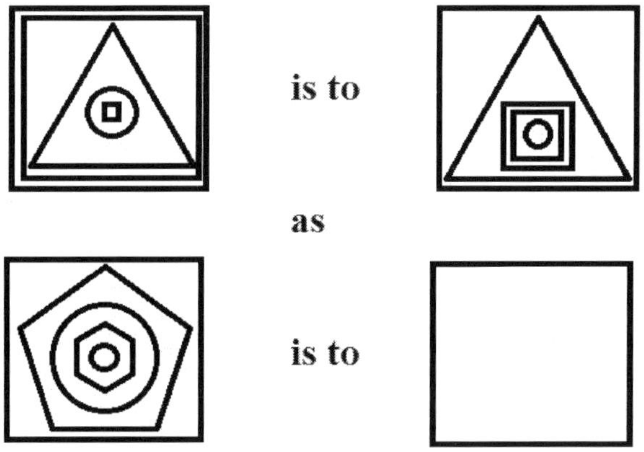

Question 29

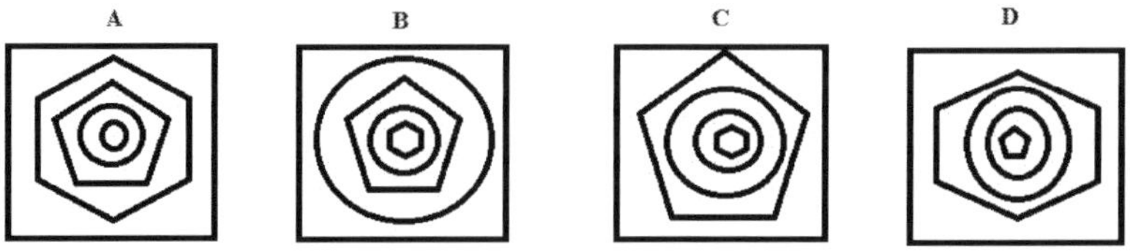

For the next set of questions, decide which of the options fits with the set stated.

Set 10:

Set A

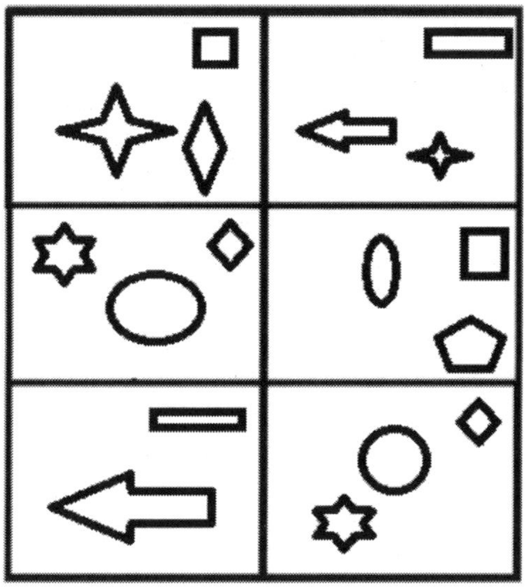

Set B

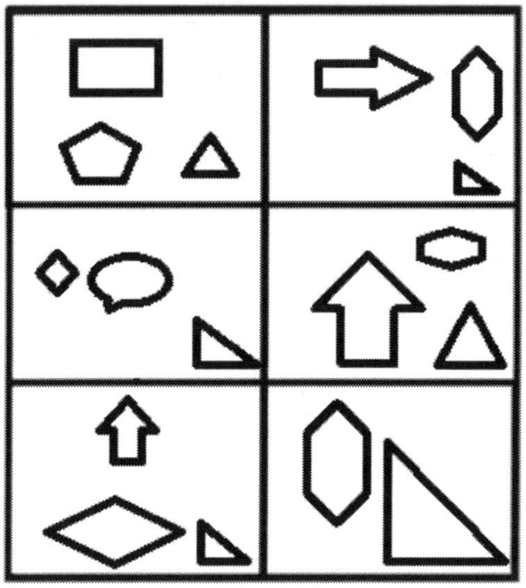

Question 30

Which of the following belongs in Set A?

A

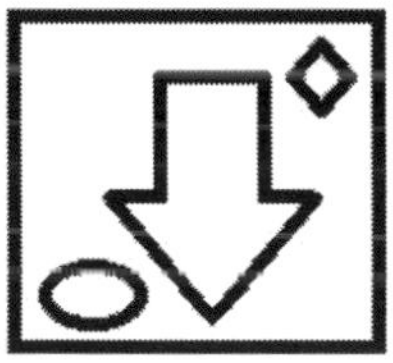

B

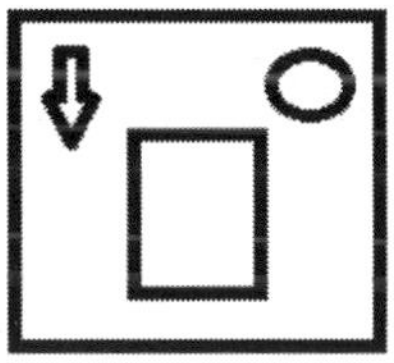

C

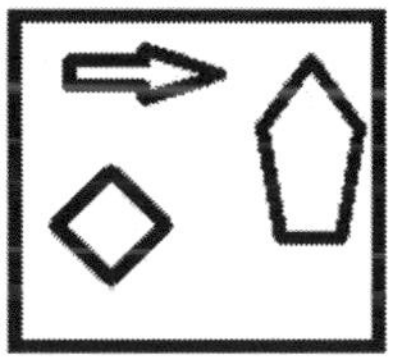

D

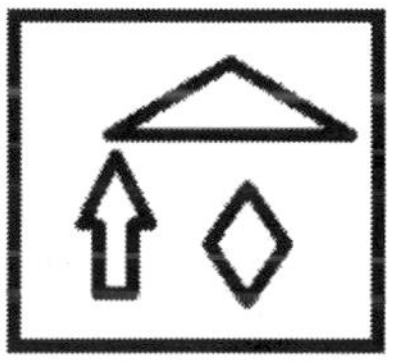

Question 31

Which of the following belongs in Set B?

A

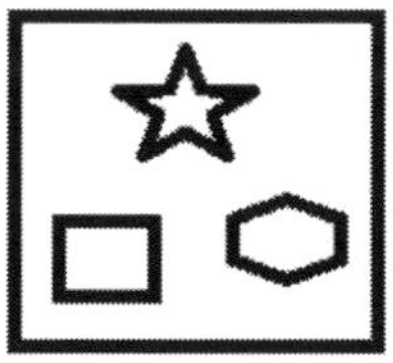

B

C

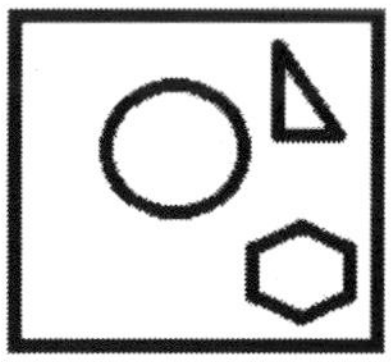

D

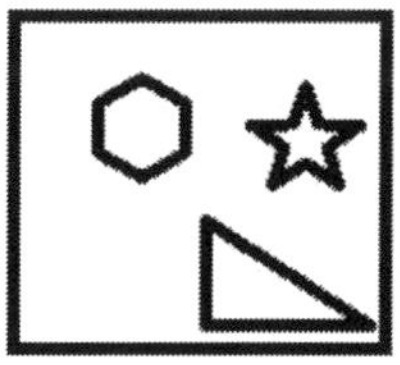

For the next set of questions, decide whether each box fits best with Set A, Set B or with neither.

Set 11:

Set A

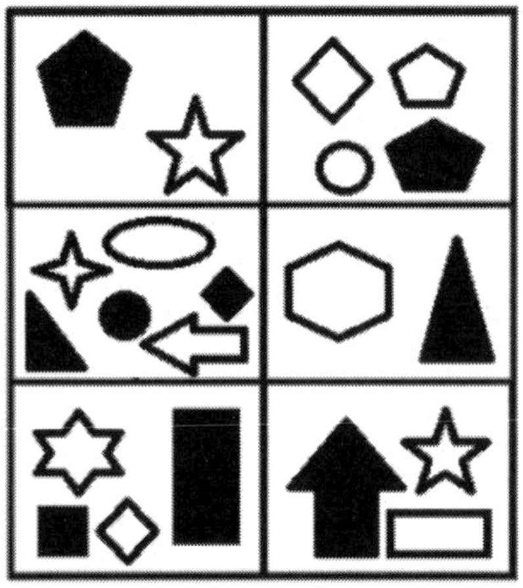

Set B

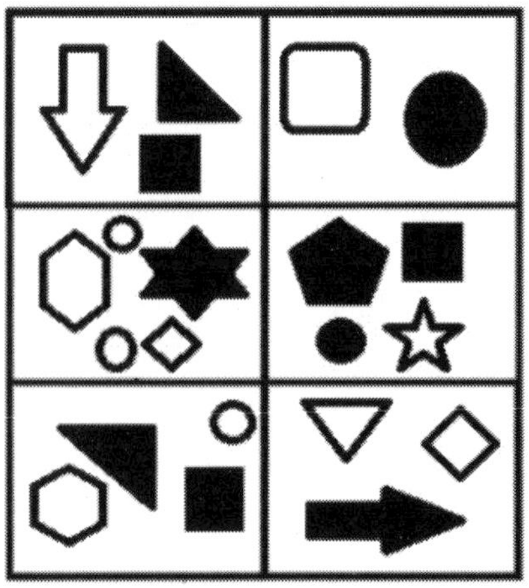

Questions 32-36

Set 12:

Set A

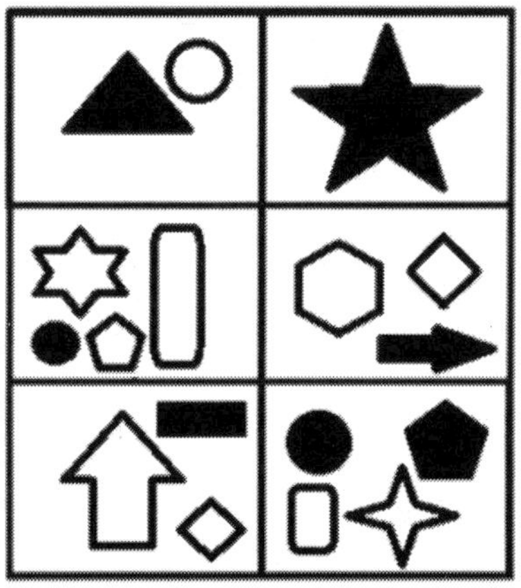

Set B

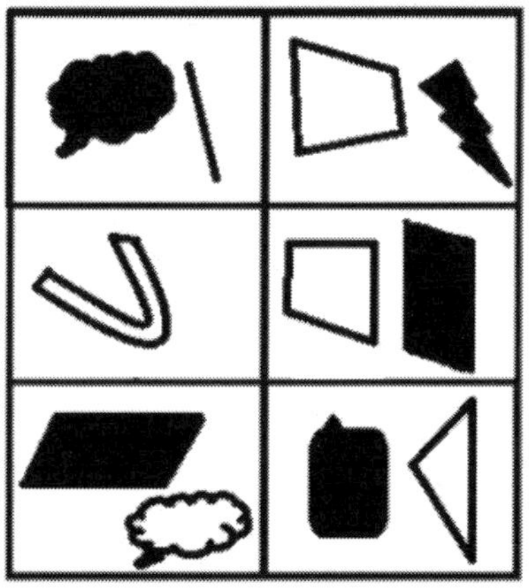

Questions 37-41

Set 13:

Set A

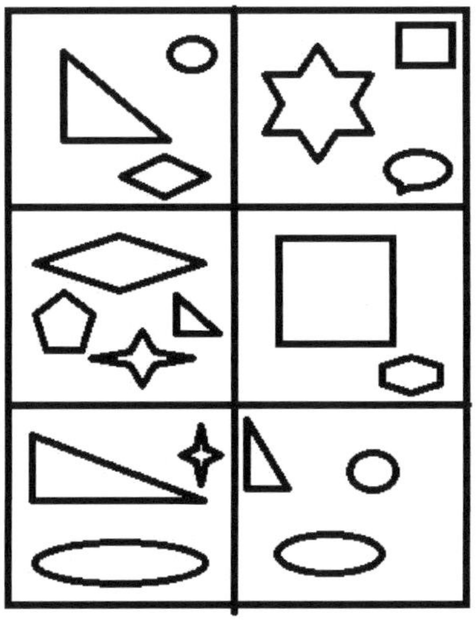

Set B

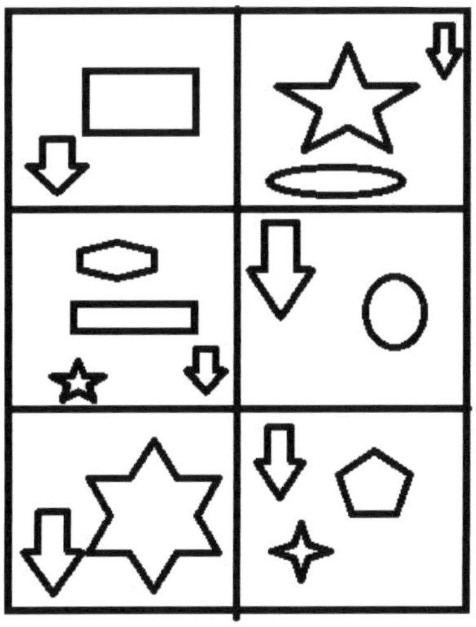

Questions 42-46

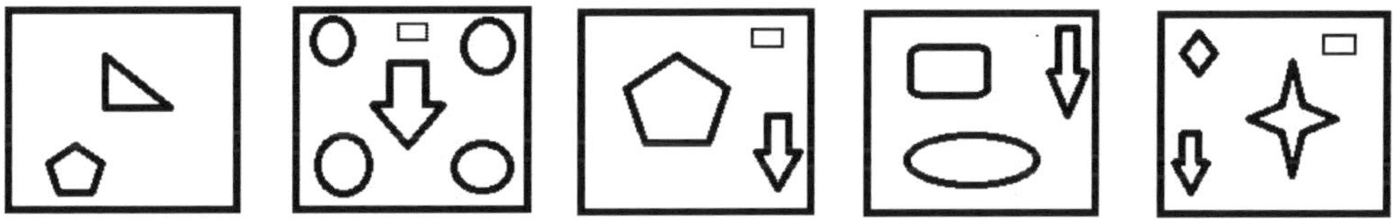

Set 14:

Set A

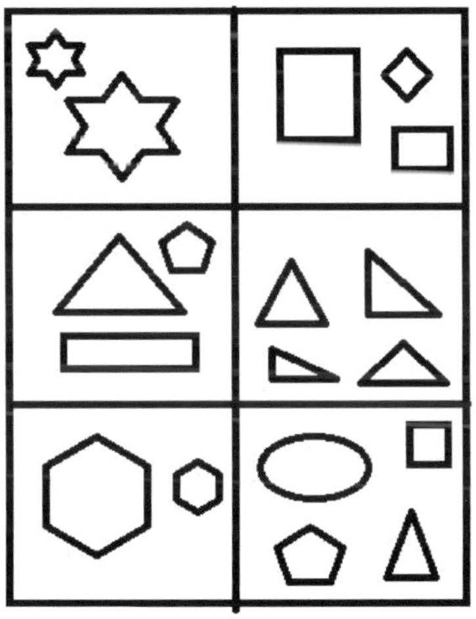

Set B

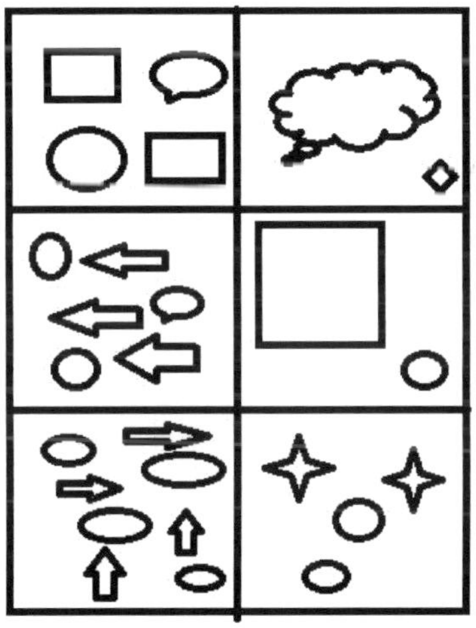

Questions 47 – 51

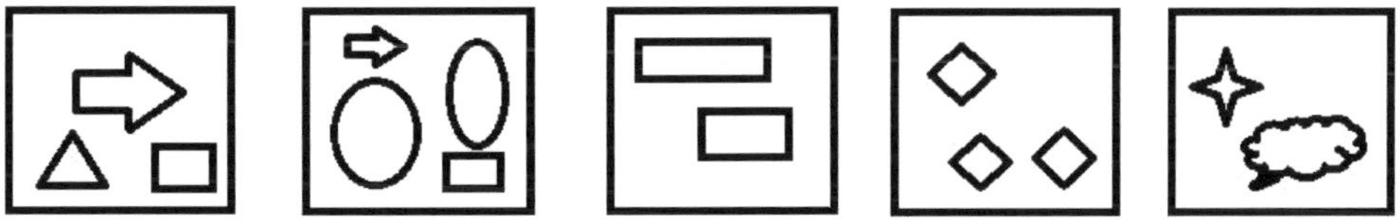

For the next set of questions, decide which figure completes the series.

Set 15:

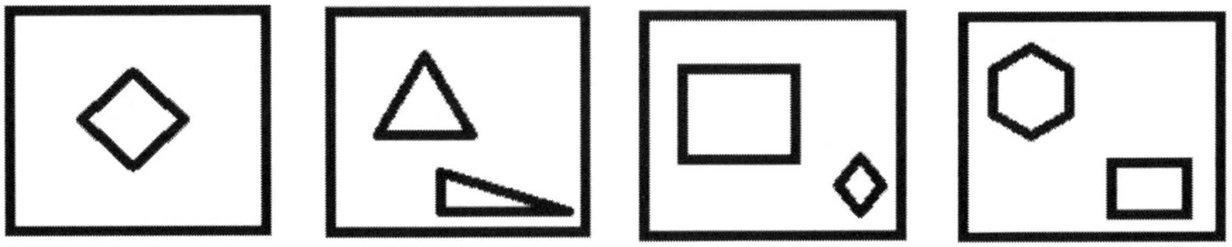

Question 52

A B C D

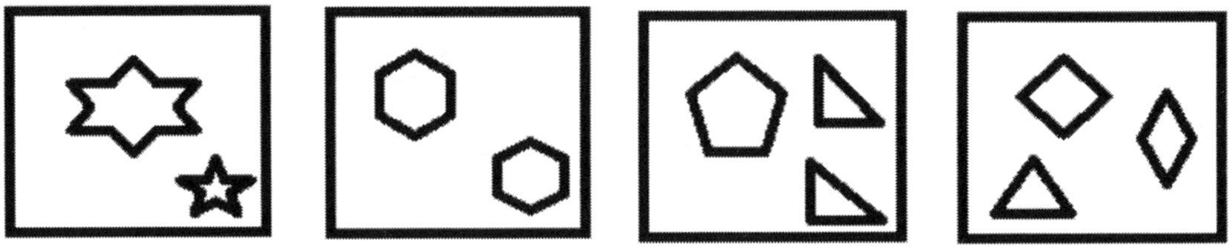

Set 16:

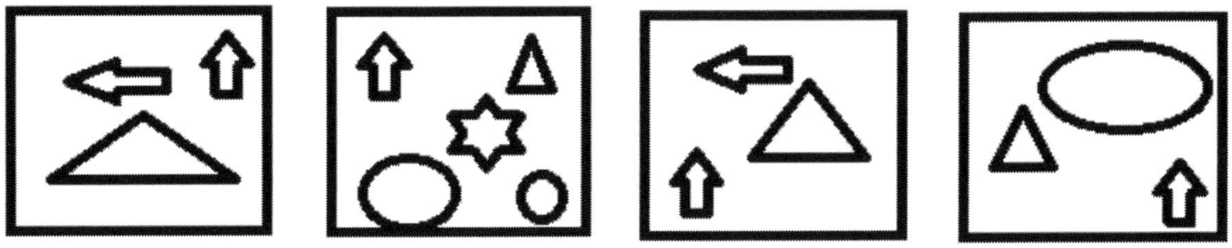

Question 53

A B C D

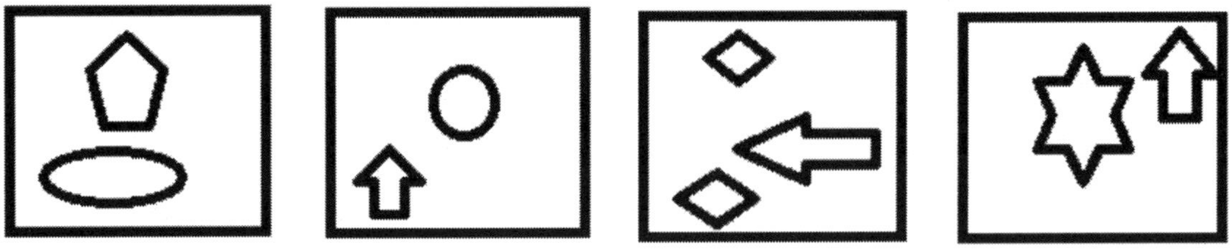

For the next set of questions, decide which of the options fits with the set stated.

Set 17:

Set A

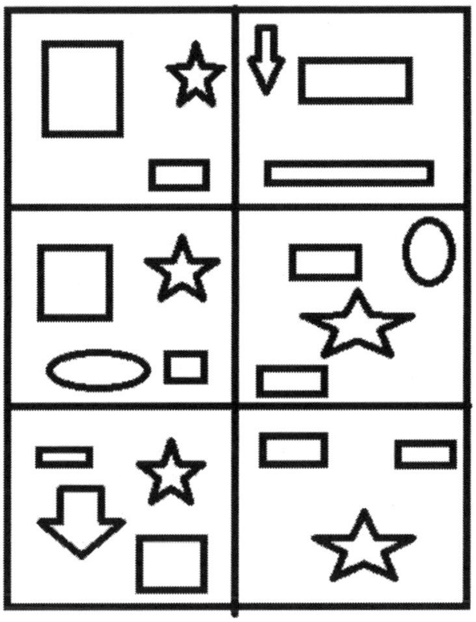

Set B

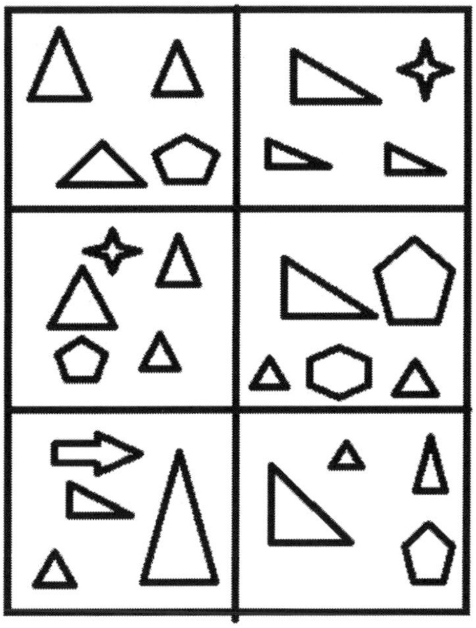

Question 54

Which of the following belongs in Set A?

A

B

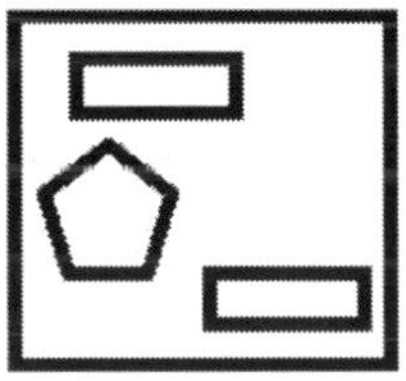

C

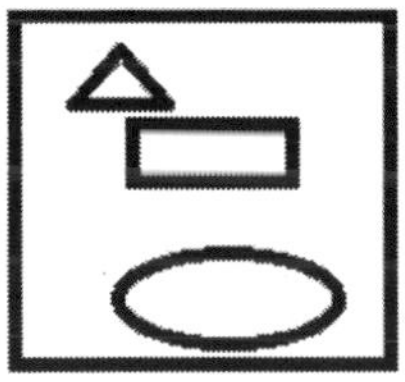

D

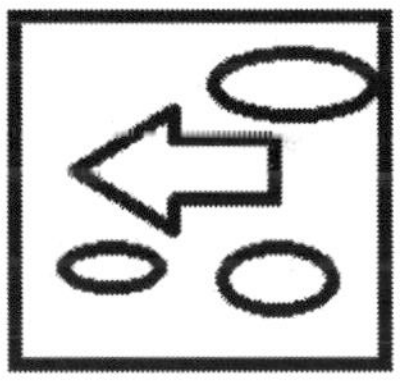

Question 55

Which of the following belongs in Set B?

A

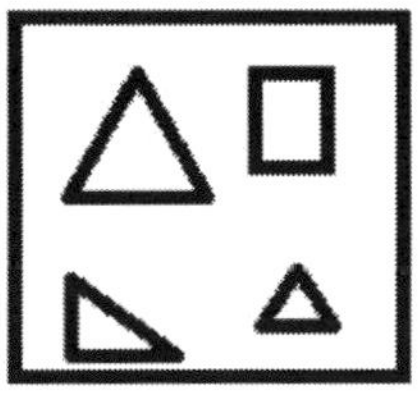

B

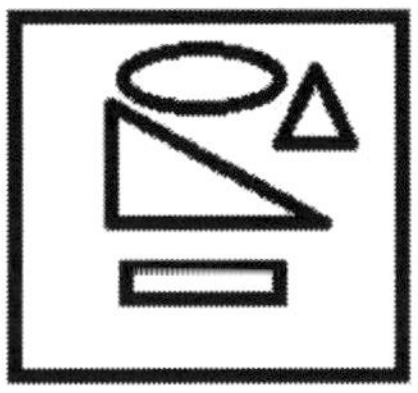

C

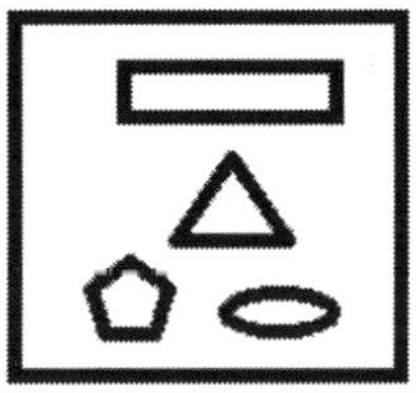

D

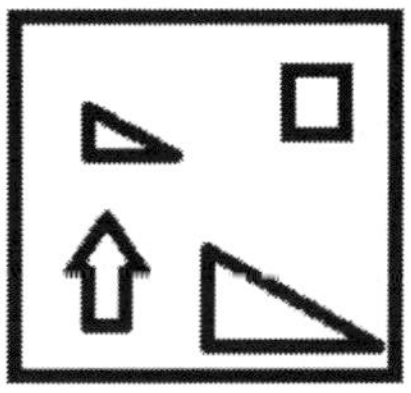

END OF SECTION

Section E: Situational Judgement Test

Read each scenario. Each question refers to the scenario directly above. For each question, select one of these four options. Select whichever you feel is the option that best represents your view on each suggested action.

For questions 1 – 30, choose one of the following options:

A **A highly appropriate action**
B **Appropriate, but not ideal**
C **Inappropriate, but not awful**
D **A highly inappropriate action**

Scenario 1
Afolarin is a first-year medical student. He plays for the university lacrosse team which has 3 training sessions a week, 1 match a week and 1 social a week. Having finished his first term, Afolarin knows he is considerably behind on work and is struggling to keep up due to his lacrosse commitments. Afolarin loves lacrosse and it is beneficial for his mental wellbeing. Afolarin has end of year exams coming and he is worried he will fail if he continues to play lacrosse.

How appropriate are the following actions to Afolarin's problem?

1. Study harder in the day time and try and fit more time to study into the day when he isn't playing lacrosse.
2. Stop playing lacrosse altogether for a month before exams.
3. Continue to play lacrosse but avoid going to the social so he has 1 more evening a week to study for his exams.
4. Speak to his coach about his concerns and try and create a new training schedule so that he has enough time to study for his exams.
5. Quit playing lacrosse as his medical degree is more important to him than his love of lacrosse.

Scenario 2
Jamal is a second-year medical student who has recently undertaken an additional project. This project will add value to Jamal and help develop his experimental technique. The project however is time consuming and the final submission for the project is 2 weeks before his 2nd year medical school exams. Jamal is keen to progress as a scientist however he does not want to jeopardise his medical exams.

How appropriate are the following responses by Jamal?

6. Quit the project and focus on his exams.
7. Continue with the project and fit preparation for his medical exams into the 2 weeks after the project submission deadline.
8. Allocate equal working hours to the project and to studying for his exams from now on.
9. Ask his peers who are also undertaking the project how they are planning to manage their time.
10. Speak to the project administrators and see if he can have an extension on the project deadline due to his upcoming exams.

Scenario 3
Jacob is a second-year medical student. He has been looking forward to the ski trip for a long time because he has booked a nice chalet with an amazing view and is staying with a group of his best friends from his course. He took out a small loan to be able to pay for this trip, and has spent a lot of time planning it. Unfortunately, the end-of-year exam results have just come out, and he has only passed 4 out of 5 exams. He only failed by 4%, but must re-sit this final exam in order to continue with his studies. The re-sit is scheduled to be only three days after his return from the ski trip.

How appropriate are the following responses to Jacob's dilemma?

11. Go on his trip and try and fit all the revision into the three days before the exam – he only failed by 4% anyway.
12. Cancel the entire trip and let his friends go without him.
13. Ask his friends if they can all reschedule for the following year.
14. Take revision with him on the ski trip – it'll be an active holiday but maybe he can study in his free time.
15. Go for part of the trip but return early to ensure sufficient time for revision.

Scenario 4

Ronit and Shloke are first year medical school students doing an experiment in biochemistry lab. They are using corrosive acids in an experiment. The professor has clearly instructed that for health and safety reasons everyone must wear lab coats and safety glasses. Shloke notices that Ronit isn't wearing his safety glasses and when prompted Ronit simply shrugs and dismisses it.

How appropriate are the following actions from Shloke?

16. Immediately alert the professor that Ronit isn't following protocol.
17. Do nothing as no harm will probably befall Ronit during the practical.
18. Tell all the surrounding classmates that Ronit isn't following protocol.
19. Explain to Ronit why following protocol is important and encourage him to wear his safety glasses.
20. Give Ronit his own safety glasses.

Scenario 5

Juan is a 4th year medical student who has just started his clinical training. During his induction he was told to just observe for the first 2 weeks of term and to not actively participate in any procedures. The following Friday is extremely busy in A&E and Juan is shadowing a nurse. She is applying pressure to a wound when she receives an urgent phone call. The nurse asks Juan to apply pressure to the wound just for a minute whilst she attends to the phone call.

How appropriate are each of the following responses by Juan in this situation?

21. Act like he didn't hear what the nurse said and go to the toilet.
22. Put on sterile gloves and immediately apply pressure to the wound.
23. Tell the nurse that he isn't allowed to and politely refuse.
24. Explain to the nurse what he was told at the induction and offer to go find someone else to cover the nurse whilst she attends to her phone call.
25. Tell the nurse okay and then ask the patient to apply pressure to their own wound.

Scenario 6

Nicolas and Jessica are first-year medical students. They are in their first anatomy class where they are observing dissected cadavers. As soon as the demonstrator removes the sheet covering the body Nicolas immediately starts to feel dizzy and becomes extremely pale but doesn't say anything. Jessica notices that Nicolas looks unwell.

How appropriate are the following actions by Jessica in this situation?

26. Say nothing as Nicolas isn't saying anything probably because he doesn't want attention.
27. Ask Nicolas if he is feeling okay and get him a glass of water.
28. Tell the demonstrator that Nicolas is unwell and needs to leave the room.
29. Open the window so Nicolas gets some fresh air.
30. Ask the demonstrator to re-cover the body and see if Nicolas feels better.

For questions 31 – 69, decide how important each statement is when deciding how to respond to the situation?

A **Extremely important**
B **Fairly important**
C **Of minor importance**
D **Of no importance whatsoever**

Scenario 7

Alvin is a 2nd year medical student. He has been offered the opportunity to interview a prominent scientist in an area of medicine he is interested in pursuing. The interview is in 2 days' time however Alvin has an essay due in for the day after the interview.

How important are the following factors for Alvin's decision?

31. The likelihood that this interview will benefit his career.
32. How quickly Alvin is able to write the essay.
33. Whether Alvin is going to have any other opportunities to interview this scientist.
34. How much this essay is going to help him in his end of year exams.
35. Alvin's reputation with the professor who will mark his essay.

Scenario 8

Damion and Phillipa are 5th year clinical medical students. They are currently collaborating on a statistical project which involves analysing patient data. Damion is one day speaking to his friend who tells him that Phillipa was explaining their project. Damion realises that Phillipa has accidentally been revealing patient data to some of her peers.

How important are the following factors for Damion in deciding what to do?

36. Completing the project before the deadline.
37. The breach of patient confidentiality by Phillipa.
38. The grade that Damion receives for the project is the same that Phillipa gets.
39. Clinical staff may find out about the breach in patient confidentiality.
40. The patient data revealed is largely harmless and will probably not be shared by Phillipa's peers.
41. The project may be invalidated.

Scenario 9

Carlos is 4th year medical student who has just started clinical school. In a clinical workshop he was lectured to about how important it is to look professional in the hospital. During his first rotation Carlos notices that the consultant he is shadowing frequently looks dishevelled and untidy when in the ward.

How important are the following factors for Carlos in deciding on what to do?

42. His rapport with the consultant.
43. His consultant will determine his final grade.
44. The consultant's appearance may reflect badly on Carlos in front of the patients.
45. The workshop on looking professional was optional to attend.
46. The consultant is extremely good at his job regardless of his appearance.

Scenario 10

Arran is a 6th year medical student. He has been invited to sit in on a rare surgical procedure that many medical students do not get to see. This is a fantastic opportunity to get experience that will stand him in good stead for the future. A day before the surgery Arran becomes ill with tonsillitis. Arran feels he is well enough to be able to attend the surgery however his illness could put the patient in the surgery at risk.

How important are the following factors for Arran to consider in deciding on what to do?

47. This opportunity will probably not arise again.
48. He has had tonsillitis before and he knows he can attend the surgery and remain focussed.
49. His illness could put the patient in the surgery at risk.
50. If he doesn't attend the surgery then the doctors may not offer similar opportunities in the future.
51. He knows that some of his friends have gone in to the hospital when they have been ill.

Scenario 11

Abraham is a 2nd year medical student. He has optional chemical pharmacology seminars on Wednesday afternoons. Abraham wants to attend these seminars so he can show his depth of knowledge in the end of year exams. Abraham is also a keen football player and football practice for the university team clashes with his chemical pharmacology seminars.

How important are the following factors for Abraham in deciding on what to do?

52. Abraham has been playing really well for his team recently and is in contention for the captaincy next year.
53. The chemical pharmacology lecturer is the examiner for the end of year exams.
54. The chemical pharmacology lecturer is a huge football fan and often comes to watch the university team play.
55. The information learned in the optional seminars will probably only improve his marks in the end of year exams a little.
56. The football team also has training sessions on other days of the week.

Scenario 12

Cameron and Brandon are 5th year medical students. One day when they are both in the clinic Cameron notices that Brandon looks extremely tired. Cameron and Brandon have suturing training later that day which involves patient contact. Cameron knows that Brandon went drinking last night and didn't get to sleep until quite late.

How important are the following factors to Cameron's situation?

57. Cameron knows that Brandon is skilled at suturing and will probably be alright.
58. Brandon's tiredness could compromise patient safety.
59. Brandon would be embarrassed if Cameron confronted him about being in hospital in an unsuitable state.
60. Brandon may look tired but maybe he feels completely fine.
61. Brandon has previously been in trouble with the medical faculty.
62. Cameron may cause problems in his friendship with Brandon if he confronts him.

Scenario 13

Jason is a 3rd year medical student currently working on a project which involves helping a research group with parts of their experiments. The research team lead offers Jason the opportunity to do some extra work during August in his summer holidays and in return he will get his name on the paper if it is published. Jason is very keen to get a publication in his name however he was planning to go on cricket tour with his teammates in August.

How important are the following factors for Jason in deciding what he should do?

63. Jason has been looking forward to this tour for a long time.
64. There is no guarantee that the paper will get published.
65. A publication in his name will help him in his future career.
66. Cricket tour occurs annually.
67. Jason's friends may be annoyed if he cancels on cricket tour.
68. Refusing to work in summer may create a bad image of Jason in the eyes of the research team lead.
69. Jason does not want to spend his summer cooped up in a lab.

END OF PAPER

Mock Paper E

Section A: Verbal Reasoning

Passage 1

"WAL, of all the dinners that ever a white man sot down to, this yere is the beat!"

The speaker was Godfrey Evans—a tall, raw-boned man, dressed in a tattered, brown jean suit. He was barefooted, his toil-hardened hands and weather-beaten face were sadly soiled and begrimed, and his hair and whiskers looked as though they had never been made acquainted with a comb. As he spoke he drew an empty nail-keg from its corner, placed a board over the top of it, and seating himself, ran his eye over the slender stock of viands his wife had just placed on the table.

The man's appearance was in strict keeping with his surroundings. The cabin in which he lived and everything it contained told of the most abject poverty. The building, which was made of rough, unhewn logs, could boast of but one room and a loft, to which access was gained by a ladder fastened against the wall. It had no floor and no windows, all the light being admitted through a dilapidated door, which every gust of wind threatened to shake from its hinges, and the warmth being supplied by an immense fire-place with a stick chimney, which occupied nearly the whole of one end of the cabin. There were no chairs to be seen—the places of these useful articles being supplied by empty nail-kegs and blocks of wood; and neither were there any beds—a miserable "shake-down" in one corner being the best in this line that the cabin could afford. Everything looked as if it were about to fall to pieces. Even the rough board table on which the dinner was placed would have tumbled over, had it not been propped up against the wall.

1. Which of the following statements is true regarding the above passage?

A. Godfrey Evans is a rich man
B. Godfrey Evans is unmarried
C. Godfrey Evans is clean-shaven
D. Godfrey Evans uses nail-kegs as chairs

2. Which of the following can be inferred from the above passage?

A. Godfrey Evans is an educated ma
B. Godfrey Evans is of Caucasian descent
C. Godfrey Evans lives in an urban area
D. Godfrey Evans has two children

3. Based on the above passage, what does Godfrey most likely do for a living?

A. Lawyer
B. Politician
C. Unemployed
D. Farmer

4. Which year is the above passage most likely to be set in?

A. 3007
B. 2018
C. 1996
D. 1878

Passage 2

William Allen, the eminent chemist, was born in London. His father was a silk manufacturer in Spitalfields, and a member of the Society of Friends. Having at an early period shown a predilection for chemical and other pursuits connected with medicine, William was placed in the establishment of Mr. Joseph Gurney Bevan in Plough Court, Lombard Street, where he acquired a practical knowledge of chemistry. He eventually succeeded to the business, which he carried on in connection with Mr. Luke Howard, and obtained great reputation as a pharmaceutical chemist. About the year 1804, Mr. Allen was appointed lecturer on chemistry and experimental philosophy at Guy's Hospital, at which institution he continued to be engaged more or less until the year 1827. He was also connected with the Royal Institution of Great Britain, and was concerned in some of the most exact experiments of the day, together with Davy, Babington, Marcet, Luke Howard, and Dalton. In conjunction with his friend Mr. Pepys, Allen entered upon his well known chemical investigations, which established the proportion of carbon in carbonic acid, and proved the identity of the diamond with charcoal; these discoveries are recorded in the 'Philosophical Transactions' of the Royal Society, of which he became a member in 1807. The 'Transactions' for 1829 also contain a paper by him, based on elaborate experiments and calculations, concerning the changes produced by respiration on atmospheric air and other gases. Mr. Allen was mainly instrumental in establishing the Pharmaceutical Society, of which he was president at the time of his death. Besides his public labours as a practical chemist, he pursued with much delight, in his hours of relaxation, the study of astronomy, and was one of the original members of the Royal Astronomical Society. In connection with this science, he published, in 1815, a small work entitled 'A Companion to the Transit Instrument.'

5. William Allen was a:

A. Scientist
B. Gardener
C. Farmer
D. Lawyer

6. Which of the following statements is true regarding the above passage?

A. William Allen always worked by himself
B. William Allen worked in a hospital
C. William Allen was only a member of one society
D. William Allen always worked by himself

7. Which of the following statements is FALSE regarding the above passage?

A. William Allen was the president of a Royal Society
B. William Allen made publications about astronomy
C. William Allen discovered carbonic acid
D. William Allen's father was a silk manufacturer

8. Based on the above passage, which of the following statements can be inferred?

A. William Allen made a significant contribution to science
B. William Allen was an only child
C. William Allen remained unmarried until his death
D. William Allen died of tuberculosis

Passage 3

Before earth and sea and heaven were created, all things wore one aspect, to which we give the name of Chaos—a confused and shapeless mass, nothing but dead weight, in which, however, slumbered the seeds of things. Earth, sea, and air were all mixed up together; so the earth was not solid, the sea was not fluid, and the air was not transparent. God and Nature at last interposed, and put an end to this discord, separating earth from sea, and heaven from both. The fiery part, being the lightest, sprang up, and formed the skies; the air was next in weight and place. The earth, being heavier, sank below; and the water took the lowest place, and buoyed up the earth.
Here some god—it is not known which—gave his good offices in arranging and disposing the earth. He appointed rivers and bays their places, raised mountains, scooped out valleys, distributed woods, fountains, fertile fields, and stony plains. The air being cleared, the stars began to appear, fishes took possession of the sea, birds of the air, and four-footed beasts of the land.

But a nobler animal was wanted, and Man was made. It is not known whether the creator made him of divine materials, or whether in the earth, so lately separated from heaven, there lurked still some heavenly seeds. Prometheus took some of this earth, and kneading it up with water, made man in the image of the gods. He gave him an upright stature, so that while all other animals turn their faces downward, and look to the earth, he raises his to heaven, and gazes on the stars.

9. Chaos is a god
A. True B. False C. Can't Tell

10. Which is the lightest part of these options?
A. The skies B. Earth C. Water D. Woods

11. Humans are made in the image of God
A. True B. False C. Can't Tell

12. The Earth was created by:
A. God B. Nature C. God and Nature D. Prometheus

Passage 4

Merlin was the son of no mortal father, but of an Incubus, one of a class of beings not absolutely wicked, but far from good, who inhabit the regions of the air. Merlin's mother was a virtuous young woman, who, on the birth of her son, entrusted him to a priest, who hurried him to the baptismal fount, and so saved him from sharing the lot of his father, though he retained many marks of his unearthly origin.

At this time Vortigern reigned in Britain. He was a usurper, who had caused the death of his sovereign, Moines, and driven the two brothers of the late king, whose names were Uther and Pendragon, into banishment. Vortigern, who lived in constant fear of the return of the rightful heirs of the kingdom, began to erect a strong tower for defence. The edifice, when brought by the workmen to a certain height, three times fell to the ground, without any apparent cause. The king consulted his astrologers on this wonderful event, and learned from them that it would be necessary to bathe the corner-stone of the foundation with the blood of a child born without a mortal father.

In search of such an infant, Vortigern sent his messengers all over the kingdom, and they by accident discovered Merlin, whose lineage seemed to point him out as the individual wanted.

13. Merlin has no human ancestry
A. True B. False C. Can't Tell

14. Based on the above passage, which of the following statements is true?
A. Merlin's father is immortal
B. Vortigern is of royal ancestry
C. There are no living heirs to the throne
D. Uther is the rightful king of Britain

15. Based on the above passage, which of the following statements is FALSE?
A. Vortigern is a superstitious king
B. Merlin's life is in danger
C. Merlin is a Christian
D. Merlin has no special abilities

16. Which correctly describes Vortigern's personality?
A. Benevolent B. Loving C. Just D. Fearful

Passage 5

My Ancestors

I was born near Thorntown, Indiana, August 21, 1834.

My father, James P. Mills, third child of James Mills 2nd and Marian Mills, was born in York, Pennsylvania, August 22, 1808. His father, James Mills 2nd, was born October 1, 1770, and died December 3, 1808.

My father's mother died in 1816, leaving him an orphan at the age of eight. He lived with his Aunt Margery Mills Hayes for about two years, when he was "bound out" as an apprentice to a tanner by the name of Greenwalt, at Harrisburg, Pennsylvania. Here he was to serve until twenty-one, when he was to receive one hundred dollars and a suit of clothes. All the knowledge that he had of books was derived from night school, Greenwalt not permitting him to attend during the day. His apprenticeship was so hard he ran away when twenty, forfeiting the hundred dollars and the clothes.

His only patrimony was from his grandfather, James Mills I, who, as father told me, sent for him on his deathbed and, patting him on the head, said: "I want Jimmy to have fifty pounds."

After running away, my father went to Geneva, New York, and served as a journeyman until twenty-two. With his inheritance of $250, he and his brother Frank started West in a Dearborn wagon, crossing the Alleghenies. He travelled to Crawfordsville, Indiana, and here, about 1830, entered eighty acres of the farm on which I was born. The land was covered with walnut, oak and ash, many of the trees being one hundred feet high and three or four feet in diameter. Felling and burning the trees, he built his house with his own hands, neighbours aiding in raising the walls.

My father had little knowledge of his ancestors, other than that they were Quakers, but, by correspondence with officials of counties where his ancestors lived, I have learned that the first of his family came over with William Penn and settled in Philadelphia.

17. The author is:
A. American
B. Chinese
C. English
D. Indian

18. Which of the following statements is true regarding the above passage?
A. The author was born after the first world war
B. James P. Mills was not an educated man
C. The author's father, grandfather and great-grandfather had the same forename
D. The author's father inherited a large sum of money from his parents

19. James P. Mills was an only child
A. True
B. False
C. Can't Tell

20. The author is female
A. True
B. False
C. Can't Tell

Passage 6

FRANK AND BEN.

"Is your mother at home, Frank?" asked a soft voice.

Frank Hunter was stretched on the lawn in a careless posture, but looked up quickly as the question fell upon his ear. A man of middle height and middle age was looking at him from the other side of the gate. Frank rose from his grassy couch and answered coldly: "Yes, sir; I believe so. I will go in and see."

"Oh, don't trouble yourself, my young friend," said Mr. Craven, opening the gate and advancing toward the door with a brisk step. "I will ring the bell; I want to see your mother on a little business."

"Seems to me he has a good deal of business with mother," Frank said to himself. "There's something about the man I don't like, though he always treats me well enough. Perhaps it's his looks."

"How are you, Frank?"

Frank looked around, and saw his particular friend, Ben Cameron, just entering the gate.

"Tip-top, Ben," he answered, cordially. "I'm glad you've come."

"I'm glad to hear it; I thought you might be engaged."

"Engaged? What do you mean, Ben?" asked Frank, with a puzzled expression.

"Engaged in entertaining your future step-father," said Ben, laughing.

"My future step-father!" returned Frank, quickly; "you are speaking in riddles, Ben."

"Oh! well, if I must speak out, I saw Mr. Craven ahead of me."

"Mr. Craven! Well, what if you did?"

"Why, Frank, you must know the cause of his attentions to your mother."

"Ben," said Frank, his face flushing with anger, "you are my friend, but I don't want even you to hint at such a thing as that."

"Have I displeased you, Frank?"

"No, no; I won't think of it anymore."

"I am afraid, Frank, you will have to think of it more," said his companion, gravely.

"You surely don't mean, Ben, that you have the least idea that my mother would marry such a man as that?" exclaimed Frank, pronouncing the last words contemptuously.

21. Frank Hunter is an only child

A. True

B. False

C. Can't Tell

22. Based on the above information, which of the following statements can be inferred?

A. Frank dislikes the idea of his mother marrying

B. Frank is a university student

C. Mr. Craven is an unpleasant character

D. Frank dislikes Ben

23. Based on the passage, which season is it most likely to be?

A. Summer

B. Spring

C. Winter

D. Autumn

24. Based on the above information, which of the following statements is most likely to be true?

A. Frank is an only child

B. Frank and Ben are brothers

C. Frank's father is absent

D. Frank's mother is a schoolteacher

Passage 7

Cynthia, Countess of Hampshire, was sitting in an extraordinarily elaborate dressing-gown one innocent morning in June, alternately opening letters and eating spoonfuls of sour milk prepared according to the prescription of Professor Metchnikoff. Every day it made her feel younger and stronger and more irresponsible (which is the root of all joy to natures of a serious disposition), and since (when a fortnight before she began this abominable treatment) she felt very young already, she was now almost afraid that she would start again on measles, croup, hoops, whooping-cough, peppermints, and other childish ailments and passions. But since this treatment not only induced youth, but was discouraging to all microbes but its own, she hoped as regards ailments that she would continue to feel younger and younger without suffering the penalties of childhood.

The sour milk was finished long before her letters were all opened, for there was no one in London who had a larger and more festive post than she. Indeed, it was no wonder that everybody of sense (and most people of none) wanted her to eat their dinners and stay in their houses, for her volcanic enjoyment of life made the dullest of social functions a high orgy, and since nothing is nearly so infectious as enjoyment, it followed that she was much in request.

Even in her fiftieth year she retained with her youthful zest for life much of the extreme plainness of her girlhood, but time was gradually lightening the heaviness of feature that had once formed so remarkable an ugliness, and in a few years more, no doubt, she would become as nice looking as everybody else of her age.

25. Based on the above passage, which of the following statements is true?
A. Cynthia is a child
B. Cynthia lives in London
C. Professor Metchnikoff is Cynthia's father
D. Cynthia eats sour milk for breakfast

26. Cynthia is 60 years old
A. True
B. False
C. Can't Tell

27. Which of the following statements correctly summarises the passage?
A. Cynthia is a countess attempting to appear more youthful
B. Cynthia is a countess looking for love
C. Professor Metchnikoff is a Psychology professor performing an experiment on Cynthia
D. The benefits and side effects of regular sour milk ingestion

28. With regards to the passage above, which of the following statements is FALSE?
A. Cynthia receives a large amount of post
B. Cynthia is a rich lady
C. Cynthia has been drinking sour milk for the past 2 weeks
D. Cynthia was good-looking in youth

Passage 8

The old writers tell how Long Island was once the happy hunting ground of wolves and Indians, the playing place of deer and wild turkeys; and how the seals, the turtles, grampuses and pelicans loved its long, quiet beaches. Seals and whales are still occasional visitors, and its coasts are rich in lore of wrecks, of pirates and of buried treasure.

A hundred years ago it could boast of hamlets only less remote from civilisation than are to-day the villages of that other "Long Island"—the group of the Outer Hebrides—which, for an equal distance, extends along the Scottish coast from Butt of Lewis to Barra Head. The desultory stage then occupied a week on the double journey between Brooklyn and Sag Harbour. Beyond the latter, Montauk Point thrusts its lighthouse some fifteen miles out into the Atlantic breakers. Here the last Indians of the island lingered on their reservation, and here the whalers watched for the spouting of their prey in the offing.

A ridge of hills runs along the island near the northern shore, rising here and there into heights of three or four hundred feet which command the long gradual slope of woods and meadows to the south, with the distant sea beyond them; to the north, across the narrow Sound, rises the blue coast line of Connecticut.

It is on the slopes below the highest of these points of wide vision that the Whitman homestead lies, one of the pleasant farms of a land which has always been mainly agricultural. Large areas of the island are poor and barren, covered still with scrub and "kill-calf" or picturesque pine forest, as in the Indian days. But the land here is productive.

29. Long Island is in Scotland
A. True
B. False
C. Can't Tell

30. Which of the following statements correctly summarises the above passage?
A. The passage describes the history of Long Island
B. The passage describes the history of Indians
C. The passage provides an account of the Scottish Coast
D. The passage describes a love story in New York

31. Which of the following statements is true regarding the above passage?
A. Montauk Point is in Scotland
B. Long Island is in Connecticut
C. There are no more Indians on Long Island
D. The Outer Hebrides are in Scotland

32. Which of the following animals have never been seen on Long Island?
A. Wolves
B. Seals
C. Whales
D. Tigers

Passage 9

In the year 2126, England enjoyed peace and tranquillity under the absolute dominion of a female sovereign. Numerous changes had taken place for some centuries in the political state of the country, and several forms of government had been successively adopted and destroyed, till, as is generally the case after violent revolutions, they all settled down into an absolute monarchy. In the meantime, the religion of the country had been mutable as its government; and in the end, by adopting Catholicism, it seemed to have arrived at nearly the same result: despotism in the state, indeed, naturally produces despotism in religion; the implicit faith and passive obedience required in the one case, being the best of all possible preparatives for the absolute submission of both mind and body necessary in the other.

In former times, England had been blessed with a mixed government and a tolerant religion, under which the people had enjoyed as much freedom as they perhaps ever can do, consistently with their prosperity and happiness. It is not in the nature of the human mind, however, to be contented: we must always either hope or fear; and things at a distance appear so much more beautiful than they do when we approach them, that we always fancy what we have not, infinitely superior to anything we have; and neglect enjoyments within our reach, to pursue others, which, like ignes fatui, elude our grasp at the very moment when we hope we have attained them.

33. The passage is set in the future
A. True
B. False
C. Can't Tell

34. The overall theme of the passage is:
A. War
B. The future
C. Human nature
D. Feminism

35. Which of the following statements is true regarding the above passage?
A. The passage is based in the USA
B. The main religion in England is Islam
C. There is no government in England in 2126
D. There is a single female leader in England in 2126

36. The author is expressing admiration for human compassion
A. True
B. False
C. Can't Tell

Passage 10

That evening at eight o'clock we met at the old Edinburgh Hotel (now no longer in existence), and after dinner he told me his very remarkable tale.

"Some years ago," he said, "I was staying in a small coast town in Fife, not very far from St Andrews. I was painting some quaint houses and things of the sort that tickled my fancy at the time, and I was very much amused and excited by some of the bogie tales told me by the fisher folk. One story particularly interested me."

"And what was that?" I asked.

"Well, it was about a strange, dwarfish, old man, who, they swore, was constantly wandering about among the rocks at nightfall; a queer, uncanny creature, they said, who was 'aye beckoning to them,' and who was never seen or known in the daylight. I heard so much at various times and from various people about this old man that I resolved to look for him and see what his game really was. I went down to the beach times without number, but saw nothing worse than myself, and I was almost giving the job up as hopeless, when one night 'I struck oil,' as the Yankees would say."

"Good," I said, "let me hear."

"It was after dusk," he proceeded, "very rough and windy, but with a feeble moon peeping out at times between the racing clouds. I was alone on the beach. Next moment I was not alone."

"Not alone," I remarked. "Who was there?"

"Certainly not alone," said Ashton. "About three yards from me stood a quaint, short, shrivelled, old creature. At that time the comic opera of 'Pinafore' was new to the stage-loving world, and this strange being resembled the character of 'Dick Deadeye' in that piece. But this old man was much uglier and more repulsive. He wore a tattered monk's robe, had a fringe of black hair, heavy black eyebrows, very protruding teeth, and a pale, pointed, unshaven chin. Moreover, he possessed only one eye, which was large and telescopic looking."

"What a horrid brute," I said.

37. The ghost in the passage had 1 eye.

A. True B. False C. Can't Tell

38. Which of the following statements regarding the above passage is true?

A. The main protagonist is called Ashton
B. The passage is set in the morning
C. The ghost is that of an old King
D. The protagonist is not fond of the ghost

39. If you had to describe the ghost in one word, what would it be?

A. Terrifying B. Worried C. Happy D. Pitiful

40. Ashton is interested in ghosts

A. True B. False C. Can't Tell

Passage 11

It was a lovely twilight evening at Lytton Springs, India. These famous springs were very high up in the Araville hills; Mandavee was the nearest city, situated on a small island in the Arabian sea. The great red sun was slowly sinking as the bells were ringing the Angelus from an ancient Hindu temple. The sacred chimes pealed forth melodiously, the sweet sounds echoing forth the harmony of those bells. Inside of this ancient temple sweet incense was burning on a beautiful golden altar. A dark, handsome prince and his family were praying around this sacred altar. Here they would often see beautiful visions of angels and their loved ones who had died in this same faith years ago. This faith was a strange, mysterious, mythical religion, handed down from the ancient Indians. It was a mixture of Catholicism and Hinduism. The Prince and his family were highly educated and great musicians; they were all great Psychics, and often spent hours in this old temple praying. They lived in constant communion with their saints, who constantly watched over them and protected them. At the other side of this altar a strange veiled princess was silently praying. After sunset they all left the temple with bowed heads. They went to their summer homes in the hills. Sita, the Prince's only daughter, felt sorry for the lonely stranger and invited her to their lovely home in the mountains.

41. Which country is the passage based in?

A. Sri Lanka B. China C. Japan D. India

42. The religion that the Princes practice is Hinduism

A. True B. False C. Can't tell

43. Which of the following statements regarding the above passage is true?

A. There are only royal characters in the passage
B. The Princes had special abilities
C. The Princes live in Mandavee
D. Sita is the Prince's wife

44. Sita is the veiled princess in the passage

A. True B. False C. Can't Tell

Section B: Decision Making

1. In 2007 AD, Halley's Comet and Comet Encke were observed in the same calendar year. Halley's Comet is observed on average once every 73 years; Comet Encke is observed on average once every 104 years. Based on this, estimate the calendar year in which both Halley's Comet and Comet Encke are next observed in the same year.

A. 9559 AD B. 2114 AD C. 5643 AD D. 3562 AD E. 1757 AD

2. "One has to be at least 18 to vote in the UK". Which statement gives the best supporting reason for this statement?

A. At 18, citizens have the right level of maturity to vote sensibly
B. One must legally be able to buy alcohol before they can vote
C. Too many people would vote in the UK otherwise
D. Citizens do not understand policies below the age of 18

3. Adam, Ben, Caitlyn, Joe, James, Simon and David are sitting around a circle facing the centre. Joe is sitting between Adam and David. Simon is second to the right of David and James is second to the right of Simon. Caitlyn is not an immediate neighbour of David. Which of the below statements is true?

A. Caitlyn is to the left of Simon
B. Simon is to the left of Adam
C. David is to the right of Simon
D. Joe is between Simon and Caitlyn
E. Caitlyn is directly opposite to David

4. In a certain Code '8 2 9' means 'how are you,' '9 5 8' means 'you are good' and '1 5 8 7 3' means 'I good and you bad'. Based on this, what is the code for 'you'?

A. 1 B. 5 C. 8 D. 7

5. 'Smoking should not be condemned because smokers pay for their healthcare through the tax on cigarettes'. Which option is the best argument against the above statement?

A. Smokers cause detrimental effects on people around them
B. Smoking should be condemned because it is bad for your health
C. That argument doesn't work if the healthcare system is private
D. Smoking makes you more likely to drink, which also causes further health problems.

6. Jason, Peter, John and Alan are four brothers. Jason is older than Peter and John. Alan is younger than John. Peter is older than John. Which of the following correctly represents the four brothers in age order (from youngest to oldest)?

A. Peter, Alan, John, Jason
B. Jason, Peter, John, Alan
C. Alan, John, Peter, Jason
D. Jason, John, Peter, Alan

7. If 'TOILET' is related to 'WDJEBW' and 'SOUNDS' is related to 'YDHILY', which of the following options is related to 'SOILED'?

A. QUDHSJQ
B. FGHDJR
C. YDJEBL
D. AJSHDG

8. 'Surgeon's mortality rates should not be available to the public'. Which of the following statements provides the best argument against this statement?

A. Surgeons are more willing to do surgery if their mortality rates are published
B. Publishing mortality rates promotes a more transparent healthcare system and embeds public trust in healthcare professionals
C. Mortality rates will increase if mortality rates are published
D. Surgeons are more likely to not leave the country if mortality rates are published

9. In a school there are 40 more girls than there are boys. The boys make up a percentage of 40% of the school. What is the number of students in the school?

A. 150 B. 200 C. 300 D. 500

10. David is 4 years older than Anna. Anna and May are in the same school year. May's younger brother Isaac is best friends with David's brother Mike.

Which of the following conclusions is true based on the above information?

A. Anna is older than Isaac
B. David is younger than Isaac
C. David and Anna are related
D. Isaac is older than Mike
E. May is older than David

11. During the school day, there are 6 lessons timetabled. Maths is never second or fifth. English always follows Science. French is not fourth and there is a lesson between French and History. There is always a break before Geography.

Which of the following statements is true?

A. Science is the second lesson of the day
B. Geography is the second lesson of the day
C. English is the third lesson of the day
D. History is the first lesson of the day
E. Maths is the fourth lesson of the day

12. 'Euthanasia should be legalised to allow people a dignified death'. Which of the following options is the best argument for this statement?

A. Elderly people may be pressured into euthanasia by their relatives
B. If euthanasia is legalised, then why not legalise murder?
C. There is no need for euthanasia; palliative patients can be kept perfectly comfortable as it is
D. Legalisation is pointless; those who want to be euthanised go abroad to do it anyway

13. If one day on Earth corresponds to 0.4 days on Mars, and there are 365 days in a year on Earth, how frequent would the Olympics be held if they were being held on Mars?

A. 10 years B. 12 years C. 32 years D. 48 years

14. There has recently been an initiative established in a developing country for schoolteachers to teach the illiterate members of society after school hours. Which of the options provides the best argument as to why the lessons are being offered after hours?

A. So that the illiterate cannot interact with schoolchildren
B. So that the schooling does not interfere with any jobs that the illiterate members of society during the day
C. So that the illiterate members of society can understand how difficult getting an education is
D. So that the streets are less crowded at night time

15. Jay either walks to school or takes the bus, depending on whether it is raining or not. If he walks to school, there is a 60% chance that he is late. If he takes the bus to school, there is a 20% chance that he is late. Given that one morning, the probability that it will rain is 70%, what is the probability that Jay will be late to school?

A. 32% B. 67% C. 23% D. 44%

16. If the number 273546 is rearranged such that the digits within the number are rearranged in ascending order (from left to right), how many digits would not change position within the number?

A. 0 B. 1 C. 2 D. 3

17. In a bank, there are 150 employees. Of these, there are 55 English employees, 58 married employees and 55 employees which PhDs. There are 19 employees who are both English and have a PhD, there are 21 employees who are both married and have a PhD, and there are 26 employees who are both English and married. Based on this information, how many employees are neither English, nor married, nor have a PhD?

A. 26 B. 38 C. 22 D. 41

18. All buses are motor vehicles. Motor vehicles include trucks. Some trucks are cars. Which of the following statements is true?

A. All cars are motor vehicles
B. All trucks are buses
C. Some cars are buses
D. All trucks are motor vehicles
E. Some buses are not motor vehicles

19. All sharks are fish. Fish, dolphins and whales are aquatic animals. Dolphins are mammals. Whales are not fish. Which of the following statements is true based on this information?

A. Whales are mammals
B. Whales and dolphins are related
C. Sharks are aquatic animals
D. Dolphins are fish
E. Sharks are mammals

20. Alex is going on a hike. He starts off in the morning walking towards the sun rise. He walks 5km, turns 90 degrees clockwise, walks 2km in that direction, then turns 180 degrees, walks 3km in that direction before turning 90 degrees anticlockwise to walk the final 4km home. Which direction is he walking for the last 4km?

A. East B. North C. South D. West

21. 'Possession of a gun should be a federal crime'. Which of the following statements provides the strongest argument in favour of this statement?

A. There would be reduced murders if possession of guns is made illegal
B. People can use knives rather than guns to protect themselves
C. Making possession illegal will reduce black market purchasing of guns
D. People will be more afraid to use guns in public if they know it is a federal crime to possess one

22. 70% of the Earth's surface is covered by water. There are 5 oceans in the world. The largest of these is the Pacific Ocean. A body of water which is partially enclosed by land is called a sea. The largest sea in the world is the Arabian Sea. Which of the following statements is true?

A. The Pacific Ocean covers 70% of the Earth's surface
B. Seas cover 70% of the Earth's surface
C. The Pacific Ocean is larger than the Arabian Sea
D. Most of the water on Earth's surface is in the oceans
E. The Arabian Sea is partially enclosed by land

23. In a medical school, 56% of the 300 students are boys. Of these, 18% are Chinese. If 25% of the girls are Chinese, how many female medical students are Chinese?

A. 33 B. 41 C. 23 D. 27

24. 'People who are obese should pay for their own healthcare'. Which of the following options provides the best argument for the above statement?

A. It is often the poorest of society who have the worst diet and therefore are most predisposed to becoming obese
B. Obesity is not an expensive morbidity
C. Obese people contribute more to the national health system than thin people
D. Obesity is a problem of genetics, it is unfair for people to have to pay for what they have inherited

25. Susan is the mother of Johnathan, Sally and Christina. Christina is married to Karl, whose brother, Sam, is married to Leanne. Sam and Leanne have 3 children-David, Nat and Liam. Which of the following statements are true based on this information?

A. Sam and Christina are related
B. Nat and Susan are related
C. Karl and David are related
D. Johnathan and Liam are not related
E. Sally and Sam are related

26. To get to school, Joanne takes the school bus every morning. If she misses this, then she can take the public bus to school. The school bus arrives at 08:15, which if she misses will come again at 08:37. The public bus comes every 17 minutes, starting at 06:56. The school bus takes 24 minutes to get to her school; the public bus takes 18 minutes. If she arrives at the bus stop at 08:25, which bus must she catch to get to school first?

A. The 08:37 school bus
B. The 08:26 public bus
C. The 08: 38 public bus
D. The 08: 31 public bus

27. Jason, Karen, Liam, Mason, Neil, Obie, Pari and Richard are sitting around a circular table facing the centre. Each of them was born in a different year-1992, 1996, 1997, 2000, 2001, 2004, 2005 and 2010, but not necessarily in the same order. Mason is sitting second to the right of Karen. Liam is sitting third to the right of Jason. Only the one born in 2004 is sitting exactly between Jason and Karen. Neil, who is the eldest is not an immediate neighbour of Jason and Mason. Richard is older than only Mason. Richard is sitting second to the left of Pari. Pari is not an immediate neighbour of Neil. Jason is younger than Liam and Obie. Karen was born before Obie but she is not second eldest. Based on this information, which of the following statements is true and which are false?

A. Neil is opposite Karen
B. Liam was born in 2000
C. Mason was born in 2005
D. Neil is between Richard and Jason
E. Obie was born in 2010

28. 'Zoos should be made illegal'. Which of the following options provides the best argument against this statement?
A. Human entertainment is more important than animal welfare
B. Children wouldn't learn about animals without zoos
C. Zoos provide an important method by which critically endangered species can be protected in conservation until their numbers recover
D. Many people would be out of a job without zoos

29. All humans are apes. The apes include the related families of chimpanzees, gorillas and orangutans. All apes are mammals. Most mammals produce live offspring. Based on this information, which of the following statements are true and which are false?

A. All humans are mammals
B. All apes are humans
C. Chimpanzees and humans are unrelated
D. All mammals produce live offspring
E. All mammals which produce live offspring are apes

END OF SECTION

Section C: Quantitative Reasoning

Data Set 1

The following graph describes the number of people visiting a store at different times of the day. Study the graph, then answer the following six questions.

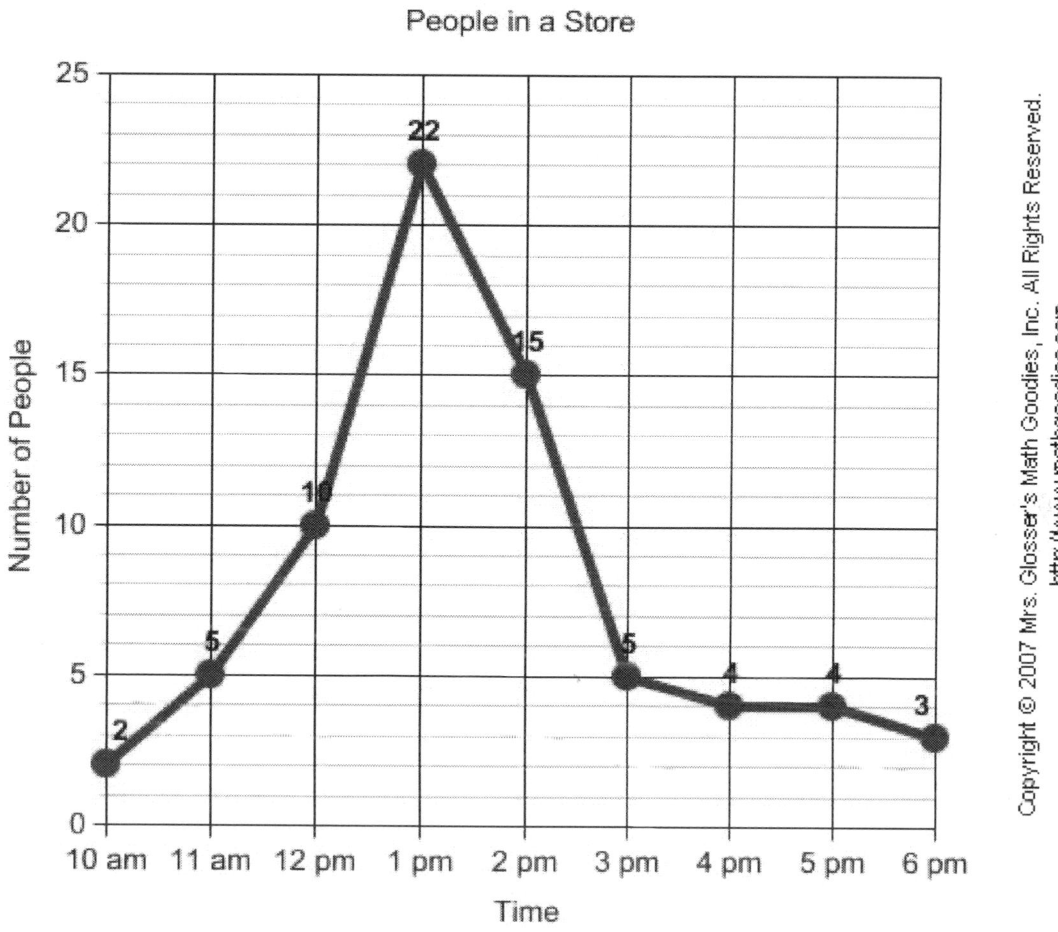

1. What is the mode number of people visiting the store over the day?

A. 22 B. 10 C. 2 D. 5 E. 4.5

2. If one was to visit the shop, what would be the best time to visit?

A. 12pm B. 4pm C. 6pm D. 10am E. 5pm

3. What is the range?

A. 15 B. 17 C. 20 D. 12 E. 9

4. If each customer spends on average £5 in the shop, what is the total income for the shop (to the nearest pound)?

A. £200 B. £176 C. £250 D. £350 E. £421

Data Set 2

The following table shows the currency exchange rates for different currencies.

	GBP	CAD	EUR	HKD	JPY	CHF	USD
GBP		0.5364	0.7470	0.0860	0.0057	0.7564	0.6667
CAD	1.8595		1.3908	0.1601	0.0105	1.4064	1.2413
EUR	1.3368	0.7178		0.1156	0.0076	1.0115	0.8922
HKD	11.6112	6.2364	8.6461		0.0658	8.7820	7.7513
JPY	176.4800	94.7300	131.9100	15.1900		133.5500	117.7500
CHF	1.3171	0.7061	0.9836	0.1132	0.0075		0.8776
USD	1.4980	0.8046	1.1204	0.1290	0.0085	1.1330	

5. Sally is planning to travel to Canada for a holiday, and wishes to convert £500 into Canadian Dollars (CAD). How many Canadian dollars can she get?

A. $836.43 B. $929.75 C. $736.44 D. $827.39 E. $283.33

6. After her trip, Sally had 150 CAD left over, which she converted back into Great British Pounds (GBP). How many pounds would she get back?

A. £80.46 B. £80.67 C. £92.18 D. £67.44 E. £81.19

7. How much money is she losing in this exchange?

A. £1.09 B. £0.89 C. £0.21 D. £1.58 E. £0.71

8. Shoko is planning to send money to her family in Japan from the USA. One travel agency is offers her a rate of 118.6300. If she is planning to send USD 700, how much more Japanese Yen (JPY) does she get from using this travel agency as opposed to the one above?

A. JPY 82425 B. JPY 83041 C. JPY 616 D. JPY 5.236 E. JPY 782

Data Set 3

The following graph shows how the Earth's surface temperature has varied with time.

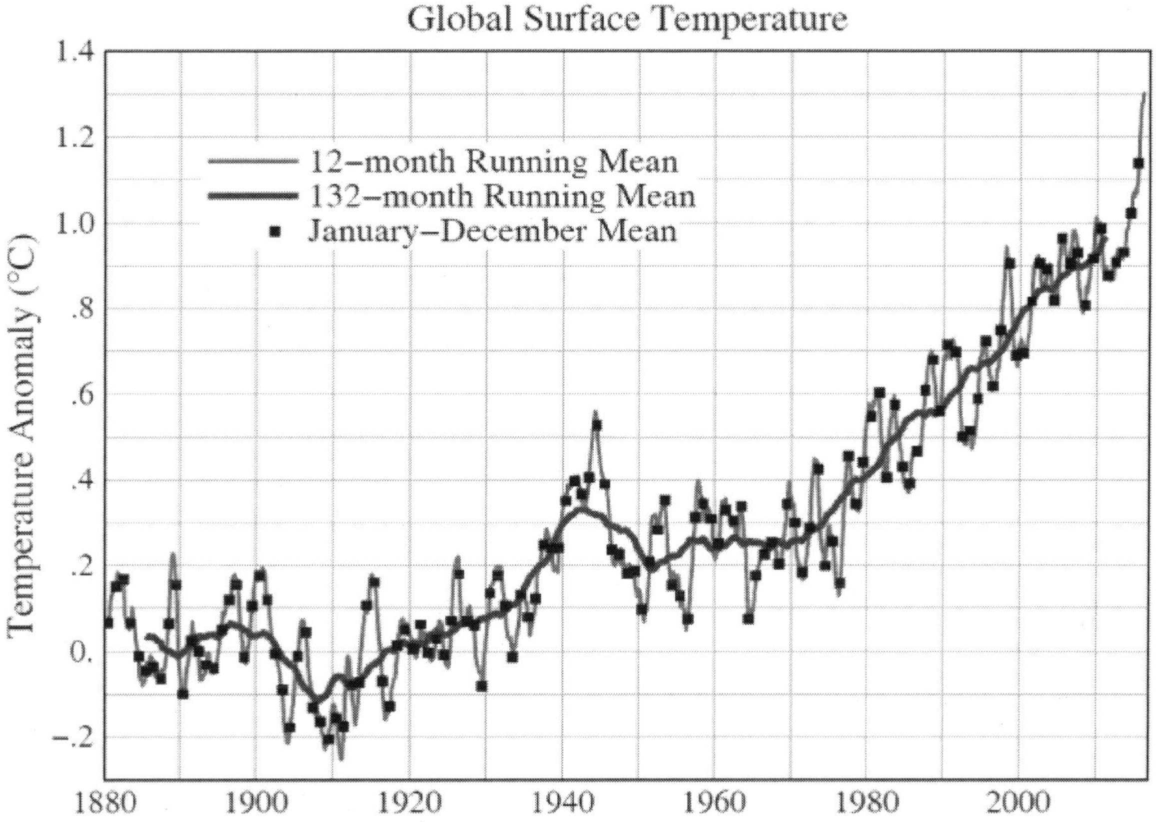

9. If the surface temperature is 22.6°C today, what was the temperature in 1940?

A. 20.4°C B. 21.6°C C. 22.0°C D. 19.8°C E. 20.7°C

10. What should the normal surface temperature be?

A. 21.3°C B. 22.1°C C. 20.8°C D. 21.1°C E. 20.2°C

11. During which period was the rate of temperature change the greatest?

A. 1880-1890
B. 1900-1910
C. 1920-1930
D. 1980-1990
E. 2010 onwards

12. What is the rate of temperature change between 1980 and 2000?

A. 0.12°C per year
B. 0.2°C per year
C. 0.06°C per year
D. 0.09°C per year
E. 0.25°C per year

Data Set 4

The following table shows how a group of students performed in their end of year examination. The number in the table gives the percentage that each student achieved in each exam

The Numbers in the Brackets give the Maximum Marks in Each Subject.

Student	Subject (Max. Marks)					
	Maths	Chemistry	Physics	Geography	History	Computer Science
	(150)	(130)	(120)	(100)	(60)	(40)
Ayush	90	50	90	60	70	80
Aman	100	80	80	40	80	70
Sajal	90	60	70	70	90	70
Rohit	80	65	80	80	60	60
Muskan	80	65	85	95	50	90
Tanvi	70	75	65	85	40	60
Tarun	65	35	50	77	80	80

13. Which student performed the best overall?

A. Muskan B. Tanvi C. Tarun D. Sajal E. Ayush

14. What mark did Rohit score in Computer Science?

A. 27 B. 25 C. 24 D. 31 E. 18

15. Which exam had the highest average score?

A. Maths
B. Chemistry
C. Physics
D. Geography
E. Computer Science

16. What mark did Sajal get in Maths?

A. 128 B. 122 C. 141 D. 135 E. 109

Data Set 5

The following graph shows how much rainfall Atlanta has been getting over the past 20 years.

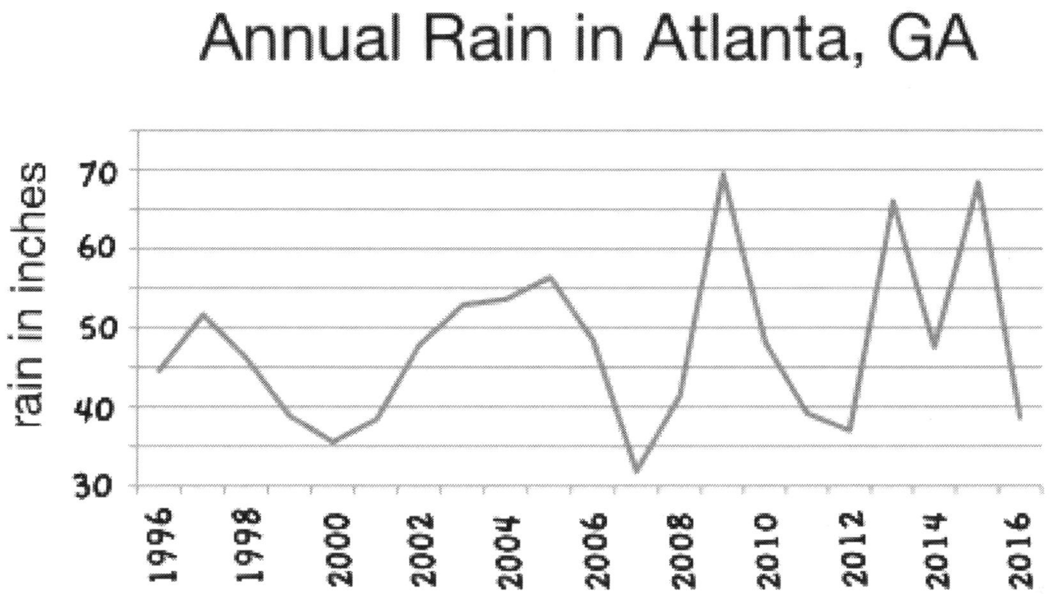

17. How much rain fell in 2010?

A. 55 inches
B. 40 inches
C. 45 inches
D. 30 inches
E. 70 inches

18. In which year did Atlanta receive the maximum rainfall?

A. 2009
B. 2003
C. 1996
D. 2016
E. 2001

19. What was the difference in rainfall between 2007 and 2009?

A. 28 inches
B. 34 inches
C. 38 inches
D. 51 inches
E. 12 inches

20. What is the average rainfall between 2012 and 2016?

A. 52 inches
B. 35 inches
C. 40 inches
D. 65 inches
E. 22 inches

Data Set 6

The following train timetable shows the times that trains reach certain stations.

	1st	2nd	3rd	4th	5th	6th
Depot	07:30	07:45	08:00	08:15	08:30	08:45
Green St	07:40	07:55	**08:10**	08:25	08:40	08:55
High St	07:45	08:00	08:15	**08:30**	08:45	?
Central Park	**07:48**	08:03	08:18	**08:33**	08:48	09:03
Railway Station	07:53	08:08	08:23	08:38	?	09:08
Shopping Centre	08:00	08:15	08:30	08:45	09:00	09:15
Brown St	08:06	08:21	08:36	08:51	09:06	09:21
Church St	08:08	08:23	08:38	08:53	09:08	09:23
St Georges School	08:15	08:30	**08:45**	09:00		
Library	08:20	08:35	08:50	09:05	**09:20**	09:35
Hospital	08:25	08:40	08:55	09:10	09:25	09:40
Friary Walk	08:33	08:48	09:03	09:18	09:33	09:48
St Marys School	**08:42**	08:57	09:12			
Forest Rd	08:48	09:03	**09:18**	09:33	09:48	10:03
Swimming Pool	09:00	?	**09:30**	09:45	**10:00**	10:15

21. If there are 5km between the depot and Green St, what speed is the train travelling in km/h?

A. 40km/h B. 30km/h C. 37km/h D. 43km/h E. 15km/h

22. If this is the average speed of the train, what is the distance between Brown St and Church St?

A. 1km B. 2.5km C. 3km D. 4.2km E. 7km

23. If Jamie misses her train from Friary Walk at 08:33 by 7 minutes, how long must he wait until the next train?

A. 9 minutes B. 7 minutes C. 12 minutes D. 8 minutes E. 6 minutes

24. Dani must walk 8 minutes to get to Central Park station from his house. He takes the train to Forest Road, from which he must walk another 12 minutes to get to his work. If he must be at work by 9am, when does he have to set out from his house?

A. 08:03 B. 07:15 C. 07:56 D. 07:28 E. 07:40

Data Set 7

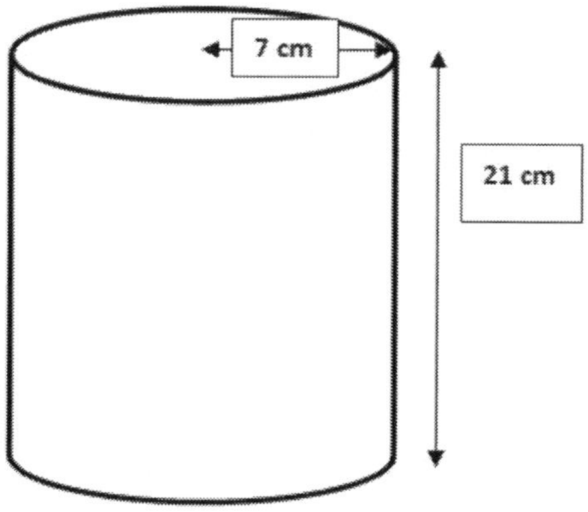

25. What is the surface area of the above cylinder to the nearest centimetre?

A. $949cm^2$ B. $1232cm^2$ C. $814cm^2$ D. $795cm^2$ E. $892cm^2$

26. What is the volume of the above cylinder to the nearest centimetre?

A. $3233cm^3$ B. $2647cm^3$ C. $4536cm^3$ D. $2222cm^3$ E. $5647cm^3$

27. What is the circumference of the cross-section to the nearest centimetre?

A. 37cm B. 28cm C. 44cm D. 50cm E. 19cm

28. If the radius increases by a factor of 2, what does the volume increase by?

A. 2 B. 4 C. 8 D. 16 E. 32

Data Set 8

Hayley buys a new car for £9000. Every year that Hayley owns the car, its value depreciates by 15%.

29. What will the value of the car be in 3 years (to the nearest pound)?

A. £5527 B. £7250 C. £6125 D. £4480 E. £8400

30. After how many years will the value of the car be £3394 (to the nearest pound)?

A. 4 years B. 3 years C. 5 years D. 6 years E. 7 years

31. As part of the cross-country race in school, the children must run 4 laps of the school field, which has a perimeter of 2.4km. If the runner in the lead is running at 12km/h, and the runner at the back is running at 8km/h, what time will the runner in the lead lap the runner in the back?

A. 20 minutes B. 25 minutes C. 36 minutes D. 24 minutes E. 17 minutes

32. James has a bag of 78 blue counters and David has a bag of 32 red counters. They must divide the counters into boxes with equal numbers of counters in each box. If there is no remainder, find the largest number of counters that can be put into a box.

A. 2 B. 4 C. 6 D. 8 E. 12

Data Set 9

The pie chart below represents a survey conducted on 300 people asking what their favourite book genre is.

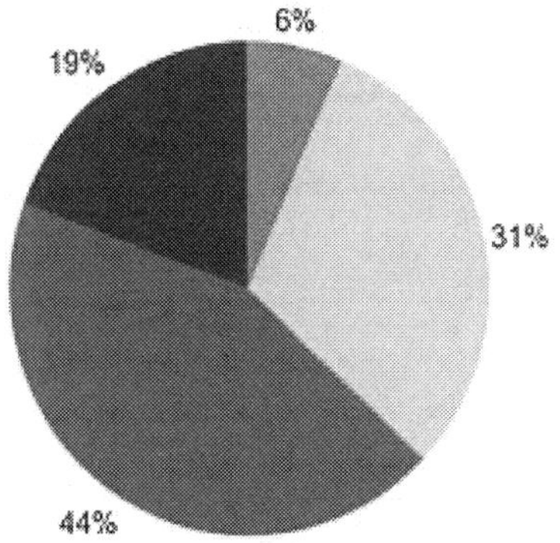

33. If the largest proportion represents romantic novels, how many people indicated this preference?

A. 44 B. 88 C. 132 D. 126 E. 182

34. If the smallest proportion represents horror, what angle does this slice of the pie make (to the nearest degree)?

A. 22° B. 18° C. 26° D. 32° E. 45°

Data Set 10

The following table shows the tax brackets for a country

Tax Rate	Single	Married (joint)/ Widow(er)	Married (separate)	Head of household
10%	$0 - $9,325	$0 - $18,650	$0 - $9,325	$0 - $13,350
15%	$9,326 - $37,950	$18,651 - $75,900	$9,326 - $37,950	$13,351 - $50,801
25%	$37,951 - $91,900	$75,901 - $153,100	$37,951 - $76,550	$50,801 - $131,200
28%	$91,901 - $191,650	$153,101 - $233,350	$76,551 - $116,675	$131,201 - $212,500
33%	$191,651 - $416,700	$233,351 - $416,700	$116,676 - $208,350	$212,501 - $416,700
35%	$416,701 - $418,400	$416,701 - $470,700	$208,351 - $235,350	$416,701 - $444,550
39.6%	$418,401 +	$470,701 +	$235,351 +	$445,551 +

35. For a single lawyer earning $176,000 a year, how much of that is deducted by tax?

A. $41461 B. $26354 C. $78263 D. $25362 E. $29283

36. If a doctor earning $200,000 gets married, what is his change in tax rate?

A. 5% increase
B. 7% increase
C. 5% reduction
D. 8% reduction
E. 3% increase

END OF SECTION

Section D: Abstract Reasoning

For each question, decide whether each box fits best with Set A, Set B or with neither.

For each question, work through the boxes from left to right as you see them on the page. Make your decision and fill it into the answer sheet.

Answer as follows:
A = Set A
B = Set B
C = neither

Set 1: **Set A** **Set B**

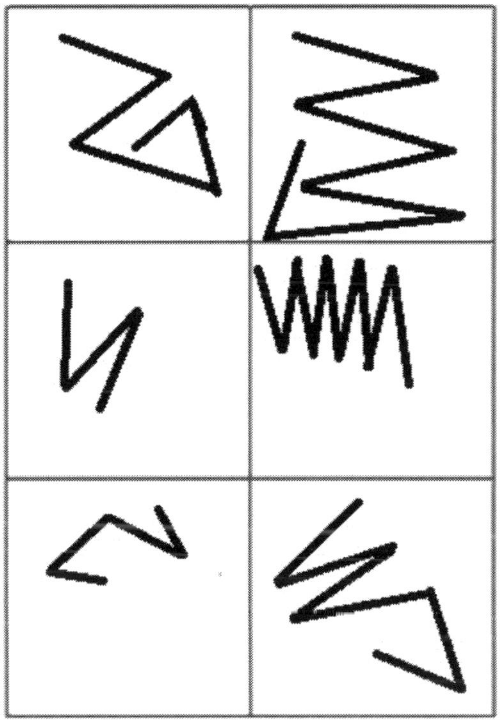

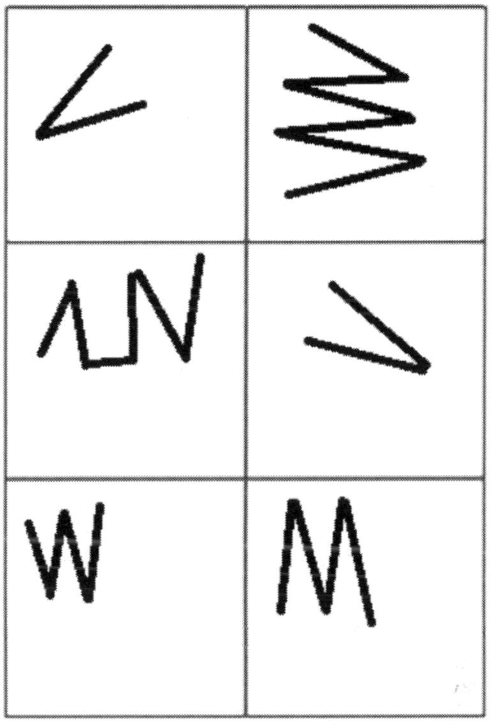

Questions 1-5:

Set 2: **Set A** **Set B**

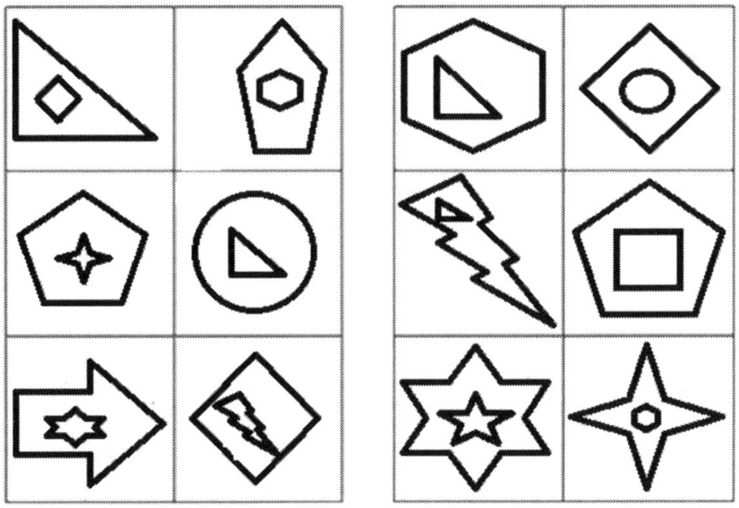

Questions 6-10:

Set 3: **Set A** **Set B**

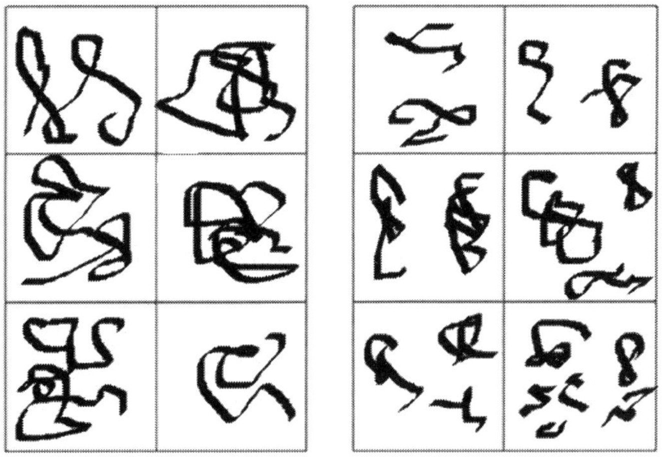

Questions 11-15:

Set 4: **Set A** **Set B**

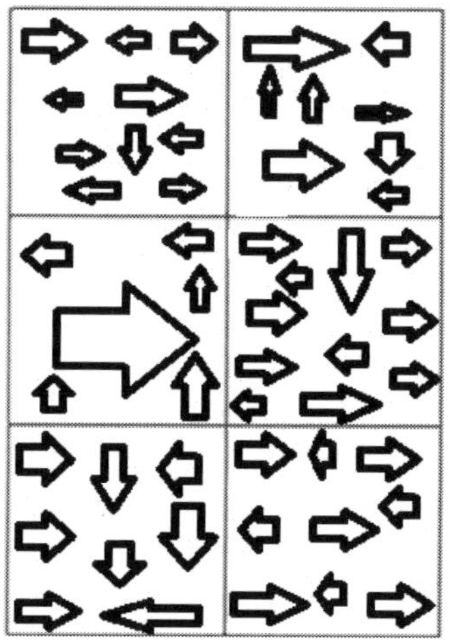

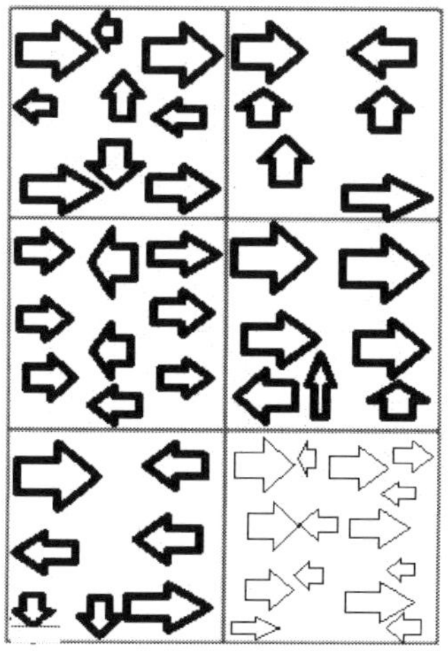

Questions 16-20:

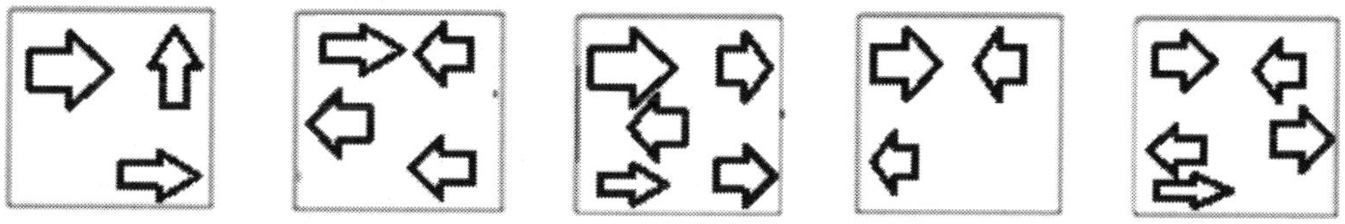

Set 5: **Set A** **Set B**

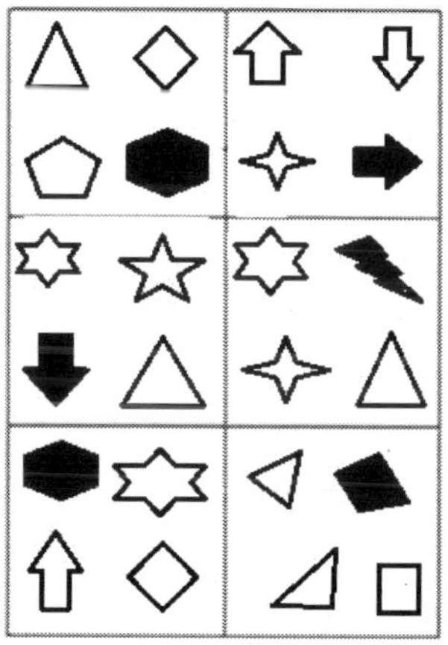

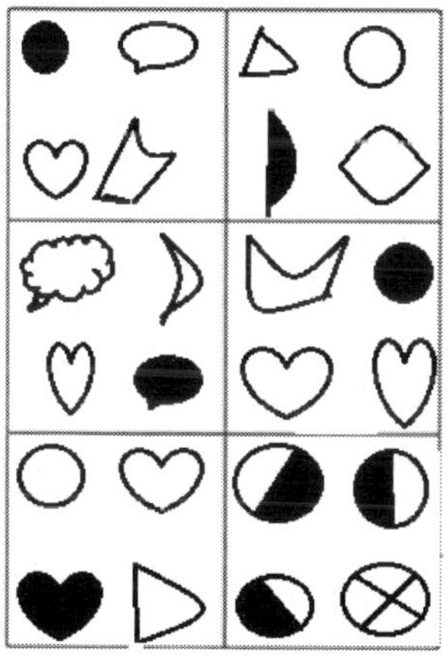

Questions 21-25:

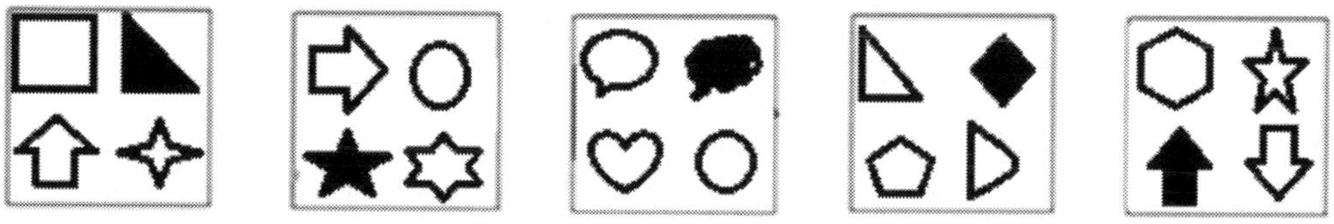

Set 6: **Set A** **Set B**

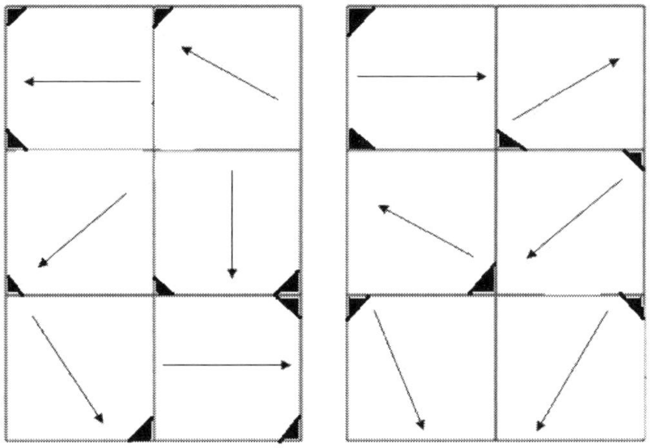

Questions 26-30:

Set 7: **Set A** **Set B**

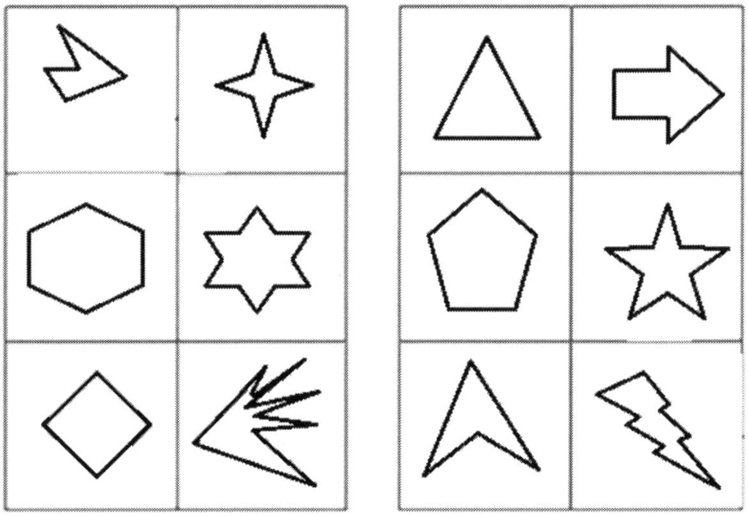

Questions 31-35:

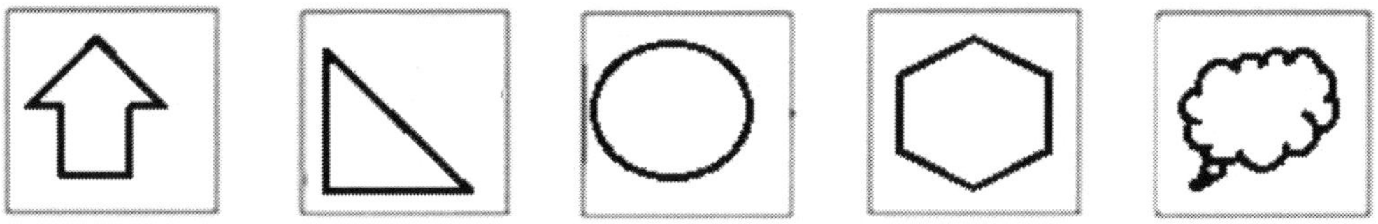

Set 8:

Set A Set B

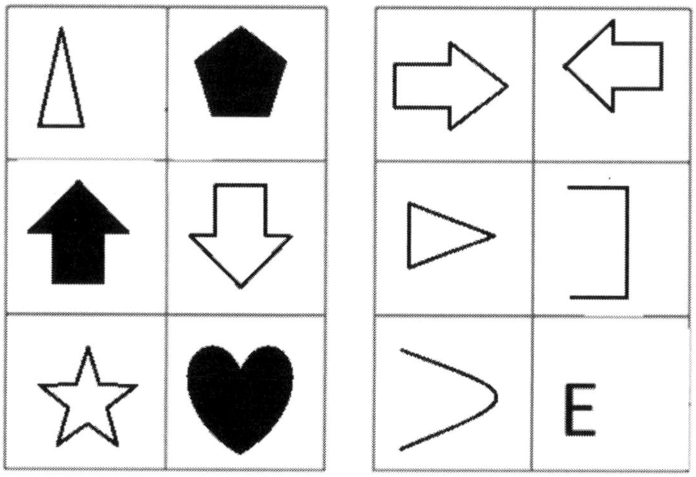

Questions 36-40:

Set 9:

Set A Set B

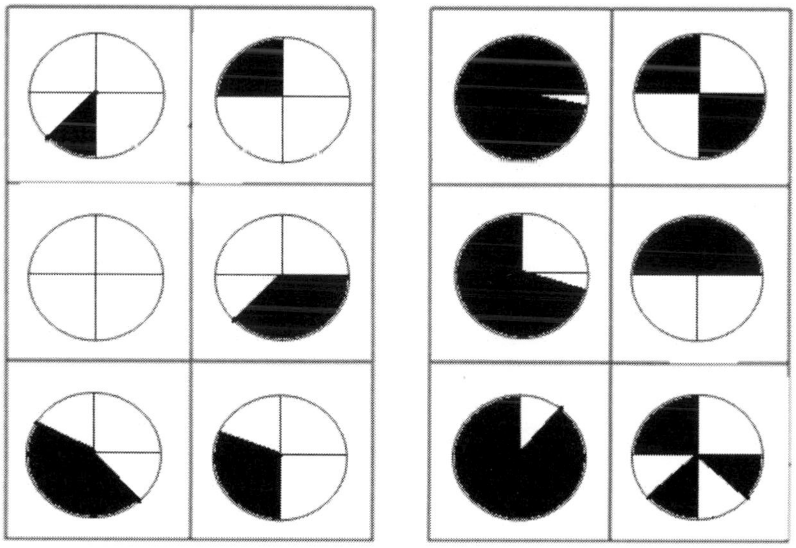

Questions 41-45:

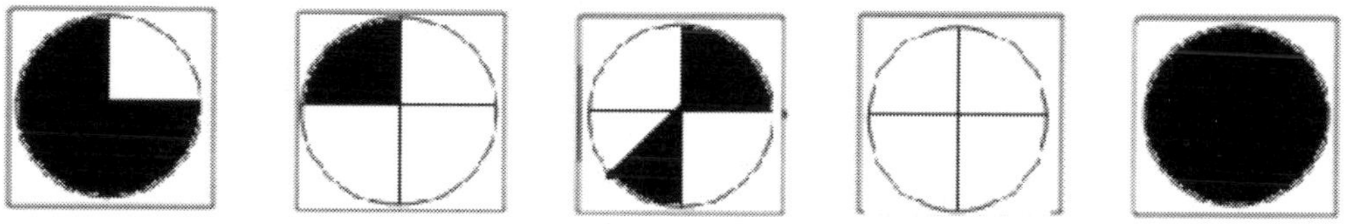

Set 10:

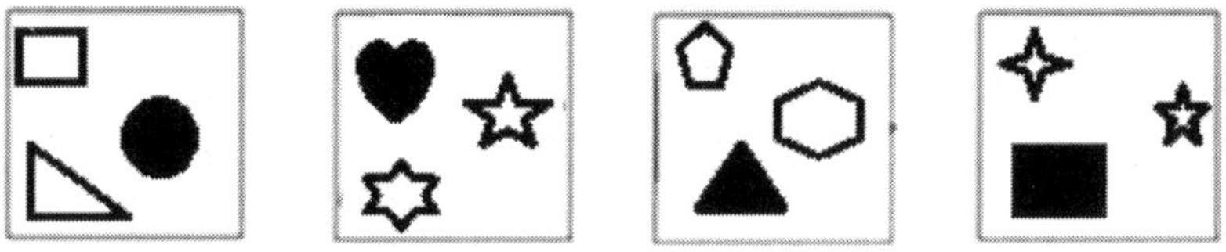

Questions 46: Which figure completes the series?

A. B. C. D.

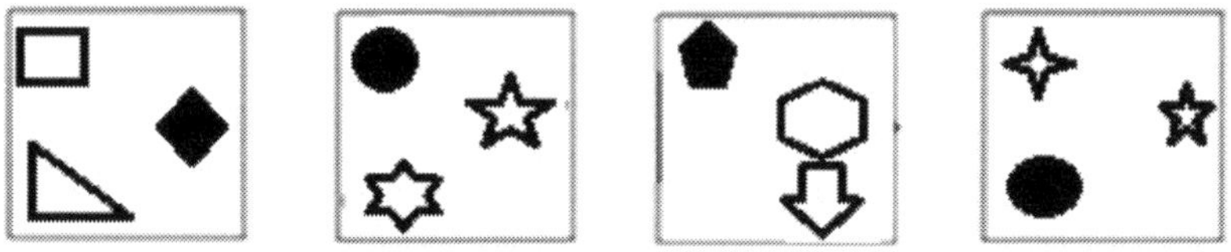

Set 11:

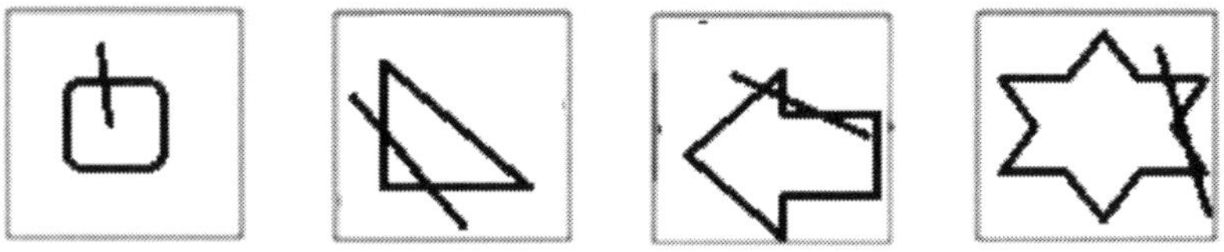

Questions 47: Which figure completes the series?

A. B. C. D.

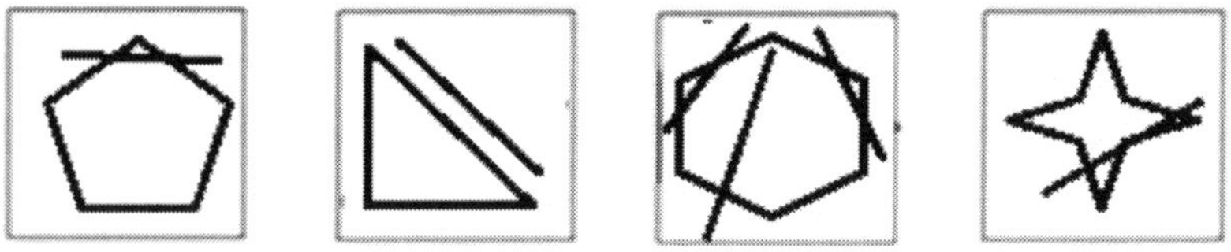

Set 12:

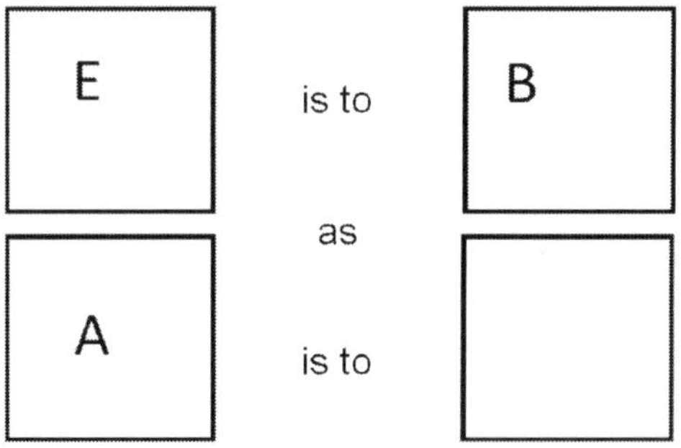

Question 48: Which figure completes the statement?

A. B. C. D.

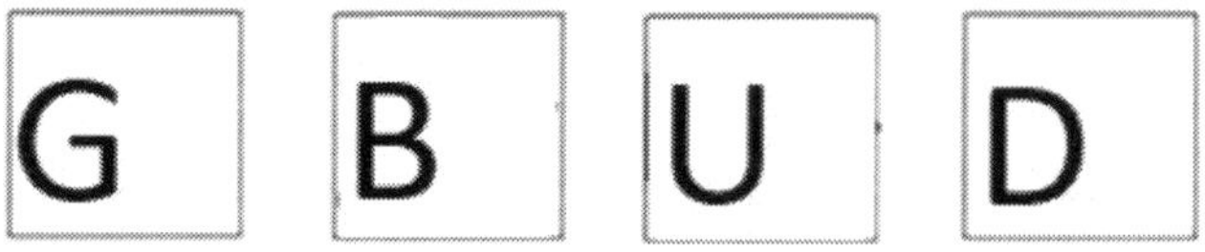

Set 13:

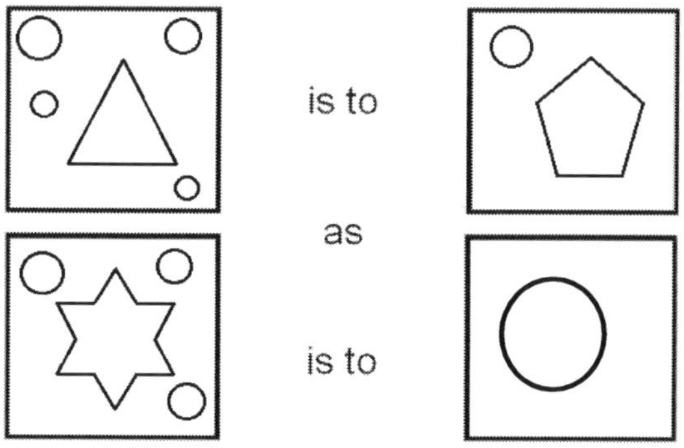

Question 49: Which figure completes the statement?

A. B. C. D.

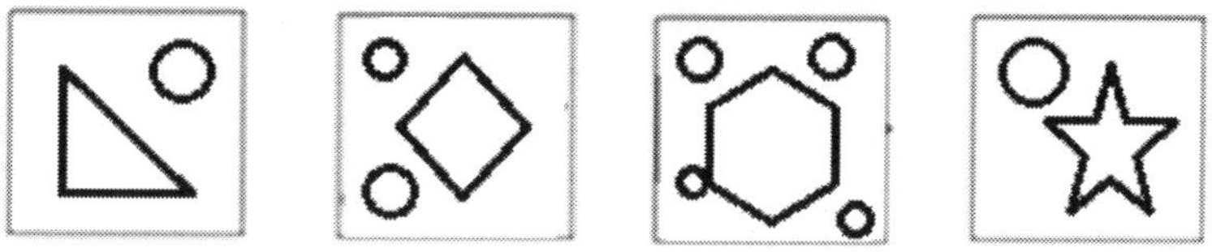

Set 14:

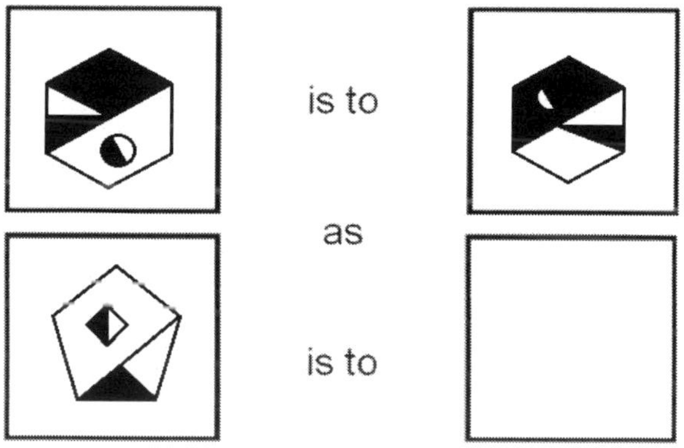

Question 50: Which figure completes the statement?

A. B. C. D.

Set 15:

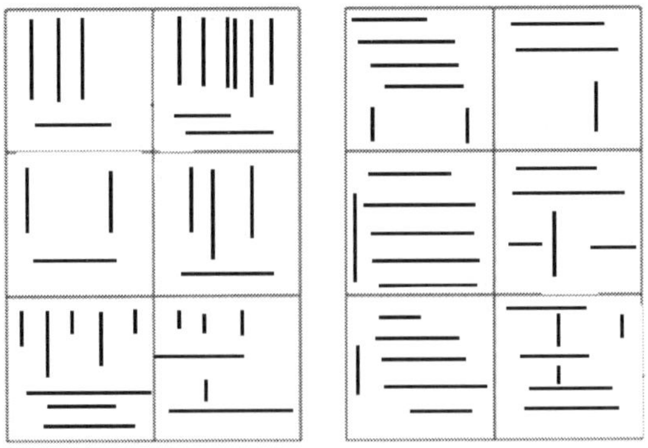

Question 51: Which of the following belongs in Set A?

A. B. C. D.

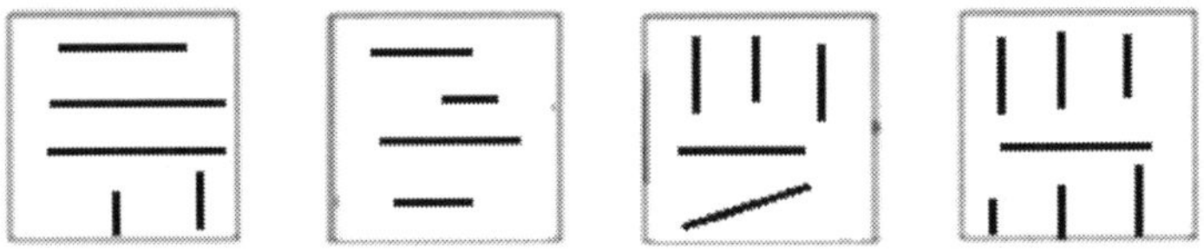

Question 52: Which of the following belongs in Set A?

A. B. C. D.

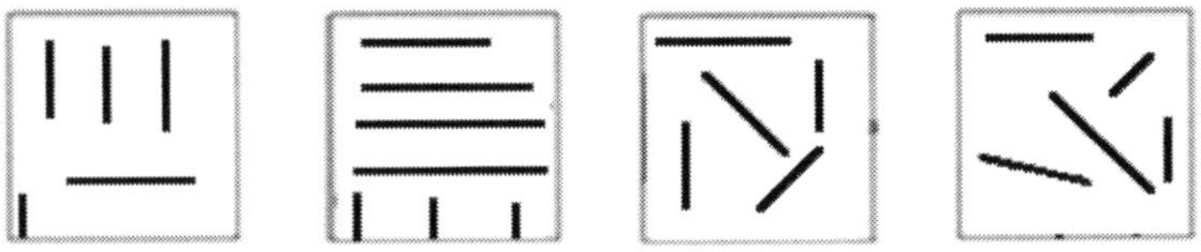

Question 53: Which of the following belongs in Set A?

A. B. C. D.

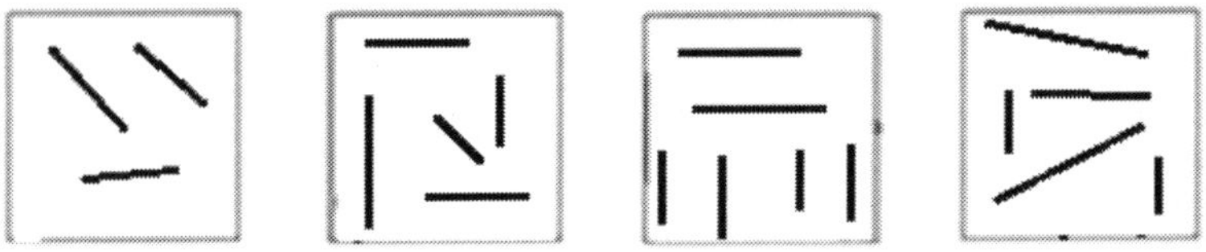

Question 54: Which of the following belongs in Set B?

A. B. C. D.

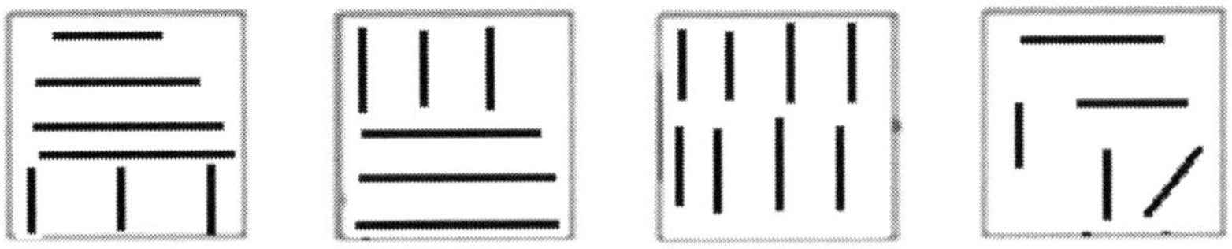

Question 55: Which of the following belongs in Set B?

A. B. C. D.

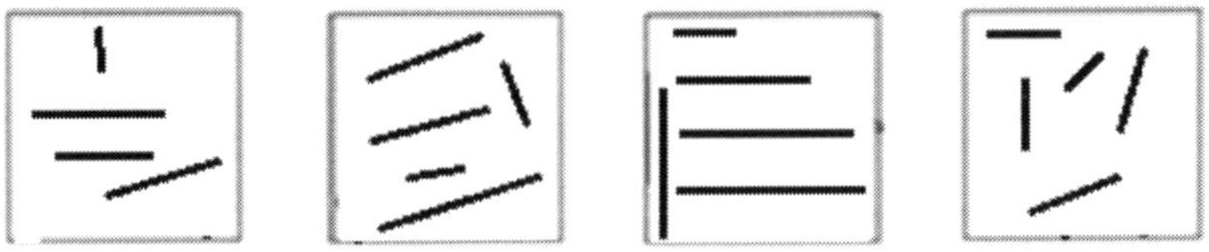

END OF SECTION

Section E: Situational Judgement Test

Read each scenario. Each question refers to the scenario directly above. For each question, select one of these four options. Select whichever you feel is the option that best represents your view on each suggested action.

For questions 1 – 30, choose one of the following options:

A A highly appropriate action
B Appropriate, but not ideal
C Inappropriate, but not awful
D A highly inappropriate action

Scenario 1

James is a fourth-year medical student. In preparation for his end of year exams, James has been asking students in the year above for questions that they had in their end of year exams, and is planning to create a question bank using these responses. Once the question bank is completed, James plans to distribute the bank to his fellow students. You are James's good friend and are aware of his plans.

How appropriate are your responses to this situation?

1. Report James to the medical school, as this is cheating
2. Don't say anything to anyone, so that you can also benefit from the question bank
3. Talk to James about what he is doing, and convey that what he is doing is technically cheating
4. Inform James's parents of his plans, so that they can intervene
5. Publicly expose James on social media, and warn your colleagues that anyone using James's question bank will be reported for cheating.

Scenario 2

Rashid is a clinical medical student. As part of his academic year, He has a 6-week research placement in which he can pursue any academic interest of his choice. During this placement, his family has arranged for him to attend a relative's wedding in Sri Lanka. This will involve a two-week trip. The trip has already been booked. Rashid wants to go, as he plays an important role in the wedding, but he is worried that if he asks permission from the clinical school then they might refuse.

How appropriate are Rashid's responses to this situation?

6. Go on the holiday without telling the clinical school
7. Ask the clinical school for permission before travelling
8. Sweet-talk his supervisor so he is more willing to pass Rashid's placement before he travels
9. Tell his parents that they should cancel his ticket
10. Tell the clinical school and go on the holiday regardless of their response

Scenario 3

Jamie is a sixth form student. As part of his A-level Chemistry, he must write a practical paper, which is worth 20% of his grade, in the classroom. However, as the paper is conducted in the classroom, different schools take the test at different times. As a result, one of Jamie's friends at another college already has done the exam, and offers Jamie the questions the week before his own exam, so that he can prepare answers beforehand.

How appropriate are Jamie's responses to this situation?

11. Take the questions-he is not cheating, his friend is
12. Take only enough questions such that he can achieve an A grade in the practical paper
13. Refuse the questions
14. Report the friend for cheating to the exam board
15. Take the questions and distribute them to all his classmates so that he is not at an unfair advantage

Scenario 4

You are a student on placement in a rural practice. Two of the patients you have been asked to see are married, and have arranged separate appointments with you to discuss the results of their STI screen. They wanted to do this to make sure both partners had no infections before they started family planning. You meet the husband first, who is clear of infections and you discuss how to optimise chances of getting pregnant with him. Later, you meet the wife, whose blood test reveals that she is HIV positive. She tells you that she does not want you telling the husband.

How appropriate are your responses to this situation?

16. Tell the wife that you have a responsibility to the husband as his doctor to tell him if he is at risk of developing HIV
17. Try to convince the wife to speak to him before they try family planning
18. Call up the husband after the wife has left
19. Call the husband into the consultation room with the wife
20. Make up an excuse for the wife as to why she has HIV so that she can tell the husband that

Scenario 5

You are a student on placement on a surgical ward. You are printing off the lists in preparation for the ward round, when your consultant walks in looking very untidy. It soon becomes obvious that he is drunk, and there is an obvious smell of alcohol on his breath.

How appropriate are your responses to this situation?

21. Consult your registrar
22. Pretend that you don't notice
23. Report the consultant to the hospital board
24. Take the consultant into a private room, make him drink plenty of water and tell him to go home
25. Tell all the patients that the consultant is too drunk to do the ward round this morning

Scenario 6

You are a fifth-year medical student approaching your finals. One of your good friends, Neil, is also preparing for his finals, but you know that every weekend Neil stays awake most of the night taking illicit drugs. It has not affected his performance at medical school so far but you've noticed that his drug use has been getting worse and worse in the run-up to finals. You are worried that Neil might go off the rails before finals and end up failing.

How appropriate are your responses to this situation?

26. Inform the university pastoral care about Neil's situation
27. Inform the medical school that Neil is taking illicit drugs
28. Try and speak to Neil, and make sure that he is ok and voice your concerns with regards to the drug use
29. Sneak into Neil's room when he is in hospital and steal his drugs
30. Inform the police that Neil is holding drugs

For questions 31 – 69, decide how important each statement is when deciding how to respond to the situation?

A Extremely important
B Fairly important
C Of minor importance
D Of no importance whatsoever

Scenario 7

Janice is a fourth-year medical student. During the ward round, the consultant on the ward offers her the opportunity to assist in a liver transplant. However, the same time that the surgery is scheduled to begin, Janice has compulsory teaching which is part of her course requirements.

How important are the following factors for Janice in deciding what to do?

31. The teaching is likely to come up in her end of year exams
32. She is unlikely to get this sort of opportunity during the rest of her time in medical school
33. Janice is very interested in transplant surgery and has been waiting for an opportunity such as this
34. The teaching is small group and it will be very noticeable is Janice is not present
35. Assisting in a transplant surgery will add to her portfolio, strengthening her application for transplant surgeon in the future.

Scenario 8

Johnathan is a second-year medical student. This year, Johnathan has been selected for the university cricket team, which involves a rigorous training schedule during the last two months of the calendar year. However, the second-year final exams are also at the end of the academic year, so most of his classmates are gearing up to sit those exams.

How important are the following factors for Johnathan in deciding what to do?

36. Second year exams determine whether Johnathan can begin his clinical training or not
37. There are prizes given for excellent achievement in the second-year final exams
38. Johnathan's father has spent a lot of money in coaching Johnathan in preparation for university cricket
39. Johnathan is only just starting to integrate into the team
40. Johnathan has a bet with his friends on who will do the best at the end of the year

Scenario 9

Hayley, a final year medical student, has been offered the opportunity to present a case report at a national conference by a consultant on the ward she is working on. Unfortunately, she has a meeting with her director of studies about elective planning the day she is flying.

How important are the following factors for Hayley in deciding what to do?

41. Her director of studies is a prestigious professor in the university, who has a very tight schedule
42. She cannot go on her elective without university funding, which must be approved by her director of studies
43. The conference is in Sydney, a city Hayley has always hoped to visit
44. The consultant is only taking one student with him
45. Hayley is guaranteed a publication if she agrees to presenting

Scenario 10

Latisha and Tim are clinical partners. Tim finds out that over the Christmas holidays, Latisha's boyfriend broke up with her. Since returning, Latisha has been arriving late to the ward round, and often leaves in a fit of tears during the middle of consultations. The doctors on the ward say nothing at the time, but Tim hears them whispering about Latisha quietly once the ward round has finished. Tim has spoken to Latisha before but she insisted that she was fine.

How important are the following factors for Tim in deciding what to do?

46. Latisha's reputation with the doctors
47. The consultant on the ward round determines whether they pass or fail that placement
48. The appearance to patients
49. Latisha may never speak to Tim again if he insists on the matter
50. Tim's friendship with Latisha's ex-boyfriend

Scenario 11

Javad is a final year medical student. One day during lunch in the hospital canteen, he overhears his friend laughing loudly about a patient he saw on the ward who is in a vulnerable position, and loudly revealing details of the patient for all to hear. Later, an emergency meeting is called with the clinical dean, who reveals that a breach of confidentiality has been reported, and it is known that it was a medical student.

How important are the following factors for Javad in deciding what to do?

51. Javad and his friend have been friends since kindergarten
52. The clinical school are sure to exclude Javad's friend if they find out it was him
53. The hospital would be heavily fined if the news got out that there was a confidentiality breach
54. This will be the first time Javad's friend has been in trouble with the clinical school
55. Javad knows that his friend has been really struggling in the run-up to finals.

Scenario 12
Ross and Alex are final year medical students currently on their Emergency Medicine rotation. One night when Ross is working, Alex comes in heavily inebriated. He takes Ross aside, and explains to him that he is working at 6am tomorrow. Alex then begs Ross to give him a bed in the Emergency Department and hook him up to an IV fluid drip, so that he can wake up sober and ready for work the next day.

How important are the following factors for Ross in deciding what to do?

56. Alex and Ross are the only students on Emergency Medicine now
57. There is a shortage of beds in the Emergency Department
58. The consultant will be doing a ward round at 5am, for which Ross will be a part of
59. IV fluids are a prescription which require inpatient admittance
60. Alex has stated that 'he would do the same' for Ross
61. Ross is going on holiday with Alex for two weeks in June

Scenario 13
Surya and Leah are two first year medical students doing their first clinical placement. When they ask the FY2 on the ward who would be a good patient to examine, the FY2 recommends a patient in one of the side rooms of the ward. He also says that the patient is MRSA positive, but that if they're quick enough then there should be nothing to worry about.

How important are the following factors for the two of them in deciding what to do?

62. MRSA requires strict isolation
63. The nurses have told them that they should not go in unless necessary
64. The junior doctor knows more about the ward than they do
65. They need to present their examination findings to the junior doctor when they're done
66. The patient is clearly unwell
67. An abdominal examination on such a patient would provide invaluable learning experience
68. It is not essential for them to examine the patient
69. Surya and Leah are going to a party later

END OF PAPER

Mock Paper F

Section A: Verbal Reasoning

Passage 1

The English Sparrow

The English Sparrow was first introduced into the United States at Brooklyn, New York, in the years 1851 and '52. The trees in our parks were at that time infested with a canker-worm, which wrought them great injury, and to rid the trees of these worms was the mission of the English Sparrow.

In his native country this bird, though of a seed-eating family (Finch), was a great insect eater. The few which were brought over performed, at first, the duty required of them; they devoured the worms and stayed near the cities. With the change of climate, however, came a change in their taste for insects. They made their home in the country as well as the cities, and became seed and vegetable eaters, devouring the young buds on vines and trees, grass-seed, oats, rye, and other grains.

Their services in insect-killing are still not to be despised. A single pair of these Sparrows, under observation an entire day, were seen to convey to their young no less than forty grubs an hour, an average exceeding three thousand in the course of a week. Moreover, even in the autumn he does not confine himself to grain, but feeds on various seeds, such as the dandelion, the sow-thistle, and the groundsel; all of which plants are classed as weeds. It has been known, also, to chase and devour the common white butterfly, whose caterpillars make havoc among the garden plants.

The good he may accomplish in this direction, however, is nullified to the lovers of the beautiful, by the war he constantly wages upon our song birds, destroying their young, and substituting his unattractive looks and inharmonious chirps for their beautiful plumage and soul-inspiring songs.

1. Which of the following statements about the English Sparrows is true:

A. The English Sparrows kills song birds
B. The English Sparrow was first discovered in the mid 19th century
C. The English Sparrow sings soul-inspiring songs
D. The English Sparrow eats canker-worms all year round

2. Which of the following statements are INCORRECT:

A. English Sparrows inhabit both the cities and countryside
B. English Sparrows accomplish more good than bad
C. English Sparrows eat seeds as well as insects
D. English Sparrows are unattractive

3. According to the above passage:

A. English Sparrows prefer insects to grains
B. Song birds are more harmonious than English Sparrows
C. English Sparrows are omnivores
D. English Sparrows eat caterpillars

4. A single pair of sparrows were observed to:

A. Convey over 40 grubs per hour to their young
B. Convey at least 40 grubs per hour to their young
C. Convey over 3000 grubs to their young per week
D. Convey over 12,000 grubs to their young per month

Passage 2

Greek Gods

In appearance, the gods were supposed to resemble mortals, whom, however, they far surpassed in beauty, grandeur, and strength; they were also more commanding in stature, height being considered by the Greeks an attribute of beauty in man or woman. They resembled human beings in their feelings and habits, intermarrying and having children, and requiring daily nourishment to recruit their strength, and refreshing sleep to restore their energies. Their blood, a bright ethereal fluid called Ichor, never engendered disease, and, when shed, had the power of producing new life.

The Greeks believed that the mental qualifications of their gods were of a much higher order than those of men, but nevertheless, as we shall see, they were not considered to be exempt from human passions, and we frequently behold them actuated by revenge, deceit, and jealousy. They, however, always punish the evil-doer, and visit with dire calamities any impious mortal who dares to neglect their worship or despise their rites. We often hear of them visiting mankind and partaking of their hospitality, and not infrequently both gods and goddesses become attached to mortals, with whom they unite themselves, the offspring of these unions being called heroes or demi-gods, who were usually renowned for their great strength and courage. But although there were so many points of resemblance between gods and men, there remained the one great characteristic distinction, that is to say, that the gods enjoyed immortality. Still, they were not invulnerable, and we often hear of them being wounded, and suffering in consequence such exquisite torture that they have earnestly prayed to be deprived of their privilege of immortality.

5. According to the above passage:

A. Gods always enjoy immortality.
B. Gods infrequently have children with mortals.
C. Gods do not need food or sleep.
D. Gods are more intelligent than humans.

6. Which of the following are not differences between gods and humans?

A. Height
B. IQ
C. Mortality
D. Emotions

7. According to the passage, which of the following statements is true of demi-gods?

A. Demi-gods are more courageous than gods.
B. Hercules is a demi-god.
C. Heroes and demi-gods can be used interchangeably to mean the same thing.
D. Demi-gods live longer than humans.

8. Which of the following statements are INCORRECT?

A. The biggest difference between gods and humans is the fact that gods are immortal.
B. Gods are taller than humans.
C. On the whole, Greeks find shorter women more attractive.
D. Gods cannot transmit illnesses between themselves.

Passage 3

The Effort of Digestion

Digestion is a huge, unappreciated task, unappreciated because few of us are aware of its happening in the same way we are aware of making efforts to use our voluntary muscles when working or exercising. Digestion begins in the mouth with thorough chewing. If you don't think chewing is effort, try making coleslaw in your own mouth. Chew up at least half a big head of cabbage and three big carrots that have not been shredded. Grind each bit until it liquefies and has been thoroughly mixed with saliva. I guarantee that if you even finish the chore your jaw will be tired, and you will have lost all desire to eat anything else, especially if it requires chewing. Making the saliva you just used while chewing the cabbage is by itself, a huge and unappreciated chemical effort.

Once in the stomach, chewed food has to be churned in order to mix it with hydrochloric acid, pepsin, and other digestive enzymes. Manufacturing these enzymes is also considerable work! Churning is even harder work than chewing but normally, people are unaware of its happening. While the stomach is churning (like a washing machine) a large portion of the blood supply is redirected from the muscles in the extremities to the stomach and intestines to aid in this process. Anyone who has tried to go for a run, or take part in any other strenuous physical activity immediately after a large meal feels like a slug and wonders why they just can't make their legs move the way they usually do. So, to assist the body while it is digesting, it is wise to take a siesta as los Latinos do instead of expecting the blood to be two places at once like los norteamericanos.

After the stomach is through churning, the partially digested food is moved into the small intestine where it is mixed with more pancreatin secreted by the pancreas, and with bile from the gall bladder. Pancreatin further solubilises proteins. Bile aids in the digestion of fatty foods. Manufacturing bile and pancreatic enzymes is also a lot of effort. Only after the carbohydrates (starches and sugars), proteins and fats have been broken down into simpler water-soluble food units such as simple sugars, amino acids and fatty acids, can the body pass these nutrients into the blood thorough the little projections in the small intestines called villi.

9. Why is digestion unappreciated?

A. Because we use voluntary muscles like when working or exercising.
B. Because we aren't conscious of the effort it takes our body to digest food.
C. Because it requires the whole digestive system.
D. Because we need food as energy for our bodies.

10. How many aspects of digestion in the passage are described as effort or hard work?

A. 2 B. 3 C. 4 D. 5

11. According to the passage, which of the following statements about digestion is true:

A. It requires blood to be diverted from muscles in the arms and legs to the stomach
B. It is as much effort as chewing half a head of cabbage and three big carrots
C. It requires amylase
D. It partially occurs in the gall bladder.

12. Which of the following statements about pancreatin is INCORRECT?

A. It is secreted into the small intestine
B. It helps with the formation of amino acids
C. It requires a lot of effort to be made
D. It only digests proteins.

Passage 4

Queen Victoria: Early years

When she was five years old the Princess Victoria began to have lessons, chiefly with a governess, Miss von Lehzen—"my dearly beloved angelic Lehzen," as she called her. These two remained devotedly attached to one another until the latter's death in 1870. The young Princess was especially fond of music and drawing, and it was clear that if she had been able to devote more time to study she would in later years have excelled in both subjects.

Her education was such as to fit her for her future position of Queen of England. The Princess did not, however, know that she was likely at any future time to be Queen. She read much, chiefly books dealing with history, and these were often chosen for her by her uncle, the King of the Belgians.

The family life was regular and simple. Lessons, a walk or drive, very few and simple pleasures made up her day. Breakfast was at half-past eight, luncheon at half-past one, and dinner at seven. Tea was allowed only in later years as a great treat.

The Queen herself said: "I was brought up very simply—never had a room to myself till I was nearly grown up—always slept in my mother's room till I came to the throne."

13. According to the passage:

A. Princess Victoria had lessons with her governess for 5 years.
B. Princess Victoria excelled in both music and drawing.
C. Princess Victoria died in 1870.
D. Princess Victoria was fond of her governess.

14. Which of the following was NOT part of Princess Victoria's day-to-day activities as a young child?

A. Breakfast, lunch and dinner at set times.
B. Lessons with her governess.
C. Tea
D. Music

15. Which of the following statements is true of Princess Victoria?

A. She was unaware that she was likely to become Queen.
B. She sometimes slept in her mother's room before becoming Queen.
C. She read about Belgian history.
D. She enjoyed music more than reading.

16. Which is INCORRECT regarding the Princesses education:

A. It was tailored to her future position as Queen
B. It involved reading history books
C. Her uncle was involved in her education
D. She was solely taught by her governess

Passage 5

Outdoor exercise in pregnancy

Outdoor exercise is indispensable to good health. It benefits not only the muscles, but the whole body. By this means the action of the heart is strengthened, and consequently all the tissues receive a rich supply of oxygen. Exercise also promotes the digestion and the assimilation of the food. It stimulates the sweat glands to become more active; and, for that matter, the other excretory organs as well. It invigorates the muscles, strengthens the nerves, and clears the brain. There is, indeed, no part of the human machine that does not run more smoothly if its owner exercises systematically in the open air; and during normal pregnancy there is no exception to this rule. Only in extremely rare cases—those, namely, in which extraordinary precautions must be taken to prevent miscarriage—will physicians prohibit outdoor recreation and, perhaps, every other kind of exertion. Under such circumstances the good effects that most persons secure from exercise should be sought from the use of massage.

The amount of exercise which the prospective mother should take cannot be stated precisely, but what can be definitely said is this— she should stop the moment she begins to feel tired. Fatigue is only one step short of exhaustion—and, since exhaustion must always be carefully guarded against, the safest rule will be to leave off exercising at a point where one still feels capable of doing more without becoming tired. Women who have laborious household duties to perform do not require as much exercise as those who lead sedentary lives; but they do require just as much fresh air, and should make it a rule to sit quietly out of doors two or three hours every day. It will be found, furthermore, that the limit of endurance is reached more quickly toward the end of pregnancy than at the beginning; a few patients will find it necessary to stop exercise altogether for a week or two before they are delivered.

17. A woman's exercise tolerance decreases throughout pregnancy.

A. True B. False C. Can't tell

18. Exhaustion can cause miscarriages.

A. True B. False C. Can't tell

19. Pregnant women should exercise until they go into labour.

A. True B. False C. Can't tell

20. Women who have household duties do not need to exercise.

A. True B. False C. Can't tell

Passage 6

Spaghetti or Macaroni with Butter and Cheese

This is the simplest form in which the spaghetti may be served, and it is generally reserved for the thickest pasta. The spaghetti are to be boiled until tender in salted water, taking care to remove them when tender, and not cooked until they lose form. They should not be put into the water until this is at a boiling point.

Take as much macaroni as will half fill the dish in which it is to be served. Break into pieces two and a half to three inches long if you so desire. The Italians leave them unbroken, but their skill in turning them around the fork and eating them is not the privilege of everybody. Put the macaroni into salted boiling water, and boil twelve to fifteen minutes, or until the macaroni is perfectly soft. Stir frequently to prevent the macaroni from adhering to the bottom. Turn it into a colander to drain; then put it into a pudding-dish with a generous quantity of butter and grated cheese. If more cheese is liked, it can be brought to the table so that the guests can help themselves to it.

The macaroni called "Mezzani" which is a name designating size, not quality, is the preferable kind for macaroni dishes made with butter and cheese.

21. Butter and cheese is the simplest accompaniment to pasta.

A. True B. False C. Can't tell

22. Only Italians can eat unbroken macaroni.

A. True B. False C. Can't tell

23. Which of the following is INCORRECT regarding the preparation of this dish?

A. If spaghetti is cooked for too long it will lose its form.
B. Spaghetti should be cooked for 12-15 minutes.
C. Stirring the pasta as it boils will prevent it from sticking to the bottom.
D. Italians eat macaroni unbroken.

24. According to the passage:

A. Pasta must be cooked in salted boiling water
B. Pasta should only be put into the water at boiling point.
C. Pasta can be drained in a colander.

D. Mezzani is the best kind of pasta for butter and cheese.

Passage 7

The Penguins of Antarctica

The penguins of the Antarctic regions very rightly have been termed the true inhabitants of that country. The species is of great antiquity, fossil remains of their ancestors having been found, which showed that they flourished as far back as the eocene epoch. To a degree far in advance of any other bird, the penguin has adapted itself to the sea as a means of livelihood, so that it rivals the very fishes. This proficiency in the water has been gained at the expense of its power of flight, but this is a matter of small moment, as it happens.

In few other regions could such an animal as the penguin rear its young, for when on land its short legs offer small advantage as a means of getting about, and as it cannot fly, it would become an easy prey to any of the carnivora which abound in other parts of the globe. Here, however, there are none of the bears and foxes which inhabit the North Polar regions, and once ashore the penguin is safe.

The reason for this state of things is that there is no food of any description to be had inland. Ages back, a different state of things existed: tropical forests abounded, and at one time, the seals ran about on shore like dogs. As conditions changed, these latter had to take to the sea for food, with the result that their four legs, in course of time, gave place to wide paddles or "flippers," as the penguins' wings have done, so that at length they became true inhabitants of the sea.

25. According to the above passage, which of the following statements is correct?

A. Penguins can fly
B. Penguins were the first land inhabitants of the Antarctic region
C. Seals benefit from the meal of penguin chicks
D. Penguin chicks cannot find food on land.

26. Penguins live in the North Polar regions

A. True
B. False
C. Can't tell

27. Penguins are safe when searching for food on land

A. True
B. False
C. Can't tell

28. Which of the following is incorrect?

A. Penguin are easy prey to foxes, bear and seals.
B. Penguins are highly adapted to the sea environment.
C. Penguins legs evolved over time into fins.
D. Seals could eat Penguin chicks.

Passage 8

Indian birds

In India winter is the time of year at which the larger birds of prey, both diurnal and nocturnal, rear up their broods. Throughout January the white-backed vultures are occupied in parental duties. The breeding season of these birds begins in October or November and ends in February or March. The nest, which is placed high up in a lofty tree, is a large platform composed of twigs which the birds themselves break off from the growing tree. Much amusement may be derived from watching the struggles of a white-backed vulture when severing a tough branch. Its wing-flapping and its tugging cause a great commotion in the tree. The boughs used by vultures for their nests are mostly covered with green leaves. These last wither soon after the branch has been plucked, so that, after the first few days of its existence, the nest looks like a great ball of dead leaves caught in a tree.

The nurseries of birds of prey can be described neither as picturesque nor as triumphs of architecture, but they have the great merit of being easy to see. January is the month in which to look for the eyries of Bonelli's eagles (Hieraetus fasciatus); not that the search is likely to be successful. The high cliffs of the Jumna and the Chambal in the Etawah district are the only places where the nests of this fine eagle have been recorded in the United Provinces. Mr. A. J. Currie has found the nest on two occasions in a mango tree in a tope at Lahore. In each case the eyrie was a flat platform of sticks about twice the size of a kite's nest. The ground beneath the eyrie was littered with fowls' feathers and pellets of skin, fur and bone. Most of these pellets contained squirrels' skulls; and Mr. Currie actually saw one of the parent birds fly to the nest with a squirrel in its talons.

29. Which of the following is incorrect?

A. Some birds of prey incorporate squirrels into their nests
B. Nests of Bonelli's eagles have been found in Jumna and Chambal
C. One is most likely to successfully find the nest of a Bonelli Eagle in January
D. The breeding season of the white-backed vulture begins in January

30. The Latin name for Bonelli's eagles is Hieraetus faciatus

A. True
B. False
C. Can't tell

31. The kite's nest is made of squirrels' skulls

A. True
B. False
C. Can't tell

32. Which is correct?

A. Bonelli's eagles build their nests on flat areas of land.
B. Kites have short and rounded tails
C. Winter is when the larger birds of prey in India breed
D. Only the highest cliffs of the Jumna and the Chambal will suit White-backed vultures

Passage 9

Argentinian history

The province of Buenos Aires, the largest in the country, has always been the most populated, and its lands have always commanded the highest prices, and these have risen tremendously, but not so much of late years in proportion as land in the northern provinces. During the years 1885, 1886, 1887, and 1888, there was a great boom in land. Foreigners were pouring in, bringing capital; great confidence was put by foreign capitalists in the country, several railways had run out new branches, new railways were built, new banks were opened, and a very large extent of land was opened up and cultivated, and put under wheat and linseed, harvests were good and money was flowing into the country. Then came a very bad year, 1889; the harvest was practically lost owing to the heavy and continuous rains which fell from December till July with hardly a clear day. This, together with a bad government and the revolution of 1890, created a great panic and a tremendous slump in all land, from which it took a long time to recover. Where people had bought camps and mortgaged them, which was the general thing to do in those days, the mortgagees foreclosed, and, when the camps were auctioned off, they did not fetch half what the properties had been bought for in the first instance, some four or five years previously. This, naturally, had a serious effect on the credit, soundness, and finances of the country, but really, the crisis was not felt until some three or four years after, and it was 1896 and 1897 which were very serious years for the country.

33. Which statement is incorrect?

A. There was a boom in land prices in the late 1880s.
B. Rain caused the land prices to fall.
C. 1889 was the worst year of the century.
D. It took a few years for the drop-in land prices to badly affect the city.

34. Which is the correct statement?

A. The government brought about the boom in land prices in the late 1880s.
B. The government foreclosed mortgages after 1890.
C. Foreign investment enables land prices to rise.
D. Many locals bought camps to try and save their land.

35. Buenos Aires is the smallest province in Argentina.

A. True
B. False
C. Can't tell

36. Monsoon season in Buenos Aires begins in December.

A. True
B. False
C. Can't tell

Passage 10

Mosquitoes

Mosquito eggs are laid in water or in places where water is apt to accumulate, otherwise they will not hatch. Some species lay their eggs in little masses that float on the surface of the water, looking like small particles of soot. Others lay their eggs singly, some floating about on the surface, others sinking to the bottom where they remain until the young issue. Some of the eggs may remain over winter, but usually those laid in the summer hatch in thirty-six to forty-eight hours or longer according to the temperature.

When the larvæ are ready to issue they burst open the lower end of the eggs and the young wrigglers escape into the water. The larvæ are fitted for aquatic life only, so mosquitoes cannot breed in moist or damp places unless there is at least a small amount of standing water there. A very little will do, but there must be enough to cover the larvæ or they perish. The head of the larvæ of most species is wide and flattened. The eyes are situated at the sides, and just in front of them is a pair of short antennæ which vary with the different species. The mouth-parts too vary greatly according to the feeding habits. Some mosquito larvæ are predaceous, feeding on the young of other species or on other insects. These of course have their mouth-parts fitted for seizing and holding their prey. Most of the wrigglers, however, feed on algæ, diatoms, Protozoa and other minute plant or animal forms which are swept into the mouth by curious little brush-like organs whose movements keep a stream of water flowing toward the mouth.

A few kinds feed habitually some distance below the surface, others on the bottom, while still others feed always at the surface. With one or two exceptions, the larvæ must all come to the surface to breathe. Most species have on the eighth abdominal segment a rather long breathing-tube the tip of which is thrust just above the surface of the water when they come up for air.

37. Mosquitoes require water to lay their eggs.

A. True
B. False
C. Can't tell

38. Eggs laid in Summer hatch thirty-six to forty-eight hours after eggs laid in Winter.

A. True
B. False
C. Can't tell

39. Select the incorrect statement.

A. Larvae are hatched wriggling.
B. Larvae must be wet when hatched.
C. The eyes of the larvae cannot see when first hatched.
D. Different groups of larvae feed at different levels underwater

40. Select the true statement.

A. All larvae feed on algae.
B. All larvae must come to the surface to breathe.
C. With a few exceptions all species of larvae have a breathing tube.
D. Larvae have a different circulatory system than mosquitoes.

Passage 11

Mites

The mites are closely related to the ticks, and although none of them has yet been shown to be responsible for the spread of any disease, their habits are such that it would be entirely possible for some to transmit certain diseases from one host to another, from animal to animal, from animal to man, or from man to man. A number of these mites produce certain serious diseases among various domestic animals and a few are responsible for certain diseases of men.

Face-mites. Living in the sweat-glands at the roots of hairs and in diseased follicles in the skin of man and some domestic animals are curious little parasites that look as much like worms as mites. Such diseased follicles become filled with fatty matter, the upper end becomes hard and black and in man are known as blackheads. If one of these blackheads is forced out and the fatty substance dissolved with ether the mites may be found in all stages of development. The young have six legs, the adult eight. The body is elongated and transversely wrinkled. In man they are usually found about the nose and chin and neck where they do no particular harm except to mar the appearance of the host and to indicate that his skin has not had the care it should have. Very recently certain investigators have found that the lepræ bacilli are often closely associated with these face mites and believe that they may possibly aid in the dissemination of leprosy. It is also thought that they may sometimes be the cause of cancer, but as yet these theories have not been proven by any conclusive experiment.

In dogs and cats these same or very similar parasites cause great suffering. In bad cases the hair falls out and the skin becomes scabby. Horses, cattle and sheep are also attacked. The disease caused by these mites on domestic animals is not usually considered curable except in its very early stages when salves or ointments may help some.

41. Select the correct statement:

A. Mites can spread diseases from one human to another.
B. Mites can spread diseases from themselves to ticks.
C. Salves prevent domestic animal infection.
D. Leprosy is caused by the bacteria lepræ bacilli

42. The main problem mites cause in humans are black heads.

A. True
B. False
C. Can't tell

43. Mites inhabit domestic animals for longer than they do humans.

A. True
B. False
C. Can't tell

44. Select the true statement.

A. Mites affect humans in a worse way than they affect domestic animals.
B. Black heads caused by mites are commonly found on extensor surfaces such as elbows.
C. Face mites cause a similar facial appearance in humans and other animals.
D. As the mites mature they develop 2 more legs.

END OF SECTION

Section B: Decision Making

1. In Manchester, a survey is done on a school. 6 children like cheese and onion crisps, 5 children like salt and vinegar crisps and 9 children like ready salted. 2 children like all three flavours, 1 child likes salt and vinegar and ready salted, 1 child likes salt and vinegar and cheese and onion, and 1 child likes cheese and onion and ready salted. All of the children like crisps. How many children took the survey?

A. 25 B. 13 C. 20 D. 15 E. 37

2. Sam is shorter than Tom who is shorter than Alex. Tom is shorter than Joseph who is shorter than Lilly. Alex is taller than Lilly. Who is the shortest?

A. Lilly B. Joseph C. Alex D. Sam E. Tom

3. All dancers are strong. Some dancers are pretty. Alexandra is strong, and Katie is pretty. Choose a correct statement.

A. Alexandra is a dancer
B. Katie is not a dancer
C. A dancer can be strong and pretty
D. A dancer can be strong and ugly

4. There is a chocolate cake. Nick takes 1/6 of the cake, then John takes 1/4 of the remainder. Alice and Jane attempt to share the rest of the cake but get full after they have eaten 2/3 of what was left. What proportion of the original cake is left?

A. 1/12 B. 1/6 C. 3/24 D. 5/24

5. At a barbecue, 1/4 of the guests are vegetarian. Of the meat eaters, 1/2 want 2 pieces of chicken each, and 1/2 want 1 piece of chicken. 50 pieces of chicken were bought, which includes 5 spare pieces for anyone who changes their mind. How many guests are at the barbecue?

A. 35 B. 40 C. 45 D. 50

6. A pig travels 5 km north then he turns to his right and walks 3 km. He then turns to his right and moves 5km forward. Now in which direction is he from his starting point.

A. North B. South C. East D. West E. North West

7. What is the next number in the following sequence: 144, 196, 256,

A. 346 B. 324 C. 289 D. 300

8. If horse A completes a job in 10 days and B completes the same work in 15 days - in how many days is the work completed if they work together?

A. 2 B. 3 C. 4 D. 5 E. 6

9. The ratio of a:b is 2:3 – if the present age of a is 20 years, find the age of b after 5 years.

A. 10 B. 15 C. 25 D. 30 E. 35

10. In a queue, Billy is 11th from the front of a queue and Amy is 22nd from the back. There are 4 people between Amy and Billy. If 3 people get money from the ATM then leave the queue, how many people are in the queue?

A. 31 B. 32 C. 34 D. 35 E. 38

11. Southampton is bigger than only Romsey. Oxford is bigger than Cambridge but not as big as London. Which is second biggest city?

A. Southampton
B. Romsey
C. Oxford
D. Cambridge
E. London

12. There are 5 giraffes, J is taller than D, but shorter than V and M. V is shorter than only R. If the height of the second tallest giraffe is 160cm and second shortest giraffe is 135cm, what is the possible height of M?

A. 130cm
B. 162cm
C. 155cm
D. Cannot be determined
E. None of these

13. All professional jobs require a university degree. Chemistry is a university degree. All lawyers are professionals. Which of the following statements is true based on this information?

A. All Chemistry teachers are professionals
B. All professionals require a chemistry degree
C. All lawyers have a degree
D. All lawyers have a chemistry degree
E. All universities offer law as a degree course

14. Read the following statements. Which of the options is correct regarding whether the conclusions drawn from the statements are true or not?

Statements:
No man is a lion.
Joseph is a man.
Conclusions:
I. Joseph is not a lion.
II. All men are not Joseph.

A. Conclusion I is TRUE and Conclusion II is TRUE
B. Conclusion I is TRUE and FALSE
C. Conclusion I is TRUE and Conclusion II is CAN'T TELL
D. Conclusion I is FALSE and Conclusion II is CAN'T TELL
E. Conclusion I is FALSE and Conclusion II is TRUE

15. The radius of a circle is 2/3 of the side of a square. The area of the square is 441 cm^2. Find the perimeter of the circle.

A. 27pi
B. 28pi
C. 29pi
D. 30pi
E. None of these

16. The sum of 2 numbers is 3430. If 12% of one of these numbers is equal to 28% of the other number, find the largest number.

A. 1029
B. 1032
C. 1041
D. 2401
E. 2453

17. Billy is James's father. 4 years ago, Billy's age was 4 times that of James. After 6 years, the ages of the Billy and James are in the ratio of 5:2. How old is Billy?

A. 12
B. 13
C. 14
D. 15
E. 16

18. Pointing to a photograph, a man said, "I have no brother or sister but that man's father is my father's son." Who owns the photograph?

A. His own
B. His nephew's
C. His father's
D. His son's
E. His sister's

19. The average marks scored by 12 students is 73. If the scores of Bea, Bay and Boe are included, the average becomes 73.6. If Bea scored 68 marks and Boe scored 6 more than Bay, what was Bay's score?

A. 75
B. 76
C. 77
D. 78
E. 79

20. Calculate the ratio of curved surface area and total surface area of a cone whose diameter is 40m and height is 21m.

A. 15:18
B. 26:28
C. 10:11
D. 2:3
E. 24:29

21. In a family, there is the father, the mother, two sons and two daughters. All the ladies were invited to a dinner. Both sons went out to play. The father is at work. Who was at home?

A. Only the mother was at home
B. All the females were at home
C. Only the sons were at home
D. Nobody was at home

22. There are five books A, B, C, D and E placed on a table. If A is placed below E, C is placed above D, B is placed below A, and D is placed above E, then which of the following books touches the surface of the table?

A. A
B. B
C. C
D. D

23. A man covers a distance in 1hr 24min by covering 2/3 of the distance at 4 km/h and the rest at 5km/h. What distance does he cover?

A. 5km
B. 6km
C. 7km
D. 8km

24. Two people starting from the same place walk at a rate of 5kmph and 5.5kmph respectively. What time will it take for them to be 8.5km apart, if they walk in the same direction?

A. 15
B. 16
C. 14
D. 18
E. 17

25. If 34 men completed 2/5th of a work in 8 days working 9 hours a day, how many more men should be employed to finish the rest of the work in 6 days working 9 hours a day?

A. 68
B. 108
C. 34
D. 36
E. 62

26. Given these statements:
Robots are Machines.
Machines are not human.

Which of the following are correct?
i) Jack is a human. Therefore, Jack is not a machine.
ii) All machines are robots.

A. True AND True
B. True AND False
C. True AND Can't Tell
D. Can't Tell AND Can't Tell
E. Can't Tell AND False

27. Artists are generally whimsical. Some of them are frustrated. Frustrated people are prone to be drug addicts. Based on these statements which of the following conclusions is true?

A. All frustrated people are drug addicts
B. Some artists may be drug addicts
C. All drug addicts are artists
D. All frustrated people are whimsical

28. Three ladies X, Y and Z marry three men A, B and C. X is married to A, Y is not married to an engineer, Z is not married to a doctor, C is not a doctor and A is a lawyer. Then which of the following statements is correct?

A. Y is married to C who is an engineer
B. Z is married to C who is a doctor
C. X is married to a doctor
D. None of these

29. 'Knowing the times tables is an important skill for a primary school child.' Which of the following statements provides the best argument against this statement?

A. Vigorously learning the times tables in primary school provides an unnecessary level of stress
B. Literacy is a more important skill than mathematics
C. Knowing the times tables provides no benefit for children in later life
D. There is no need for mental arithmetic when calculators are so readily available

END OF SECTION

Section C: Quantitative Reasoning

Data Set 1

John purchases a 360g box of chai latte powder. The label states the following:

	Per 100g (dry powder)	Per 18g serving (with 200g whole milk)
Energy (kJ)	1555	845
kCal	372	200
Protein (g)	8.9	8.0
Carbohydrate (g)	65.2	20.4
Fat (g)	8.4	9.6

INSTRUCTIONS
Put 3 heaped teaspoons (18g) into a mug, Add 200ml of hot milk and stir well. For a diet drink, use semi-skimmed or skimmed milk. Semi-skimmed milk contains 1.7g fat per 100ml. Skimmed milk contained 0.3g of fat per 100ml.

1. How much fat is contained in 200ml whole milk (to the nearest 0.1g)?

A. 1.2g B. 3.4g C. 6.8g D. 8.1g E. 9.6g

2. John is on a diet so decides to use a combination of semi-skimmed milk and water instead. He then adds 200ml of the mixed liquid to 18g of the chai powder. The total fat content of the resulting drink is 2.464g. Given that water does not contain any fat, what volume of semi skimmed milk did he use?

A. 56.0ml B. 81.5ml C. 144.9ml D. 118.5ml E. 170.4ml

3. John uses up the whole box of chai latte powder, making hot drinks according to the instructions. How many pints of milk will he have used (1pint = 570ml)?

A. 0.35 B. 4.4 C. 7.0 D. 14.1 E. 20.0

4. John buys semi-skimmed milk with a label that says its protein content is 3.3g per 100ml. What is the total amount of protein that he will have drunk once he has made chai latte with the entire box using standard proportions and semi-skimmed instead of whole milk (to the nearest gram)?

A. 66g B. 160g C. 164g D. 244g E. 272g

5. The calories of food is measured in kCal and it calculated by adding the calorific values of fat, protein and carbohydrate. The calorific value of 1g of protein is 4kCal and of 1g carbohydrate is 4kCal. What is the calorific value of 1g fat to the nearest gram?

A. 4 kCal B. 6 kCal C. 9 kCal D. 21 kCal E. 44 kCal

Data Set 2

Parking at Great Ormond Street Hospital

Parking Fees
This car park uses three separate changing time zones
Time zone 1: Monday – Friday
9:00am-1:00pm: 20p for each period of 10 minutes
1:00pm-6:00pm: 30p for each period of 10 minutes
Time zone 2: Saturday, Sunday and Bank Holiday
9:00am-6:00pm: 15p for each period of 20 minutes
Time zone 3: 6:00pm-9:00am any day
£1 standard fee regardless of the duration

NOTICE

1. Payment is made as you exit the car park
2. Any period stated should be paid for in full e.g. if a driver stays in the car park for 15 minutes on a Monday afternoon they should pay for a full 20 minutes (i.e. 2 x 10-minute periods)
3. If a car is parked in the car park over several charging zones then a calculation will be made separately for each zone, each being subject to its own minimum charge. For example, if a driver arrived at 12:59pm on a Monday and stayed 20 minutes, they would be charged 20p for the period between 12:59pm and 1:00pm and 60p for the period for 1:00pm to 1:19pm, a total of 80p.

6. A driver parks his car on Monday morning at 9:00am and leaves it in the car park until Sunday evening 6:00pm. How much will it cost him?

A. £59.10 B. £65.10 C. £71.10 D. £77.10 E. £83.10

7. A driver enters the car park at 5:55pm on a Monday afternoon and leaves the car park at 6:15pm. How much will he be charged?

A. 40p B. 60p C. £1 D. £1.15 E. £1.30

8. A driver arrives at the car park at 9am on a Monday and stay in the car park for 37 minutes. How much will he be charged?

A. 20p B. 50p C. 74p D. 80p E. £1

9. A driver uses the car park all year round and contacts the council to obtain a weekly season ticket. The season ticket he requires is for commuters and only allows him to use the car park Monday to Friday between 8:30am and 6:00pm. The cost of the weekly season ticket is £54. How much money will be save in comparison to paying full price for that period?

A. £5 B. £10 C. £15 D. £20 E. £25

10. A driver comes into the car park at 12:58pm and leaves 4 minutes later at 1:02pm on a Monday lunch time after having dropped his wife and son off at the hospital. How much will he be charged?

A. 10p B. 20p C. 30p D. 40p E. 50p

11. A driver only has £4.90 in his pocket to pay for car park fees. He enters the car park on Friday afternoon at 5pm. Until when can he stay in the car park?

A. Friday 9:00pm B. Saturday 9:00am C. Saturday 11:00am D. Saturday 11:40am E. Saturday 1:40pm

Data Set 3

The following table shows the gold price per 10 grams of cold in India from 1925-2011. The price is given in Indian Rupees.

Gold Prices in India from 1925 - 2011 (per 10 gm)

Year	Price	Year	Price	Year	Price	Year	Price	Year	Price
1925	18.75	1943	51.05	1961	119.35	1979	937	1997	4725
1926	18.43	1944	52.93	1962	119.75	1980	1330	1998	4045
1927	18.37	1945	62	1963	97	1981	1800	1999	4234
1928	18.37	1946	83.87	1964	63.25	1982	1645	2000	4400
1929	18.43	1947	88.62	1965	71.75	1983	1800	2001	4300
1930	18.05	1948	95.87	1966	83.75	1984	1970	2002	4990
1931	18.18	1949	94.17	1967	102.5	1985	2130	2003	5600
1932	23.06	1950	99.18	1968	162	1986	2140	2004	5850
1933	24.05	1951	98.05	1969	176	1987	2570	2005	7000
1934	28.81	1952	76.81	1970	184.5	1988	3130	2006	8400
1935	30.81	1953	73.06	1971	193	1989	3140	2007	10800
1936	29.81	1954	77.75	1972	202	1990	3200	2008	12500
1937	30.18	1955	79.18	1973	278.5	1991	3466	2009	14500
1938	19.93	1956	90.81	1974	506	1992	4334	2010	18500
1939	31.74	1957	90.62	1975	540	1993	4140	2011	26400
1940	36.04	1958	95.38	1976	432	1994	4598		
1941	37.43	1959	102.56	1977	486	1995	4680		
1942	33.05	1960	111.87	1978	685	1996	5160		

12. What is the price of 1kg of gold in 2010?

A. 1 750 000 Rupees
B. 1 850 000 Rupees
C. 18500 Rupees
D. 1850 Rupees
E. 18 500 000 Rupees

13. If there are 85 rupees in 1 Great British pound, what is the price of 1kg of gold in 2010 in Great British Pounds (to the nearest pound)?

A. £22547
B. £24536
C. £26534
D. £22981
E. £21765

14. How much gold would £25000 buy in 1940 (to the nearest kilogram)?

A. 625kg
B. 590kg
C. 716kg
D. 821kg
E. 678kg

15. In 1940 however, £1 was worth 110 Indian Rupees. Based on this, how much gold would £25000 buy in 1940 (to the nearest kilogram)?

A. 783kg
B. 779kg
C. 763kg
D. 634kg
E. 921kg

16. During school break, Aaron and Mason must arrange 46 blue pens and 38 red pens in equal quantities into pencil cases. If there is no remainder, what is the maximum number of pens that can go into each pencil case?

A. 2
B. 4
C. 6
D. 5
E. 7

Data Set 4

The following graph shows how the value (in US dollars) of the crypto-currency, Bitcoin, has varied over the past 8 years.

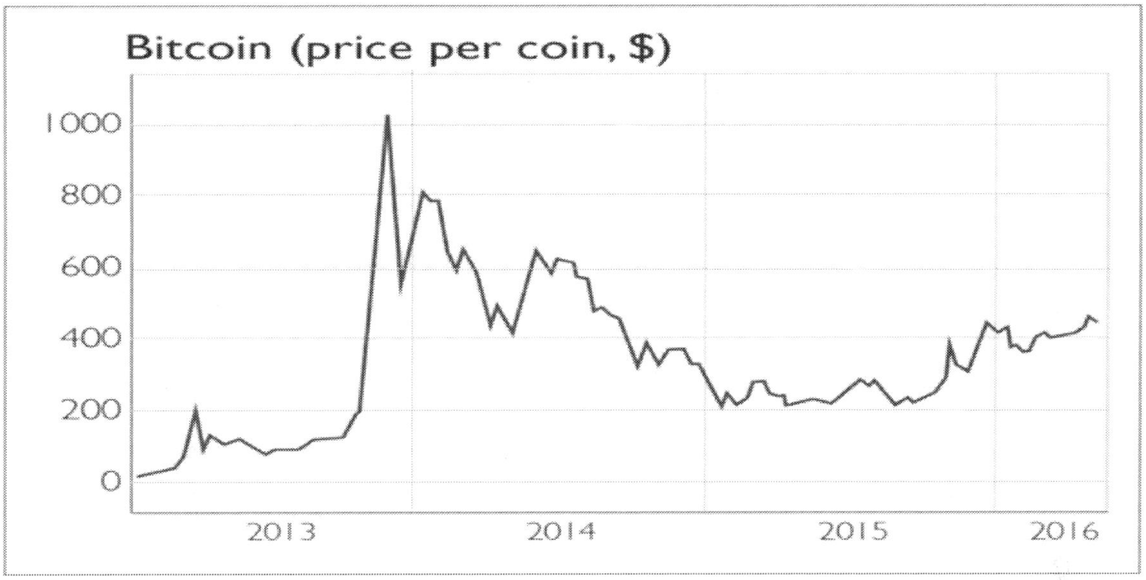

17. At what point did Bitcoin's price reach its peak?

A. July 2013
B. September 2013
C. Decemeber 2013
D. July 2015
E. July 2016

18. What was the price of Bitcoin at this stage?

A. $1020
B. $1350
C. $1256
D. $1789
E. $898

19. What is the rate of increase of the value of Bitcoin between July 2013 and December 2013 (to the nearest dollar)?

A. $150 per month
B. $230 per month
C. $143 per month
D. $184 per month
E. $350 per month

20. Jamil is a young entrepreneur who believed that Bitcoin would rapidly increase its value at some point. As a result, he invested $1000 into Bitcoin shares in January 2013, when the price of a Bitcoin share was 50 cents. He sold the shares in March 2013.How much more money would he have made had he sold it in December 2013?

A. $364537
B. $1600000
C. $2736281
D. $271928
E. $17728

Data Set 5

The following cone has radius (r) of 19cm and perpendicular height (h) of 65cm.

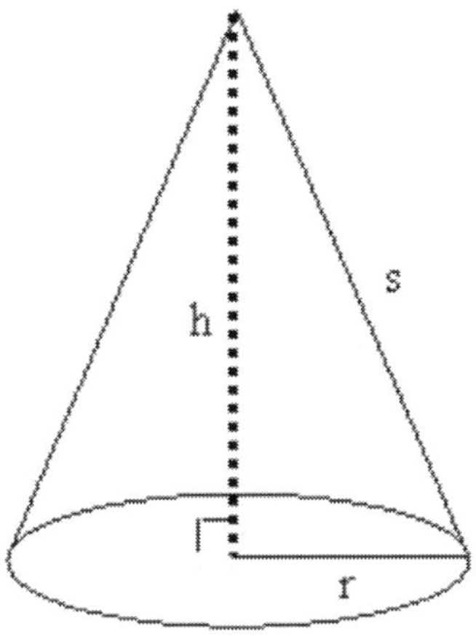

21. What is the volume of the above shape (to the nearest metre cubed)?

A. 1.79m³ B. 1.25m³ C. 1.40m³ D. 0.25m³ E. 2.34m³

22. Given that the value s=79cm, what is the surface area of the above shape (to the nearest metre squared)?

A. 0.79m² B. 0.92m² C. 0.28m² D. 0.33m² E. 0.58m²

23. If the angle made between h and s=34°, what is the angle between s and r?

A. 64° B. 56° C. 23° D. 39° E. 51°

Data Set 6

The following bar chart shows how many deaths are caused by several cancers.

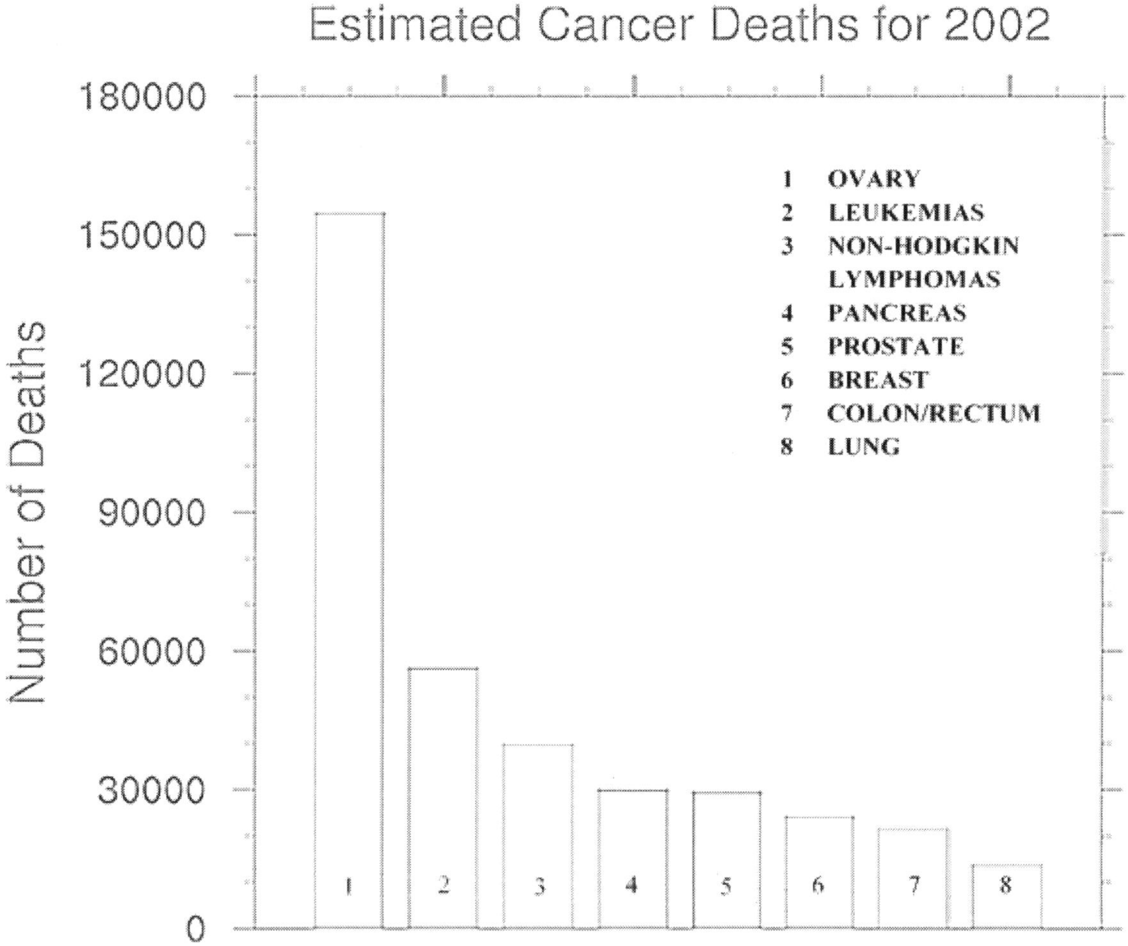

24. What is the mode of the above data set?

A. Ovary cancer
B. Breast cancer
C. Colon/rectum cancer
D. Lung cancer
E. Pancreas cancer

25. What is the mean of the above data set?

A. 46250 B. 78350 C. 87290 D. 17350 E. 22350

26. What is the range of the above data set?

A. 120 000 B. 130 000 C. 150 000 D. 140 000 E. 200 000

Data Set 7

The following graph shows how the human population has changed since 1750.

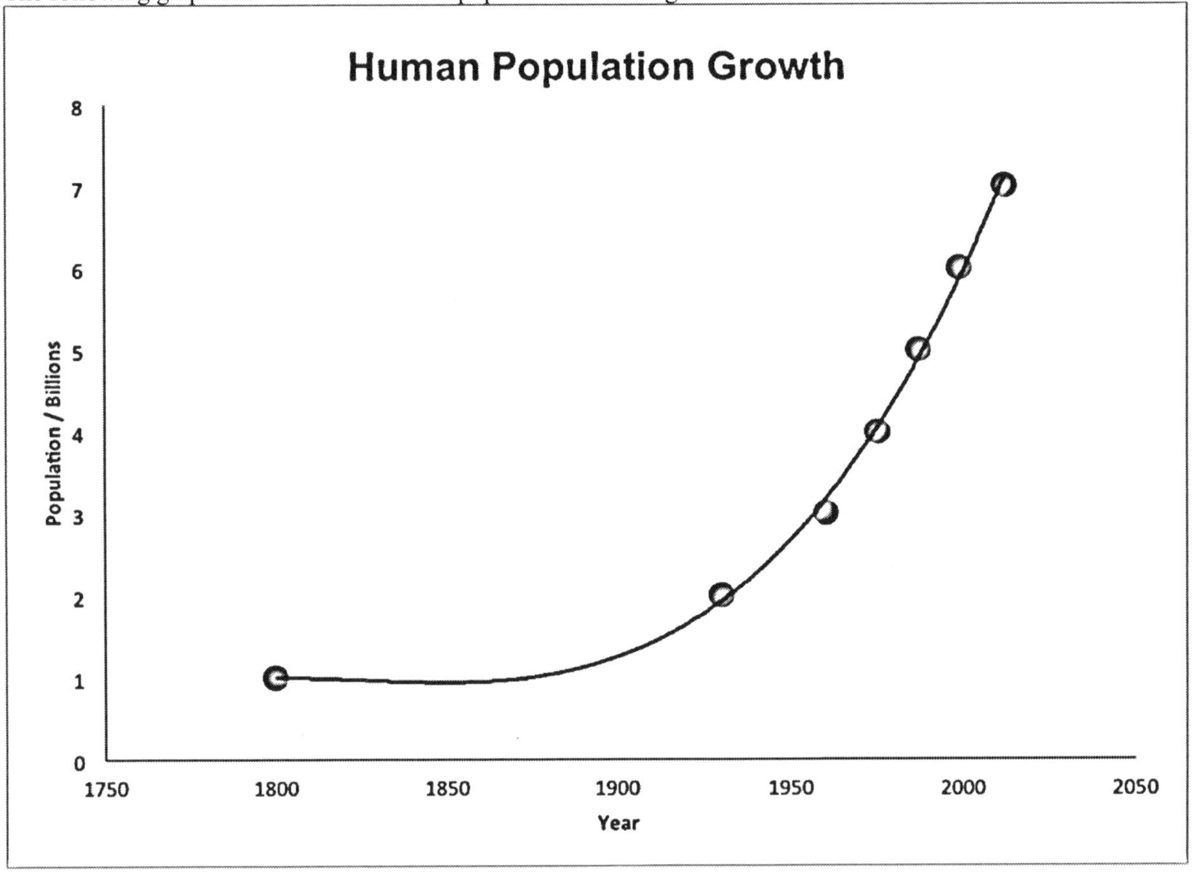

27. Estimate the human population in 1900

A. 1 billion
B. 1.5 billion
C. 1.2 billion
D. 800 million
E. 1.8 billion

28. What is the rate of population increase between 1960 and 2010?

A. 40 million per year
B. 50 million per year
C. 60 million per year
D. 70 million per year
E. 80 million per year

29. Assuming the same rate of increase, what will the population be in 2125?

A. 14.5 billion
B. 15.9 billion
C. 16.2 billion
D. 17.8 billion
E. 20.2 billion

Data Set 8

Ali is the CEO of an accounting firm. In 2016, the company had 3600 accounts. In 2017, their business saw a massive drop, falling to 2250 accounts.

30. What percentage drop does this represent?

A. 37.5% B. 21.5% C. 31.5% D. 41.2% E. 67.5%

31. If each client contributes a revenue of $150 000 to the firm, how much money did the firm lose between 2016 and 2017?

A. $390 million
B. $420 million
C. $215 million
D. $202.5 million
E. $512 million

32. If the firm must pay each employee between $30 000 and $100 000, what is the minimum number of employees that Ali must fire because of the revenue loss in 2017?

A. 5675 B. 7275 C. 1465 D. 265 E. 2025

Data Set 9

The following table is a bus timetable for Ludlow Town

701 Ludlow Town Service Saturday Schedule commences 27 January 2014

Service No	701	701	701	701	701	701	701	701	701	701	701	701
Ludlow, Tourist Info Centre	..	0740	0840	0940	1040	1140	1240	1340	1440	1540	1640	1740
Ludlow, Railway Station	..	0745	0845	0945	1045	1145	1245	1345	1445	1545	1645	1745
Ludlow, Henley Road	..	0749	0849	0949	1049	1149	1249	1349	1449	1549	1649	1749
Ludlow, Rocks Green Estate	0705	0751	0851	0951	1051	1151	1251	1351	1451	1551	1651	1751
Ludlow, Weyman Road, Potters Close Jct	0707	0753	0853	0953	1053	1153	1253	1353	1453	1553	1653	1753
Ludlow, Bringewood Road, opp Bringewood Close	0709	0755	0855	0955	1055	1155	1255	1355	1455	1555	1655	1755
Ludlow, Sandpits Road, Whitefriars Jct	0711	0759	0859	0959	1059	1159	1259	1359	1459	1559	1659	1759
Ludlow, Clee View	0712	0800	0900	1000	1100	1200	1300	1400	1500	1600	1700	1800
Ludlow, Sidney Road	0716	0804	0904	1004	1104	1204	1304	1404	1504	1604	1704	1804
Ludlow, Sheet Road, Kennet Bank Jct	0717	0805	0905	1005	1105	1205	1305	1405	1505	1605	1705	1805
Ludlow, Eco Park & Ride	0720	0810	0910	1010	1110	1210	1310	1410	1510	1610	1710	1810
Ludlow, Tollgate	0723	0814	0914	1014	1114	1214	1314	1414	1514	1614	1714	..
Ludlow, Parys Road, opp Vashon Close Jct	0725	0816	0916	1016	1116	1216	1316	1416	1516	1616	1716	..
Ludlow, Greenacres	0729	0820	0920	1020	1120	1220	1320	1420	1520	1620	1720	..
Ludlow, Steventon New Road, Churchill Close Jct	0732	0823	0923	1023	1123	1223	1323	1423	1523	1623	1723	..
Ludlow, Weeping Cross Lane, Friarfields Jct	0733	0824	0924	1024	1124	1224	1324	1424	1524	1624	1724	..
Ludlow, Upper Galdeford, Cooperative Store	0735	0826	0926	1026	1126	1226	1326	1426	1526	1626	1726	..
Ludlow, opp Railway Station	0737	0828	0928	1028	1128	1228	1328	1428	1528	1628	1728	..
Ludlow, Tourist Info Centre	0740	0831	0931	1031	1131	1231	1331	1431	1531	1631	1731	..

33. If the bus is driving at a speed of 40 miles per hour between Sidney Road and Tollgate, what is the distance between these two stops?

A. 9 miles B. 10 miles C. 6 miles D. 4.66 miles E. 3 miles

34. If the total distance between Henley Road and Greenacres is 34 miles, what is the average speed of the bus?

A. 50mph B. 60mph C. 36mph D. 42.5mph E. 68mph

35. Susan catches the 0733 bus from Weeping Cross Lane to the Railway station every day, in order for her to get to work by 8. One morning, Susan misses her bus by 2 minutes. If there is a 1.5 mile walk to the station from Weeping Cross Lane, how fast does she have to walk to make the 0752 train?

A. 4.8mph B. 3.2mph C. 5.3mph D. 6.4mph E. 8mph

36. Tom and Jack have a bag of skittles, which have 53 skittles in them. If there 12 blue skittles, 13 red skittles and 14 yellow skittles, what is the probability that they take out a purple skittle, given that skittles come in either blue, red, yellow or purple?

A. 0.284 B. 0.298 C. 0.217 D. 0.264 E. 0.156

END OF SECTION

Section D: Abstract Reasoning

For each question, decide whether each box fits best with Set A, Set B or with neither.

For each question, work through the boxes from left to right as you see them on the page. Make your decision and fill it into the answer sheet.

Answer as follows:
A = Set A
B = Set B
C = neither

Set 1 **Set A** **Set B**

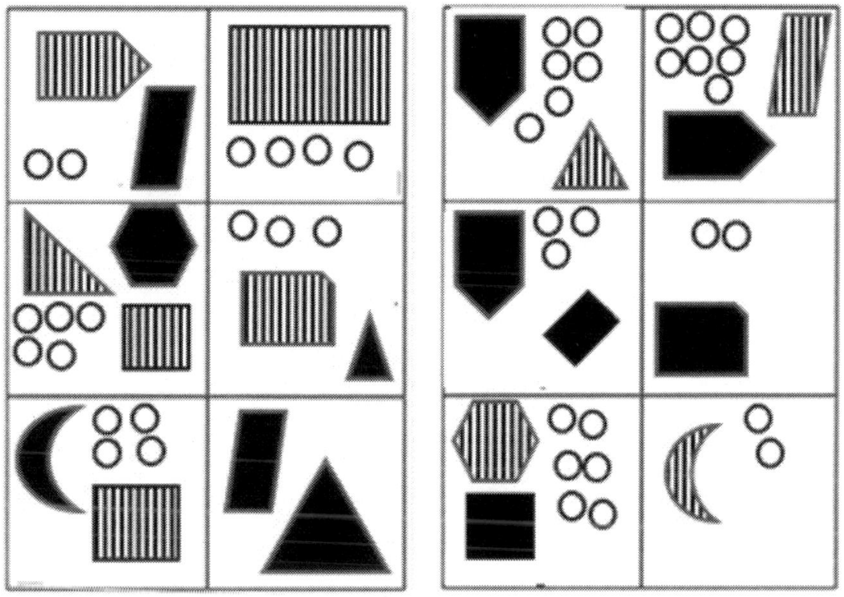

Questions 1-5:

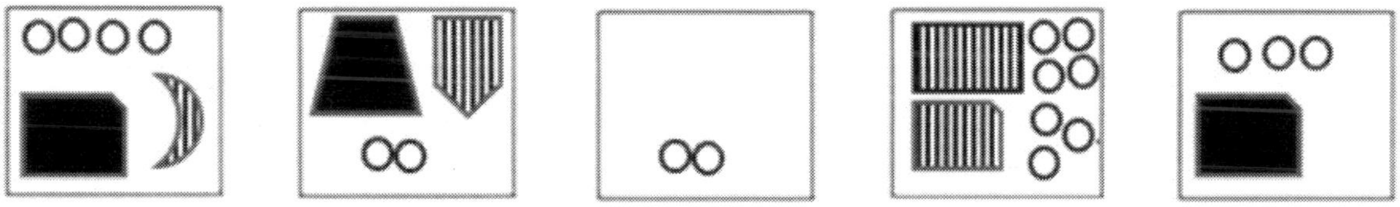

Set 2

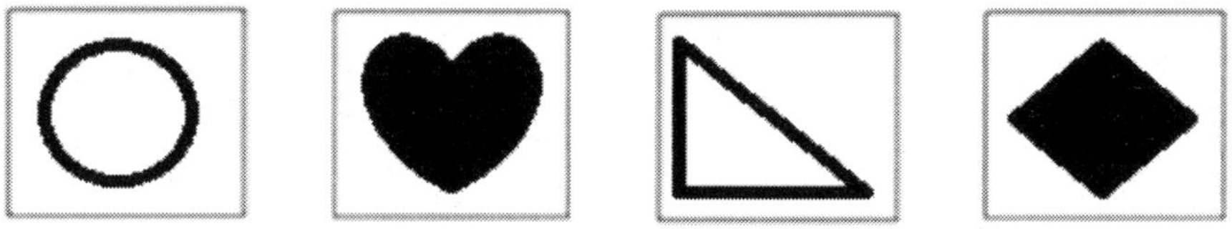

Question 6: Which figure completes the series?

A. B. C. D.

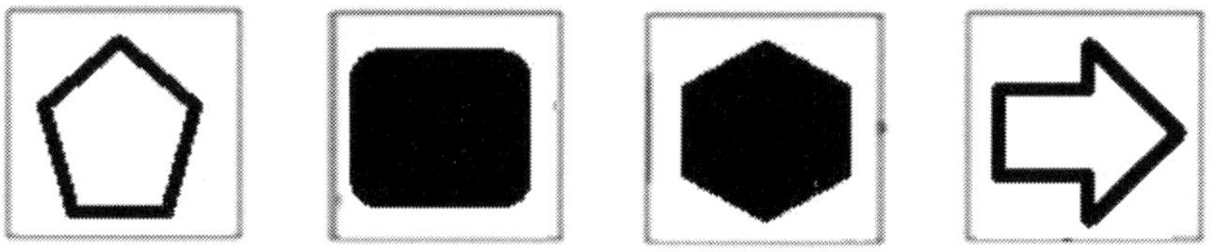

Set 3

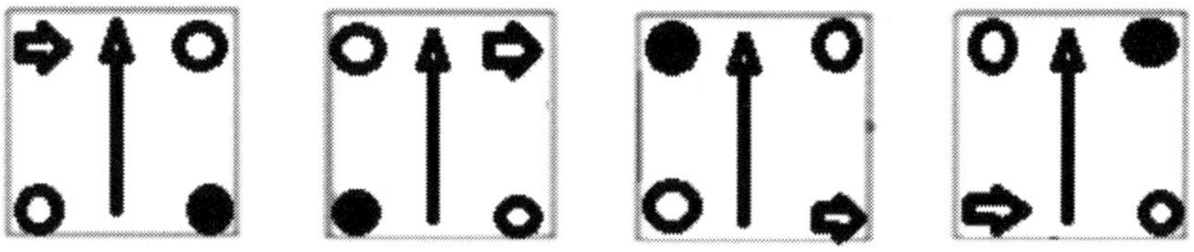

Question 7: Which figure completes the series?

A. B. C. D.

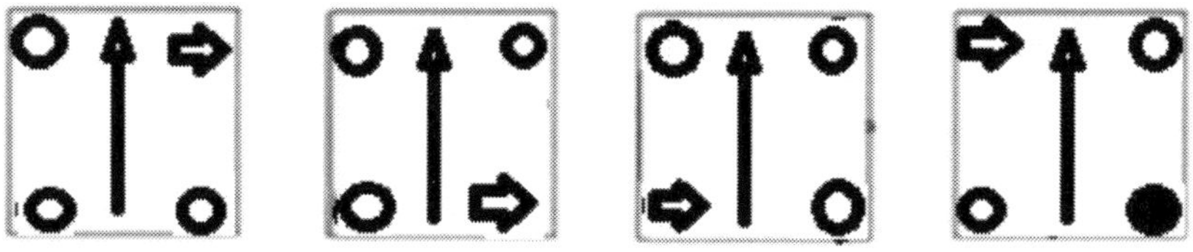

Set 4

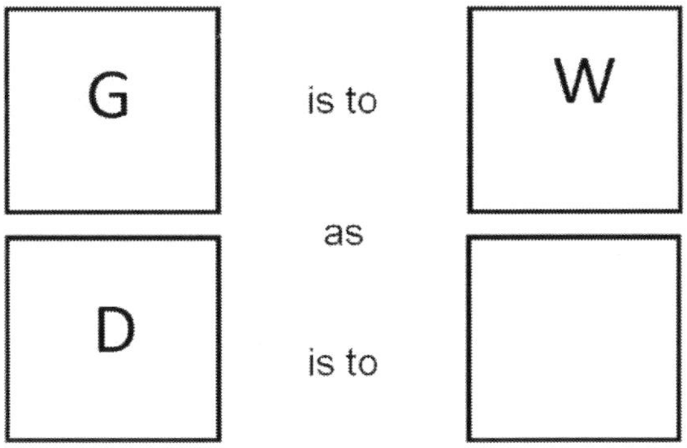

Question 8: Which figure completes the statement?

A. B. C. D.

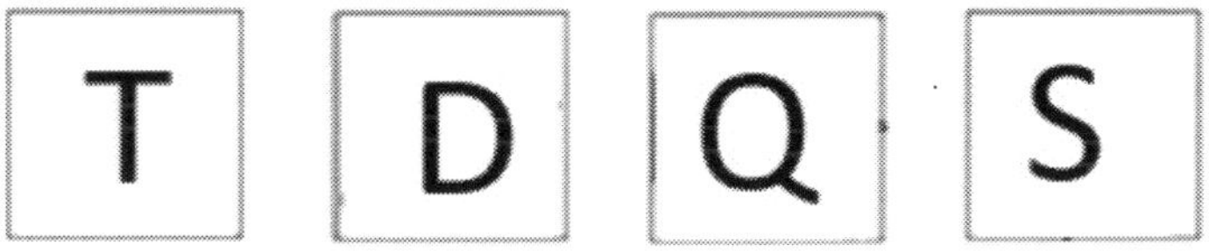

Set 5

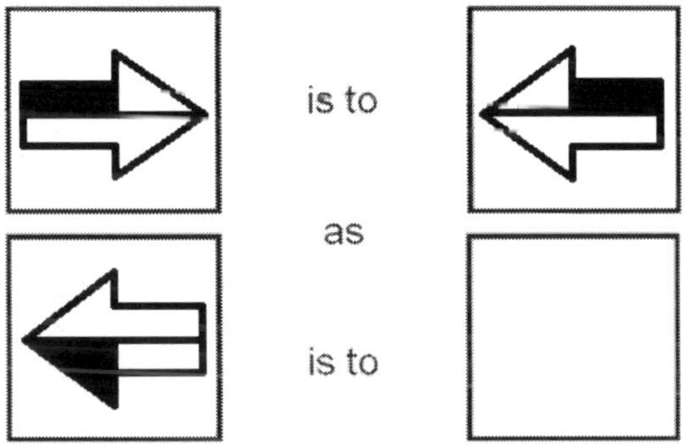

Question 9: Which figure completes the statement?

A. B. C. D.

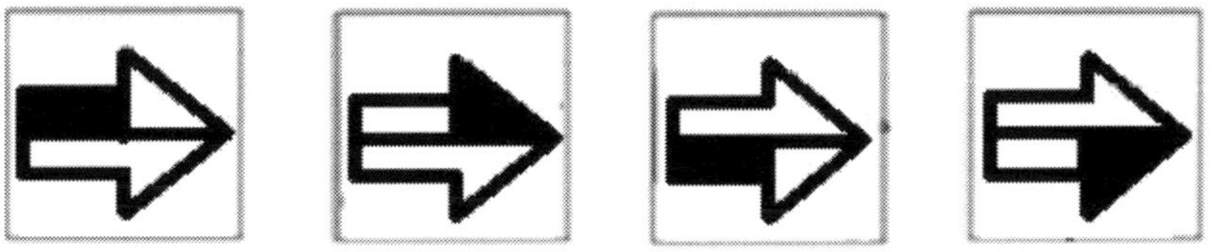

Set 6

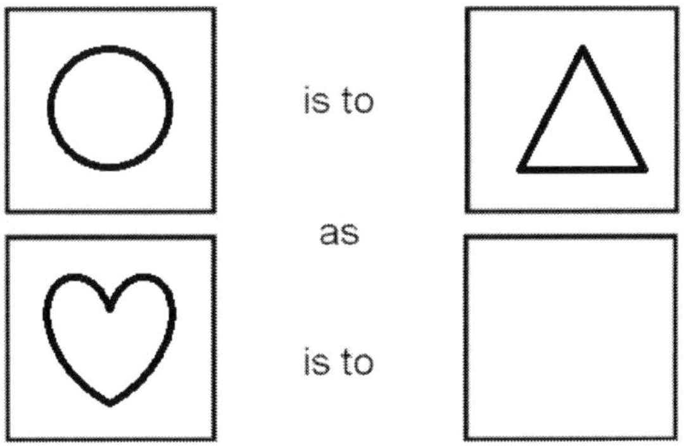

Question 10: Which figure completes the statement?

A. B. C. D.

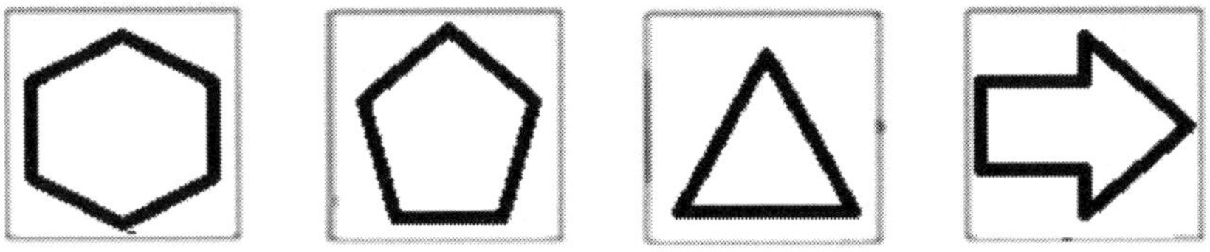

Set 7

Set A **Set B**

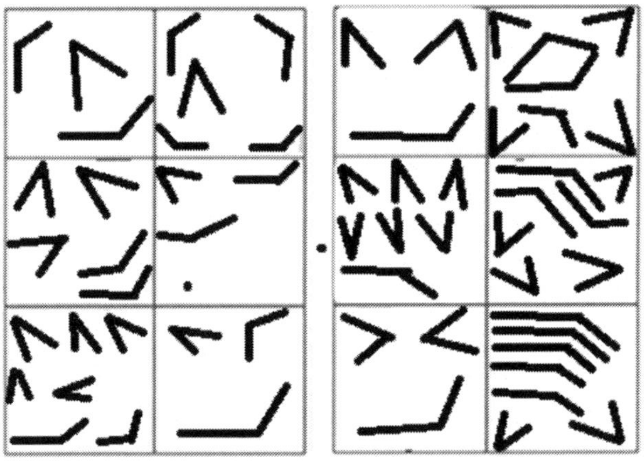

Question 11: Which of the following belongs in Set A?

A. B. C. D.

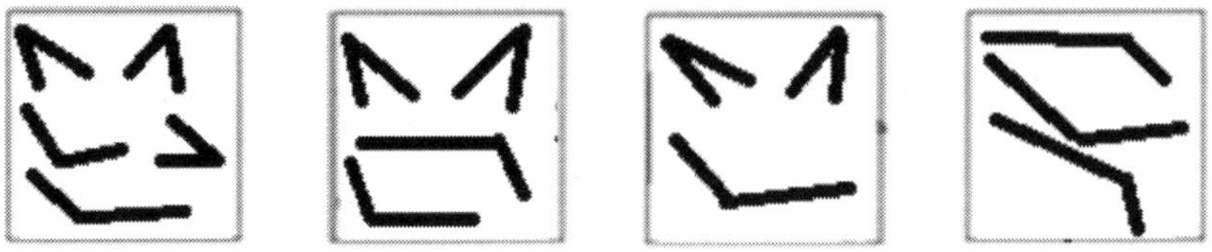

Question 12: Which of the following belongs in Set A?

A. B. C. D.

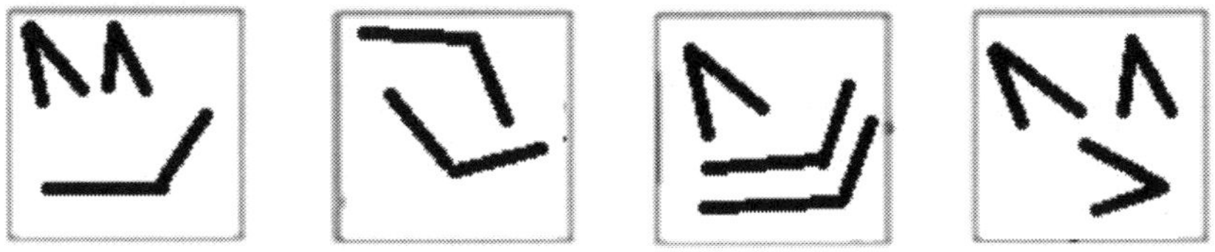

Question 13: Which of the following belongs in Set A?

A. B. C. D.

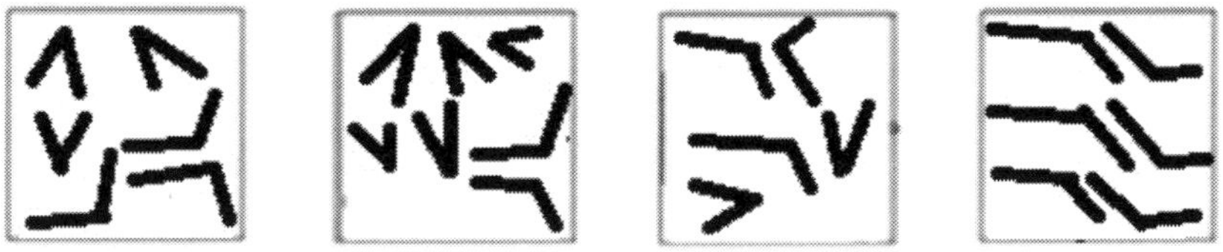

Question 14: Which of the following belongs in Set B?

A. B. C. D.

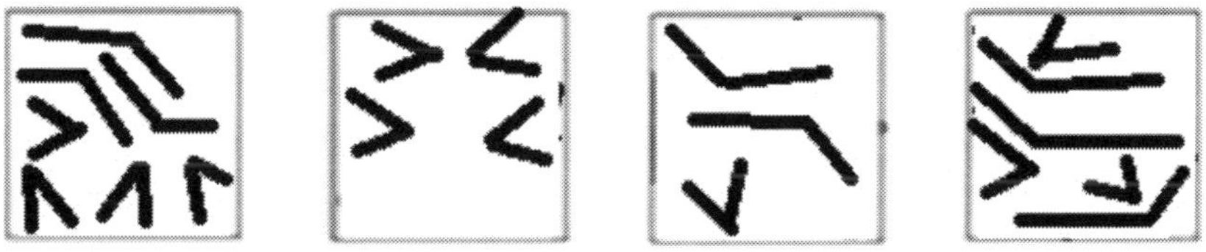

Question 15: Which of the following belongs in Set B?

A. B. C. D.

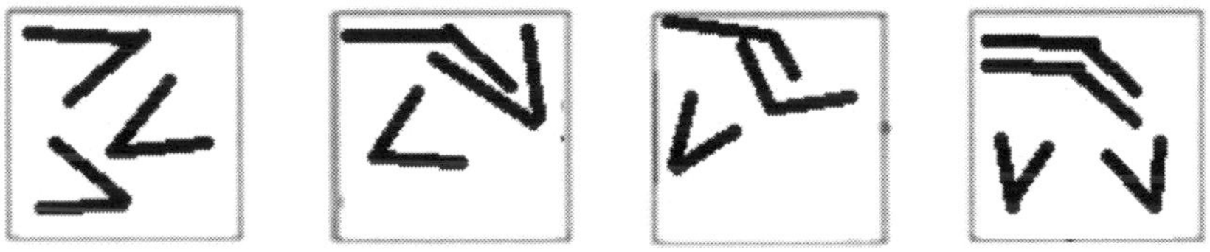

Set 8 **Set A** **Set B**

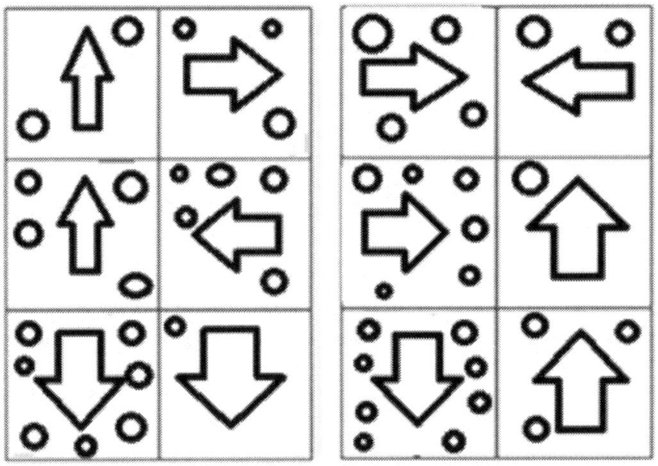

Questions 16-20:

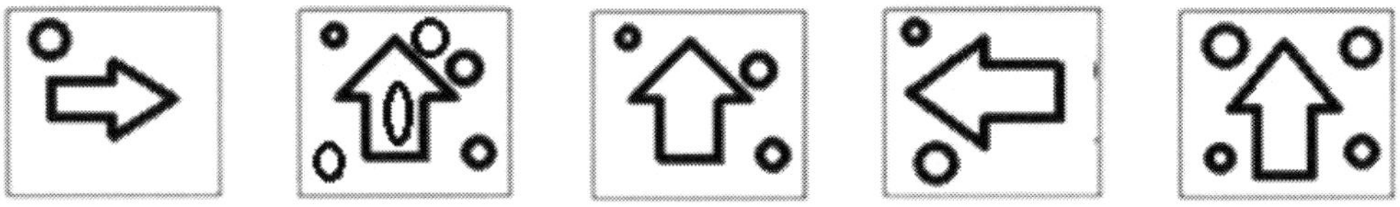

Set 9 **Set A** **Set B**

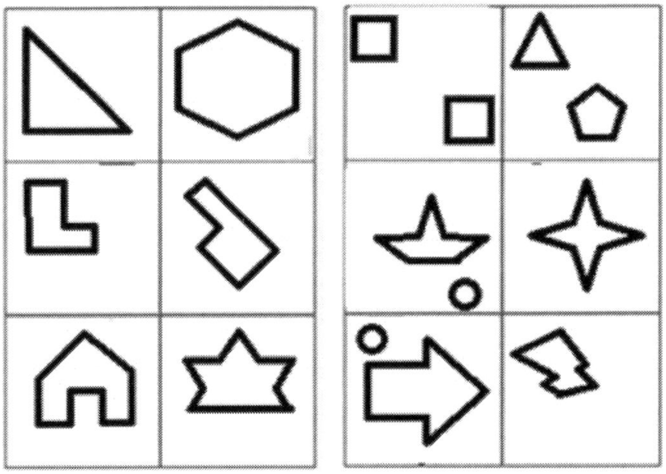

Questions 21-25:

Set 10 **Set A** **Set B**

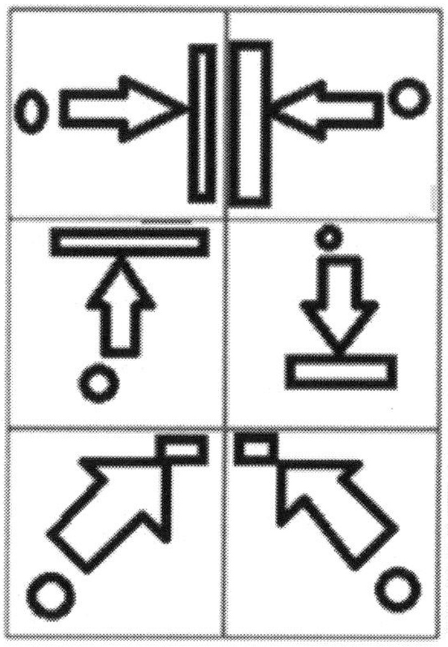

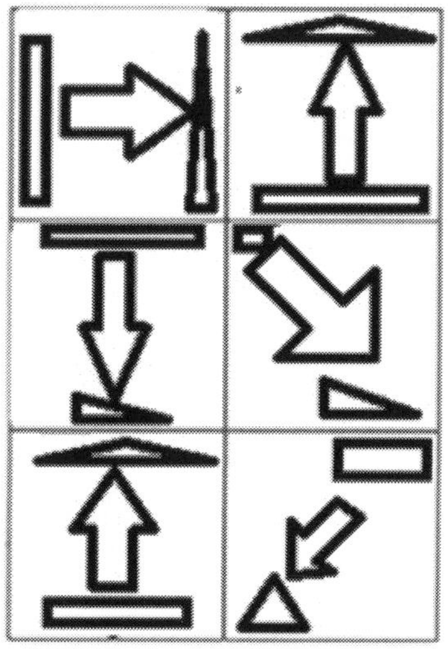

Questions 26-30:

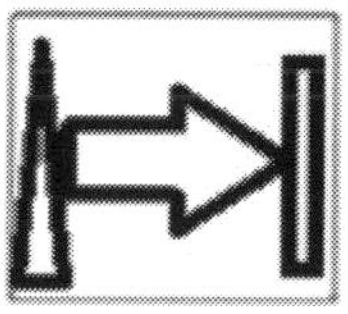

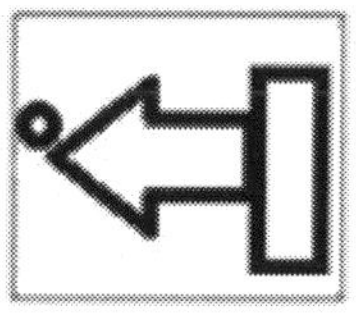

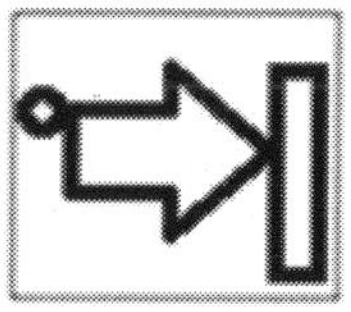

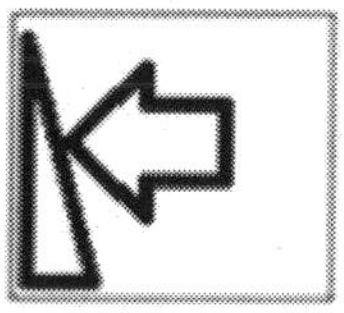

Set 11 **Set A** **Set B**

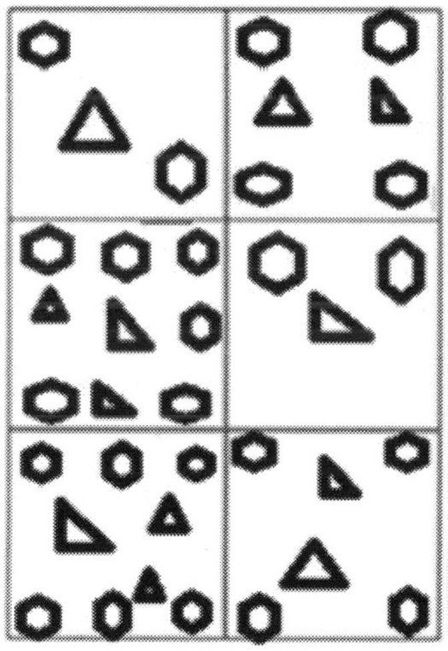

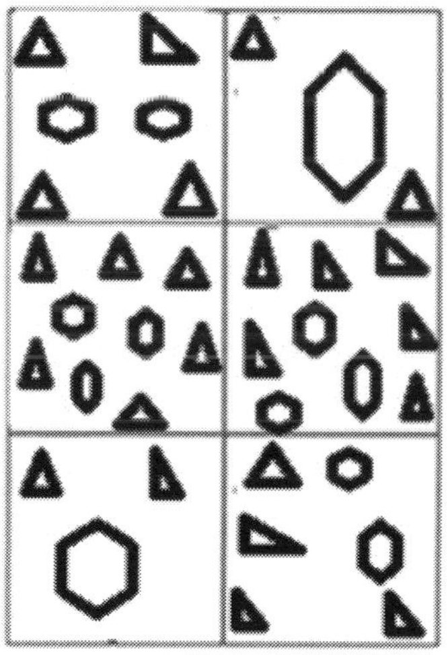

Questions 31-35:

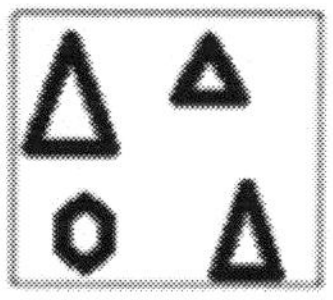

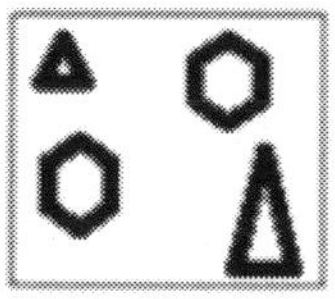

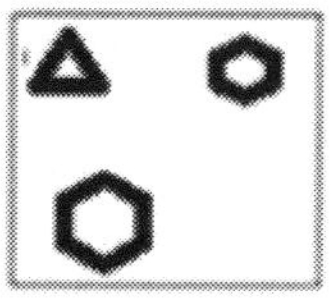

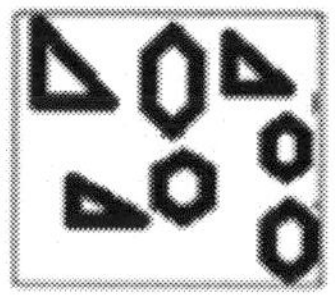

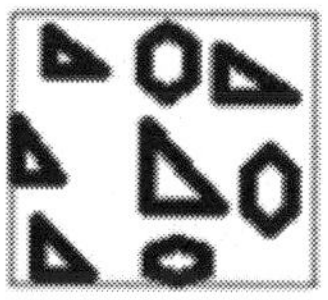

Set 12 Set A Set B

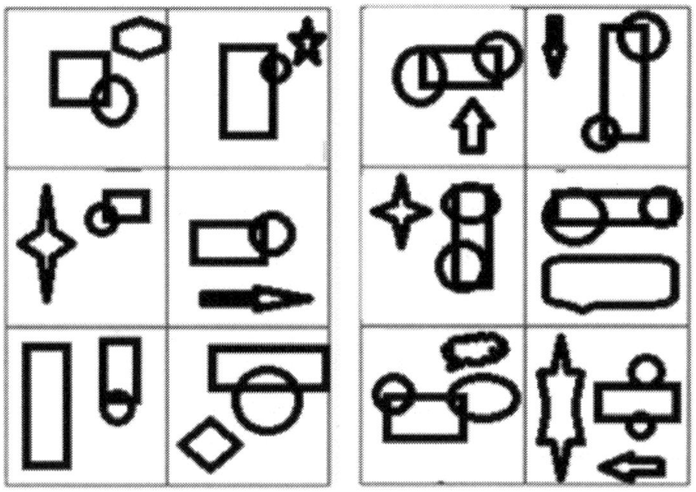

Questions 36-40:

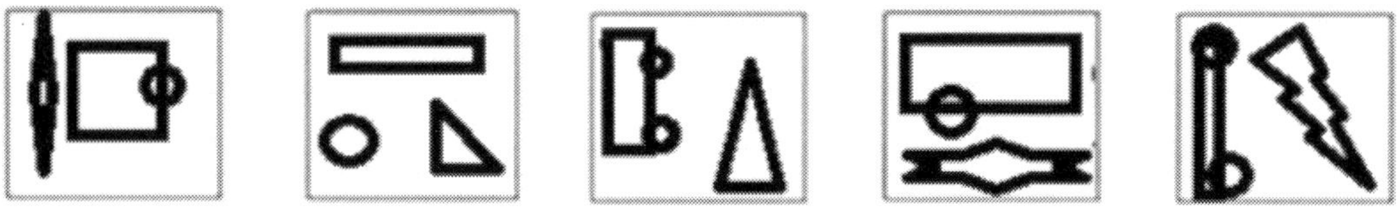

Set 13 Set A Set B

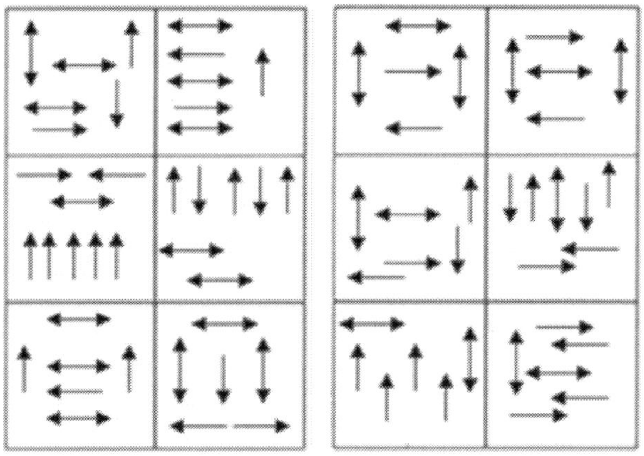

Question 41-45:

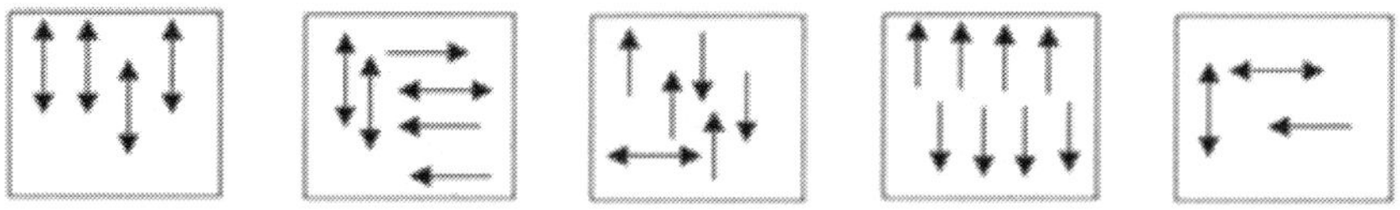

Set 14 **Set A** **Set B**

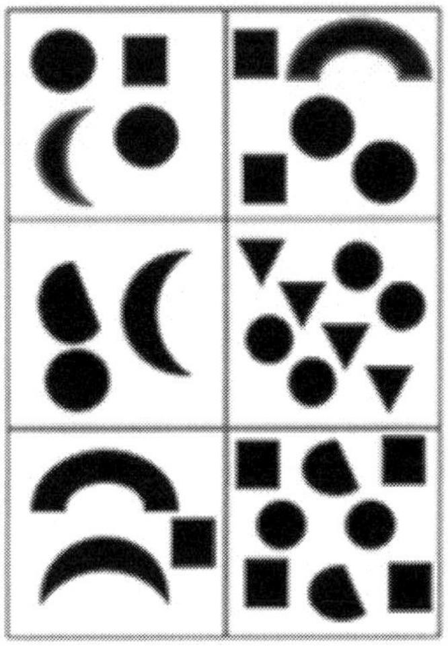
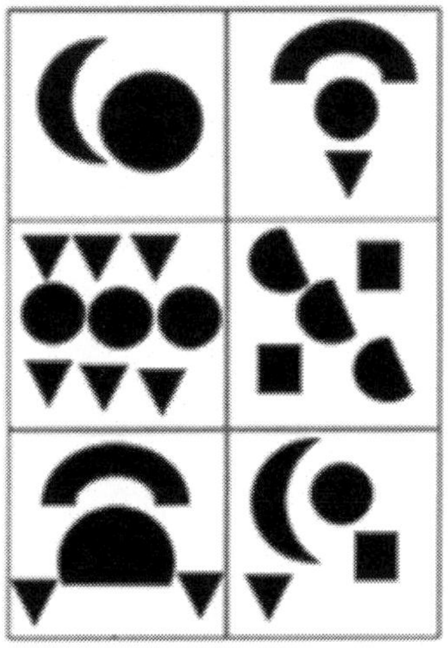

Question 46-50:

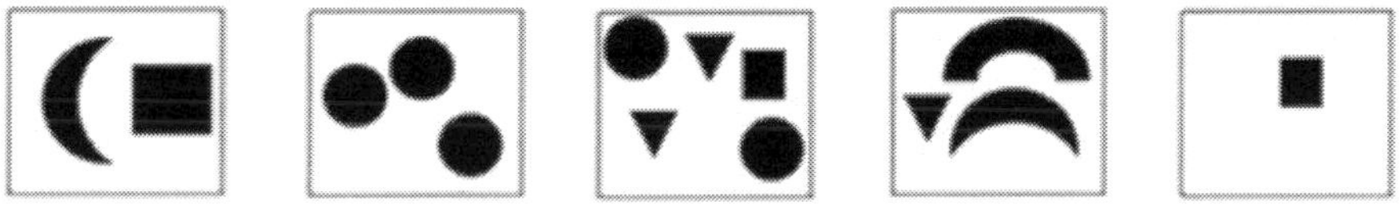

Set 15 **Set A** **Set B**

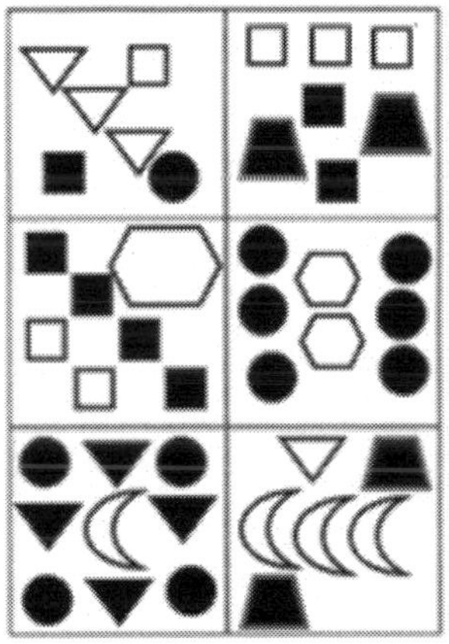
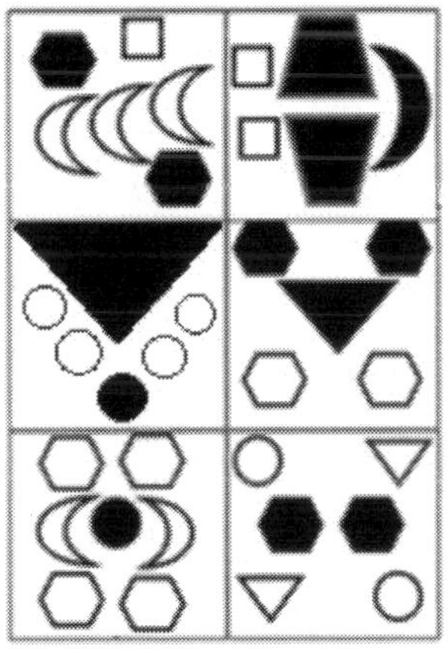

Question 51-55:

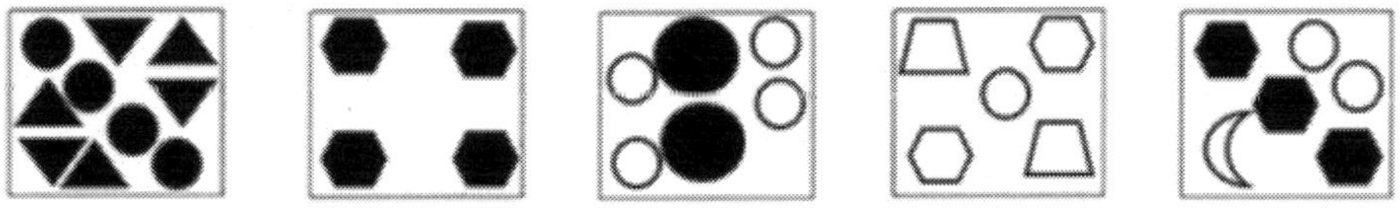

END OF SECTION

Section E: Situational Judgement Test

Read each scenario. Each question refers to the scenario directly above. For each question, select one of these four options. Select whichever you feel is the option that best represents your view on each suggested action.

For questions 1 – 30, choose one of the following options:

A A highly appropriate action
B Appropriate, but not ideal
C Inappropriate, but not awful
D A highly inappropriate action

Scenario 1
John is a 4th year medical student doing a placement on a general medical ward. One morning he notices that his fellow medical student, Tom, has slightly slurred speech. He can also smell alcohol on Tom's breath.
How appropriate are the following responses to this situation?

1. Do nothing, it is not your responsibility.
2. Report him to the head of the medical school.
3. Speak to Tom and express your concerns, and that you think it is not appropriate for him to be on the ward round today. Let him open up to you about any problems he may be having, and encourage him to seek help if he needs it.
4. Discuss this occurrence with your fellow medical students and seek their advice on how to manage the situation.
5. Discuss this occurrence with your medical supervisor and seek their advice on how to manage the situation.

Scenario 2
Jacob is a 3rd year medical student, who has a compulsory communications skills session about 'breaking bad news' to patients next week. His mother was diagnosed with cancer a month ago and this feels very close to home. He is not keen on attending the session.
How appropriate are the following responses to this situation?

6. Don't show up even though it was compulsory, it is too difficult for him to cope with a session like this right now.
7. Show up and tolerate the session even though he doesn't feel comfortable with the idea of it.
8. Speak to the doctor running the session and inform them of his circumstances and why he will not be able to attend the session.
9. Tell his friend, who knows about his mother, to tell the doctor he cannot come for personal reasons.
10. Show up to the session and leave half way when he thinks that he can't cope with being there anymore.

Scenario 3
Lucy, a third year medical student, is captain of the University hockey team but is also very interested in paediatrics. A week before the final hockey match she realises that an interesting looking paediatrics conference is being held in the university on the same day in the afternoon. She is unsure what to do.
How appropriate are the following responses to this situation?

11. Inform the members of the hockey team that she can't attend the match and attend the conference instead.
12. Let the team members know about the conference, and see if there is a way for her to play in the majority of the match and be subbed in for the time when the conference begins.
13. Attend the match fully and sign up for the conference, and turn up to the conference mid-way through once the match is over.
14. Don't attend the conference, she is only a third year after all and there will be one next year when she is no longer captain of the team.
15. Pretend to be ill and attend the conference instead.

Scenario 4
Tara is a 4th year medical student on the consultant-led ward round on a medical ward. Yesterday on the ward round, the consultant shouted at her in front of a patient for turning up two minutes late. She tried to brush it off, but today she was shouted at again, for not writing in the notes quickly enough. Tara found both experiences very unpleasant and distressing.
How appropriate are the following responses to this situation?

16. Report the consultant to the head of the medical school.
17. Speak to her clinical supervisor about her concerns and how to proceed.
18. Speak to the consultant about how uncomfortable she felt in this situation.
19. Do nothing about it and continue the placement on the ward.
20. Stop attending the placement and pretend to be sick.

Scenario 5
Alice is a second year medical student. She failed one of her exams and has to retake them in the beginning of September. However, her sister's wedding is two days before her retake and as the maid of honour she will have a lot of wedding-related work to do in the weeks approaching the wedding.
How appropriate are the following responses to the situation?

21. Don't revise for the exams until two days before (when the wedding is over), she didn't fail by much and won't have time before her sister's wedding.
22. Hand over some of the maid of honour responsibilities to another family member, giving her more time to focus on her retake at the same time.
23. Attempt to take on the responsibilities of both being maid of honour (and all this entails) whilst also revising for the retake.
24. Ask her sister if she could move the date of her wedding.
25. Ask her sister if she would be happy for another family member/friend to be maid of honour.

Scenario 6
Luke is a final year medical student. On the way out of the hospital, in the lift, he overhears a student on the phone speaking loudly about a patient in the hospital, using the patient's name.
How appropriate are the following responses to the situation?

26. Report the student to the head of the medical school.
27. Ignore the student and pretend not to know them.
28. Speak to his supervisor about the most appropriate action to take.
29. Speak to the student and explain that he should not be talking about patients publically.
30. Tell the student that he should not be speaking about patients whilst still in the hospital.

For questions 31 – 69, decide how important each statement is when deciding how to respond to the situation?

A Extremely important
B Fairly important
C Of minor importance
D Of no importance whatsoever

Scenario 7
Eva is a final year medical student, who has her finals coming up in a month. She has a mock OSCE (clinical examination) this week, which is the only one before the exam. However she comes down with the flu, she does not feel too well but is determined not to miss this opportunity. The medical school states that you should not attend if you are unwell.
How important are the following factors for Eva in making her decision?

31. This mock OSCE is a good opportunity to practice on real patients before finals.
32. Eva having the flu could put the patients at risk.
33. There are no further mocks after this one.
34. The patients participating in the mock are not going to be extremely unwell.
35. The medical school has stated that if ill you should not take part.
36. Eva's finals are in a month, so if she allows herself to recover she will still have time to go on the wards and practice on patients for the exam.

Scenario 8

Lucy is a 5th year medical student. She was lucky to get first choice in the ballot for GP placement and so has chosen a GP surgery because it is a 10 minute walk away. Alice is near the bottom of the ballot and so had to choose a practice which is either 30 minutes driving or 1 hour 30 minutes by bus, and she cannot drive. Lucy can drive. Alice has asked to swap with Lucy in exchange for the top place in the ballot for psychiatry placements.
How important are the following factors for Lucy in making her decision?

37. The medical school would reimburse Lucy for petrol so she would not be losing out financially by driving to the further GP practice.
38. The half an hour drive Lucy would have to do is much more convenient than the 1.5 hour bus ride Alice would have to take.
39. She would be higher in the psychiatry placement in return.
40. Lucy would be compromising her morning by giving up the GP placement.
41. There are other people in nearby GP practices who can drive and swap places with Alice.
42. Lucy prefers GP as a speciality to psychiatry.

Scenario 9

Nick is a second year medical student. He struggles with bad insomnia whereby he is wide awake through most of the night but then falls asleep in the morning. He has missed many morning lectures because of this and is unsure of what to do.
How important are the following factors for Nick in making his decision?

43. Whether he learns better by going to lectures or by reading a textbook.
44. If he attends the lectures in the morning, he will either fall asleep during them or compromise his concentration for the teaching in the afternoon.
45. Whether the other students say the lectures are useful.
46. Whether the lectures are available online.
47. Whether someone is able to record the lectures for him.
48. He has a medical problem, so should not be afraid to seek help from the medical school

Scenario 10

Lorna is a 3rd year medical student on her paediatrics placement. She really enjoys paediatrics and really likes her consultant - and her consultant has offered to give her extra teaching sessions on Thursday evening. However, she is also a member of the hockey team and this is when they have their practice.
How important are the following factors for Lorna in making her decision?

49. The consultant is only free on a Thursday evening.
50. The teaching may not be useful for the exams.
51. Hockey practice is only on a Thursday evening.
52. Lorna is considering paediatrics as a speciality.
53. Lorna's team mates will be disappointed if she doesn't show up to practice.
54. Lorna does not carry out any other extracurricular activities.

Scenario 11

Chris has written an essay for assignment. When handed back their essays, he notices that Joe's essay is an exact replica of an essay they were both sent by a medical student in the year above. He is unsure as to what to do.
How important are the following factors for Chris in making his decision?

55. Chris and Joe are good friends.
56. Plagiarism is against University rules.
57. It is unfair to the medical student in the year above that Joe copied his essay word for word.
58. Joe's essay was very good.
59. This essay only counts for 5% of the grade this year.
60. Plagiarism is inevitable - has occurred in the past and will occur in the future.

Scenario 12

Chen is a final year student on his medical elective in Swaziland. He is assisting surgery on a girl who has a deeply infected hand. If her fingers are not amputated, the infection will spread and could make her very unwell. The surgeon asks Chen to assist him in amputating the girl's fingers with scissors, as this is the only equipment available. The surgeon wants Chen's assistance as it is a difficult task. Chen is not sure whether he is comfortable with this situation.
How important are the following factors for Chen in making his decision?

61. The girl will become very ill and possibly die if her fingers are not amputated.
62. Chen is likely to find the procedure psychologically traumatic.
63. The UK and Swaziland have very different resources (e.g. only scissors for amputation) to the UK, as well as policies regarding how much students are allowed to do.
64. Chen is the only person available to help the surgeon with this procedure.
65. In the UK, Chen would not be allowed to do anything of this calibre as a medical student.

Scenario 13

Jasmine is a third year medical student. She has completed a poster for the genetics project she has been working on. Her supervisor says that if she continues coming to the labs three times a week for the next 2 months, she will have enough data for a publication. However, her exams are also coming up in a couple of months.
How important are the following factors for Jasmine in making her decision?

66. Going to the lab three times a week could interfere with her upcoming exams.
67. A publication will be useful on Jasmine's CV and application for jobs.
68. A publication also benefits the lab – Jasmine does not want to let them down.
69. Jasmine also plays university level netball and hockey.

END OF PAPER

PRACTICE PAPER

ANSWERS

Answer Key

PAPER A

VR	DM	QR	AR		SJT	
1. B	1. D	1. B	1. C	46. C	1. D	46. B
2. D	2. B	2. B	2. C	47. B	2. B	47. B
3. D	3. A	3. A	3. B	48. C	3. C	48. A
4. B	4. A	4. D	4. A	49. B	4. C	49. C
5. D	5. E	5. C	5. B	50. D	5. A	50. D
6. C	6. E	6. B	6. A	51. C	6. C	51. A
7. D	7. C	7. C	7. B	52. A	7. C	52. B
8. A	8. B	8. D	8. C	53. B	8. C	53. B
9. C	9. D	9. C	9. A	54. A	9. B	54. C
10. C	10. A	10. C	10. C	55. D	10. D	55. A
11. D	11. A	11. B	11. B		11. D	56. D
12. B	12. B	12. C	12. C		12. B	57. C
13. A	13. D	13. E	13. C		13. D	58. A
14. C	14. B	14. C	14. C		14. D	59. A
15. D	15. E	15. C	15. C		15. A	60. A
16. D	16. C	16. C	16. B		16. C	61. D
17. A	17. C	17. C	17. B		17. A	62. D
18. C	18. B	18. A	18. C		18. D	63. D
19. D	19. C	19. D	19. C		19. C	64. A
20. C	20. E	20. B	20. A		20. A	65. D
21. A	21. A	21. C	21. A		21. C	66. D
22. A	22. A	22. E	22. A		22. A	67. D
23. C	23. B	23. B	23. A		23. C	68. D
24. D	24. E	24. D	24. A		24. C	69. A
25. B/A	25. A	25. A	25. B		25. D	
26. C	26. D	26. D	26. C		26. B	
27. D	27. C	27. C	27. C		27. A	
28. C	28. A	28. E	28. A		28. B	
29. B	29. B	29. C	29. B		29. D	
30. A		30. A	30. A		30. C	
31. C		31. D	31. B		31. D	
32. A		32. E	32. N		32. A	
33. B		33. C	33. A		33. B	
34. A		34. D	34. A		34. B	
35. C		35. C	35. C		35. C	
36. C		36. D	36. B		36. C	
37. C			37. C		37. D	
38. C			38. C		38. B	
39. C			39. C		39. A	
40. C			40. A		40. B	
41. C			41. A		41. A	
42. D			42. B		42. B	
43. C			43. A		43. A	
44. B			44. C		44. A	
			45. B		45. A	

PAPER B						
VR	DM	QR	AR		SJT	
1. A	**1.** C	**1.** B	**1.** A	**46.** A	**1.** A	**46.** B
2. B	**2.** E	**2.** B	**2.** B	**47.** B	**2.** C	**47.** C
3. D	**3.** B	**3.** A	**3.** C	**48.** A	**3.** B	**48.** C
4. A	**4.** B	**4.** B	**4.** C	**49.** C	**4.** D	**49.** B
5. A	**5.** B	**5.** D	**5.** B	**50.** B	**5.** C	**50.** A
6. B	**6.** A	**6.** B	**6.** B	**51.** D	**6.** A	**51.** C
7. D	**7.** B	**7.** C	**7.** C	**52.** B	**7.** D	**52.** B
8. D	**8.** C	**8.** A	**8.** B	**53.** C	**8.** A	**53.** B
9. C	**9.** D	**9.** C	**9.** A	**54.** B	**9.** D	**54.** B
10. D	**10.** E	**10.** A	**10.** N	**55.** A	**10.** D	**55.** A
11. C	**11.** C	**11.** B	**11.** C		**11.** A	**56.** D
12. C	**12.** A	**12.** B	**12.** B		**12.** C	**57.** B
13. C	**13.** A	**13.** C	**13.** C		**13.** D	**58.** A
14. C	**14.** D	**14.** C	**14.** A		**14.** C	**59.** A
15. A	**15.** D	**15.** A	**15.** B		**15.** A	**60.** B
16. D	**16.** B	**16.** B	**16.** B		**16.** D	**61.** A
17. B	**17.** D	**17.** B	**17.** B		**17.** C	**62.** A
18. D	**18.** B	**18.** A	**18.** B		**18.** A	**63.** C
19. D	**19.** A	**19.** C	**19.** A		**19.** C	**64.** B
20. B	**20.** D	**20.** C	**20.** A		**20.** D	**65.** D
21. C	**21.** D	**21.** D	**21.** C		**21.** B	**66.** A
22. D	**22.** C	**22.** C	**22.** A		**22.** A	**67.** C
23. B	**23.** A	**23.** B	**23.** B		**23.** D	**68.** D
24. C	**24.** B	**24.** C	**24.** A		**24.** C	**69.** C
25. C	**25.** B	**25.** A	**25.** C		**25.** D	
26. D	**26.** D	**26.** C	**26.** C		**26.** D	
27. C	**27.** B/D	**27.** A	**27.** A		**27.** C	
28. B	**28.** C	**28.** B	**28.** B		**28.** A	
29. D	**29.** B	**29.** A	**29.** A		**29.** C	
30. C		**30.** B	**30.** C		**30.** D	
31. D		**31.** C	**31.** C		**31.** D	
32. D		**32.** B	**32.** B		**32.** A	
33. A		**33.** D	**33.** C		**33.** B	
34. C		**34.** C	**34.** C		**34.** D	
35. A		**35.** C	**35.** A		**35.** D	
36. A		**36.** B	**36.** A		**36.** D	
37. A			**37.** A		**37.** A	
38. C			**38.** B		**38.** B	
39. D			**39.** B		**39.** D	
40. C			**40.** C		**40.** B	
41. C			**41.** B		**41.** A	
42. B			**42.** B		**42.** B	
43. C			**43.** A		**43.** B	
44. C			**44.** D		**44.** B	
			45. C		**45.** D	

PAPER C

VR	DM	QR	AR		SJT	
1. B	**1.** A	**1.** C	**1.** N	**46.** N	**1.** D	**46.** D
2. D	**2.** D	**2.** B	**2.** N	**47.** A	**2.** D	**47.** B
3. C	**3.** C	**3.** C	**3.** A	**48.** A	**3.** B	**48.** A
4. B	**4.** A	**4.** D	**4.** N	**49.** A	**4.** A	**49.** B
5. C	**5.** B	**5.** E	**5.** B	**50.** B	**5.** D	**50.** C
6. C	**6.** D	**6.** E	**6.** N	**51.** B	**6.** D	**51.** B
7. B	**7.** C	**7.** D	**7.** B	**52.** N	**7.** A	**52.** C
8. C	**8.** B	**8.** D	**8.** A	**53.** N	**8.** B	**53.** B
9. B	**9.** C	**9.** B	**9.** B	**54.** N	**9.** C	**54.** A
10. C	**10.** A	**10.** D	**10.** A	**55.** A	**10.** B	**55.** A
11. A	**11.** C	**11.** B	**11.** B		**11.** C	**56.** A
12. C	**12.** C	**12.** C	**12.** B		**12.** C	**57.** D
13. C	**13.** D	**13.** D	**13.** A		**13.** A	**58.** A
14. C	**14.** B	**14.** A	**14.** B		**14.** D	**59.** B
15. A	**15.** C	**15.** D	**15.** A		**15.** D	**60.** A
16. A	**16.** B	**16.** A	**16.** B		**16.** C	**61.** A
17. A	**17.** D	**17.** C	**17.** N		**17.** D	**62.** A
18. A	**18.** B	**18.** B	**18.** N		**18.** A	**63.** A
19. C	**19.** C	**19.** B	**19.** N		**19.** B	**64.** C
20. C	**20.** D	**20.** C	**20.** A		**20.** D	**65.** A
21. B	**21.** C	**21.** A	**21.** A		**21.** D	**66.** B
22. A	**22.** D	**22.** C	**22.** N		**22.** A	**67.** D
23. A	**23.** C	**23.** B	**23.** B		**23.** D	**68.** D
24. C	**24.** B	**24.** D	**24.** N		**24.** D	**69.** D
25. B	**25.** D	**25.** C	**25.** B		**25.** A	
26. B	**26.** C	**26.** A	**26.** B		**26.** D	
27. B	**27.** D	**27.** D	**27.** D		**27.** A	
28. C	**28.** C	**28.** C	**28.** A		**28.** C	
29. C	**29.** A	**29.** D	**29.** C		**29.** D	
30. B		**30.** B	**30.** B		**30.** A	
31. B		**31.** B	**31.** A		**31.** D	
32. C		**32.** C	**32.** D		**32.** D	
33. A		**33.** D	**33.** A		**33.** A	
34. D		**34.** E	**34.** C		**34.** C	
35. A		**35.** E	**35.** D		**35.** D	
36. B		**36.** C	**36.** A		**36.** C	
37. C			**37.** A		**37.** C	
38. A			**38.** D		**38.** C	
39. A			**39.** C		**39.** B	
40. B			**40.** B		**40.** A	
41. A			**41.** N		**41.** D	
42. C			**42.** N		**42.** A	
43. C			**43.** A		**43.** A	
44. A			**44.** B		**44.** C	
			45. B		**45.** D	

PAPER D

VR	DM	QR	AR		SJT	
1. **B**	**1.** E	**1.** B	**1.** N	**46.** B	**1.** B	**46.** D
2. **C**	**2.** B	**2.** C	**2.** A	**47.** N	**2.** A	**47.** C
3. **A**	**3.** C	**3.** E	**3.** B	**48.** B	**3.** B	**48.** D
4. **C**	**4.** B	**4.** B	**4.** A	**49.** N	**4.** A	**49.** A
5. **D**	**5.** A	**5.** D	**5.** A	**50.** A	**5.** C	**50.** C
6. **A**	**6.** D	**6.** C	**6.** B	**51.** B	**6.** C	**51.** D
7. **A**	**7.** C	**7.** C	**7.** N	**52.** B	**7.** C	**52.** C
8. **A**	**8.** A	**8.** A	**8.** A	**53.** D	**8.** B	**53.** C
9. **B**	**9.** A	**9.** E	**9.** A	**54.** B	**9.** C	**54.** C
10. **B**	**10.** A	**10.** C	**10.** N	**55.** A	**10.** B	**55.** B
11. **B**	**11.** E	**11.** D	**11.** B		**11.** D	**56.** A
12. **A**	**12.** D	**12.** A	**12.** B		**12.** C	**57.** D
13. **A**	**13.** B	**13.** E	**13.** A		**13.** B	**58.** A
14. **C**	**14.** C	**14.** E	**14.** A		**14.** C	**59.** C
15. **C**	**15.** C	**15.** B	**15.** A		**15.** A	**60.** D
16. **D**	**16.** B	**16.** B	**16.** A		**16.** C	**61.** B
17. **D**	**17.** C	**17.** A	**17.** N		**17.** D	**62.** C
18. **B**	**18.** C	**18.** D	**18.** N		**18.** C	**63.** C
19. **D**	**19.** C	**19.** B	**19.** B		**19.** A	**64.** B
20. **C**	**20.** E	**20.** E	**20.** A		**20.** D	**65.** A
21. **A**	**21.** C	**21.** C	**21.** B		**21.** D	**66.** A
22. **A**	**22.** C	**22.** D	**22.** A		**22.** C	**67.** C
23. **A**	**23.** C	**23.** C	**23.** A		**23.** B	**68.** D
24. **C**	**24.** E	**24.** B	**24.** N		**24.** A	**69.** A
25. **C**	**25.** A	**25.** C	**25.** B		**25.** D	
26. **C**	**26.** C	**26.** B	**26.** B		**26.** C	
27. **C**	**27.** B	**27.** A	**27.** D		**27.** A	
28. **D**	**28.** D	**28.** E	**28.** C		**28.** B	
29. **C**	**29.** E	**29.** D	**29.** B		**29.** C	
30. **C**		**30.** C	**30.** A		**30.** D	
31. **D**		**31.** C	**31.** D		**31.** A	
32. **A**		**32.** B	**32.** N		**32.** A	
33. **B**		**33.** A	**33.** A		**33.** B	
34. **C**		**34.** C	**34.** N		**34.** B	
35. **A**		**35.** D	**35.** A		**35.** C	
36. **B**		**36.** D	**36.** B		**36.** D	
37. **C**			**37.** B		**37.** A	
38. **C**			**38.** A		**38.** D	
39. **D**			**39.** N		**39.** B	
40. **B**			**40.** A		**40.** D	
41. **A**			**41.** B		**41.** D	
42. **B**			**42.** A		**42.** C	
43. **D**			**43.** N		**43.** C	
44. **D**			**44.** B		**44.** D	
			45. B		**45.** D	

PAPER E

VR	DM	QR	AR		SJT	
1. D	**1.** A	**1.** E	**1.** A	**46.** C	**1.** C	**46.** B
2. B	**2.** A	**2.** D	**2.** N	**47.** C	**2.** D	**47.** A
3. C	**3.** E	**3.** C	**3.** B	**48.** C	**3.** A	**48.** A
4. D	**4.** C	**4.** D	**4.** N	**49.** D	**4.** B	**49.** C
5. A	**5.** A	**5.** B	**5.** B	**50.** C	**5.** D	**50.** D
6. B	**6.** B	**6.** A	**6.** A	**51.** D	**6.** D	**51.** D
7. C	**7.** C	**7.** C	**7.** A	**52.** A	**7.** A	**52.** A
8. A	**8.** B	**8.** C	**8.** B	**53.** C	**8.** C	**53.** A
9. B	**9.** B	**9.** B	**9.** N	**54.** A	**9.** B	**54.** D
10. A	**10.** A	**10.** A	**10.** A	**55.** C	**10.** D	**55.** D
11. A	**11.** E	**11.** E	**11.** A		**11.** D	**56.** B
12. C	**12.** A	**12.** B	**12.** B		**12.** D	**57.** A
13. B	**13.** A	**13.** A	**13.** A		**13.** A	**58.** A
14. A	**14.** B	**14.** C	**14.** B		**14.** C	**59.** A
15. D	**15.** A	**15.** A	**15.** A		**15.** D	**60.** D
16. D	**16.** C	**16.** D	**16.** N		**16.** B	**61.** D
17. A	**17.** D	**17.** C	**17.** N		**17.** A	**62.** A
18. C	**18.** D	**18.** A	**18.** B		**18.** D	**63.** A
19. B	**19.** C	**19.** C	**19.** A		**19.** D	**64.** D
20. C	**20.** D	**20.** A	**20.** A		**20.** C	**65.** C
21. C	**21.** A	**21.** B	**21.** A		**21.** A	**66.** A
22. A	**22.** E	**22.** A	**22.** N		**22.** D	**67.** D
23. A	**23.** A	**23.** D	**23.** B		**23.** C	**68.** A
24. C	**24.** A	**24.** E	**24.** N		**24.** B	**69.** B
25. B	**25.** C	**25.** B	**25.** A		**25.** D	
26. C	**26.** C	**26.** A	**26.** N		**26.** B	
27. A	**27.** A	**27.** C	**27.** A		**27.** D	
28. D	**28.** C	**28.** B	**28.** A		**28.** A	
29. A	**29.** A	**29.** A	**29.** A		**29.** D	
30. A		**30.** D	**30.** B		**30.** D	
31. D		**31.** C	**31.** B		**31.** A	
32. D		**32.** A	**32.** B		**32.** B	
33. A		**33.** C	**33.** N		**33.** C	
34. C		**34.** A	**34.** A		**34.** D	
35. D		**35.** A	**35.** N		**35.** B	
36. C		**36.** C	**36.** N		**36.** A	
37. A			**37.** A		**37.** D	
38. D			**38.** N		**38.** B	
39. D			**39.** B		**39.** C	
40. A			**40.** A		**40.** D	
41. D			**41.** B		**41.** C	
42. B			**42.** A		**42.** A	
43. B			**43.** A		**43.** D	
44. C			**44.** N		**44.** C	
			45. B		**45.** B	

PAPER F

VR	DM	QR	AR		SJT	
1. A	1. B	1. D	1. B	46. N	1. D	46. A
2. B	2. D	2. A	2. N	47. B	2. D	47. A
3. C	3. C	3. C	3. A	48. N	3. A	48. A
4. B	4. D	4. C	4. A	49. A	4. C	49. A
5. D	5. B	5. C	5. N	50. N	5. B	50. D
6. D	6. C	6. E	6. A	51. A	6. D	51. A
7. C	7. B	7. E	7. D	52. B	7. D	52. A
8. C	8. E	8. D	8. A	53. A	8. A	53. B
9. B	9. E	9. D	9. D	54. A	9. B	54. B
10. C	10. C	10. E	10. A	55. N	10. B	55. C
11. A	11. C	11. E	11. A		11. D	56. A
12. D	12. C	12. B	12. C		12. C	57. A
13. D	13. C	13. E	13. B		13. A	58. D
14. C	14. C	14. B	14. A		14. B	59. D
15. A	15. B	15. C	15. B		15. D	60. D
16. D	16. D	16. A	16. A		16. C	61. A
17. A	17. C	17. C	17. A		17. A	62. B
18. C	18. D	18. A	18. B		18. C	63. A
19. B	19. C	19. D	19. A		19. D	64. A
20. B	20. E	20. B	20. A		20. D	65. C
21. C	21. D	21. C	21. A		21. D	66. A
22. C	22. B	22. E	22. N		22. A	67. B
23. B	23. B	23. B	23. B		23. C	68. C
24. C	24. E	24. A	24. A		24. D	69. A
25. D	25. C	25. A	25. N		25. B	
26. C	26. C	26. D	26. N		26. C	
27. B	27. B	27. C	27. N		27. D	
28. C	28. D	28. E	28. A		28. A	
29. D	29. A	29. C	29. B		29. A	
30. A		30. A	30. N		30. D	
31. C		31. D	31. N		31. B	
32. C		32. E	32. N		32. A	
33. C		33. D	33. A		33. A	
34. C		34. C	34. N		34. C	
35. B		35. C	35. N		35. A	
36. C		36. D	36. A		36. A	
37. B			37. N		37. A	
38. B			38. B		38. B	
39. C			39. A		39. A	
40. C			40. B		40. C	
41. A			41. B		41. C	
42. B			42. A		42. D	
43. C			43. N		43. B	
44. D			44. B		44. A	
			45. N		45. C	

Mock Paper A Answers

Section A: Verbal Reasoning

Passage 1

1. **B** The passage states that the existence of atoms 'has been suggested since ancient Greece'. Though there have been recent developments in our understanding of atoms, the idea of its existence is not recent or 19th century but 'ancient', and so, old.

2. **D** It was 'concluded' that the nucleus was 'positively charged' (and so *not* negatively charged) in 1909, so well within the 20th century. Dalton only theorised about tiny units, he did not prove their existence, and Thomson's and Bohr's ideas described in **B** and **C** are stated in the passage to have been proved false.

3. **D** Quarks make up neutrons, protons and electrons (not the other way round, so **B** is false), and so must be smaller than atoms, which are made up of these three things. It is said we will discover more on atomic structure, so **C** is incorrect, and that 'no less than six' types of quark have been discovered - not 'more than six', so **A** is also false.

4. **B** It is said that electrons' behaviour is 'difficult to predict'. The other statements are verified by information in the passage. Quarks make up electrons, so electrons contain quarks. Electrons 'do not behave like other particles'. Electrons orbit the positively charged nucleus.

Passage 2

5. **D** The passage simply states the powers were 'at odds' after WWII, but does not at any point explicitly state why.
6. **C** The Soviet Union were the first to launch a man-made satellite into space, and so achieved the first success. There is no stated 'winner' of the Space Race, nor are there comments made on which side was superior/inferior - they each received different 'victories' in the race, so A and D are false. B is not stated anywhere in the passage: no link is drawn explicitly between the two in this manner.
7. **D** The president of the US campaigned for the moon-landing, giving it a political element. Spacewalks happened before a man landed on the moon, so **C** is incorrect, and the reasons the Soviet space program was 'plagued by difficulties' is not stated, so **A** and **B** are also incorrect.
8. **A** Only one man is explicitly mentioned in the passage to have landed on the moon, and there is no mention of a political truce or research *achieved*, only the potential for research. That 'humans' orbited the moon is stated, and the plural 'humans' equates to 'multiple humans', making **A** the only correct statement.

Passage 3

9. **C** The service is important for 'most' families, and parents 'generally' cherish their kids above all else, but these statements allow for there to be exceptions to this general trend, so **A** and **B** are incorrect. Both physical and emotional safety is stated as something parents need to feel assured of when entrusting their child to someone else, and as the emotional safety is not stated to be preeminent, **D** is wrong.
10. **C** Physical needs including food are mentioned, as are emotional needs and the desire for a child to feel respected. A tidy appearance is not stated as something to keep in mind when caring for a child.
11. **D** If the carer suspects abuse, they should contact the appropriate authority, and this is a 'procedure'. Unusual aggression and depression, as well as bruises, may suggest serious problems at home (including abuse) but they are not said to directly prove them.
12. **B** Holiday camps are not mentioned in the above passage. The other statements are all corroborated by the passage.

Passage 4

13. **A** Original settlers were criminals, and if they reproduced, modern Australians may be able to trace back to their criminal ancestors.
14. **C** The English settled, and so spread their language. The Dutch did not, and so could not spread theirs. The English did not steal the land, nor did the natives show a distaste for the Dutch or a preference for the English language.
15. **D** The passage states nothing about the effect this has on England, Great Britain or native Australians, only that Australia was then a major world power, and so the creation of an independent Australia created a 'new' major world power.
16. **D** The fictional character Sweeney Todd's fate is not to be seen as proof of many falsely-convicted men being forced to move to Australia. There is no mention about the reproduction habits of immigrants or natives, and neither **B** or **C** necessarily explain the current population demographic. 250 years has changed this country from predominately Aboriginal to predominately European decedents, so **A** is correct.

Passage 5

17. **A The theory of** Spontaneous Generation is said to be 'ancient', and so before the middle ages, and not conclusively disproved until 1859, so **C** and **D** are incorrect. The passage states that spontaneous generation was the idea that "certain types of life could appear on their own, without coming from a parental source." Therefore, A is correct.

18. **C** Pasteur is referred to as 'he', is said to be French, and is known as the 'father of microbiology' (and who conducts biological experiments, and who is implicitly called a biologist in the phrase 'Pasteur and other biologists'), so **A, B** and **D** are not the answers. The passage does not ever call him a genius, it simply states he made important discoveries.

19. **D** The methods are explicitly stated to be 'preservation' methods, and so stopped food from going off. The other statements may be true, but are not stated in the passage.

20. **C** The drinks are ruined by boiling, not pasteurisation. Pasteurisation gets rid of many microbes in a fluid, but the passage does not state it gets rids of them all- and the guarantee mentioned in **D** is not mentioned in the passage, so **A, B** and **D** are incorrect. The structure of the fluid is said to remain 'intact', so **C** is correct.

Passage 6

21. **A** The passage states few innovations took hold even though 'Farming has been common in Europe for thousands of years', so the practice remained roughly the same.
22. **A** The passage states changes in agriculture spurred an industrial revolution, linking agriculture and industry.
23. **C** Medieval farmers were practicing leaving lands fallow, but the passage states it was not until the 1700s farmers knew to plant crops to help return nutrients to the fields. It does not state when the discovery was made that crops could leech fertilisers and nutrients from the soil, and though we may assume Medieval farmers knew this as they knew to leave their lands fallow, it would not be relevant to the question unless the opposite was stated as true, which it is not.
24. **D** Both help restore the soil, but they do not do this in the same way: turnips are said to get nutrients from the Earth and improve the topsoil, whereas clover does not get nutrients from the atmosphere and we are not told what it does to the topsoil.

Passage 7

25. **B & A** The passage clearly states that advances in agricultural technology allowed farms to be operated by fewer labourers, creating a surplus of labour. This means there were fewer jobs for *farm* labourers, although many of these individuals found work in mills and mines. Arguably, C & D are also correct, as increased food production is linked, albeit indirectly, to the improvement of mills and migration to the colonies. B may be the *most* correct, but strictly speaking, they are all true according to the passage.
26. **C** Though it helped, the passage does not state if this was the main factor which led to colonisation - there could be other, unmentioned but more important causes.
27. **D** The passage does not make an explicit positive or negative judgment as to the Industrial revolution, it just states what happened because of it. It similarly does not say things got 'simpler', and the increased poverty described sounds like a complication. It says that overpopulation in the city led to 'disease, poverty and crime', a higher population thus led to problems and so **D** is correct.
28. **C** The passage states employers could 'overwork and underpay their employees', an exploitative act, making **C** correct. They are not described as possibly doing anything kind, nor is anxiety mentioned, nor is it stated they would cause pain in others for their own pleasure, so **A, B** and **D** are wrong.

Passage 8

29. **B** For 'most' of 100,000 years does not equate to for 'all' of them.
30. **A** What is now known as Scotland *used* to be covered by the sheet, but is not now.
31. **C** A piece of ice left to melt caused Loch Fergus, not ice-water that was flowing, or newly deposited sand, gravel or rocks.
32. **A** 'Sea levels rose to separate…the British Isles from Europe' means that the British Isles were once *not* separate from Mainland Europe.

Passage 9

33. **B** Germany is a 'republic' and so cannot be a monarchy.

34. **A** Over 100 million people are 'native speakers', whereas the other 80 million speakers learned it as a foreign language. The passage does not state it is the dominant language in Austria and Switzerland, only that it is widely spoken there. The possibility of **D** is not mentioned anywhere in the passage.

35. **C** It is ranked the 'fourth largest economy in the world', well within the top ten. Migrants are attracted to the strong economy, but that does not mean A or D are true - migrants may not strengthen the economy and there may not be jobs for all those who seek them. B is not mentioned. The strong economy does not necessarily guarantee each individual's income.

36. **C** Although the Croatians are excluded from the EU's Freedom of Movement treaty Article 39, there is not enough information on their migration rights comparative to Middle Easterners in the text to confirm or deny the statement.

Passage 10

37. **C** There is only a short extract from the book, and we can't tell whether the rest of the text might speak on Biblical matters.

38. **C** The passage does not state Hobbes' thoughts on war from birth, nor does he explicitly state a dislike of the Spanish. His father being a clergyman does not mean he was meant to be a clergyman. The conditions of his birth are described as stressful (premature birth upon hearing of a frightening invasion), so **C** is correct.

39. **C** Hobbes was born in the sixteenth century, so **A** and **B** cannot refer to him, and the passage does not speak of any other political philosopher. Though the extract is downbeat, one cannot necessarily deduce Hobbes is depressed at this point. *Leviathan* was published in 1651, so **C** is the correct answer.

40. **C** The enemy or war's necessity are not mentioned, just how war impacts negatively on society, so that there is 'no society' - it has been shut down. The illiterate poor are not mentioned: the stopping of literature and arts is not limited to the poor.

Passage 11

41. **C** The passage does not describe the entire century, so we cannot know the state of affairs after 1913.

42. **D** The passage states they fought for 'male and female equality', not female superiority. There is no mention of either the vote or alternative sexualities.

43. **C** The passage does not state whether hunger strikes did or did not have an effect on how the public saw feminism, nor does it state when they ended, so **A** and **D** are wrong. They may well have gained something, despite being countered with force-feeding (for example, publicity for the feminist movement), and as there is nothing to state the contrary **B** is an incorrect answer for this question. Force-feeding was awful treatment that answered hunger strikes, so **C** is correct.

44. **B** We do not know if she was pre-eminent, suicidal or a genius from the passage: only that she sacrificed much fighting for her cause.

END OF SECTION

Section B: Decision Making

1. **D** The question asks what the largest number you CANNOT make is, therefore work through the numbers from the largest. 52 = 20 + 20 + 6 + 6. Correct answer is d as there is no combination that will add up to 43.

2. **B** Statement a is wrong because although it gives a reason as to why some people may not apply, it does not give a reason why 18 is the optimum age to start medical school. Statement c does not relate directly to the statement. It is possible to live at home and go to medical school in the same city. Statement d is close but it assumes that 18 is the age of an adult and we know that in certain situations different ages can assume a more mature role, e.g. contraception for 16 year olds. Statement b is the only statement that directly addresses the statement and provides a reasonable answer.

3. **A** Dr Smith can prescribe antidepressants.

4. **A** Lucas goes to school on Monday – Friday. Last week there were two sunny days, and three rainy days. Therefore, the probability he walks on a sunny day with an umbrella is 0.3 x 0.4 x 2 = 0.24, and the probability he walks to school in the rain without an umbrella is 0.2 x 0.6 x 3 = 0.36. He is more likely to walk to school in the rain without an umbrella.

5. **E** Statement a - Karen is a musician so she must play an instrument but we do not know how many instruments she plays. Therefore statement a is incorrect. Although all oboe players are musicians, it does not mean all musician play the oboe. Similarly, oboes and pianos are instruments but that does not mean that they are the only instruments. So statements b and c are incorrect. Karen is a musician but that merely means that she plays an instrument, we do not know if it is the oboe. So statement d is incorrect.

6. **E** The key to this question is *most likely* to be correct. There is a possibility that any one of these statements could be true or all could be false but one is most likely. There is no information to suggest that we can predict the baby's eye colour based on past babies. Each one presents a new event and probability so statement a is wrong. There is no information on the parents' eye colours and how it is linked to the baby's so we cannot be sure statement b is correct. We are not told how many boys/girls James has so we can't work out probability and statement c and d are incorrect.

7. **C** If Millie starts the game with 4 pennies, she is guaranteed a loss. If she takes 1 penny, then Ben will take 3. If she takes 2, then Ben will take 2. If she takes 3, then Ben will take 1. In each scenario, Ben takes the last penny. This works for all multiples of 4. No matter how many Millie takes at the start, Ben can take enough to reach a multiple of 4. This rules out a, b and d. For statement c, Millie can take one penny and this will leave 12. This is a multiple of 4 so now Ben is in the situation where any number he chooses will lead to loss - as explained above.

8. **B** Statement B directly rejects the assumption of the statement and so is the strongest answer.

9. **D** A sky view of the arrangement leads to:

C	A	B	*or*	A	C	B
D		E			D	E

In both, D is to the left of E, thus is the only correct answer.

10. **A** If Arnold is correct then their father owns at least 4 cars, this would also make Eric right because he would own at least 1 car. If Eric is correct then their father owns at least 1 car, this would make either Carrie (less than 4 cars) or Arnold (at least 4 cars) also correct. Therefore, Carrie must be the correct one and their father owns less than 4 cars. If Eric is incorrect then he must own less than 1 car so therefore, zero cars.

11. **A** Statement a clearly states that there is an increase in a carbon monoxide to harmful levels with traffic which provides a clear link to poor health and traffic. Statements b and c rely on assumptions; that people will use their spare time to exercise, and that road tax reduces traffic, respectively. This makes them weaker supporting statements than statement a. Acid rain damages buildings and the environment so is not directly damaging to health so statement d is incorrect. Statement e weakens the conclusion.

12. **D** Work from the worst-case scenario – Fred initially picks one sock of each colour. When Fred picks his 5th sock, it must make a pair. The worst case would be that this, and every other sock Fred picks, is an orange sock. This is because he cannot make all three pairs from any other colour, and therefore would require only one sock to complete the second and/or third pair. If you work this through: when Fred picks 1r 1g 1b 2o = 1pair, he next gets a pair when he takes out one green or blue, or two orange socks so must take 7 socks to guarantee 2 pairs, again for the third pair he needs one green or blue, or tow orange socks thus meaning he needs 9 socks to guarantee three pairs.

13. **D** We know how old Tom is in relation to the others so we cannot say who is oldest or youngest. So statements a and e are incorrect. We do not know is Olivia wins more or less than anyone else other than Tom and Gabby so statement b is incorrect. No opinions can be made from the statements so statement c is incorrect. Tom loses most often so everyone wins more than Tom so statement d is correct.

14. **B** There are two directions: clockwise and anticlockwise and rats will only collide if they pick opposing directions Rat A - clockwise, Rat B - clockwise, Rat C - clockwise = 0.5 x 0.5 x 0.5 = 0.125 Rat A - anticlockwise, Rat B - anticlockwise, Rat C - anticlockwise = = 0.5 x 0.5 x 0.5 = 0.125 0.125 + 0.125 = 0.25. So the probability they **do not** collide is <u>0.25</u>.

15. **E** Statement a is clearly wrong. "Plums are not sweets." We do not know the correlation with sweet and tasty. It is never explicitly said that sweet and tasty coexist or are interchangeable. Therefore, we cannot make a statement on the taste of plums. This makes statements b, c and d incorrect. If only *some* plums are sweet, then there must be a subset that are not sweet, so statement e is correct.

16. **B** The info as a Venn diagram is shown right. Remember the children can make numerous responses so ensure each is only counted once. Start with the total number of children who like each ice cream in the large circle, then minus the number who also like other ice cream when they are placed in the overlapping parts of the Venn diagram. You will end up with the above, and finally add in the 2 children who don't like ice cream, giving 12.

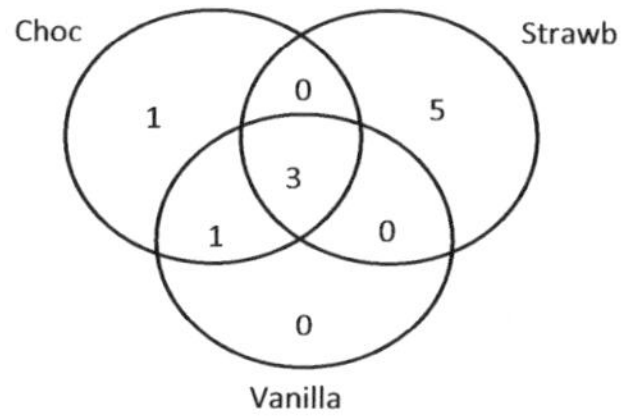

17. **C** We start by working backwards so filling in the centre first with 4 children liking all types. We also know that 4 like vanilla only so we can put that in. We know 1 child likes chocolate and vanilla and 4 children like strawberry and vanilla. That leaves 12 that like chocolate. 12 - (4+1) = 10. We have no information on strawberry by itself.

18. **B** "Every dress she bought was blue." Do not be distracted by the extra information and the different sentence structure. Statement a and e - blue dresses were not necessarily the only dress she saw. She could have seen but not bought other dresses. Statement c - there were not necessarily no other dresses there. Statement d - Tasha bought all the blue dresses she saw, not every dress she saw.

19. **C** Scenario 1: John picks Kelly, Kelly picks Lisa, Lisa picks John Scenario 2: John picks Lisa, Kelly picks John, Lisa picks Kelly Any other scenario will result in starting the game over. As it is not possible to pick one's own name, there is a 50/50 chance of picking each other person. So statement c is correct.

20. **E** Helpful to draw a tree diagram and build up from the information. The woman's brother's father is also her father. As the father is the ONLY son of her grandfather, it follows that this must also be Mary's father. The woman is therefore Mary's sister and so her daughter's aunt.

21. **A** If society disagree that vaccinations should be compulsory, then they will not fund them. So Statement a is correct. It attacks the conclusion. Statement b - society does not necessarily mean local so this does not address the argument. Statement c strengthens, not weaken, the argument for vaccinations. Statement d – the wants of healthcare workers do not affect whether vaccinations are necessary.

22. **A** Statement a - if the pain is from a blood test, Tim assumes needles will cause pain. Statement b - This can only be true via the mechanism of the needle, hence answer (a) is a more proximal cause and therefore a better response Statement c - experiencing pain with this doctor before doesn't mean Tim always will. Statement d - leaving a bruise does not necessarily inflict pain. Statement e - similar to (b), trying different needles is not the primary cause of pain - using the needle in the first place is.

23. **B** The runners aren't apart at a constant distance; they get further apart as they run. Xavier and Yolanda are less than 20m apart at the time William finishes. Each runner beats the next runner by the same distance so they must have the same difference between speeds. When William finishes at 100m and Xavier is at 80m. When Xavier crosses the finish line then Yolanda is at 80m. We need to know where Yolanda is when Xavier is at 80m. William's speed = distance/time = 100/T. Xavier's speed = 80/T. So Xavier has 80% of William's speed. This makes Yolanda's speed 80% of Xavier's and 64% (80% x 80% = 64%) of William's. So when William is at 64m when William finishes. 100m - 64m = 36m, thus William beats Yolanda by 36m.

24. **E** The statements can be written as: E > C, E > M > J, and N > E > J. Therefore, Naomi is the tallest.

25. **A** Erica: Ferrari/Mercedes/BMW. Chris: Audi/BMW. Harry: Ferrari/Ford. Lily: Volkswagen. Michael: Ford/BMW

26. **D** At 99% water, the watermelon is 99g water and 1g matter. After drying, the watermelon still has 1g matter but now 98% water. So 1g is now worth 2%. This means that the total weight is 50g (1 / 0.02 = 50)

27. **C** We only have information of Emmanuel's time. We know that Jon and Saigeet are faster but we do not know the definitive times so we cannot make statements on their ability to qualify. Emmanuel's best time is greater than the qualifying time so he will not qualify. Though statement e could be true, it is not necessarily so.

28. **A** Statement a - all doctors are handsome and some are popular so some must be handsome and popular. Statement b and d - We are not told that Francis and Oscar are doctors. We are not told about the general public, only doctors, so statement c is wrong. We do not know who Oscar is popular with so statement e is incorrect.

29. **B** Lucy must live between Vicky and Shannon, as we know Vicky and Shannon are not neighbours. Either Lucy or Shannon have a blue door, however as Vicky lives next to someone with a red door, Lucy must have the red door. This leaves Shannon with the blue door and Vicky with the white. There is a house with a green door is across the road, which is the forth house on the street and so does not belong to any of them.

END OF SECTION

Section C: Quantitative Reasoning

Data Set 1

1. B 10 m/s. Speed is distance/time, which will be the slope of the car line on the graph. Distance/time = (20 meters – 10 meters)/(1 second – 0 seconds) = 10 m/1 s = 10 m/s.

2. B 25 m/s. Speed is distance/time, which is the slope of the motorcycle curve on the graph. The maximum speed will be at the point of maximum slope. The slope is steady and greatest between 4 and 5 seconds or 50 and 75 meters. Speed = distance/time = (75 meters – 50 meters)/(5 seconds – 4 seconds) = 25 m/ 1 s = 25 m/s.

3. A 0 m/s^2. The car keeps a steady speed throughout, as seen by its unchanging slope on the graph. Therefore the car never accelerates and the acceleration is 0 m/s^2.

4. D True – but only initially. The car travels at a constant speed throughout, and thus has no acceleration. The motorbike decreases its speed in the first few seconds, as seen by the increasing slope of the curve, indicating it has a positive acceleration. It reaches a steady speed and zero acceleration like the car at about 3 seconds.

Data Set 2

5. C £ 3.19. A seven minute call is in the 1-10 mins category, so in peak time will be charged at £ 0.42 per minute. The UK-France connection charge is £ 0.25. Cost = £ 0.25 + 7 min x £ 0.42 = £ 3.19.

6. B £ 0.10. There is no per minute or connection charge on an unanswered call, but there is a £ 0.10 surcharge on Europe-Australia unanswered calls.

7. C 11**%.** 463 seconds = 7.72 minutes, which rounds up to 8 minutes. 15:43 is a peak time. The per minute charge of a 1-10 mins call is £ 0.42. Duration charge = 8 min x £ 0.42 = £ 3.36. No surcharges apply to this call. The USA-China connection charge is £ 0.43. Percentage of fixed charges/overall cost = 100% x (£ 0.43)/(£ 0.43 + £ 3.36) = 100% x 0.11 = 11%.

8. D £ 14.37. 1935 is off peak. The 75 minutes will include minutes charged at 4 different per minute rates.

(10 min x £ 0.25) + (10 min x £ 0.18) + (40 min x £ 0.16) + (15 min x £ 0.15) = £ 2.50 + £ 1.80 + £ 6.40 + £ 2.25 = £ 12.95.

There is an off peak over-an-hour surcharge of £ 0.88 and a China-France connection charge of £ 0.54. Total cost = £ 12.95 + £ 0.88 + £ 0.54 = £ 14.37.

9. C £ 6.09. This is a peak time call that is 763/60 = 12.72 minutes long, which rounds up to 13 minutes. No surcharges apply, but there is a France-Australia connection charge of £ 0.78. The first 10 minutes will be charged at a per minute rate of £ 0.42 and the 3 final minutes at a per minute rate of £ 0.37. Total cost = £ 0.78 + (10 minx £ 0.42) + (3 min x £ 0.37) = £ 0.78 + £ 4.20 + £ 1.11 = £ 6.09.

Data Set 3

10. C 155%. From the graph, in January 2004 the price of gold is approximately $ 400 per ounce and $ 620 in January 2007. Percentage change = 100% x new price/old price = 100 x ($ 620 per ounce/$ 400 per ounce) = 100% x 1.55 = 155%.

11. B £ 486. In January 2004 gold cost $ 400 per ounce. The conversion rate is $ 1=£ 0.68, so $ 1 x 400 per ounce = £ 0.68 x 400 per ounce = £ 272 per ounce. 1 ounce = 28g, so 50g gold = 50g/28g per ounce = 1.785 ounces. 50g gold costs 1.785 ounces x £ 272 per ounce = £ 485.52.

Data Set 4

12. C 31.5 g/kg. A lasagne has 190 g sugar per 450 g total mass. 1 kg lasagne therefore has 1000 g/450 g x 19 g sugar = 42 g sugar. The beef noodle dish contains 35 g sugar per 475 g total mass. 1 kg beef noodles has 1000 g/475 g x 35 g sugar = 73.5 g sugar. 73.5 g/kg sugar is 31.5 g/kg more than 42 g/kg sugar.

13. E More information required. To answer this question the energy content of sugar and the other ingredients per weight would need to be known. If the rest of the meal is made of high calorie ingredients, the relative proportion of sugar calories will be smaller than if the rest of the mass is comprised of low calorie ingredients.

Data Set 5

14. C £5.80. Average error = (|wine 1 retail value – estimate respondent 1| + |wine 1 retail value – estimate respondent 2| + |wine 1 retail value – estimate respondent 3| + |wine 1 retail value – estimate respondent 4| + |wine 1 retail value – estimate respondent 5|)/5 = (|8-13| + |8-17| + |8-11| + |8-13| + |8-15|)/5 = (5 + 9 + 3 + 5 + 7)/5 = 5.80.

15. C Respondent 3. Average error = (|wine 1 retail value – estimate 1| + |wine 2 retail value – estimate 2| + |wine 3 retail value – estimate 3|)/3. Respondent 1: (|8-13| + |25-16| + |23-25|)/3 = (5 + 9 + 2)/3 = 5.33. Respondent 2: (|8-17| +|25-16| + |23-23|)/3 = (9 + 9 + 0)/3 = 6. Respondent 3: (|8-11| + |25-17| + |23-21|)/3 = (3 + 8 + 2)/3 = 4.33. Respondent 4: (|8-13| + |25-15| + |23-14|)/3 = (5 + 10 + 9)/3 = 8. Respondent 5: (|8-15| + |25-19| + |23-29|)/3 = (7 + 6 + 6)/3 = 6.33. Respondent 3 has lowest average error and thus highest average accuracy.

Data Set 6

16. C £ 252.00. Weekly profit per product = (Sale price – Cost per unit) x Number sold per week.
Weekly profit Gobstopper = (£ 0.40 - £0. 22) x 150 = £ 27.00.
Weekly profit Bubblegum = (£ 0.50 - £ 0.35) x 180 = £ 27.00.
Weekly profit Everton mints = (£ 0.90 - £ 0.45) x 300 = £ 135.00.
Weekly profit = (£ 0.65 - £ 0.50) x 420 = £ 63.00.
Total weekly profit = £ 27.00 + £ 27.00 + £ 135.00 + £ 63.00 = £ 252.00.

17. C £ 267.00. Value of sales per product per week = Sale price x Number sold per week.
Value of sales Gobstoppers per week = £ 0.40 x 150 = £ 60.00.
Value of sales Everton mints per week = £ 0.90 x 300 = £ 270.00.
Purchase price per product per week = Cost per unit x Number sold per week. Purchase price Bubblegum per week = £ 0.35 x 180 = £ 63.00.
Gobstopper sales + Everton mint sales – Bubblegum purchase price = £ 60.00 + £ 270.00 - £ 63.00 = £ 267.00.

18. A Gobstopper. Gobstoppers and Bubblegum both generate the same profit of £27.00, which is the lowest of the sweets in his shop. However Bubblegum requires half the shelf space that either Gobstoppers or the new product require.

Data Set 7

19. D 38.6 million. Country A : 140% Country B. Country C : 70% Country D. Country D : 120% Country B.
Population Country A/1.40 = Population Country B = 45 million/1.40 = 32.1 million people.
Population Country B x 1.20 = Population Country D = 32.1 million people x 1.20 = 38.6 million people.

20. B $ 1.45 bn. Country A : 140% Country B. Population Country A/1.40 = Population Country B. 45 million people/1.40 = 32.1 million people. Health initiative cost = $ 45 per capita x 32.1 million people = $ 1.45 billion.

21. C 12.3 million. Country C : 70% Country D.
Population Country C/0.70 = Population Country D. 25 million people/0.70 = 35.7 million people.
48 % population are men = 0.48 men x 35.7 million = 17.1 million men. 72% men are adults = 0.72 adults x 17.1 million men = 12.3 million adult men.

Data Set 8

22. E 393 euros. Difference in advertising costs = Most expensive advertising costs – least expensive advertising costs = 576 euros – 183 euros = 693 euros.

23. B Civil service.
Trade and industry = 447 euros/5370 euros = 0.083.
Civil service = 431 euros/4380 euros = 0.098.
Liberal professions = 75 euros/3001 euros = 0.025.
Crafts and skilled trades = 139 euros/2895 euros = 0.048.
Agriculture = 168 euros/2311 euros = 0.073.
Civil service has the greatest proportion lost working hours/overall recruitment cost = 0.098.

Data Set 9

24. D 207. Y321 had 230 offences in 2011. 2013 is 10% lower than 2011 rate = 2011 rate x 0.90 = 230 offences x 0.90 = 207 offences.

25. A 373. There were **more than** 1837 Y offences in 2012 – 210 Y321 offences – 490 Y632 offences – 754 Y230 offences = **less than** 383 Y115 offences in 2012. The only option lower than 383 is 373.

26. D Y632. Percentage change per crime type = number of 2013 offences/number of 2012 offences.
X632 = 2670/2453 = 1.088 = 8.8% increase.
X652 = 3231/3663 = 0.882 = 21.8% reduction.
Y321 = 207/210 = 0.986 = 1.4 % reduction.
Y632 =432/490 = 0.881 = 21.9% reduction.
Y115 = 431/383 = 1.125 = 12.5% increase.
Y230 = 714/754 = 0.947 = 5.3% reduction.
Y632 has the greatest reduction of 21.9% between 2012 and 2013.

Data Set 10

27. C 38 minutes. The arrival times for each bus stop listed in the left-hand column are shown in that grey or white row. The bus moves forward in time, down the column of stops, starting at the station at the top of the column at each of the times listed in that row, and going toward its end station listed at the bottom of the column. Different times apply on Saturdays. On Monday the 1225 bus to Winchester Bus Station from Petersfield Tesco stops at East Moon All Saints Church at 1247 and Itchen Abbas Trout Inn at 1325. There are 38 minutes between these stops.

28. E 165 minutes. At 1321 on Tuesday the bus to Winchester Bus station from Petersfield Tesco has just left at 1306. The next bus at 1506 only goes one stop further to New Alresford Perins School. The 1606 bus goes all the way to Winchester Bus Station past Winchester City Road at 1638. There are 165 waiting minutes between 1321 and 1606, 2 hours and 45 minutes.

Data Set 11

29. C 7%. July 1987 saw 66 mm of precipitation. The long-term July average is 71 mm precipitation. The percentage difference = 100% x (long-term average – 1987 value)/long-term average = 100% x (71 mm – 66 mm)/71 mm = 100% x 0.07 = 7%

30. A 1985. Average seed moisture content = (slight + moderate + severe)/3. By visual appraisal the answer is clearly 1985, as it has the lowest value for each of the three rows. By calculation: 1985 = (22.6 + 24.8 + 24.7)/3 = 24.03.
1986 = (22.7 + 26.0 + 25.9)/3 = 24.87.
1987 = (26.5 + 25.9 + 27.2)/3 = 26.53.
1988 = (26.0 + 25.1 + 31.3)/3 = 27.47.
1989 = (31.6 + 30.4 + 31.6)/3 = 31.2.
1985 has the lowest average of 24.03%.

31. D 1760. Corn grain yield in slightly eroded Marlette soil in 1986 was 8150 kg/ha. Corn grain yield in moderately eroded Marlette soil in 1989 was 9910 kg/ha. Difference = 1989 – 1986 = 9910 kg/ha – 8150 kg/ha = 1760 kg/ha.

32. E September. Average monthly precipitation = (monthly precipitation 1985 + monthly precipitation 1986 + monthly precipitation 1987)/3.
May = (69 mm + 89 mm + 38 mm)/3= 65.3 mm.
June = (56 mm + 119 mm + 64 mm)/3 =79.7 mm.
July = (51 mm + 71 mm + 66 mm)/3 = 62.7 mm.
August = (104 mm + 99 mm + 127 mm)/3 = 110 mm.
September = (89 mm + 203 mm + 102 mm)/3 = 131.3 mm.
September has the highest average precipitation of 131.3 mm.

33. C 1684 cm^2. In lightly eroded Marlette soil in 1986 there were 59 400 plants/ha. 1 ha = 10 000 m^2 = 10 000 x 100 x 100 cm^2. 100 000 000 cm^2 x 1 ha/59 400 plants/ha = 1684 cm^2/plant.

Data Set 12

34. D 25th. The point on the lower weight versus age plot on the vertical 2 month line (2nd point from bottom left) also lies on the 25th percentile line.

35. C 71.5 cm. This point lies in the upper length section of the graph on the vertical 24 month line, just below the intersection with the 72 cm line.

36. D 19.2 lbs. The three final weight measurements in pounds are 18.2 lbs, 18.5 lbs and 20.8 lbs as read off the table in the bottom right corner for 17.5, 24 and 36 months of age. Average weight = (18.2 lbs + 18.5 lbs + 20.8 lbs)/3 = 19.2 lbs.

END OF SECTION

Section D: Abstract Reasoning

Rules:

Set 1: Edges in Set A= 14; edges in Set B = 15.

Set 2: Sum of Arrow directions; Set A -Point left/right, Set B- point Up/down. N.B. – the double headed arrows 'cancel out', which is why the answer to 7 is B

Set 3: In Set A there are two points of intersection between the lines in total; in set B there is one point of intersection between the lines in total

Set 4: Set A has at least one White triangle. Set B has at least one Black Quadrilateral.

Set 5: Number of shapes is Odd in Set A and even in Set B.

Set 6: Number of corners in shaded shapes is 8 in Set A and 9 in Set B.

Set 7: Arrow points to corners in set A, arrows point to edges in set B.

Set 8: Number of edges Inside circle minus number of edges outside circle = 4 in set A and 3 set B.

Set 9:

41. A white shape with an increasing number of sides is added each time. The colour of each shape alternates between white and black each tile.
42. Central pentagon rotates 90° clockwise. Dots rotate one space clockwise.
43. Tiles alternate between reflecting in the horizontal and rotating 90° clockwise
44. Number of triangles increases by 1 each time. Colour and size of shape is irrelevant.
45. Number of black circles increases by 1. Number of white circles decreases by 2.

Set 10:

46. Shapes with an even number of sides turn black and gain 1 side. Shapes with an odd number of sides turn white and decrease number of sides by 1.
47. White shapes turn to grey with the number of black circles = the difference in number of sides between the grey and white shape.
48. The number of white shapes is double the number of black shapes. 2 white shapes are added.
49. The grid rotates 45° clockwise. The are n+1 black circles opposite n grey circles in the first tile; the number of grey circles decreases by 1 and the number of black increases by 2 (so n grey = n+3 black).
50. The image is reflected in the horizontal.

Set 11: Set A; the number of white circles = number of edges of black shapes. Number of black circles = number of edges of white shapes. Set B, the number of white circles = number of edges of white shapes. Number of black circles = number of right angles in black shapes.

END OF SECTION

Section E: Situational Judgement Test

Scenario 1

1. **Very inappropriate.** This is too much of a risk – she may end up doing worse than the original exam because of the time elapsed.
2. **Appropriate but not ideal.** Given the time and money spent on the trip, cancelling would mean she would lose a lot. However, she would have plenty of time to study.
3. **Inappropriate but not awful.** Her best friends might understand as they are all on the same course. However, this would also compromise their trips.
4. **Inappropriate but not awful.** This is a risky option – she may not enjoy the holiday because she is studying, or she may have very little time to study. However, bringing work is better than not doing any.
5. **Very appropriate**. This option ensures she gets to enjoy some of the trip whilst leaving enough time to revise for her exam properly.

Scenario 2

6. **Inappropriate but not awful.** His friends have to fund their own tours, but may be willing to contribute if they really want him there.
7. **Inappropriate but not awful** It is not really worth the debt just to go on a sports tour.
8. **Inappropriate but not awful**. It is probably better to ask his parents rather than his friends/the bank and they may be willing to help, however it is not a really important reason to ask for money.
9. **Appropriate but not ideal** He will have other numerous opportunities to make friends and have an active role within the club. He is only in his first year so there will be many other tours throughout his university career.
10. **Very inappropriate.** His medical studies should definitely not be sacrificed just for sports tour.

Scenario 3

11. **Very inappropriate.** If he were to be successful with his application, he would not have given his parents any warning about the costs. If they are unable to help him he will then be letting the other students down.
12. **Appropriate but not ideal**. This way he avoids the financial aspect of living away from home, but still has opportunities to make friends.
13. **Very inappropriate.** Clearly Ade is unhappy, so he should make an effort to rectify his situation.
14. **Very inappropriate.** It is unreasonable to put this pressure on his parents.
15. **Very appropriate.** This will allow Ade and his family to plan and make appropriate financial decisions.

Scenario 4

16. **Inappropriate but not awful.** This is risky and would have to be very carefully worded.
17. **Very appropriate.** This means that she can both inform a superior and take action.
18. **Very inappropriate.** Doing nothing would mean that the doctor would continue to upset patients in the future and no change would happen.
19. Inappropriate but not ideal. It could be deemed inappropriate to go behind the doctor's back and encourage patients to report him. It would be better to gain some advice first.
20. **Very appropriate.** This action means that a superior has been informed and they can decide whether or not to take the matter further.

Scenario 5

21. **Inappropriate but not awful** It would most likely make the patient uncomfortable to sit in silence, so some kind words should be offered. If the patient then says they don't want to talk, silence is appropriate.
22. **Very appropriate.** It is difficult to word this correctly, but the patient is likely to appreciate kind words.
23. **Inappropriate but not awful.** Although the doctor shouldn't really have left the room at such a poignant moment either, it would be inappropriate to leave the patient on his own at a time like this.
24. **Inappropriate but not awful.** Given the little knowledge she has about prostate cancer, this could do more harm than good. However, if the patient wishes to know the information and it is beneficial to them, it might be acceptable to share.
25. **Very inappropriate.** It is a good idea to offer support. However, the patient has been told he is terminal and thus saying he will be Okay seems like empty words.
26. **Appropriate but not ideal.** It is true that often talking to a medical student is less daunting for a patient and after receiving such shocking news the patient may wish to express themselves. However should she then proceed to answer any prognostic questions she would then be being inappropriate.

Scenario 6

27. **Very appropriate.** If she has not been taught how to complete the procedure, she should definitely not attempt it alone for the first time on a patient without any one to help.
28. **Appropriate but not ideal.** This way a trained professional can talk her through the procedure and be on hand if anything goes awry. However, this introduces a delay for a time pressured procedure and so it would be preferable for Larissa to go and directly seek a member of staff to assist, rather than wait.
29. **Very inappropriate.** There is no way of knowing if the skills she has learnt elsewhere are transferable. This is putting the patient at considerable risk.
30. **Inappropriate but not awful.** Whilst it is necessary to inform the patient that it would be the first time, it is still dangerous to carry out the procedure alone for the first time.
31. **Very inappropriate.** It would be very unprofessional to just leave without ensuring someone else can carry out the ABG, especially seeing as Larissa knows the patient needs it done ASAP.

Scenario 7

32. **Very important.** He has been told the chances of publication are very likely, and currently he has no other chances for publication. It is too much of a risk to reject the offer.
33. **Important.** A publication would make him more competitive when it comes to applying to jobs. Many of his friends already have publications.
34. **Important.** It is important for Romario to make the most of his last year as a student before the reality of becoming a junior doctor.
35. **Of minor importance.** It is important to continue to look professional, especially as his consultant could influence his grades.
36. **Of minor importance.** There is a group of friends going so no one would be left in the lurch. All of his friends already have publications so should understand his decision to stay.

Scenario 8

37. **Not important at all.** He has been told that if he is at all unwell he should not come in. Even a cold could put high dependency respiratory patients at risk.
38. **Important.** This would be a great learning opportunity for Mahood and probably his only chance to see such interesting cases.
39. **Very important.** This instruction has been given for a reason, as a minor illness could put such sick patients at serious risk. Mahood should follow these explicit instructions.
40. **Important.** As above, this is a one-off learning opportunity for Mahood.
41. **Very important.** It is part of Mahood's responsibility as a medical student to be professional and not put patients at risk.

Scenario 9

42. **Important.** The captain is responsible for organising the team. Theodore may be letting the rest of the team down if he is absent.
43. **Very important.** Extra-curricular activities should not compromise medical studies, especially if this will impact on Theodore's final grades.
44. **Very important.** Although important, Theodore's rugby matches should not count for more than his medical career.
45. **Very important.** This is Theodore's only chance to learn from his consultant and also impress him.
46. **Important.** Theodore has the chance to show leadership skills beyond medicine.

Scenario 10

47. **Important.** Both the essay and the clinic seem to be important to Malaika. Therefore, if she allocates an appropriate amount of time to her essay, she may be able to do both.
48. **Very important.** The essay should be her priority if it contributes towards her final mark, as the clinic is not compulsory and would be being attended out of interest.
49. **Of minor importance.** Malaika cannot tell how much she will gain from the clinic. The fact that she is interested in the field suggests she will learn something useful.
50. **Not important at all.** Although Malaika is interested in the field, this clinic is optional and so she will not look unprofessional for not attending. Not handing in her essay in time and getting a poor grade would be worse for her academic reputation!
51. **Very important.** If it is possible for her to attend another clinic, she need not worry.

Scenario 11

52. **Important.** It is important for students to look and act professional around both the staff and the patients.
53. **Important.** As they are clinical partners, it is important that they are on good terms so they continue to work well together. However, if they are good friends, Franklin should realise that Jean means well and is not trying to insult him.
54. **Of minor importance.** Franklin should realise this is not a personal attack and that Jean is ensuring they look professional as a pair.
55. **Very important.** It is important to look and act professional around patients, even as a student.
56. **Not important at all.** If Jean remains tidy and professional herself, there is no reason why the appearance of her colleague should influence opinions about her.

Scenario 12

57. **Of minor importance.** Although the project may feel important to Rory, taking patient notes home without permission breaks patient confidentiality and is unprofessional.
58. **Very important.** This is a serious breach of confidentiality and hospital policy, and Priya could get in a lot of trouble.
59. **Very important.** Lack of access to the notes could compromise patient care.
60. **Very important.** A member of staff is very likely to report the issue. Both Rory and Priya could then both be at risk of being in trouble, as the staff may not know who took the patient notes.
61. **Not important at all.** The project is not worth breaching patient confidentiality for.
62. **Not important at all.** Despite this, Rory has an obligation to put a stop to Priya's actions, which should not be ignored.

Scenario 13

63. **Not important at all.** Patient safety cannot be compromised for the sake of Nelson's embarrassment!
64. **Very important.** This is the most important factor of all – patient safety. Contaminated equipment could have devastating effects.
65. **Not important at all.** The duration/site of the contact is irrelevant – if the equipment is contaminated it cannot be used.
66. **Not important at all.** The staff would much rather carry out a safe and clean procedure than put their patient's life at risk.
67. **Not important at all.** Horatio and Nelson's learning experience is not worth risking the life of the patient.
68. **Not important at all.** We know that Nelson did touch the trolley and so the equipment is already contaminated. If the procedure shouldn't be carried out because of this then Horatio needs to inform them.
69. **Very important.** If Nelson were scrubbed in a sterile surgical gown then there would be no chance of contamination, indeed had he not been told to stand back he may have been expecting to participate in the surgery and handle the equipment regardless.

END OF PAPER

Mock Paper B Answers

Section A: Verbal Reasoning

Passage 1

1. **A** The Scottsboro boys case shows another example of racism in the USA, showing how race could lead to false indictments.
2. **B** The law did not state black people had to vacate seats, but conductors did. It is not mentioned if she was arrested at a previous protest, nor does it state how long she had been working - it may not have been for years.
3. **D** It treated white people and black people as different due to their skin colour, determining a 'coloured section' and a 'white' one, but it did not consider different members within the races. Rather, African-Americans were treated as one uniform group and white people as a (superior) other.
4. **A** The passage clearly states that Rosa was arrested "for her refusal [to move]". Therefore, the answer is A.

Passage 2

5. **A** He wanted prostitutes to leave their trade, not stay in it with better conditions. He is neither said to be in a romantic engagement, nor to have used prostitutes. The advert at the end, which he wrote, considered the condition of prostitutes, and so **A** is correct.
6. **B** He originally tried to 'dissuade' her, so initially opposed it, and **A** is incorrect and **B** correct. His general opinion of Burdett-Coutt, whether positive or not, is not mentioned, nor is his behaviour to her described as 'patronising'.
7. **D** It would be unlike other institutions with their harsh ways. It would actively be 'kind', so 'sympathetic', and not neutral, so **A** and **B** are wrong. No mention is made of religious behaviour within the refuge.
8. **D** The advert promises women they can gain back what they lost, so **A** is false, and it also states he does not see himself as 'very much above them' . He does not mention the 'devil', but promises that deserving women can gain back 'friends, a quiet home, means of being useful to yourself and others, peace of mind, self-respect, everything you have lost', making **D** correct.

Passage 3

9. **C** The passage states that values are relative, and does not claim objective right or wrong (so **D** is incorrect.) It does not tell as not to act charitably or that all attempts at doing good end up hurting the do-er, so **A** and **B** are incorrect.
10. **D** The passage does not state **A**, **B** or **C**, as there is nothing to link one view of happiness/morality to the entirety of the poor population or to all prostitutes. Dickens' expectations may have equalled some prostitutes, and not others, and the passage does not state what expectations are 'higher' than others. Instead, the passage states people are contented by different things.
11. **C** The passage states the unnamed writer was 'angered by those who would actively try to get rid of her means of earning', and so she accused 'do-gooders' of depriving those in her trade of work, not of making conditions worse. Conservatism and prudishness are not explicitly stated as accusations.
12. **C** It does not mention either social reformer by name, and was written in the 19th century (1858). She does not call on reformers to be ashamed, but questions their self-perception of being 'pious' with the phrase 'as you call yourselves', suggesting they merely *think* they are, not that they *truly* are, and thus questioning what piety is.

Passage 4

13. **C** The passage does not state the specific contents of either novel, only that they are dystopias. They may not be set in the future.
14. **C** The passage does not state how Orwell would feel about this, it simply states one may wonder how he would feel.
15. **A** The constant surveillance is not specified to be *camera* surveillance. The other three statements are contained within the passage ('children informing on parents', truth being rewritten corroborates and 'love being sacrificed to fear' shows how **B, C** and **D** are all described in the passage.)
16. **D** Concerns of the different dystopias are not stated, and though 'many' audiences are drawn to them, that does not mean all are. The passage does not state that dystopias can be used to make us feel better about the current state of things, but it does say that many are 'drawn' to dystopias, and so these horrible fictional realities 'do not necessarily repel people'.

Passage 5

17. **B** Though Wilde is a playwright who lived during the Victorian era and wrote comedy, none of this is mentioned in the passage. The fact he wrote a novel is mentioned, so he is a writer of fiction.
18. **D** The critic is not denounced as a 'beast', and Wilde does not state how a critic should react to things that aren't beautiful. He describes two types of critic: one who is 'corrupt', the other 'cultivated', so **D** is correct.
19. **D** Books cannot be 'moral' or 'immoral', and books are not specified as being the 'highest form of art'. As a book is either simply 'well written or badly written', a beautifully written book is simply beautifully written.
20. **B** There is no claim that the writer himself will be able to produce a 'well-written' book, or that he will be able to achieve the aim of 'concealing the artist'. There is no guarantee either that critics will like this work. However, as 'all art is useless', this book, as art, must be useless and so **B** is correct.

Passage 6

21. **C** It is said 'Eugenists seem to be rather vague' about what Eugenics is, not that they are too blunt/pithy or badly define their opponents.
22. **D** Though he states he would be justified in his actions, Chesterton acknowledges 'I might be calling him away from much more serious cases, from the bedsides of babies whose diet had been far more deadly'.
23. **B** The passage states 'we know (or may come to know) enough of certain inevitable tendencies in biology' that we can understand an unborn baby as we would an existent person. This mention of the use of science to predict the reality of 'the babe unborn' supports **B** as the correct answer.
24. **C** The passage states that 'The baby that does not exist can be considered even before the wife who does. Now it is essential to grasp that this is a comparatively new note in morality.' So, the baby who is not yet born can be considered more important than a woman who exists, making **C** correct. The other statements are not mentioned in the passage as ethical truths belonging to anyone.

Passage 7

25. **C** The source of the curiosity is not explicitly stated, and may or may not have anything to do with the gender of the individuals working there.
26. **D** She states 'one's first thought' of seeing the workers in the kitchen is of 'some possibly noxious ingredient that might be cunningly mixed in the viand'. She does not make a mention of their safety of comfort whilst working in a kitchen, but only of the potential for poisoning.
27. **C** They call out 'fie! A dirty skirt!', but we are not told about them at work, nor does the passage discuss the other inmates' apparel. No reference is made to them cleaning the writer's skirt.
28. **B** She wonders about their 'intellects; particularly as some of them employed in the grounds, as we went out, took off their hats, and smiled and bowed to us in the most approved manner.' Her specific reason is that they show politeness, not that they speak well or demonstrate particularly high intelligence.

Passage 8

29. **D** She has self-immolated by the writing of the passage, and so was dead.
30. **C** Hydrophobia (fear of water) and being next to a river is the cause stated for his agony.
31. **D** He was to light the pile, and so burn his father and enable his mother to jump into the flame. He was to lose both his parents, and so become an orphan. But the passage does not state he would go on to support his siblings.
32. **D** She was 'apparently', but not definitely, praying, and though she did not move that does not mean she was unable to. She was 27 years younger than her husband, which is less than three decades. She had, however, chosen to leave her children: a choice which is registered by the fact she prepared for her suicide by leaving her children in her mother's care.

Passage 9

33. **A** The passage states many qualities and actions a boy must have and do to be 'respected'.
34. **C** There is no mention of what girls can achieve in terms of respect.
35. **A** He should 'never get into difficulties and quarrels with his companions'.
36. **A** These boys, who will be respected, will 'grow up and become useful men'.

Passage 10

37. **A** The revenge tragedy genre in which Shakespeare wrote was very popular, and so populist.
38. **C** Though the other revenge tragedies are not named after characters, there may be unmentioned ones that are.
39. **D** Biting off one's own tongue, a raped woman and a poisoned skull are named, meaning **A, B** and **C** are not the correct answers for this question. Suicide is not explicitly mentioned, so **D** is correct.
40. **C** One play involves an act of cannibalism, but this does not mean all others of the genre are 'obsessed' with it. We can't tell for certain where all plays are set, as this is not mentioned as a general rule. The tragedies are described as 'dramas', but not as poems. The ethical code, where killers die, is mentioned and described as a general rule for the genre, so **C** is correct.

Passage 11

41. **C** The passage makes no reference to the modern existence of wild cats, but nor does it deny their existence.
42. **B** Cats may have been originally used to hunt rodents, have a gut and tongue suited for raw meat consumption and may find food outside their owner's home. The passage does not state that cats are still used to kill things.
43. **C** 'Washington University's Wesley Warren' states a relationship between the academic body and the individual, so **C** is correct. The passage does not state the individual's gender, whether they are a student or whether they are an acclaimed professor.
44. **C** The passage does not talk in terms of all humanity: though humans are said to have affection towards cats, and previously humans wanted rats dead, it does not state that all humans are unified in affection or loathing. Though originally the relationship with cats might have been one of gratitude for a job well done, this does not mean that human love is predicated on this exchange. For thousands of years, however, cats have been domesticated and kept as pets, so **C** is correct.

END OF SECTION

Section B: Decision Making

1. **C** We are not told whether any of the chemistry exams constitute the paper double sided exams, so I is not correct. Likewise, we are not told whether non-chemistry papers can make up paper exams, but it is likely they can. Therefore, only statement III is true.

2. **E** The Government wants to improve health by encouraging walking so we can conclude that walking is a good form of exercise. The other statements do not explain the Government's initiative.

3. **B** Our Venn diagram should look like the one shown to the right. The total is 30 and we have (6+5+3=) 14 people represented. We need to account for 16 students. We know 14 like Pharmacology and 19 Biochemistry. From the data already on the Venn diagram, there are 11 students who like biochemistry +/- Pharmacology, and 9 who like Pharmacology +/- Biochemistry, however as we know there are only 16 student in total, there must be an overlap of 4. (11+9=20, 20-16=4)

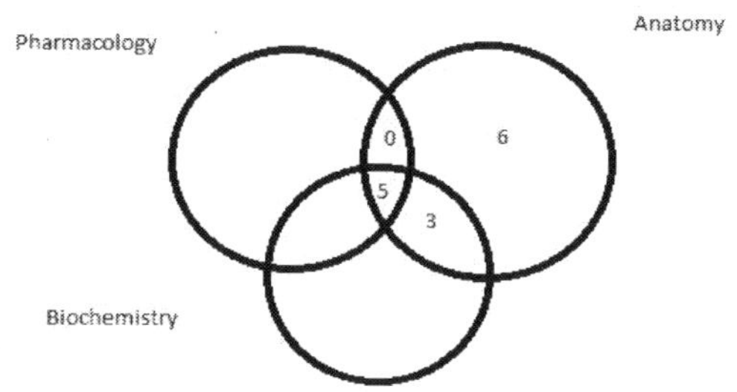

4. **B** The conclusion is: "developing countries need better medical care". Supporting statements must directly affect the conclusion. Statements a, c, and d are not the focus of the conclusion and are not mentioned in the question. Statement e may be true but it does not address the conclusion which is about developing countries.

5. **B** All mothers are women, but not all women are mothers, therefore:

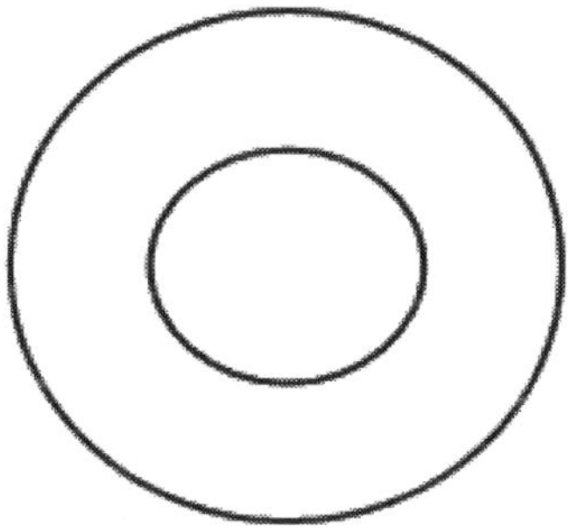

Some women and mothers are doctors but not all doctors are women, which looks like:

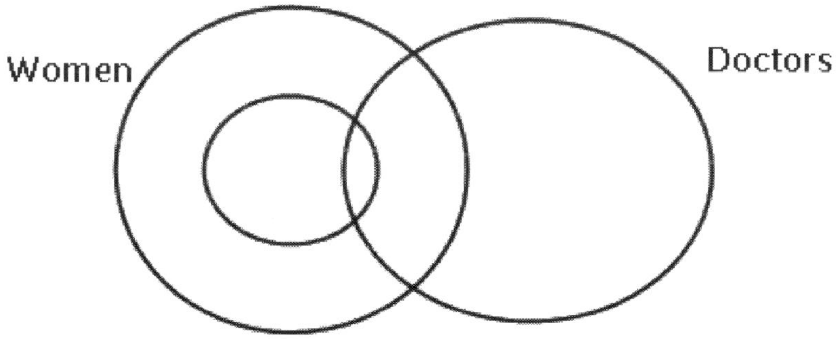

6. **A** Statement a - Percentage change = percentage difference/original percentage so 20-15/20 = 5/20 = 25%. So it is correct.

   Statement b - we are not given any information on food costs. Although there are more dogs we do not know how expensive it is to feed one.
   Statement c - dogs + rabbits + cats = 65% but some reptiles have four legs so they must be included.
   Statement d - Although the same number of reptiles and rodents are purchased, it does not mean that they are purchased together.
   Statement e - rabbits were the most owned animals at 25% and dogs are at 20%

7. **B** Statement b – The formula is: (difference in amounts/ original amount) x 100% So Jake has the greatest percentage change at 40%.
   Statement a - 2012-2013: The overall loss is £15. 2010-2011: The overall loss is £35. 2010 - 2011 has the greatest loss.
   Statement c - we can see that Lauren earns more than Nathan in 2010, 2013, 2014 and 2015. So she earns more than him for 4 years.
   Statement d is clearly wrong.

8. **C** Statement c - Anna's average is (90+35) 62.5, Emily (65+75) 70, Isabelle (20+55) 37.5, Olivia (75+40) 57.5, and Uri (55+35) 45. Emily has the highest average.
Statement a - Anna beats Olivia by 50 marks and Olivia beats Anna by 35.
Statement b and e - There is no way of knowing this from the data given. Statement d - Isabelle and Uri's combined score - 35+55 = 90. Anna also scored 90 so they share the highest score.

9. **D** Statement d - BMWs contribute the greatest percentage of annual revenue but have the least number of cars sold. This means that each car must have high value. Mazda cars are the opposite contributing the least to total annual revenue but sold the most so they must be cheaper.
Statement a - Audi is included in the total revenue so Millie has made money.
Statement b - there is no data that suggests a change in price during the year.
Statement c - BMW and Ford sold (10 + 20+40 +35) 105. Audi sold (60+35) 95 cars

10. **E** There are 20 students in Y10 and Y11 and 160 in Sixth Form. We convert the table from proportion to numbers. Remember that being female and being a swimmer are not mutually exclusive.

	Female	Swimmers
Year 10	0.3 x 20 = 6	0.65 x 20 = 13
Year 11	0.7 x 20 = 14	0.5 x 20 = 10
Sixth form	0.45 x 160 = 72	0.3 x 160 = 48
Total	92	71

We can see from the table that this is correct

A - 10 swimmers in Y11 and 71 swimmers in total gives a percentage of 10/71 = 14%. Even if you cannot work this out, we can see that 65% is the percentage of people in Y11 that can swim and not the percentage we want.
B - there are 71 swimmers in the school (0.355 x 200)
C - there are (20 - 14) 6 males in Y11 and (160 - 72) 88 in Sixth Form.
D - being female and a swimmer are not mutually exclusive so cannot be worked out from the data present.

11. **C** If we work back from the final totals of all having 32p. Queenie loses the first, Rose the second, and Susanna the third game. Each time, they keep half their money, and the other two get one quarter each. Therefore at the beginning of the round they lose, they will have double the money.
Start game 3: Q 16 R16 S 64 – Susanna has double (64p) as she has lost half her money, and therefore Q and R 16p less. The 32p lost is split equally
Start game 2: Q 8 R 32 S 56 – Rose has double (32p), so the other two 8p less
Start game 1: Q 16 R 28 S 52 – Queenie has double (16p), so the other two 4p less

Queenie therefore has the lowest starting amount and Susanna the most.

12. **A**
A. Correct as it addresses the fundamental challenge to the communist social idea.
B. Correct, but not necessarily a problem of communism.
C. Correct, but also not necessarily a problem of communism.
D. Irrelevant for this question.

13. **A**

Peter	Pat	Dave	Lauren	Joe

Although we are not told about Joe by name, we can exclude the other options from the information available to conclude the name of the last place finisher is Joe.

14. **D**
A. False – we are not told her profession
B. False – no information regarding this
C. False – he only wears white shirts with black trousers, but we can't assume he doesn't wear other colours of shirt with black trousers
D. True – he owns white shirts as per the text

15. **D**
A. False – we are not told about the healthcare directly but are told that injury and disease posed a threat

B. False – the terrain was difficult and mapping was poor
C. False – outlaws were a significant threat
D. True – as the text states, there was a marked lack of bridges.

16. B
A. Potentially correct, but extreme sports also carry higher risks of injury.
B. True.
C. True, but irrelevant for the question.
D. Potentially correct, but irrelevant to the question.

17. D
A. Incorrect. The text clearly states that the exercise routine is resistance training based.
B. False. Both groups contain equal numbers of men and women per the text.
C. False. Both groups are age matched in the range of 20 to 25 years.
D. Correct. As the only difference between the two shakes is the protein content.

18. B
A. Incorrect. As the text states, often lead animals are the only ones to mate, not always.
B. Correct answer.
C. False as per text – they are born in late summer in order to be stronger by the winter.
D. False.

19. A
From weakest to strongest:

Fisher's Ale	Knight's Brew	Monk's Brew	Ferrier Ale	Brewer's Choice

Even though Brewer's Choice is not mentioned in the question, as none of the beers mentioned are the strongest, this must be the strongest. We are not told enough information about which beers are German or are made from spring water to deduce any correlation.

20. D
A. False, there are total 80 plants
B. False, he plants the same amount of potatoes as heads of salad.
C. False. There must be 40 tomato plants
D. True. There are 40 tomato plants and 10 salad heads.

21. D
A. Incorrect. According to the text, the majority is due to inhaled substances and due to food intolerances.
B. Incorrect. The majority of diagnoses are being made from 5 and younger.
C. False as irrelevant for the question.
D. Correct. The study demonstrates that this increase has occurred.

22. C
A. Incorrect - the text describes the technical skills required.
B. Incorrect – the text explains the physical forces that need to be optimised.
C. Correct – the text describes both aspects of rowing.
D. Incorrect as per text.

23. A
A. Correct. By piecing together the two pieces of information about restaurant density and its relation to obesity, it can be deduced that obesity is higher in low-income neighbourhoods.
B. Incorrect as per text, there are more around schools.
C. Irrelevant for the question.
D. Beyond the scope of the question.

25. B
Three friends only support the dress, so this must stand alone. Adding in the other preferences you see that the 5 represents recommending earrings, overlapping also with 3 necklace and 4 shoes, and 1 handbag.

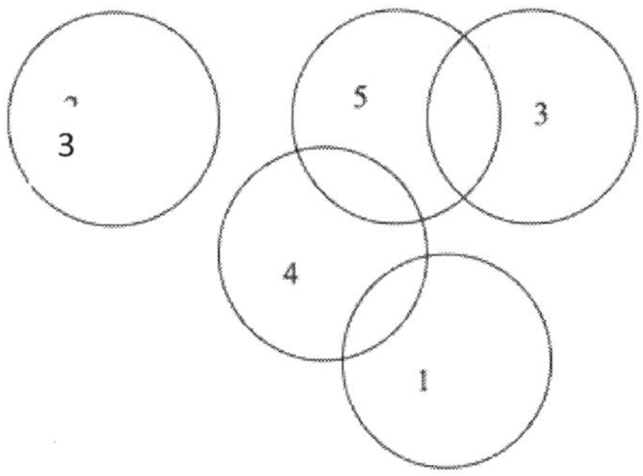

26. B
A. Correct, but irrelevant for the question.

B. Correct answer, it provides a sound rationale for the policy.
C. Depends on the perception of moral responsibility, so weaker than (B).
D. Irrelevant for this question, it argues in the wrong direction.

27. D
A. Incorrect, the text states it is an important problem.
B. Incorrect, this is described in the text.
C. Incorrect, this is described in the text.
D. Correct.

28. B & D
A. False – he has Canadian stamps
B. True – as Germany is in Europe Stan may have German stamps
C. False – Half a dozen = 6 and therefore this is more than the 3 Canadian stamps
D. True – as France is in Europe Stan may have French stamps

29. C

Communication skills	Mental flexibility	Intelligence	Dependa-bility	Empathy

Communication skills: 5%
Mental flexibility: 15%
Intelligence: 18%
Dependability: 28%
Empathy: 34%

We can see from that diagram that A and B are incorrect. Although empathy is not mentioned, we can conclude it is 34% so D is incorrect.

30. B
A. True, but not far-reaching enough.
B. Correct answer. Sugar does indeed have an addictive potential as it causes the release of endorphins and the health concerns are well known. This characteristic makes it like alcohol and smoking and potentially suitable for similar policies.
C. True, but similar to option a) and thus too limited.
D. Potentially true, but also too limited.

END OF SECTION

Section C: Quantitative Reasoning

SET 1

1. **B** The cost of the order is (£2.00x2)+ £5.00 + £4.30 + £6.00 + £3.40 = £22.70. The rice comes to £9.00, so the proportion is 9:22.7 = 1:2.5.

2. **B** The most expensive option is to buy the Roast Pork and the Sichuan pork, for £11.60, and then two egg fried rice for £4.00, so the cost is £15.60 without the deal.
She thus saves £5.60, giving the proportion: 5.6/15.6 = 36%.

3. **A** The cost of Anne's order is £20, and the cost of the items separately is £24.60. So, she saves nothing on delivery, as for both orders the delivery charge is a flat rate of £3.50.

4. **B** Her previous bill would have come to £39.4x1.10 = £43.34. Her new bill comes to £41.40 with free delivery, so she saves £1.94: 1.94/43.34 = 4.5%.

SET 2

5. **D** Bob would pay £300 with Red Flag; with Chamberlain he has a 12% discount, so would pay £308; with Meerkat Market he has a £40 discount so would pay £260, and with Munich he pays £250. Therefore Munich is the cheapest insurance provider for Bob.

6. **B** Normally it would cost £300 per year. With the 10% discount this comes to £270, and with the two free months this comes to (10/12) x£270 = £225.
225/300 = 75%. If 75% of the original cost is paid, the total saving is 25%.

7. **C** Laura has 3 years of no claims discount so she has a 3 x 3% = 9% discount. The cost with 3 years no claims discount from Chamberlain is £350 x 0.91 = £318.50
The cost with 3 years no claims discount from Meerkat Market is £300-£30 = £270, so the saving = £318.50 - £270 = £48.50.

8. **A** Delia's current policy is £270 and Elliot's current policy is £350x0.85 = £297.50. The total old cost = £270 + £297.50 = £567.50 Together their new cost will be £500x0.90 = £450, thus, the proportion is 450:567.5 = 0.79:1.

SET 3

9. **C** The number of students playing at least one game = 341 (the sum of every individual box)
Therefore the number of students playing none of the games = 500 – 341 = 159
The number of students playing exactly one game = 27+23+31+18 = 99
The number of students playing at most one game
= number playing none + number playing one
= 159 + 99 = 258

10. **A** This includes only students who play cricket or basketball, not both. Therefore the number of students who play either cricket or basketball but not football = 27 + 18 + 16 + 31 = 92.

11. **B** Students playing at least three games = students playing exactly three + student playing exactly four
= 8 + 13 + 36 + 31 + 37 = 125.

12. **B** The number of students playing at most one game = 258
Therefore the number of students playing at least two games = 500 – 258 = 242
Difference = 258 – 242 = 16

13. **C** The number of students who do not play cricket, football or hockey is the number of students who play only basketball plus the number of students who play no sports at all = 31+ 159 = 190.

14. **C**
The number of students playing at least one game = 341
The number of students playing none of the games = 159
The number of students playing exactly one game = 27+23+31+18 = 99
The number of students playing none of the games **outnumber** the number of students playing exactly one game by = 159 – 99 = 60

SET 4

15. **A** Number of daily train users = 300,000. Since 41.67% use trains, the total number of travellers is 300000/0.4167 = 719,942 people. Since 16.67% use private cars, the number is 719,942 x 0.1667 = 120,000 people

16. **B** In 1999, number of people using taxis = (150000 x 0.0833)/0.4167 = approximately 30,000 people.

17. **B** Number of people using public transport in 1998 = 200,000/0.25 = 800,000
Number of people using public transportation in 2000 = 300,000/0.4167 = 720,000
Therefore, there is a decrease of 80,000 passengers per day from 1998 to 2000
Percentage decrease = 80,000/800,000 = 0.1 = 10%

18. **A** Number of people using taxis as a means of transport in 2000 = percentage using taxis x total travelling = 0.0833 x 720,000 = 60,000. Therefore, the number of people using taxis as a means of transport in 1998 = 60,000/1.5 = 40,000. Percentage of total in 1998 = number using taxis/total travelling = 40,000/800,000 = 0.05 = 5%

19. **C** Number of people using buses in 2000 = 0.33 x 720,000 (total travelling) = 240,000
Therefore, the number of people travelling by buses in 1999 = (240,000 x 5)/6 = 200,000
And the number of people travelling by buses in 1998 = (240,000 x 8)/6 = 320,000
So the total fare collected is the sum of the total fares for each of the two years of interest (1998 & 1999), which is the daily fare multiplied by the number of passengers multiplied by the number of days.
1999: 200,000 x £1.5 x 358 = £107,400,000
1998: 320,000 x £1 x 358 = £114,560,000
Total amount collected in 1998 and 1999 together = £221,960,000

20. **C** In 1999, the percentage using private cars and buses combined is 16.67 + 33.33 = 50%
Therefore the number this corresponds to is the total number travelling in 1999 multiplied by 0.5
= (720,000 x 0.5) x 0.5 = 180,000 people

SET 5

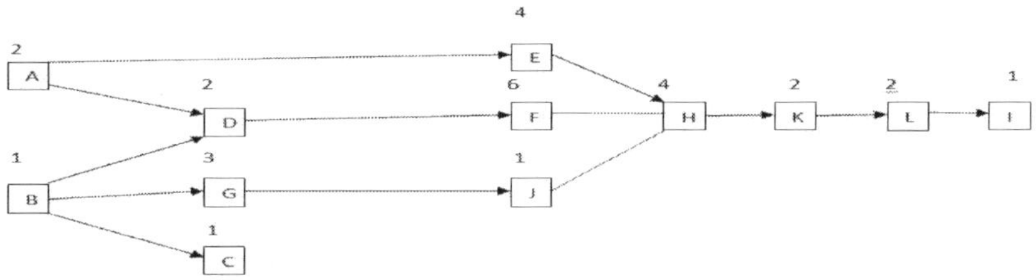

21. **D** The network from the given data is:

False ceiling (H) can start at earliest in the 11th week. Before this work begins, E, F, J, A, D, G and B must be completed, as shown by the flowchart. Work can take place simultaneously, so simply adding these durations is not the correct solution. The longest individual path is A > D > F which takes 2+2+6 weeks = 10 weeks. Therefore, the false ceiling work can begin in the 11th week.

22. **C** J must start before H. The latest it can start is by the 10th week. It could start as early as week 5 once G and B are completed, but in order not to hold up construction work it doesn't have to begin until week 10, so it is completed at the same time the air conditioning system is finished, allowing the false ceiling work to begin in week 11.

23. **B** If no more than one job can be done at any given time, the minimum time all the work can be done, one after the other, is in a total of 29 weeks. Simply add together the duration totals to arrive at this figure.

24. **C** Maximum time gap between F and L is F+E+G+C+J+H+K = 21 weeks.

25. **A** F must finish before H can start. Since F takes 6 weeks and must be completed by the end of week 10, the latest it can start is by week 5 to keep the building work on schedule.

SET 6

26. **C** Target food grain production in 1999-2000 = 1989 production x 1.2 = 175 x 1.2 = 210 million tons
Actual food grain production = 190 + 13 = 203 million tons
Therefore the absolute deficit = 210 – 203 = 7 million tons
Deficit as a percentage of total production target = 7/210 = 3.3%

27. **A** Firstly calculate the percentage decrease in the production of pulses from 1989-90 to 1999-2000
= (15 – 13)/15 = 13.33%
Therefore the average price of pulses for the given years increase by the same 13.33%
Therefore the price in 1999-2000 = 1.8 x 1.133 = £2.04, approximately £2.00

28. **B** Relative percentage = 1999-2000 production/1989-90 production = 190/160 = 1.1875 = 118.75%

SET 7

29. **A** To solve this you need to calculate the time taken by each team to complete the race. Whilst it might be tempting to attempt to find the average speed of each team, this cannot be done arithmetically as different runners run for different durations depending on their speed.
Time to complete = time per metre x number of metres = 1/speed x distance
USA = (1/8 + 1/12 + 1/9 + 1/11) x 400 = 164 seconds
Kenya = (1/9 + 1/14 + 1/6 + 1/11) x 400 = 176 seconds
Russia = (1/10 + 1/15 + 1/9 +1/6) x 400 = 178 seconds
Australia = (1/10 + 1/13 +1/10 +1/7) x 400 = 168 seconds
Therefore USA finishes in the shortest time and is therefore the winner.

30. **C** Once again calculate the time each team takes to complete the course.
Time to complete = time per metre x number of metres = 1/speed x distance
USA = (1/8 + 1/12 + 1/9 + 1/11) x 400 = 164 seconds
Kenya = (1/9 + 1/14 + 1/6 + 1/11) x 400 = 176 seconds
Russia = (1/10 + 1/15 + 1/9 +1/6) x 400 = 178 seconds
Australia = (1/10 + 1/13 +1/10 +1/7) x 400 = 168 seconds
The Russian team took the greatest length of time to complete the course and therefore finished last.

31. **B** The third Runner from Russia and Kenya did not meet. The first, second and third Russian runners were all faster than their corresponding Kenyan runners, so the Russian is ahead at the start of the third runner and the gap only increases during the third leg.

32. **B** This is a simple case of adding up the lap times:
First Runners: 8 + 9 +10 +10 = 37
Second Runners: 12 + 11 + 15 +13 = 51
Third Runners: 9 + 6 + 9 + 10 = 34
Fourth Runners: 11 + 14 + 6 + 7 = 38
Thus, the second runners were the slowest on average.

SET 8

33. **D** In 1999, the total weight of exports = overall cost/cost per tonne = 140000000/7000 = 20 000 tonnes
Total weight of imports = overall cost/cost per tonne = 180000000/6000 = 30 000 tonnes
Exports are less than imports by = (30 – 20)/30 = 33.33%

34. **C**
Trade surplus in 1998 = Exports – Imports = 130 – 110 – 20 Million USD
Trade surplus in 2001 = Exports – Imports = 160 – 150 = 10 Million USD
Therefore the percentage decrease = (20 – 10) / 20 = 50%
Trade surplus in 2002 = 50% of 2001 value = 0.5 x 10 = 5 Million USD
Imports in 2002 = 150 + (0.2 x 150) = 180 Million USD
Exports in 2002 = Imports + Trade surplus = 180 + 5 = 185 Million USD

35. **C** This question tests compound growth – the 2001 value must be increased by 10% three times.
Imports in 2004 = Imports in 2001 x $(1.1)^3$ = 150 x $(1.1)^3$ = 199.65, approximately 200 Million USD

36. **B** The compound annual growth rate is the rate that describes the growth when applied each year.
Therefore 2001 exports = 1996 exports x $(CAGR)^5$
Substitute the numbers in: 160 = 100 x $(CAGR)^5$
Rearrange: CAGR = $(160/100)^{(1/5)}$ = 1.098
Therefore the compound annual growth rate is 9.8%, approximately 10%

END OF SECTION

Section D: Abstract Reasoning

Set 1: In Set A there is always a quadrilateral that is cut by two circles. In Set B there is always a quadrilateral cut by one circle.

Set 2: In set A all the triangles have a black dot above them; in set B all the circles have a black dot below them

Set 3: In Set A, there is at least one circle that is cut by two lines. In Set B there is always at least one circle that has 2 tangents.

Set 4: In set A the sum of the dots is always odd, whilst in set B it is always even.

Set 5: In Set A there is always one more dot than there are rhomboids; in set B there is always one more rhomboid than there are dots.

Set 6: In Set A, the number of rhomboids and crosses are equal; In Set B, the number of rhomboids and black dots are equal

Set 7: In set A there is always one more black shape than white shape. In set B there is always one more white shape than black shape.

Set 8: In Set A there is always one square that overlaps with a circle. In Set B there is always a circle inside a larger square.

Set 9:

41. Black shapes increase number of sides by 1 and white shapes decrease number of sides by 2. There is at least one grey shape.
42. If a shape has an odd number of sides, it turns black in the next tile and stays black for subsequent tiles. Size and orientation is irrelevant.
43. Number of sides increases by 1 each time. Colour, shape and size is irrelevant.
44. Total number of right angles increases by 1 each time. Colour is irrelevant.
45. Number of intersections increases by 1 each time.

Set 10:

46. The number of intersections decreases by 1.
47. The total number of sides increases by 2. Size and colour of shape is irrelevant.
48. The number of acute angles increases by 2.
49. Each shape rotates 90° anticlockwise. Positions are irrelevant.
50. There is an added curved line.

Set 11: Set A; total number of white edges = even. Total number of black edges = odd. Always 1 grey shape. Set B; total number of black edges = even. Total number of grey edges = odd. Always 1 white shape.

END OF SECTION

Section E: Situational Judgement Test

Scenario 1

1. **Very appropriate.** This way Arthur is not speaking for the patient but inviting him to share his feelings so that they can be resolved.
2. **Inappropriate but not awful.** Suicidal thoughts are a 'red flag' and so need to be mentioned to the doctor. However, going against the patient's request in front of them jeopardises their future engagement with the GP.
3. **Appropriate but not ideal.** Although this is good to inform the doctor, and true that confidentiality can be broken in this instance, Arthur should not have let the patient go home without exploring the matter further.
4. **Very inappropriate.** Although the patient has asked Arthur not to say anything, suicide risk is a very serious matter and one that needs to be reported, even if it risks breaking patient confidentiality.
5. **Inappropriate but not awful.** Although this is better than doing nothing, Arthur needs to explicitly tell the doctor the issue, there is no point just hinting about something so serious.

Scenario 2

6. **Very appropriate.** His personal tutor is there to help him out in difficult situations and together they may be able to come up with a solution.
7. **Very inappropriate.** Nico cannot break the rules of the medical school simply because he is feeling underprepared.
8. **Very appropriate.** It is important that Nico maximises the remaining time he has, all he can do is his best! He should not be embarrassed at the prospect of failing.
9. **Very inappropriate.** As a medical student, this would be very unprofessional and not solve Nico's problem.
10. **Very inappropriate.** Nico should not hide from the problem, he must make the most of the time he has left and put in as much effort as he can.

Scenario 3

11. **Very appropriate.** This is a very polite and appropriate way of acknowledging the patient.
12. **Inappropriate but not awful.** Encountering patients can be a difficult situation to navigate. If Mrs Hamilton has not spotted Alan there might not be an issue – Alan is not obligated to approach her.
13. **Very inappropriate.** This would be a breach of patient confidentiality. Mrs Hamilton's health issues are private and she most likely wouldn't want them broadcast on the bus.
14. **Inappropriate but now awful.** This may be seen as rude and unprofessional of Alan. However, he is not obligated to talk to her.
15. **Very appropriate.** Again Alan is not obligate to talk to her, nor may she even want to talk to him. Alan should follow her lead, not actively seek conversation, but respond politely and professionally if confronted.

Scenario 4

16. **Very inappropriate.** Sabrina should put a stop to the obvious breach in patient confidentiality. As an older student she should remind the younger students of their professionalism.
17. **Inappropriate but not awful.** Sabrina should talk to the girls before reporting them. Perhaps if they had behaved in this way before then reporting them straight away would be more appropriate.
18. **Very appropriate.** Discussions about patients should occur in a private and professional manner, and Sabrina should remind her fellow students of this.
19. **Inappropriate but not awful.** This may slightly help the situation, however it is still a public environment and they could easily be overhead.
20. **Very inappropriate.** This leaves the problem unresolved and the patient's confidentiality is still at risk. Observations of wrongdoing should be stopped if possible.

Scenario 5

21. **Appropriate but not ideal.** This may be unfair to the rest of the group who are prepared, however it is not Maxine's fault that she did not receive the email.
22. **Very appropriate.** The best option is for Maxine to be honest to the doctor.
23. **Very inappropriate.** It would appear as though Maxine had just not bothered to prepare if she does not turn up – she needs to be honest to her consultant.
24. **Inappropriate but not awful.** Although she may gain some information, this does not give Maxine adequate or equal time to understand the contents of the test and she may not achieve her full potential or achieve a safe level of understanding.
25. **Very inappropriate.** Copying another student's work does not achieve anything for Maxine, as she will not have learnt from preparing for the test. Cheating is not the solution!

Scenario 6

26. **Very inappropriate.** This is not Marcus' position as a student. The consultant may have had valid reasons for phrasing it how he did. It is also an entirely inappropriate way for the patient to hear such news.
27. **Inappropriate but not awful.** This could come across very rudely, so would need to be phrased differently. As above, the consultant may have had a valid reason.
28. **Very appropriate.** This will give Marcus' a greater understanding as to why the consultant did what they did, and he may gain greater insight into the skill of delivering bad news.
29. **Inappropriate but not awful.** Marcus should not ignore something that he strongly believes in, however as a student it is not necessarily his place to ensure the patient understands everything the doctor tells them.
30. **Very inappropriate.** Marcus should not go behind the doctor's back, especially as he is likely to have a limited understanding of the patient's condition. This also has implications for patient confidentiality.

Scenario 7

31. **Very inappropriate.** Tunde himself should not lie.
32. **Very appropriate.** This answer is honest, and does not put the other student's marks at risk.
33. **Appropriate but not ideal.** Whilst he is being honest to the other students, it does not provide them sufficient time to adequately prepare for the test.
34. **Very inappropriate.** This again is dishonest and it is likely that the consultant would give all of the students the test anyway.
35. **Very inappropriate.** This does not solve the problem in any way.

Scenario 8

36. **Very inappropriate.** This would be very inappropriate given Delilah's position as a medical student in a clinic that he is a patient of.
37. **Very appropriate.** This is a polite way of refusing the patient's offer whilst maintaining professionalism.
38. **Appropriate but not ideal.** If Delilah feels uncomfortable because of the patient's behaviour, she should inform her seniors as she does not have to put up with him. However, initially a simple polite refusal to the patient may end the situation there without the need for escalation via a complaint.
39. **Very inappropriate.** Despite what she may be feeling, Delilah must remain composed and maintain her professionalism in the face of adverse patient behaviour.
40. **Appropriate but not ideal.** Whilst this solves the solution for Delilah, this could put another student at risk of the patient's behaviour.

Scenario 9

41. **Very important.** Medical studies should be prioritised over extra-curricular activities.
42. **Important.** Chad has only been offered a trial and should recognise that, although this is a good opportunity, it by no mean guarantees him becoming a professional footballer. Therefore this may not be worth compromising his exams for.
43. **Important.** Conversely to the above factor, although a small step in a long process, if this is something Chad wants to pursue this may be a very good opportunity for him.
44. **Important.** Chad may have ample time to study for his exams as well as trial for the team.
45. **Not important at all. Whilst ideally Chad's parents would agree with his chosen profession, the final decision should remain with Chad.**

Scenario 10

46. **Important.** Although the situation is unpleasant, Troy must consider the underlying reasons for the patient's actions, as he does not know the patient's reason for being there. However whilst explaining why this has occurred it does not excuse aggressive and verbally abusive behaviour towards members of the medical team.
47. **Of minor importance.** Whilst the patient's diary is not Troy's responsibility, and there is nothing Troy can do about the delay, he must consider that this could be a very important reason as to why the patient has become aggressive.
48. **Of minor importance.** All of the other patients have to wait too yet have remained calm, suggesting this patient is being unreasonable.
49. **Important.** Although it has inconvenienced the patient, the doctor was delayed due to an emergency, so Troy can explain this to the patient.
50. **Very important.** Troy needs to maintain his professionalism in front of the patients who he will later be seeing.
51. **Of minor importance.** Troy is there to help out but should be supported by other professionals in the clinical environment.
52. **Important.** There is no excuse for violence towards healthcare professionals but those patients who have a diagnosis that pre-disposes them to violence should be treated differently as it is expected.

Scenario 11

53. **Important.** This factor will greatly influence Leroy's decision even though to an impartial person the answer may seem obvious. He must balance the implicit trust in a relationship with his duty to prevent plagiarism.
54. **Important.** Although he does not want to betray Bryony's trust, he now knows she has done something wrong and should do something about it.
55. **Very important.** Plagiarism is a serious offence and if Leroy has the chance to put a stop to it he should.
56. **Not important at all.** Plagiarism should be reported no matter how prestigious the environment in which it occurs.
57. **Important.** This could cast an embarrassing light on the university, which could make Byrony's punishment more severe.

Scenario 12

58. **Very important.** Benson should do all he can to do his best in his studies.
59. **Very important.** If Benson is able to borrow the books from the library he does not necessarily need his own copies.
60. **Important.** Students tend to get into lots of debt in these scenarios, which could create extra stress for Benson and compromise his studies.
61. **Very important.** It is not worth putting his studies at risk for a job, as there are other ways of obtaining funds for medical books.
62. **Very important.** A contribution from his parents could make all the difference when buying these books.
63. **Of minor importance.** His medical studies should be put before going on a sports tour. However, this may be a meaningful part of his University experience, and so should not be completely discounted.

Scenario 13

64. **Important.** As Albert-Clifford placed this as his first choice, whilst Anna-Theresa put it as her last choice, it seems there may have been some sort of irregularity in the allocation system which may be worth querying as part of an appeal.
65. **Not important at all.** Anna-Theresa was not allocated her first choice of project either, so it does not seem fair that Albert-Clifford should be re-allocated and no one else.
66. **Very important.** Albert-Clifford should realise that he is not the only one who wanted this project and it may be unfair of him to demand his place on the project over other people.
67. **Of minor importance.** He has put extensive time and resources into the project and has the opportunity to take this further. However, unfortunately putting in that amount of effort prior to a random allocation process was always going to be a risk.
68. **Not important at all.** Albert-Clifford should commit to whichever project he has been allocated. Many other students are likely to be in a similar position.
69. **Of minor importance.** This may help Albert-Clifford if he decided to appeal as he has demonstrated enthusiasm to the project supervisor. However, similarly to above, demonstrating enthusiasm does not have any influence in a random allocation process.

END OF PAPER

Mock Paper C Answers

Section A: Verbal Reasoning

Passage 1

1. **B** The text states that the pest-control business as a whole profits $6.7 billion of which bird-control only comprises one offshoot. Therefore, this statement is false.
2. **D** The text states that cryptococcosis is exceedingly rare and the $1.1 billion a year of excrement damage is the reason there is a need for pest-control in the first place irrespective of bird lover views. C is difficult to evaluate but it can be assumed to be false due to the "lucrative" bird control industry, leaving the correct answer D which is directly implied through the trade journal article the text mentions.
3. **C** The text states that pigeons can spread more than 60 diseases among humans however it does not offer any insight on how the significance of this issue compares with say the $1.1 billion a year due to excrement damage. Therefore, more information is needed to appraise this statement.
4. **B** The text explicitly states that culling remains a common fall-back method in response to public complaints. Our growing concern for pigeon welfare questions the ethics of culling but the text does not imply that it has caused its outlaw.

Passage 2

5. **C** At no point does the author categorically state or imply that he is or isn't the creator. He makes several vague references to time throughout the passage but without knowing the date the text was written/age of the author it is impossible to make any definitive conclusions.
6. **C** We know that the gun can hit a toy soldier at 9 yards 90% of the time but that doesn't necessarily mean that the accuracy deteriorates 1 yard further away. More information is needed.
7. **B.** The author states that the breechloader supersedes spiral spring makes thus implying it uses an alternative mechanism.
8. **C** This is the only conclusion which has direct evidence within the text. In the middle of the second paragraph where the author explains how the breechloader shoots wooden cylinders about an inch long. B seems like it could be an answer, however the text states 'the game of Little war, as we know it, became possible with the invention...' which may imply that the game is only possible with this gun however only states that the game at its current form needs the gun. This doesn't rule out the possibility that an inferior version of "little wars' was played prior to the invention of the spiral spring breechloader.

Passage 3

9. **B** Whilst much of the article describes the benefits to trading vessels, the second sentence states that the canal was opened to strengthen Germany's navy.
10. **C** The article does directly imply that bypassing the difficult navigation at Kattegat and Skager Rack would avoid the half million moneys loss of trading vessels each year. It doesn't, however, state a currency for that amount. Therefore the statement in the question may or may not be true.
11. **A** Recall that Germany's primary motivation for opening the canal was to strengthen their navy, trade benefits are just a coincidence, which is what the article is trying to demonstrate.
12. **C** Benefits to the navy are not described in the article therefore more information is needed. Furthermore, the text describes the potential future benefits of the new canal and doesn't describe any benefits that have come from the new canal (as it has only just opened).

Passage 4

13. **C** The statement in the question implies that each of the books in the trilogy was discussing the geology of South America. If you look back at the text you will see that the author only states that one specific volume of the trilogy focused on South America. It is of course possible that the other two volumes discussed South America as well but it is not mentioned.
14. **C** It is in a quote that Darwin himself calls his work dull. In the very first sentence the author describes Darwin's work as remarkable which we can assume does not mean boring. However, the author presents no opinion of whether they find Darwin's work boring or not so we are unable to answer this question with any certainty.
15. **A** The author states that there was a year delay in the completion of Darwin's work and the publishing of his manuscript. In a subsequent quote from Darwin himself the author implies ill health as a reason.
16. **A** In the last quote Darwin refers to his 240 pages much condensed. Implying that initially his draft was much longer.

Passage 5

17. **A** There is not a single argument in the text to argue against this, indeed one could argue that this is the main argument of the text through the examples that it uses.
18. **A** The article not only states that cattle are not indigenous to America, it also describes how the Conquistadores first introduced them to South America. Whilst you're not expected to know the Conquistadores nationality, references to the Spanish national sport and old Madrid certainly imply that they were Spanish.
19. **C** Whilst all of the conclusions are to a certain extent true on inference C is the most important. Indeed, answers A, B and D are actually all used to exemplify answer C in the text.

20. **C** The text states that was uptake of the Spanish national sport in all these locations. That does not however mean necessarily that the Conquistadores landed in each of those locations.

Passage 6

21. **B** The author explicitly states that in his opinion this belief is a fallacy.

22. **A** The author states that white pine has grown in New England "from time immemorial", which does not necessarily mean it grows best there. However, the use of the author's rhetorical question in conjunction with this statement suggests a degree of sarcasm and as such heavily implies that the statement in the question is true. The phrase 'Where do you find white pines growing better' also supports this statement.

23. **A** All the other answers are used as part of the authors argument towards A. Using examples such as the English oak and white pine to demonstrate that soil nutrient depletion is not sufficient to prevent the growth of established forests, unless the entire population is destroyed in which case new species move in.

24. **C** Although almost word for word this is the concluding sentence of the passage there are subtle differences in the wording which means it is used more as an observation or metaphor in the text. It is therefore impossible to know whether the author believes this.

Passage 7

25. **B** The only thing the text states about conflict is that in the event of war the cables may be cut by each of the aggressors with no implication that America has the right to seize overall control.

26. **B** The text states that "seven are largely owned, operated or controlled by American capital". As there are nine cables in the question it is impossible for America to own them all.

27. **B** Although if taken on face value this statement is not 100% true with the cables also residing above 40 degrees north, it is in itself not false – just half the truth. A and C directly conflict with passages of the text and D is not mentioned at all.

28. **C** The passage tells us that France owns only one of the cables, that however does not allow for any inference of usage. More information is required.

Passage 8

29. **C** The author presents this as one possible theory whereas the question presents it as fact. There is not enough evidence in the text to either accept or reject the statement.

30. **B** The text explicitly states that the excavations occurred during winter 1894-95, i.e. December of 1894.

31. **B** The text states that Libyans may have resided in Egypt between the old and middle kingdoms, i.e. before the middle kingdom ended not after it.

32. **C** The text refers to 3,000 "graves". 3,000 bodies is therefore a good estimate however one cannot assume that there was exactly one body to every grave and as such more information is needed.

Passage 9

33. **A** The text opens with "the best feed" and at no point does it mention any meat, so this statement can therefore be assumed to be true.

34. **D** At first glance B may appear the correct answer but note the text only describes a change in diet depending on wet/damp and cold weather and does not specify a specific time of year. The sentence "water and boiled milk, with a little lime water in each occasionally, is the best drink…" directly implies a turkey's need for distinct items of food and drink.

35. **A** The text directly states not to combine water and rice since the chicks are unable to swallow the paste, which therefore may cause them to choke.

36. **B** The author writes that the whites should only be added after the chicks are several days old.

Passage 10

37. **C** The author writes the passage from a relatively neutral standpoint, describing Lintner's opinion on the matter. We cannot be sure the author believes this himself.

38. **A** The text directly implies this in the penultimate line where it states the closed system labours under the disadvantage of making it difficult to maintain cleanliness.

39. **A** The text describes one of the flaws of the current malting system being a problem with the removal of carbonic acid, thus implying that carbonic acid has a negative impact on the malting process. As germination ceases at 20% carbonic acid, we can thus assume that 30% carbonic acid, which is greater than 20% and would occur if you can't remove the carbonic acid, would also make germination not possible.

40. **B** Although this sentence is not explicitly reiterated in the text it is implied through the mentioning of at least two types of pneumatic malting apparatus: closed vs. open.

Passage 11

41. **A** The question does not state that it ONLY flows north of Cork and is therefore at least in part true.

42. **C** Whilst the final paragraph does describe how the new bridge displays many features dictated by local conditions, it does not mention anything about practicality or difficulty.

43. **C** The new Angelsea bridge is certainly a swing bridge however the mechanism adopted by the previous bridge is not mentioned.

44. **A** In the second paragraph the text states that Cork train station is on the southern back of the southern branch of the river Lee.

Section B: Decision Making

1. **A** The statement currently presented demonstrates a jump of logic. The only way to establish logical flow is if a reason is given for not reading biased journals. It does not matter whether President Trump or the magazine are "good" or not.

2. **D** If a Venn diagram is drawn with the above information, such a picture should emerge. 25-13= 12, which is the number of students who like Beer/Spirits but not Wine. 12- 6 (Students who like spirits) = 6. Thus the number of students who liked beer alone is 6.

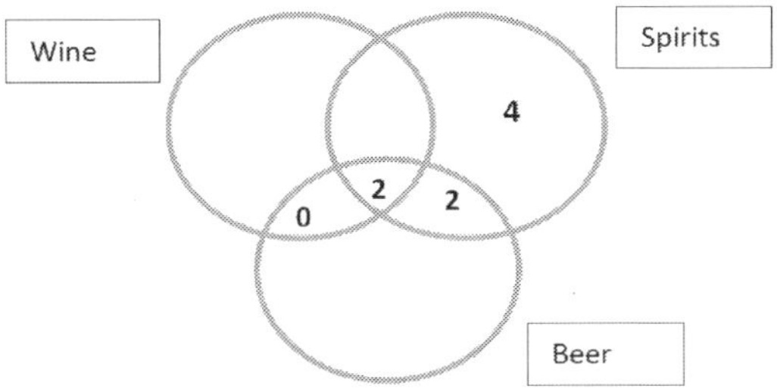

3. **C** Statements A and D are unrelated to the need for sleep, (which refutes the lack of sleep statement) and thus can be eliminated. Statement B is wrong because the functionality of the immune system is not a logical indicator of life/death.

4. **A** This argument contains the slippery slope fallacy. Statements B and C are irrelevant to the argument because they would not change the logic within it. Statements A and D are quite similar, however the focus of the statement is on gay marriage in particular, not gays and thus A is the answer.

5. **B** The word to focus on in this passage is that the factory "claimed" …. This indicates that none of the conclusions about the casualties can be confirmed, but also this does not indicate that there is some ulterior motive as in statement A.

6. **D** With the information given to us, it is impossible to work out the probability of full attendance of students, hence the answer is D.

7. **C** Pervill's number cannot be formed by adding multiples of 7, 28 or 16. 7 and 28 are both divisible by 7. As 7 and 28 are divisible by 7, and thus we can get to any total in the 7x table, the easiest method is to keep subtracting 16 from the potential answers to see if we reach a number in the 7x table which indicates that this total number of marbles can be achieved. 55-3x16=7, so this total can be reached. 51-16=35. 67-2x16=35. The odd one out therefore is C, as taking multiples of 16 away from 63 gives us 47, 31 and 15, thus this total is impossible to reach with combinations of 7, 16 and 28.

8. **B** Within the Venn Diagrams, reading the information should make it obvious that 17% fulfils all three categories and is placed at their intersection. Since this is included in the 60% of students who get into medical school, to find those that ax§re not included in the middle should be 60-17=43%. The 8% should be obsolete of any junctions as these are the students who do not "get in". Option B fulfils all these categories.

9. **C** If a diamond is drawn with all of the names placed as described, Hans is eliminated for standing in the front. Amelia can be eliminated because she stands at the very back, being 2 steps behind Hans in the diamond. That leaves Jake, Lola and Macy. Jake has been positioned to the far left and thus can be eliminated. As Lola is right next to Jake, she is the one in the middle. The formation is shown below.

	Amelia	
Jake	Lola	Macy
	Hans	

10. **A** The total number of shoe pairs available is 14. The probability that Stan smiths are selected is $\frac{4}{14}$ and the probability that BAIT are selected is $\frac{3}{14}$. To select both we can either have Stan Smiths AND BAIT or BAIT AND Stan Smiths. Thus $\frac{4}{14}$ X $\frac{3}{14}$ X 2= $\frac{6}{49}$

11. **C** The candidate has to identify which of the options would support the statements in the question. They have to choose the answer that explains which lung cancer patients should be charged. Options A and B do not explain why the smokers are charged, but rather introduces new patient categories. Thus option C is the right answer.

12. C There are n+1 people at the conference so hugs given = 1+2+3+ ... + n. Since this sum is n(n+1)/2, we need to solve the equation n(n+1)/2 = 28. This is the quadratic equation n2+ n -56 = 0. Solving for n, we obtain 7 as the answer and deduce that there were 8 people at the party.

13. D It is important to realise that the past does not predicate the present, thus decisions of the past will not affect establishment of deals now. Thus answers A and B are unlikely. Option C can be ruled out because there is not enough information to draw such a conclusion about Trump's negotiating abilities from the question.

14. B Statement A & C refers to individuals whom we cannot assume from the question are in any other category than those assigned to them (good grades/ party hard). The problem with statement D is that it generalises to include everybody, but not all medical students get good grades. Thus B which states the possibility of being in the good grades and party hard category is the right answer.

15. C It is important to realise that the Swimmers aren't a constant distance apart. They get further apart as they swim. Holly and Alex are less than 15m apart when Jon wins. Since they beat each other by the same distance, the difference between speeds must be equal.
When Jon reaches 200m, Alex is at 185m. When Alex finishes, Holly is at 185m. We need to know where Holly is when Alex is at 185m.
Alex is at has 92.5% $(\frac{185}{200})$ of Jon's speed. Holly's speed is 92.5% of Alex's and 85.5% (92.5% x 92.5% = 85.5%) of Jon's.
Thus 85.5% of 200 = 171m

16. B While option A might be true, it does indicate not why action is better than inaction.
Option B refers to improvement, the result of an action which is better than inaction, and is thus the correct answer.
Option C refers to success but the question only refers to betterment or improvement and is thus wrong

17. D The concept of greater good is irrelevant to whether medicolegal services should be hired and thus option A can be eliminated. The expense of the services does not directly explain why doctors do not need to hire them thus eliminating B. It is true that hospital lawyers can protect the doctors but that does not automatically exclude the need for medicolegal services. D is the only option that gives a reason and fits between the two statements in the question.

18. B All four of the options could be considered true facts. The question is looking for the assumption associated with the cybersecurity which gives reason for pornography being banned. Only statement 2, about pornography being a risk factor explains why it should be banned.

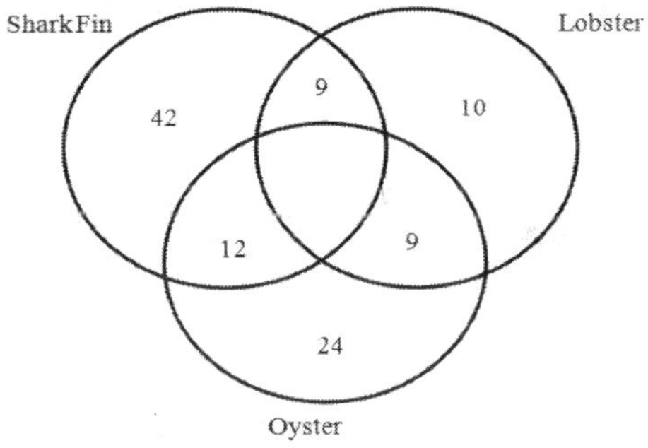

19. C A Venn diagram can help to calculate how many restaurants keep only one of each seafood type.

As n=130, adding up all the numbers in the Venn diagram (=106) and subtracting from 130 should give us 24.

20. D From the information given, the hexagon represents the group that can use most rooms but within a larger group. The only one at the intersection of all the groups is Women and thus D is the answer.

21. C The question might seem like a probability calculation, but actually just requires careful reading. The probability of completing the assignment if the brain stem is dissected is not given, while the probability of finishing the assignment or even completing 85% is quite high if the cerebellar cortex is dissected. Thus the *best* reason for choosing the cerebellar cortex as the region of choice is option C.

22. D Several snippets of information are provided but many of the options have a gap in logic. The question does not talk about all Dalmatians, so concluding anything about the whole group would be wrong. The same applies for the statement on all dogs, because the question only refers to dogs that bark loudly. Thus options A and B can be eliminated. Option C could be a solution in a real life situation, however according to the question we only know about one Dalmatian and cannot generalise it to even a few others in the breed. Thus option D is the most accurate answer.

23. C From the question, on Saturday, airline F is the cheapest. On Thursday, airline F is not the cheapest but airline B is the cheapest. That should already allow us to conclude that option C is wrong. With option D, we know airline N has good service. The first statement in the question says that Airlines F, N and B provide cheap fares so option D is not wrong.

24. B The number of students who get to watch the play is 0.6 X 83 = 50. Since the probability of them not winning the voucher is 1-0.25 =0.75, the chance of both of these instances occurring is 0.75 X 50 = 37.5 (rounded up to 38)

25. D Methane is a subset of greenhouse gases. It shares all characteristics of greenhouse gases but not the other way around. Thus options A and B can be eliminated for generalising flammability and pollution to all greenhouse gases. Option C may be correct but the question does not state a link between flammability and pollution, thus the answer would be a reach. Since greenhouse gases are released in cow faeces, and methane is one of them, it has to be released in cow faeces too.

26. C Any answer that is a multiple of 4 will lead to her losing.
If she starts with 4 marbles, she is guaranteed a loss. If she takes 1, Tim will take 2, leaving the last for her. If she takes 2, then Tim will take 1, again leaving the last one.

For statement c, Jess takes one marble, leaving 12. This is a multiple of 4 so the opposite of what has been happening before will take place, allowing Jess to win.

27. D Armstrong's probability of doing all three actions was 0.14 = 0.7 X 0.4 X P(NASA communication)
Thus P(NASA communication) = 0.5
Thus Buzz Aldrin too has a 50% chance of communicating with NASA.

28. C Option A is wrong because of the false generalisation. While it is true as a fact, the focus of the question is the logic, where Aspirin is a subset of NSAIDs. The discussion of herbal medicines does not arise in the questions and is thus irrelevant to the answer.

29. A
If three columns are drawn like below:

Tuesday	Fish	Leia
Wednesday	Lentiles	James
Thursday	Noodles	Carrie

Leia and Mike can be ruled out as they do not make noodles. Option D can be ruled out because it exactly contradicts the sentence 4 "*On Monday, chicken was cooked but not by Carrie*". Lentils were not cooked on Thursday, so the only day left for them is Wednesday. This leaves only the option A.

END OF SECTION

Section C: Quantitative Reasoning

SET 1

1. **C** There are multiple ways to approach this question but the most important step is recognizing that Chris is cooking 10 portions when the recipe only provides 6. Therefore calculate the amount of squid per portion (450/6 = 75g per person) and multiply by 10 giving the correct answer of 750g. Alternatively the problem can be solved in one step using the ratio of desired portions to the actual number provided by the recipe (10/6 x 450).

2. **B** In this question it is easiest to total up the cooking time before subtracting from 8.30pm. Which is a total of (10 x 7) 70 minutes plus the required 10 minutes early. Subtracting 80 minutes from 8.30pm leaves Chris needing to start his preparations at 7.10pm or 19:10.

3. **C** There are a few ways of approaching this question; the quickest is probably noting that a single portion is a quarter of Chris' recommended daily intake and therefore he must first eat 4 whole portions to exceed it. Leaving the calorific content of the remaining 6 portions in excess (6 x 575 = 3450). Alternatively it is possible to calculate the total calorific content of the meal (10 x 575) and subtract Chris' recommend daily intake like so: 5750 – (4 x 575).

4. **D** In this situation it is first necessary to calculate the total cost of the meal, which for 10 portions is £18.00. Then divide this amongst the remaining 8 friends giving the correct answer of £2.25. Or, total up the cost of the uneaten portions (2x £1.80) and divide this by the 8 remaining friends (3.60/8=£0.45). Now add that to the normal cost (£1.80 + £0.45 = £2.25

5. **E** At this stage it is important to look back to the recipe and recall that it only serves 6. Therefore the recipe requires 12/6 = 2 prawns per person. Meaning for the now 11 people eating the email 22 prawns are required.

SET 2

6. **E** In this question there is lots of information to consider. To achieve the correct answer the full £3 surcharge (£2 for premiere and £1 for 3D) must be added to peak prices for each ticket. Hence the new prices are £14 for an adult and £10 for a child or concession. Adding up these cumulative charges (2 x 14) + (2 x 10) + 10 gives the correct total of £58.

7. **D** Although on a Tuesday all tickets are £5, the 3D surcharge must still be added making each individual ticket £6. Therefore 3 admissions out of the £50 leaves 50 – (3 x 6) = £32 change.

8. **D** As a standard non 3D film Joe pays the basic rate of £5 per ticket, therefore 4 x 5 = £20 in total. Next the interest must be considered at 30%. For Joe's transaction this is calculated as 0.3 x 20 = £6. As the question asks for the total cost to Joe this must be added onto his initial expenditure of £20 producing the correct answer of £26. A quicker method would be to simply calculate 20 x 1.3.

9. **B** First ascertain the price per child: 5.50 + 2 = £7.50. Next divide this into the total amount of money available giving 100/7.50 = 13.3333. As it is not possible to take a third of a child to the cinema this number must be rounded down to the correct answer of 13.

10. **D** Once again recall that all tickets are £5 on a Tuesday but the correct surcharges (of £3) must be applied. Therefore the total cost on a Tuesday would be (5 + 3) x 5 = £40. Alternatively the total cost at peak time can be calculated as 11 + 3 + [2 x (7 + 3)] + [2 x (5 + 3)] = £50. Hence this leaves the correct difference of £10.

SET 3

11. **B** First recognize that the 1 bedroom flat has 0kWh gas usage and the same electricity usage as the 2 bedroom flat. Therefore it is not necessary to calculate the household electricity rate just yet. Instead isolate the gas component of the 2 bedroom flat bill like so (700 – 300 = £400). The question asks for the answer as per kWh therefore 400/8,000 = £0.05 is the correct answer.

12. **C** First calculate the household electricity rate from the 1 bedroom flat (300/2000 = £0.15). Next use the given business gas rate of £0.03 per kWh in any of the business rows to isolate a business electricity component – probably easiest with the microbusiness like so: 635 – (4,500 x 0.03) = £500. Therefore per kWH the business electricity rate is 500/5,000 = £0.10. Finally remember to calculate the difference as asked in the question 0.15 – 0.10 = £0.05

13. **D** Recall the gas rates for both businesses (£0.03) and households (£0.05) are now known. Therefore Kate's expenditure on business gas is £270 (0.03 x 9,000) and on household gas is £900 (0.05 x 18,000). Giving a total gas expenditure of £1170 per year. Notice the question asks "every two years" so don't forget to double your answer to give £2340.

14. **A** First calculate Luke's share of medium business energy costs as 0.5 x 3360 = £1680. Add on the energy costs of his 1 bedroom flat giving a total annual cost of 1680 + 300 = £1980. Here however the question asks for a monthly expenditure so divide by 12 to give the final answer of 1980/12 = £165

15. **D** Recall that household and business electricity rates were £0.15 and £0.10 respectively. Business rates are 0.1/0.15 or two thirds the cost of household rates. With a difference in price of a third, business rates are approximately 33% cheaper. As 1m^2 of photovoltaic cells equates to a 1% saving, 33m^2 are required.

SET 4

16. **A** Note that both quantities are less than 99 and therefore taking pricing from the first category it is £9 for a rugby ball and £5 for a pack of 3 tennis balls. Therefore although 60 tennis balls are being purchased in total this equates to only 60/3 = 20 packs. As such the correct answer is given as (50 x 9) + (20 x 5) = £550. As this is collection in store there is no delivery charge to add on.

17. **C** As 8 footballs costs (8 x7) £56, that leaves a remaining £19.01 to cross the minimum spend figure for free delivery. As footballs can only be sold as a whole this must be rounded up to the nearest integer number of footballs – in this case to £21 and the correct answer of 3 footballs.

18. **B** Recall that the data set says "home delivery is free on orders *exceeding* £75" and that therefore with a budget of £75 exactly the delivery charge must be paid. For a home 36 miles away this is £20 leaving a remaining £55 for tennis balls. Assuming this cannot purchase more than 99 items use the price of £5 per pack allowing for a total of 55/5 = 11 packs to be purchased. Recall that these are packs of 3 tennis balls and therefore the correct answer is 11 x 3 = 33 tennis balls.

19. **B** Notice here that when the quantities of items are halved the individual pricing of items changes and therefore one unfortunately cannot simply calculate the total price and halve it. Instead each order must be calculated separately and the difference taken as so: [(1000 x 4) + (500 x 7)] – [(500 x 5) + (250 x 8)] = £3,000

20. **C** First calculate the actual number of tennis ball packs being purchased (6,000/3 = 2,000). From the graph we know this equates to a price of £2 per item before the inflation. The new unit price can be calculated as 2 x 1.2 = £2.40. Therefore 2,000 tennis ball packs cost £4,800. At this point do not forget to add the cost of delivery which is also subject to the 20% price increase (20 x 1.2 = £24) Giving a total cost of 4,800 + 24 = £4,824.

SET 5

21. **A** The quickest way to solve this problem is to recognise that the plan illustrated effectively consists of 3 squares (with one broken into two right angle triangles). Secondly note the use of different units in the question and answer so straight away convert 200m to 0.2k to avoid a more difficult conversion later. Calculate the length of a square's side as 0.2/2 = 0.1km. Then calculate the total field area as 0.1 x 0.1 x 3 = 0.03km^2.

22. **C** For this question it is quickest to calculate the area of field A in metres as follows 100 x 100 = 10,000 m^2. As each cow requires 2m^2 the correct answer is given by 10,000/2 = 5,000 cows.

23. **B** First ascertain the total number of cows within the fields. As described previously this can be achieved using the idea that the total area is three times that of field A or D. Therefore there are 3 x 5,000 cattle present. First consider water expenditure per day as 3.5 x 15,000 x 0.02 = £1050. Next it is simplest to convert the pellet food price given into a per kg form like so 10/20 = £0.50. Daily food expenditure is therefore given by 4 x 15,000 x 0.5 = £30,000. Leaving a total of 30,000 + 1050 = £31,050 per day.

24. **D** First calculate the total volume of milk produced upon milking as 200 x 1.5 = 300L. As a cow can be milked only once every two days, if milking were to begin on Monday, milking could then only occur on Wednesday, Friday and Sunday. Thus there is the opportunity for 4 milking periods giving a total of 4 x 300 = 1,200L.

25. **C** Note the new daily cost of feed at £2.93 per cow. However don't forget that each cow also required 3.5L of water (3.5 x 0.02 = £0.07 per day). Therefore on the new feed (with water) the new daily cost of keeping a cow is £3. On a £1,000 daily budget this leaves the farmer able to house 1,000/3 = 333.33 cattle. As it is impossible to keep a third of a cow this must be rounded down to the nearest integer of 333.

SET 6

26. **A** In this question the first important thing to notice is that although the track time has been given in minutes; all other units use hours. Therefore begin by converting the lap time into an hourly figure like so: 3/60 = 0.05 hours. Next recall that distance = (average) speed x time. Therefore the correct length of the race track is given by 150 x 0.05 = 7.5 miles.

27. **D** As we are given the cost of fuel in terms of pence per litre, first convert car C's fuel consumption into a value in terms of miles per litre. Given that one gallon = 4.5 litres, a fuel consumption of 36mpg is therefore the equivalent of 36/4.5 = 8mpL. As the distance required is 10 miles, car C therefore requires 10/8 or 1.25 L of fuel which costs a total of 1.25 x 102 = 127.5 pence.

28. **C** The use of the term "average track speed" is a red herring in this question; it is actually not necessary to use car D's average car speed in any calculation. Instead the question is telling us that we can assume car D's fuel consumption will remain constant at 13.5mpg as it is driving at its average track speed. As the fuel tank capacity is given in litres first convert fuel consumption to miles per litre like so: 13.5/4.5 = 3 miles per litre. With a total fuel tank capacity of 40 litres, on a full tank car D can travel a total of 3 x 40 = 120 miles

29. **D** Assuming both cars at travelling in the same direction as it is a race track, car B has a speed of 180 – 150 = 30mph relative to car A. That is car B is gaining on car A at a speed of 30mph. As car B must first travel the 1.8 miles, and time = distance/speed, it will take car B 1.8/30 = 0.06 hours to overtake car A. As speed is given with units miles per hour, the correct answer has units of hours.

30. **B** As fuel tank capacity is given in litres, first convert the fuel consumption into units of miles per litre like so: 54/4.5 = 12 miles per litre. Therefore on a full tank car A can drive a total distance of 60 x 12 = 720 miles. On a track 8 miles long this equates to 720/8 = 90 laps

SET 7

31. **B** From the graph 4 bedroom house prices have risen by £40,000 pounds between 2010 and 2015 (240,000 – 200,000 = £40,000). As the question asks for the percentage RISE, we need to calculate what percentage this difference is out of the original house price in 2010. Which is (40,000/200,000) x 100 = 20%.

32. **C** First note the difference in price between 2 and 4 bedroom houses in 2014: 225,000 – 115,000 = £110,000. As they are able to save a total of £50,000 in the first 10 years this leaves them with a remaining £60,000 to save. By saving £10,000 a year this should take them 6 years. Leaving a total of 10 + 6 = 16 years to reach their minimum savings to upgrade. Don't forget to subtract these 16 years from 2014 giving the correct answer of 1998.

33. **D** After the price increase a 4 bedroom house in 2010 now costs 125% of the 2009 price. Therefore 1% is the equivalent of 200,000/125 = £1,600 and the price of a 2009 4 bedroom house can be calculated as 100 x 1,600 = £160,000. A quicker method is to spot that the 2010 house is 125% (1.25x) the price of the 2009 house so 200000/1.25=160000.

34. **E** The quickest method here is to first calculate the difference in 2 bedroom house prices in 2012, 3 bedroom house prices in 2013 and 4 bedroom house prices in 2014 compared to 2010 prices. Then calculate the sum like so: (105,000 – 95,000) + (135,000 – 125,000) + (225,000 – 200,000) = £45,000

35. **E** First calculate the maximum price that a 2010, 3 bedroom house could be let for each year: 125,000 x 20% = £25,000. Now consider the profit that would be received from selling the house in 2014 as 145,000 – 125,000 = £20,000. However when letting the house, the initial cost of the house must be first paid off before an investor would start making any profit. Therefore the total amount of money that must be earned to equate to a profit of £20,000 when letting is in fact 125,000 + 20,000 = £145,000. When receiving £25,000 a year this would therefore take 145,000/25,000 = 5.8 years.

36. **C**
(2 x 120) + (3 x 150) + (3 x 240) = 1,410
240/1,410 = 0.17 = 17%

END OF SECTION

Section D: Abstract Reasoning

Rules

Set 1: In set A number of white edges = 2(black edges); in set B number of white edges = 3(black edges). → quite a hard rule compared the standard ones you see in the test?

Set 2: In set A black edges > white edges; in set B white edges > black edges. There is always a grey arrow – its orientation/size is not relevant.

Set 3: In set A the angle is acute when total number of sides is even, whereas the angle is obtuse when the total number of sides is odd. In set B the converse is true – in both sets the colours are irrelevant.

Set 4: In set A the number of grey edges = the sum of black and white edges; in set B grey edges = the difference between black and white edges.

Set 5: In set A the number of edges within the largest shape is less than the number of edges of the largest shape; in set B the converse is true. Colours are irrelevant.

Set 6:

26. With each progressive frame the central star rotates 90º clockwise whereas the outer arrows individually rotate 90º anticlockwise.
27. Black shapes decrease by one side whereas white shapes increase by one side. Each progressive frame rotates 90º clockwise as well.
28. The number of black shapes increases by 2 each time. The number of white shapes is half the number of black shapes.
29. Shapes transform until they contain a right angle. Once a right angle shape is reached the shape alternates between white and black.
30. Each frame is rotated 45º clockwise and then flipped 180º along an alternating horizontal/vertical axis.

Set 7:

31. The number of grey sides is equal to the product of the number of black and white shapes.
32. If an arrow points to a shape it turns black. If an arrow points away from a shape, the shape transforms and the arrow itself becomes black.
33. The number of white shapes added is equal to half the number of black sides.
34. Shapes with an odd number of sides move inside those with an even number of sides and change colour. Size, orientation, and position within the second frame is not relevant.
35. Black shapes change colour to white. White shapes disappear. The size and position of the remaining shapes is not relevant, but their orientation is.

Set 8: Set A has more black shapes than white shapes. In set B the converse is true.

Set 9: All the frames are divided in half. In set A in any half there must be an even number of white shapes and an odd number of black shapes. In set B the converse is true with an odd number of white shapes.

Set 10: In set A there are less black and white shapes than there are grey sides; in set B there are more black and white shapes than there are grey sides. The ratio of black to white shapes does not matter.

Set 11: In set A when there is one grey shape there are more black than white shapes; when there are two grey shapes there are more white than black shapes. In set B the rule is reversed with more white than black shapes in the presence of one grey shape.

END OF SECTION

Section E: Situational Judgement Test

Scenario 1

1. **Very inappropriate** – although the patient has asked her not to say anything, it is something that is a cause for concern and would be better discussed with the GP, who may be able to persuade the patient to go to the police and therefore resolve the issue.
2. **Very inappropriate** – this breaches confidentiality and in this case, although domestic abuse is apparent, it is not in the student's remit to escalate this to the police without the patient's consent. Only the patient can escalate the issue (unless children are involved, then confidentiality can be broken).
3. **Appropriate but not ideal** – this reassures the patient that anything she says won't leave the practice walls, but also makes her aware of the fact that the GP may come to know of her situation and thus she is less likely to be surprised if the GP calls her in and talks to her about abuse. It is not ideal, however, as Maya has a duty to report all reports of abuse to her senior.
4. **Very appropriate** – the GP is likely to know of the protocols available in this kind of situation and how to go about discussing this issue with the patient. They will be able to take matters further if required.
5. **Very inappropriate** – this is a breach of confidentiality and it does not help the patient in any way. Maya's parents are unlikely to be able to help or provide any advice on this matter as they are not involved in the patient's care.

Scenario 2

6. **Very inappropriate** – there are still things he can do and people he can see and as it is a timetabled day, he should attend his activities, regardless of who is and isn't there.
7. **Very appropriate** – other members of staff on the ward are equally as helpful to observe or to tell him what to do and see. There are many things you can learn on a ward if you search hard enough.
8. **Appropriate but not ideal** – although Abdul is still doing something in his timetabled slot, there is a reason the university has given him that particular placement and so it would be better if he found something to do in the paediatric ward.
9. **Inappropriate but not awful** – The supervisor, while good to email, is not likely to be able to do anything as they may not be able to arrange an alternative option for placement with such short notice.
10. **Appropriate but not ideal** – This is a good idea, as Abdul can practice his communication skills, but it is often best to ask the doctors or nurses on the ward which patients would be the best to go and see as they are more likely to know which patients will be happy to have histories taken from them.

Scenario 3

11. **Inappropriate but not awful** – This is not the best way to deal with the situation. It is embarrassing for the students and doesn't address the problem of the upset relative. However, their supervisor has been alerted of their behaviour and this will allow them to deal with the students.
12. **Inappropriate but not awful**– This doesn't immediately stop the students talking about the patient, and they may say more in Mike's absence which may upset the relative even more, but their supervisor will be informed and thus further action can be taken.
13. **Very appropriate** – This reprimands the students and also makes sure that they apologise to the family member.
14. **Very inappropriate** – it is not Mike's responsibility to apologise for the students and does not stop the students from doing it again.
15. **Very inappropriate** – it doesn't address the situation and the students may continue with this behaviour.

Scenario 4

16. **Inappropriate but not awful** – although Alisha is has alerted someone else of the man, there is no guarantee that they will help and it is unlikely that they will be able to help in this situation better than Alisha can with the clinical skills she may have learnt. She will be able to administer CPR if needed and give the correct information to the paramedics when they arrive.
17. **Very inappropriate** – Alisha is likely to be trained in CPR and thus, is likely to be able to help until the ambulance arrives. It is also unmoral to leave an injured person in the middle of the road without stopping to help.
18. **Very appropriate** – Although Alisha may know CPR, it always helps to have a trained paramedic on the line who can guide her through the first aid, until the ambulance arrives, and by calling her date, she can explain the situation, and hopefully they will understand.
19. **Appropriate but not ideal** – although the ambulance is on the way, Alisha still has to wait for the paramedics so they find the right area and so that she can tell them what she knows.
20. **Very inappropriate** – the friend does not know where the patient is, and what has happened. The paramedics also need someone to guide them to the right place and may be able to tell Alisha what to do until they arrive.

Scenario 5

21. **Very inappropriate** – George is not competent enough to do the procedure and he may put the patient at harm.
22. **Very appropriate** – He has explained why he cannot do the procedure and has also not put the patient at risk.
23. **Very inappropriate** – it is likely the FY1 doctor is busy and it is unprofessional to both push a job onto someone else and leave without letting the nurse know.
24. **Very inappropriate** – this is not very professional as the nurse will return with the equipment and have to spend time finding someone else to do the procedure. She may be very busy, which is why she asked someone else to take the bloods in the first place.
25. **Very appropriate** – this means the nurse can get back to other jobs that she may have, and it means that the patient will have his bloods taken.

Scenario 6

26. **Very inappropriate** – although the patient does not know English, it is not very professional to make such a joke in a busy ward, where others can hear them. It reflects badly on the hospital and the rest of the staff working there.
27. **Very appropriate** – a senior has been alerted of this behaviour and it will be dealt with appropriately.
28. **Inappropriate but not awful** – It is best to lodge a complaint immediately, as action needs to be taken.
29. **Very inappropriate** – this joke should not be spread around, and a canteen is a very public place which means more people can hear it. This would damage the reputation of not only herself, but the entire organisation.
30. **Very appropriate** – This deals with the situation immediately, the FY2 will most likely apologise, and a senior can take this further if required.

Scenario 7

31. **Very inappropriate** – this could be harmful or even fatal to the patient if they have an allergic reaction to the drugs.
32. **Very inappropriate** – as a student, he should not be writing in or changing drug records unless told to do so and the patient has been prescribed the medication for a reason, so it is important a doctor knows so they can prescribe an alternative.
33. **Very appropriate** – an alternative can be proscribed for the patient.
34. **Inappropriate but not awful** – although the drug chart will be changed eventually, it may be signed off and the medication given to the patient in the space between they make that change, which could result in harm to the patient.
35. **Very inappropriate** – the drug chart will contain other medications that the patient needs so removing it may mean that they don't get the rest of the medication.
36. **Inappropriate but not awful** – patients should be aware of their medical treatment, however there is no guarantee the patient is fit to remember to inform the doctors. It is much better to alert the medical team directly as this poses a significant danger to the patient.

Scenario 8

37. **Of minor importance** – although the deadline is important, patient confidentiality and professionalism is more important.
38. **Of minor importance** – whilst this is obviously likely to be on Meena's mind, she should challenge Tom's inappropriate behaviour regardless of any potential repercussions for herself or Tom.
39. **Fairly important** – if their supervisor finds out, it could bring their marks down which could impact them on the final grade.
40. **Extremely important** – if Tom loses his phone, or shares the pictures, then patient confidentiality is broken. Patient information should be stored in a secure place and only be sent through encrypted pathways. It is unprofessional to take patient information out of the hospital without permission.
41. **Of no importance** – Tom does not have permission to take pictures of the notes.

Scenario 9

42. **Extremely important** – the hospital has a reputation to uphold and this post reflects badly on its values. It is a public post that anyone can access.
43. **Extremely important** – as stated above this is a public post and it can be linked back to Maria which can impact on her future.
44. **Of minor importance** – she has been linked to the post and therefore people can easily find out who she is.
45. **Of no importance whatsoever** – Maria has a responsibility in terms of her reputation and the hospital's reputation.
46. **Of no importance whatsoever** – the post will be available indefinitely so regardless of where she is placed, it will always affect her.

Scenario 10

47. **Fairly important** – this means that Muhammed will be able to go next year.
48. **Extremely important** – This is an avoidable situation, as there are many other opportunities to go to this conference.
49. **Fairly important** – supervisors are often busy and it is best not to rearrange too often, unless there is no other option.
50. **Of minor importance** – there are other ways to get work experience in those laboratories e.g. emailing the researcher.
51. **Fairly important** – Muhammed may not be able to get to the conference easily, if it is out of London

Scenario 11

52. **Of minor importance** – the patient can continue and resume her story.
53. **Fairly important** – if Melissa asks politely enough, the patient should be able to understand that it would take two minutes to return the sheet to the front desk.
54. **Extremely important** – patient confidentiality is very important
55. **Extremely important** – the person may not be a staff member and that would compromise patient confidentiality.
56. **Extremely important** – the nurse may need it to give medicines to the patient and thus without it, it will cause a delay.
57. **Of no importance** – The reason for the patient's admission to hospital doesn't affect the importance of listening to their story over the dropped documents.

Scenario 12

58. **Extremely important** – As they are clinical partners, it is important on good terms so they work well together, but if they are good friends then Tariq should not take offence.
59. **Fairly important** – Tariq may take offence at Jeremy's comments but he should realise that this is not a personal attack.
60. **Extremely important** – if they are to have so much contact with patients, they must look professional.
61. **Extremely important** – If Tariq is to make a good impression then he must remain professional.
62. **Extremely important** – professionalism is very important in medicine and must be maintained at all times.

Scenario 13

63. **Extremely important** – the patient must be treated immediately, or they could die.
64. **Of minor importance** – it is an inconvenience, but patient safety is extremely important.
65. **Extremely important** – if the patient contracts an infection, this could be more fatal than the initial reason for the surgery. It will also mean that the patient has to stay in hospital for longer which could have been avoided.
66. **Fairly important** – it is not fair to make others wait, but safety of the patient currently on the operating table is paramount.
67. **Of no importance** – as a student he is still part of the team and has a duty of safety to the patient.
68. **Of no importance** – everyone and everything in the room must be sterile, as even the smallest chance of infection could have big consequences for the patient.
69. **Of no importance** – she may touch the surgical equipment, or other utensils that come into contact with the patient.

END OF PAPER

Mock Paper D Answers

Section A: Verbal Reasoning

Passage 1

1. **B** The passage states that children have temporary teeth which appear in the 6th or 7th months. That means their teeth begin to appear before the age of one hence B is the correct answer.
2. **C** The second paragraph states that no teeth that come after the sixth year are ever shed. This means that all teeth that come after that age are permanent hence C is correct.
3. **A** The final sentence of the first paragraph states that temporary teeth require the same care that is exercised towards permanent teeth. Thus, statement A is correct.
4. **C** Statement A is correct as the third paragraph states that wisdom teeth appear in between 18 and 24 years of ages. Statement B is correct due to the answer for question 2. Statement D is correct as it states in the third paragraph that parents mistakenly suppose molars are temporary teeth. Hence C is the answer.

Passage 2

5. **D** The second paragraph states that magnetism may be cultivated and is inherent in every human being hence statement D is correct.
6. **A** The second sentence in the third paragraph states that self-preservation is the first law of nature hence statement A is correct.
7. **A** In the second paragraph when describing a person being hypnotized the first step mentioned is that the patient experiences a soothing influence which relaxes their muscles. Hence, statement A is correct.
8. **A** In the second paragraph it states that a pleasant, drowsy feeling is followed by a refreshing sleep. Hence A is the correct statement.

Passage 3

9. **B** The author states that coffee if rightly used is the most valuable addition to the morning meal. Hence statement B is correct.
10. **B** Tea and its active constituent theine is stated to be a pain destroyer, nerve stimulant and can produce hysterical symptoms. Thus by elimination B is the correct answer.
11. **B** It is stated in the text that when coffee is taken strongly in the morning is often produces dizziness and muscae volilantes hence statement B is correct
12. **A** The passage states that excess caffeine can cause a peculiar vision symptom whose name when translated is read as dancing flies, this is distinctly different from actual flies dancing making statement A incorrect and thus the answer.

Passage 4

13. **A** The first sentence states that pianos should avoid being exposed to atmospheric changes. Thus pianos must be exposed to similar atmospheres in winter and summer thus making the statement true.
14. **C** The passage states that the absence of frost in zero degrees weather is positive proof of a dry atmosphere. From this the converse can be humidity causes frost in cold temperatures hence C is correct.
15. **C** The passage states that an entirely dry atmosphere can cause physical effects which consequently puts the piano seriously out of tune. Hence C must be correct.
16. **D** The passage states that loosening of the glue joints produces clicks and rattles. Hence the converse is that's stiffening of these joints will make the clicks and rattles subside hence D is correct.

Passage 5

17. **D** The passage states that theosophy excludes all reasoning processes as they are considered imperfect. Therefore statement D is correct.
18. **B** In the passage it states that of the sects which practiced theosophy, one is the Hesychasts off the Greek Church. The Greek church is distinct to the Roman church hence statement B is correct.
19. **D** The passage states that the leader of the Theosophists had become fascinated with the doctrine of Buddhism. Hence statement D is correct.
20. **B** The passage states that the object of theosophical study is to understand the nature of divine things. This is synonymous with statement B.

Passage 6

21. **A** The first sentence of the last paragraph states that the dream must occur during healthy and tranquil sleep for it to have any significance. Hence the answer is true.
22. **A** The 3rd paragraph recites a passage about dreams written in the Holy Scripture. From this we can deduce that the answer is true.
23. **A** In the third paragraph it is written that Hippocrates said the body is asleep hence statement A is the answer.
24. **C** The passage says that modes of worship have been founded upon the interpretations of dreams which means statement C is correct.

Passage 7

25. **C** The passage states that deep sunken eyes are selfish. Selfishness is the opposite of selflessness, therefore a lack of selflessness is synonymous with selfish hence C is correct.
26. **C** The passage states that the normal distance between the eyes is the width of one eye and a distance greater than this intensifies the character of the person. Since the person could have any number of characteristics. Due to the ambiguity we cannot tell if erraticism is the characteristic that would be intensified.
27. **C** The passage states that eyes that are far apart and open indicate frankness. Frankness is synonymous to honesty therefore C is the correct answer.
28. **D** The passage states that long, almond-shaped eyes are indicative of genius, thus the answer is D

Passage 8

29. **C** The second paragraph says that probably the most important appliance for gym work is the wooden dumbbell. Due to the use of the word probably, we cannot be sure this is a fact. Hence the answer is C.
30. **C** The passage states that increasing circulation is done by exercising the extremities, the arms, the head and the feet. The abdomen is not mentioned hence C is the answer.
31. **D** The passages states that oxygen-hunger is only satisfied by breathing exercises hence statement D is correct.
32. **A** The passage states that strengthening the muscles of the back holds the body erect. This is synonymous with maintaining posture hence the answer is A.

Passage 9

33. **B** The passage states that a sponge in its natural state is different from what we see in commerce. Therefore the statement is false.
34. **C** The passage states that types of sponges are found in the Mediterranean Sea and are numerous in variety. Thus, the answer is C.
35. **A** The passage states that definite channels are constantly maintained and are essential to life of the sponge. A is therefore the correct answer.
36. **B** The passage states that the composition of the skeleton varies in different kinds of sponges. Hence B is the answer.

Passage 10

37. **C** Nowhere in the text is osteopathy defined as the study of bones, but also nowhere in the text is it said that osteopathy could be something else as a result of which it cannot be the study of bones. Since there is no evidence, the answer is C.
38. **C** In the text it says that what Dr Still asserted about osteopathy is not now maintained to any great extent by his followers. Hence C is the answer.
39. **D** The passage states that the constriction of an artery may be caused by a very slightly displaced bone. Thus the answer is D.
40. **B** The passage states that osteopathists do generally claim that all diseases arise from some maladjustment of the bones and ligaments that form the skeleton. This is synonymous with the answer B.

Passage 11

41. **A** The passage states that going over the body with a dry brush after bathing for two to three weeks will soften the skin. From this we can deduce that softening of the skin requires rubbing hence the answer is A.
42. **B** The passage states that the duty of pores is to carry waste matter off. Hence B is the right answer.
43. **D** The passage states that if you should quietly sit down in a tub of water and as quietly get up and dry off without rubbing, your skin wouldn't be much benefited. This supports answer D.
44. **D** The passage states that a little ammonia or any alternative should be used during bathing which makes the water soft.

END OF SECTION

Section B: Decision Making

1. **E** A is wrong because (18 x 10) + 8 =188. B is wrong because (18 x 2) + 8 = 44. C is wrong as 5 + 8 = 13. D is wrong because (8 x 2) + 5 = 21. This leaves answer E, which you can't reach using any combination of 5, 8 and 18.

2. **B** Statement A assumes all teenagers are immature. It also makes the argument that immaturity means that a person is unsafe at driving. Statement C does not provide an argument for why it is best for teenagers to start driving at 17. It simply provides a reason why most teenagers do not drive until they are 17. Statement D provides an argument as to why teenagers should drive at 17, however it is unknown what other factors are necessary to drive a car. Statement B provides a reason why it is illegal for teenagers to drive before the age of 17 and thus supports that 17 is the best age to start driving as this is when they are legally allowed to.

3. **C** Statement A is false as we know professor Moriarty can only lecture on physics. Statement B is false because identity is a philosophy topic and we know that professor Moriarty cannot lecture on philosophy. Statement D is a statement we can't say is true or false as no information has been given regarding this. Statement E is false as we know that professor Moriarty can only lecture on physics. Statement C is correct as we know all philosophy lectures are given by physics lecturers.

4. **B**
Table listing cars and their properties:

Colour of Car	Yellow	Red	Blue	Unknown
Seats	Fluffy pink cotton	Shiny black leather	Green cotton	
Tires	Orange	Silver	White	Gold

Table which indicates position of cars with regards to each other:

Red	Yellow	Blue
	Unknown	

By creating 2 tables and filling in information only when possible we can list all of the information and then can see clearly that the yellow car has orange tires.

We know that the yellow red and blue cars are adjacent and that the red car is not next to the blue car. From this we know that the yellow car is in the middle. We are told that a car opposite the yellow car has gold tires thus we know that this 4th car is not next to the red or blue cars. We know that a car next to the red car has orange tires, and since we know that the only car that can be next to the red car is the yellow car, we deduce that the yellow car has orange tires.

5. **A** It is never stated that Derek is intelligent so B is wrong. It is never stated that all funny people are intelligent. We can only infer that some funny people are intelligent as some engineers are funny and all engineers are intelligent. This makes C a wrong answer as well. It is never stated that Jamal is an engineer and it is never stated that all intelligent people are engineers hence D is wrong. A is proven correct as we know some engineers are funny. This makes E wrong as well, hence A is the answer.

6. **D** A is not correct as Prakash and Harry could still be faster than Ryan but set a time of above 12 seconds (e.g. both set a time of 12.1 seconds). B is not correct as Ryan's fastest time is 12.2 seconds which is above the qualifying time. C is incorrect as Prakash and Harvey may set a time of below 12 seconds, we do not know. D is correct as we know Ryan's fastest time is above the threshold time for qualification. Hence E is also incorrect and D is the right answer.

7. **C** If the coffee weighs 100g and it is 95% water and 5% coffee granules, then the water weighs 95g and the coffee weighs 5g. After drying the water content of the coffee is 75%. Assuming the weight of coffee granules has not changed, the 5g of coffee granules constitute 25% of the coffee. Therefore the total weight of coffee including the water is 20g. This added to the 10g weight of the cup make the total weight of the cup of coffee 30g. Hence C is the answer.

8. A

Table listing people and shops that they own.

	Julia	Polly	Fred	James	Harrison	Holly
Sweet shop	X	X	X			
Bakery			X	X		
Grocery store					X	
Pharmacy	X	X				
Sports shop						X
Shoe Shop		X		X	X	
Total	2	3	2	2	2	1

We can clearly see that Polly owns the most shops hence A is the answer.

9. **A** This question can be easily answered if written in inequalities and then the inequalities are combined.
Br<A.
Cl<M<A
A<Bi
Ch<Bi
From looking at these we know that Archith weighs more than Brian, Clarissa and Mike so these 3 can be discounted. We also know that Billy weighs more than Archith and Christy so those two can be discounted. Therefore, the answer is A – Billy.

10. **A** Sanjay thinks that a certain series of events (which we will call A) is more likely than a certain series of events which we will call B. Therefore, the probability for A is higher than B is what we are testing. The probability of A is 0.3 x 0.5 x 3 = 0.45. This is the probability of losing the match on a cold day (0.3) x probability of not eating ice cream (0.5) x the number of cold days (3). The probability of B is 0.1 x 0.5 x 4 = 0.2. This is the probability of losing the match on a hot day (0.1) x probability of eating ice cream (0.5) x number of hot days (4). Since 0.45>0.2, Sanjay is correct hence the answer is A.

A (much) quicker way to answer this is to look at the answer options before doing any maths. Without doing any calculations; answer a is possible, answer b is wrong (as the chance of winning the match when it's cold is lower than winning when higher, not lower, c is incorrect as he doesn't eat ice cream most days (only on half the number of days) and d is incorrect as he doesn't have an almost certain chance of losing his match on a hot day. Therefore, without needed to do any probability calculations, we know the answer MUST be A.

11. **E** A is false as we know all athletes play sports but we do not know which sports. B is false as we only know that Drogba is an athlete. C is false as we don't know which sports athletes play. D is false as we only know that Drogba is an athlete. Therefore, the answer is E.

12. **D** A is false as all events are independent and we can never be certain of the outcome as either outcome is equally probable. The same reasoning means B is also wrong. There is no information given to support C. D is correct as we know homer is flipping regular 10 pence coins thus both outcomes are equally probable. Hence, E is wrong and D is the correct answer.

13. **B** The cyclists aren't apart at a constant distance; they get further apart as they cycle. David and Alex are less than 50m apart at the time Alaric finishes. Each cyclist beats the next cyclist by the same distance so they must have the same difference between speeds. When Alaric finishes at 500m, David is at 450m. When David crosses the finish line then Alex is at 450m. We need to know where Alex is when David is at 450m.

Alaric's speed = distance/time = 500/T. David's speed = 450/T. So David has 90% of Alaric's speed. This makes Alex's speed 90% of David's and 81% (90% x 90% = 81%) of Alaric's. So, when Alaric finishes, Alex is at 0.81 x 500 = 405m. 500 – 405 = 95. Therefore, Alaric beats Alex by 95m.

14. **C** A is false as we are not given any information about maths questions. B is false as we are not given any information about cheating. D is false as we are not given any information regarding how well Corrine is going to do in this exam. C must be correct as Corrine is assuming this exam will make her cry.

15. **C** The argument never states that only the local public should pay for the ceremony hence A is wrong. The fact that the MPs support Jed is completely irrelevant to the argument hence B is wrong. The fact that many politicians think the ceremony is outdated is irrelevant to the argument hence D is wrong. C directly challenges the fact that not all the public voted for Jed and thus not all of the public should have to pay for the ceremony. Hence C is the right answer.

16. **B** The only daughter of Isabella's grandmother is Isabella's mother. The person's sister's mother is the same as the person's mother. Therefore, the person's mother is the same as Isabella's mother. Therefore, the person depicted in the family tree must be Isabella's sister.

17. **C** We know that 5 children like all types of cake therefore B is wrong as the central overlapping segment is empty. We know that 2 like banana cake only so this also means that B is wrong. We know that only 1 child like all flavours except chocolate, therefore the region overlapping between carrot and banana must have 1 in it. This eliminates A and D as potential answers. C is the only diagram which satisfies all conditions hence C is the correct answer.

18. **C** If Harold says 1 number, then Fletcher can say "2 and 3". From this point onwards, Harold cannot win no matter what. If Harold says 4, then Fletcher will say 5,6,7 and Harold will only be able to say either 8, 8 and 9, or 8, 9 and 10. All of these result in Fletcher saying 11. If Harold says 4, 5 then Fletcher will say 6, 7 and the same outcome is achieved. If Harold says 4, 5, 6 then Fletcher will say 7 and once again the same outcome is achieved. Using this reasoning, the same can be said if Harold says 2 numbers as Fletcher will simply say 3 and thus win again. The only way for Harold to guarantee a win is to say 1, 2 and 3 when he starts. Whoever is able to say 3 is the person that can guarantee a win regardless of what the other person says. Hence C is the correct answer.

19. **C** Scenario 1: Imogen picks Lucy, Lucy picks Norden, Norden picks Imogen.
Scenario 2: Imogen picks Norden, Lucy picks Imogen and Norden picks Lucy.
All other scenarios result in the game restarting as Norden will have to pick himself. Since each person cannot pick themselves, they each have a 50:50 chance of dancing with either of the two-other people. Hence C is correct.

20. **E** Table depicting the position of each person:

Eric	**David**	
Andrew	Charlie	Barry

From this we can see that David is sat to the right of Eric. This is synonymous with Eric being sat to the left of David. Hence E is the correct answer.

21. **C** A is wrong as it simply states having more than 1 child is expensive, it does not state that this does not discourage people from having children. B is wrong as it talks about a certain group of the population which is not relevant to the argument. Statement D is wrong because it does not state why benefitting a certain group of people is bad. Statement C is correct as it disproves the assumption made I the argument that increasing cost discourages people from having children.

22. **C** If Peter is telling the truth, then Edwin is also telling the truth. If Edwin is telling the truth then either Max is also telling the truth, or Peter is also telling the truth. The only way that just 1 of them is telling the truth is if Max is telling the truth. If Max is being honest and both Peter and Edwin are lying, then they must have been to the swimming pool 0 times. Hence C is the answer.

23. **C** Statement A simply suggests that people living in cities are less fit than people living in rural areas. This does not necessarily mean that they are unhealthy or that living in a city is injurious to health. Statement B is incorrect since it doesn't necessarily mean that all people will buy unhealthy amounts of junk food if it is cheaper in cities. Statement D is incorrect as some vehicles may not produce as much pollution as others and we are not told if pollution is harmful. Statement E contradicts the conclusion; hence it is incorrect. High levels of carbon monoxide are dangerous to health and living in cities could be injurious if there are harmful amounts present. So, statement C is correct.

24. **E** There is a total of 17 shoes. In the worst-case scenario, Will picks 1 blue, 1 black, 3 orange and 3 red. That is 8 shoes in total. The next shoe he picks will be either black, orange or red and will complete his 3rd set. Therefore, Will has to pick at least 9 shoes to guarantee 3 matching pairs.

25. **A**

A.	Bob is better at basketball than Chris.		**True**
B.	Gerard is better at basketball than Bob.	**False**	
C.	Bob is the shortest.		**False**
D.	Chris is the tallest.		**False**
E.	Felix is the worst at basketball.	**False**	

The height of the 4 boys can be written as: G > F > B. Statements B and C are incorrect as no information is given on Chris' height in relation to the others.
According to the given information, the level of proficiency in basketball can be written as: F > G > C. Statement B is incorrect as we cannot infer if Bob fits in between Felix and Gerard or Gerard and Chris in the above statement. Statement E is incorrect as Chris is the worst at basketball and Felix is better than Gerard. The question states that Chris is the worst at basketball, hence, statement A must be correct.

26. **C** The probability of the mice colliding is equal to 1 minus the probability of the mice not colliding. The probability of the mice not colliding is if all the mice travel in the same direction. If each mouse can travel either clockwise or anticlockwise, the probability of the mouse travelling in 1 direction is 1/2. Since there are 4 mice, the probability of all the mice travelling in the same direction and not colliding is: 1/2 * 1/2 * 1/2 * 1/2 = 1/16. Since there are 2 directions that the mice can travel, the probability of them not colliding is: $2 * (1/2)^4 = 1/8$. The probability of the mice colliding is: 1 – 1/8 = 7/8. 7/8 > 1/8, therefore, the mice are more likely to collide than not.

27. **B** We only have information about whether lizards are poisonous, but we do not know any definitive facts about lizards and their offspring. Therefore, statements A, D and E are incorrect. The facts in the question clearly state that lizards are not mammals, therefore statement C is incorrect. We are told that some lizards are poisonous, therefore some are not poisonous. Hence, statement B is correct.

28. **D** Statement A is incorrect as we do are not told about all the goals scored in the match. We are only told about the goals Jacob scored. Statement B is also wrong based on this reasoning. Statement C is also wrong based on the reasoning. We are not told what goals Jacob saw during the match apart from the ones he scored so statement E is wrong. Statement D is correct as we are told every goal Jacob scored was from a free kick

29. **E** If 30 people liked all 3 sports and 80 people said they liked football, then 50 of these 80 people must like only football. If 10 people liked only rugby and cricket and 50 people said they liked rugby, then 10 of these 50 people must like only rugby (50 - (30 + 10) = 10). Out of the 40 people that said they liked cricket, 30 of these people said they liked all 3 sports and 10 liked rugby and cricket only. Therefore altogether, 50 people liked football, 10 people liked rugby and 40 people liked cricket, giving a total of 100.

END OF SECTION

Section C: Quantitative Reasoning

Data Set 1

1. **B** 98.4 miles per hour. Convert Jake's travel time into minutes: (2 x 60) + 8 = 128 minutes. Speed = distance/ time = 210/ 128 = 1.64 miles per minute. Convert this back into miles per hour: 1.64 x 60 = 98.4 miles per hour.
2. **C** 336 km. The conversion of kilometres to miles is given: 1.6 km = 1 mile. 210 x 1.6 = 336 km.
3. **E** 66%. To calculate this, convert both Jake and Martha's travel time into minutes. Jake: (2 x 60) + 8 = 128 minutes. Martha: (3 x 60) + 32 = 212 minutes. Martha's journey was 84 minutes longer than Jake's (212 - 128 = 84). Percentage change = difference/original so the percentage difference in travel time is calculated as follows: (84/ 212) x 100 = 66%, to the nearest whole number.

Data Set 2

4. **B** 16000m^2. Area = Length x Width. Area = 200m x 80m = 16000m^2

5. **D** 5min 36 sec. The distance Helen jogs is the perimeter of the field, which is calculated as follows: Perimeter = 2L x 2W. Perimeter = (2x200) + (2x80) = 560m. Time is distance/ speed, which will be how fast it takes Helen to jog the perimeter of the field. Time = (560/ 6000) x 60 = 5.6 mins. Remember to multiply .6 by 60 to give the answer in minutes. .6 x 60 = 36 so 5.6 mins = 5 min 36 sec.

6. **C** 161 rows. As the row intervals are given in cm, convert 80m into cm and divide by the given interval value: 8000/ 50 = 160. The question states that the first and last rows grow on the WX and YZ edges of the field. The trap to avoid is not to miss the final row; hence, there are 161 rows of cabbages on Sam's field.

Data Set 3

7. **C** 29300. Number of people older than 65 years = 7500 + 6450 + 6000+ 5700 + 3650 = 29300.
8. **A** 18.76%. If 65 years is the retiring age, then a person must be 51 years or above to be within 14 years of this age. The population of town X that is between 51-65 years = 8400 + 7850 + 8350 = 24600. Total population = 6900 + 6750 + 8200 + 7150 + 6350 + 6400 + 8750 + 7750 + 9950 + 9050 + 24600 + 29300 = 131150. 24600/131150 = 18.76% so A
9. **E** 80000. The working population consists of those aged 16-65, inclusive. 7150 + 6350 + 6400 + 8750 + 7750 + 9950 + 9050 + 8400 + 7850 + 8350 = 80000. A quicker way to do this is to subtract those not working age from the total population worked out previously i.e. 131150 – (6900 + 6750 + 8200 + 29300) = 80,000
10. **C** Approximate population under 30 years: 6900 + 6750 + 8200 + 7150 + 6350 + 6400 = 41750. Total population = 131150 so 41750/131150 = 0.318 so ~1/3 so C

Data Set 4

11. **D** 11:4. From the pie chart, it can be derived that the ratio of popularity between badminton and basketball is 22:8. This is 11:4 in its simplest form.
12. **A** 6/19. The difference between the popularity of tennis and football is 6%. Therefore, as a fraction, football is less popular than tennis by 6/19.
13. **E** 295. The racquet sports at this leisure centre consist of tennis, badminton and squash. If 570 people play a sport at the leisure centre a week, 108 play tennis (570 x 0.19), 125 play badminton (570 x 0.22) and 62 play squash (570 x 0.11), all calculated rounding down to a whole number. Therefore, the total number of people that play a racquet sport each week is 295.

Data Set 5

14. **E** 23000. From the graph, it can be read that the hot chocolate sales were £5000 in August and £28000 in December. The difference in the hot chocolate sales between these months is calculates as: 28000 – 5000 = 23000. Hence, the sales increase by £23000 from August to December.
15. **B** £17045. The sales of hot chocolate in October is £15000. £15000 represents 88% of company D's expected sales in October. The sum: 15000/ 88 gives the value of 1% of the expected sales. This can be multiplied by 100 to give the total expected sales in October: (15000/ 88) x 100 = £17045, to the nearest whole number. A quicker way to do this is to divide 15000 by 0.88.
16. **B** 10800. Company D made £27000 from the sales of hot chocolate during the month of January. The number of hot chocolates they made during this month is calculates as: 27000/2.50 = 10800.

Data Set 6

17. **A** 3/20. In focus group B, a total of 85% (55% + 30%) made some pronouncement, so 15% did not have a preference. This expressed as a fraction is: 15/100 = 3/20.
18. **D** 60. The number of people who preferred mango juice 2 in focus group A was 27 (108 x 0.25) and 33 in focus group B (110 x 0.30). Therefore, the total number of people who preferred mango juice 2 was: 27 + 33 = 60.

Data Set 7

19. **B** 67.7%. Average percentage obtained by the students = The sum of the students' percentages scored / the number of students. Average = (64 + 75 + 48 + 79 + 33 + 71 + 87 + 50 + 76 + 57 + 82 + 93 + 67 + 45 + 88)/ 15 = 67.7%.

20. **E** 88%. There are 15 students in the class. 15% of this is 2.25. This means that only the 2 students with the top scores will be able to obtain the maximum grade. From the bar chart, the 2 highest scores are 93% and 88%. Therefore, the minimum threshold mark value for this exam would be 88%.

21. **C** 4 students. The 2 lowest scores are 33 and 45, which combined = 78. If all the marks go up by 2% then 78 x 1.02 = 79.56.. If everyone else's marks went up by 2%, only 5 students would have marks greater than 79.56. Their marks would be (rounding to the nearest integer) 81, 89, 84, 95 and 90.

Data Set 8

22. **D** 15/17. Company R's April and September share prices are 85p and 75p, respectively. The calculation is as follows: 75/ 85 = 15/ 17.

23. **C** 96.05 p. Company R's share price in December 2007 was 85p. The new price in January 2008 would be: 85 x 1.13 = 96.05p.

Data Set 9

24. **B** B. BMI = Weight in kg / (Height in m)^2. The calculated BMI for each person is as follows: A: 24.9/B: 20.4/C: 27.6/D: 21.0/E: 22.3 (however, you could have a reasonable educated guess by just eyeballing the data if you're low on time).

25. **C** 3kg. BMI = kg / m^2 so m^2 = kg/ BMI. m^2 = 45/ 17.6= 2.56. To have a BMI just within the normal range, a value of 18.5 is needed. BMI = kg / m^2 so kg = BMI x m^2. kg = 18.5 x 2.56 = 47.36 kg. Person F needs to gain just under 2.5kg.

26. **B** 1/10. BMI = kg / m^2 so kg = BMI x m^2. Person G's original weight is: 28 x 1.7^2 = 80.92 kg. The weight at a BMI of 24.9 is 71.96 kg. 80.92 – 71.96 = 8.96 kg needs to be lost. 8.96/ 80.92 is approximately 1/10.

Data Set 10

27. **A** 3x + 4y = 20.95 ; 4x +5y = 27.10. In these simultaneous equations, x represents portions of chicken and y represents portions of chips, which equates to the price of the combined portions in £.

28. **E** £6.65. Multiply the first equation by 4 and the second equation by 3 to give 12x (12 portions of chicken) in both equations. Then subtract the two equations to eliminate x (chicken) and leave y (chips).
4(3x + 4y = 20.95) ; 3(4x +5y = 27.10) = 12x + 16y = 83.80 ; 12x + 15y = 81.30
y = 2.50. Use the calculated value of y and plug it into one of the equations to give the value of x (chicken): 3x + 4y = 20.95, 3x + 4(2.50) = 20.95. x = 3.65.
A 10% increase in the price of chicken would be 3.65 x 1.1 = £4.02, and a 5% increase in the price of chips would be 2.50 x 1.05 = £2.63. Therefore the cost of a chicken and chips would be 4.02 + 2.63 = 6.65

29. **D** $27.52. At the original prices, a portion of chicken is £3.65, and a portion of chips is £2.50. The total cost of the order in £ is: 2(3.65) + 5(2.50) = £19.80. This converted into $ is: 19.80 x 1.39 = $27.52.

Data Set 11

30. **C** 180.4. The conversion factor for kg to lb is: 1kg = 2.2 lb. Thus, Kyran'a weight in lb is: 82 x 2.2 = 180.4 lb.

31. **C** 12 stone 4 lb. Alex weighs 78kg and the conversion factors are: 1kg = 2.2 lb, 1stone = 14 lb. Alex's weight in stones and lb is calculated as: 78 x 2.2 = 171.6 lb, 171.6/ 14 = 12.26 stone. 0.26 stone is approximately 4 lb (rounded up).

32. **B** 417.9kg. To calculate this, the weight of Jay and Thomas needs to be converted firstly into lb and then to kg. Jay: (13 x 14) + 7 = 189 lb, 189/ 2.2 = 85.9 kg. Thomas: (11 x 14) + 11 = 165 lb. 165/ 2.2 = 75 kg.
The sum of the boys' weights can now be calculated: 78 + 85.9 + 75 + 82 + 97 = 417.9 kg.

33. **A** 1/5. Alex weighs 78kg and James weighs 97kg. 78/ 97 is approximately 4/5. Therefore, Alex is approximately 1/5 lighter than James.

Data Set 12

34. **C** 65%. The production of weed killer in 1998 and 1999 was 200,000 and 330,000, respectively. The increase in the production of weed killer from 1998 to 1999 was: 330,000 – 200,000 = 130,000. Hence, the percentage increase is calculated as: (130,000/ 200,000) x 100 = 65%. (Hint: using the data from the table in 10,000s simplifies the calculations by making the numbers simpler to use).

35. **D** 4 years. The average production of weed killer in 10,000 litres between the years 1998- 2005 is: (20 + 33 + 40 + 36 + 35 + 44 + 48 + 51)/ 8 = 38.4. The years in which the production of weed killer was higher than the average calculated were: 2000, 2003, 2004, and 2005. Therefore, the answer is 4 years. (Hint: if short of time, you can take a fairly good guess by looking at the graph that the data is fairly evenly distributed around the mean so there's likely to be an even split between years above and years below the average so 4 would be a well-informed guess).

36. **D** The production of weed killer in 2005 and 2006 was 510,000 and 350,000, respectively. The difference in production between 2005 and 2006 is: 510,000 – 350,000 = 160,000. The decrease in production as a decimal is therefore: 160,000/ 510,000 = 0.314.

END OF SECTION

Section D: Abstract Reasoning

Rules:

Set 1: Set A: Circle intersects 1 shape. Set B: Circle intersects 2 shapes.

Set 2: Set A: At least 1 black square. Set B: Circle intersects 2 shapes.

Set 3: Set A: Even number of shapes. Set B: Odd number of shapes.

Set 4: Set A: Total number of sides is 16. Set B: Total number of sides is 11.

Set 5: Set A: Only curved shapes. Set B: Only shapes with straight edges.

Set 6: Darkly shaded segment rotates anticlockwise by one position and the lightly shaded segment rotates clockwise by one position.

Set 7: Number of shapes increases by 1 and the new shape is always shaded black.

Set 8: Shapes inside small square and big square swap. Position of shapes in big square rotates clockwise by 1 position after swap. Position of shapes in small square changes to the opposite position after swap.

Set 9: Outermost shape switches with second outermost shape. Innermost shape switches with second innermost shape.

Set 10: Set A: There is always a 4-sided shape in the top right corner. Set B: There is always a 3 sided shape in the bottom right corner.

Set 11: Set A: The total number of sides on white shapes is double the total number of sides on black shapes. Set B: The total number of sides on white shapes is equal to the total number of sides on black shapes.

Set 12: Set A: All the shapes have at least one line of symmetry. Set B: There are no lines of symmetry in any of the shapes.

Set 13: Set A: There is always one shape with one or more 90° angles. Set B: There is always a downwards pointing arrow in one of the 4 corners.

Set 14: Set A: Total number of sides of all shapes is 12. Set B: The number of straight edged shapes always equals the number of curved edge shapes.

Set 15: Number of sides increases by 2.

Set 16: Upward pointing arrow is always in a corner and moves anticlockwise through the corners.

Set 17: Set A: There are always 2 rectangles present. Set B: There are always 3 triangles present.

END OF SECTION

Section E: Situational Judgement Test

Scenario 1

1. **Appropriate but not ideal.** This is with good intention and will likely improve his performance in the exams, but it does not guarantee that he will pass.
2. **Very Appropriate.** This will ensure Afolarin has plenty of time to prepare for exams, and he will only miss out playing lacrosse for a month which is a short period of time.
3. **Appropriate but not ideal.** This is good as it will free more time for him to study however just 1 extra evening of work a week may not be sufficient.
4. **Very appropriate.** This is arguably the best option as it may enable him to still have time to play lacrosse as much as he wants whilst still finding enough time to study so his end of year exams are not compromised.
5. **Inappropriate but not awful.** This is not appropriate as lacrosse is important to him and maintaining a good work life balance is key to success in all parts of his life in the long term. This would however still ensure success in the exams so it is not extremely inappropriate.

Scenario 2

6. **Inappropriate but not awful.** This is inappropriate as it means he misses out on the opportunity of the project and the development it will grant him in his experimental technique. It will not jeopardise his exams however.
7. **Inappropriate but not awful.** This is not good as it risks Jamal not doing well in his exams as he may not have enough time to prepare. Although he will be able to continue with the project, it is not worth jeopardising his exams.
8. **Appropriate but not ideal.** This is a sensible approach to ensure equal work is done for both the exam and his project and that both will be done to an equal standard. The issue here lies with the fact that although a certain amount of time on the project will mean it is done well, the same amount of time spent preparing for exams may not guarantee passing.
9. **Inappropriate but not awful.** This will not necessarily cause any harm to Jamal's preparation for his exam or project however, it is unlikely to help either as there is no guarantee his peers have come up with a good solution and what may work for his peers may not necessarily work for Jamal.
10. **Appropriate but not ideal.** This would provide a solution as it would mean Jamal has enough time to prepare for his exams as well as work on his project. This is not ideal however because if Jamal receives an extension then it is unfair on his peers. It also may make Jamal look unprofessional in the eyes of his peers.

Scenario 3

11. **Very inappropriate.** The fact he failed by only 4% is largely irrelevant as the time between Jacob taking his exams and taking his resits means he may not be as prepared as he was when he took the exams as he may have forgotten some information. Thus, allocating only 3 days to prepare the exam is very inappropriate as it makes failing a likely outcome and will prevent him continuing with his studies.
12. **Inappropriate but not awful.** This is not an awful choice as he will have enough time to revise for exams, but it means he will not get a holiday. A holiday could be beneficial so he can relax and have some time off before diving into preparation for his resits. He has also taken a loan out so no going on the trip will cause financial issues too.
13. **Appropriate but not ideal.** This is good for Jacob as it means he can prepare for his exams and not miss out on the trip as he will be able to go the next year. This is not ideal however as it means his friends will have to miss out on going this year.
14. **Inappropriate but not awful.** Although this means Jacob is able to go on the trip and do some revision whilst there, this is not a great plan. Getting a lot of revision done on the trip is unlikely and after he returns home he only has 3 days to prepare further.
15. **Very appropriate.** This ensures that Jacob gets a break and is able to attend the trip with his friends which he has been looking forward to for a long time. It also means he will return home with enough time to prepare for his exam.

Scenario 4

16. **Inappropriate but not awful.** This is not helpful as it gets Ronit into trouble with the professor and this is a matter that can easily be managed by Shloke himself. Escalation of the issue is unnecessary.
17. **Very inappropriate.** This is very bad as it is compromising Ronit's safety and by doing nothing Shloke is responsible for any harm that may befall Ronit.
18. **Inappropriate but not awful.** This provides no help in resolving Ronit's safety and although this may pressure Ronit to wear his glasses it also embarrasses him in front of his peers.
19. **Very appropriate.** This will inform Ronit why it is important to take the proper safety precautions and will encourage him to wear the glasses.
20. **Very inappropriate.** This will compromise Shloke's own safety in the process of resolving Ronit's therefore this is completely inappropriate.

Scenario 5

21. **Very inappropriate.** This is terrible as it is compromising care of the patient as well as being very unhelpful to the nurse.
22. **Inappropriate but not awful.** This will likely help the patient and the nurse however this goes directly against strict protocol which Juan has been told to follow. This is inappropriate as it may result in Juan having disciplinary proceeding against him if the medical faculty find out.
23. **Appropriate but not ideal.** This communicates to the nurse why Juan shouldn't actively participate in care of the patient however it does not in any way help the nurse's dilemma
24. **Very appropriate.** This is ideal as it explains to the nurse why Juan can't do as she says, but also provides an alternative solution to the nurse's problem.

25. **Very inappropriate.** This involves directly lying to the nurse and compromising patient care which is a serious offence.

Scenario 6

26. **Inappropriate but not awful.** This is of no aid to Nicolas if he is unwell and thus is irresponsible of Jessica.
27. **Very appropriate.** This directly allows Nicolas to communicate what is wrong as well as providing water for him which may be beneficial if he needs it.
28. **Appropriate but not ideal.** This is good for Nicolas as it ensures that if he isn't feeling well that he will get the attention and care he requires, however it is unknown whether Nicolas requires help from the demonstrator and may be attracting unwanted attention. Jessica should see if she can help Nicolas before asking others to assist.
29. **Inappropriate but not awful.** This may cause no harm to Nicolas however this doesn't help Jessica find out more about what is wrong with Nicolas and thus opening the window may be of no benefit.
30. **Very inappropriate.** This would attract attention to Nicolas as well as stop the teaching session for other participants. This is an overreaction and Jessica needs to first assess how Nicolas is feeling herself by speaking to him.

Scenario 7

31. **Extremely important.** This is directly tied to Alvin's motivation for conducting the interview thus is of utmost importance.
32. **Extremely important.** This is an essential factor in Alvin deciding whether he can conduct the interview and write the essay as both require time for preparation.
33. **Fairly important.** If Alvin is likely to have another opportunity like this then that may sway him to focus on his essay and conduct the interview at another point, however there is no guarantee whether he will get another opportunity. Hence, this is a fairly important factor in his decision
34. **Fairly important.** This influences his motivation to write the essay however Alvin's assessment of the importance of writing the essay is probably not as accurate as his professor's assessment. Also, even if the essay does not help him much in his end of year exams, not handing it in on time will displease his professor.
35. **Of minor importance.** This factor partially motivates Alvin to write his essay however the benefit it provides him in terms of his academic development is the main driving factor. Thus, this factor is not very important.

Scenario 8

36. **Of no importance whatsoever.** With regards to the breach in patient confidentiality, completion of the project before the deadline isn't important, especially since stopping this breach of patient confidentiality shouldn't impact on their ability to complete the project. The most important factor is the breach in confidentiality and ensuring this doesn't happen again.
37. **Extremely important.** This is the most important factor for Damion to consider as this is a serious issue and needs to be resolved urgently.
38. **Of no importance whatsoever.** The breach in confidentiality is far more important than the grade that Damion and Philippa receive. This should not factor into Damion's decision at all.
39. **Fairly important.** This is important for Damion to consider as this may cause Phillipa to undergo disciplinary proceedings. It also means that how the breach occurred may be misconstrued and Damion may also then also be blamed. This factor is important in Damion understanding how urgently this must be resolved.
40. **Of no importance whatsoever.** The assessment of how important the data revealed is completely subjective and is not relevant to Damion at all. The breach in patient confidentiality is a very serious issue and thus needs to be addressed as such.
41. **Of no importance whatsoever.** Patient safety must be placed above any of his own personal gains and so the risk of losing all the time invested in the project is not important.

Scenario 9

42. **Of minor importance.** Although Carlos may care about his rapport with the consultant, being professional and looking professional in front of patients is more important.
43. **Of minor importance.** This is not very important is it is unlikely that the consultant will give Carlos a bad grade based on the decision Carlos makes.
44. **Of no importance whatsoever.** The consultant's appearance does not reflect on how presentable and professional Carlos looks himself. This should not be the reason why Carlos wants the consultant to look professional. The image displayed to patients should be his primary concern.
45. **Of no importance whatsoever.** Simply because the workshop was optional does not mean that the advice offered is any less important and that it should not be followed in a clinical setting.
46. **Of no importance whatsoever.** There is no relationship between the consultant's ability to do his job and his appearance.

Scenario 10

47. **Of minor importance.** Patient safety should be Arran's primary concern. The fact that this opportunity may not arise again is minor to compromising patient safety.
48. **Of no importance whatsoever.** His experience with tonsillitis is irrelevant when considering a breach in patient safety. Simply because he could focus with tonsillitis last time does not mean he is not compromising patient safety.
49. **Extremely important.** This is the main factor that Arran needs to consider when deciding whether to attend the surgery.
50. **Of minor importance.** Patient safety is far more important than whether the doctors conducting the surgery will ask Arran to sit in on other surgeries in the future.
51. **Of no importance whatsoever.** This fact is completely irrelevant. Simply because his peers have compromised patient safety does not mean it is okay and that Arran should do it himself.

Scenario 11

52. **Of minor importance.** Although being awarded the captaincy is something Abraham would like, this is not as crucial his scientific development which will assist him in his career.
53. **Of minor importance.** Simply attending the seminars will not mean the examiner will mark Abraham's papers more favourable and this should not be a driving factor in why Abraham chooses to attend the workshops. It is of minor importance however as it means that it is likely that the information taught in the seminars will translate into information that can be used in the exam.
54. **Of minor importance.** This is not a major factor in deciding whether Abraham should attend the seminars or play football. This is of minor importance as it may enable Abraham to build a better rapport with the lecturer which may the assist him his studies.
55. **Fairly important.** This is an important factor to consider as attending the seminars is largely motivated by the benefit it will grant Abraham in his exams. Although this is not the most important factor as the academic benefit derived from the seminars may not outweigh the benefits (e.g. mental wellbeing) derived from playing football.
56. **Extremely important.** This is extremely important to consider as it means that Abraham has the option of attending the seminars and still playing football on alternative dates thus reducing the proportion of training and football he is missing out on.

Scenario 12

57. **Of no importance whatsoever.** Although Brandon is more skilled at suturing and thus may perform alright in a tired state, this is not a valid factor when it may cause a breach in patient care and safety.
58. **Extremely important.** This is the main factor that needs to be considered and patient care is the upmost priority.
59. **Of minor importance.** Although embarrassing Brandon is unfortunate and not something Cameron wants to do, it is overshadowed by the importance of ensuring patient safety is not compromised.
60. **Of no importance whatsoever.** Assuming that Brandon is fine even though the information presented to Cameron suggests that Brandon isn't, is an irresponsible thing to do and thus this factor is irrelevant.
61. **Fairly important.** This is important in considering how to resolve the situation. Cameron needs to consider this factor because if he gets Brandon into further trouble he may risk Brandon undergoing severe disciplinary procedures. This matter can be resolved without alerting medical faculty to Brandon's tired state.
62. **Of minor importance.** Although this is unfortunate, it is overshadowed by the fact that patient safety could be compromised if Cameron does nothing.

Scenario 13

63. **Of minor importance.** This factor is directly involved with Jason's motivation for going on the trip, however it does not consider the negative impact it may have on his academics when considering the opportunity cost of a publication in his name.
64. **Fairly important.** This factor is key to Jason's decision as missing out on the tour may bring no benefit to Jason and thus would have been a wasted opportunity to go abroad with his peers.
65. **Extremely important.** A publication in his name is likely to be of tremendous use to Jason in his career and this factor may be far more beneficial to Jason than attending the tour.
66. **Extremely important.** This is a crucial factor for Jason to consider as it provides him with a solution of attending tour on an alternative year and still being able to undertake the extra work needed for the project this year. Although this may delay the tour, it still enables him to reap the benefits of both opportunities in the long term.
67. **Of minor importance.** This is important to Jason as he does not want to cause issues with his friends, however this is not so important when compared to the benefits granted by having a publication in his name. It also does not consider the fact that some of his friends may have publications already in their names which is why they are so keen to go on tour.
68. **Of no importance whatsoever.** The image Jason has in the eyes of the research team lead is irrelevant. The key factors at play are the benefits granted by either opportunity to Jason, not impressing the team lead is unlikely to have any negative consequences for Jason,
69. **Very important.** There is no obligation for Jason to work through his summer holidays and so the decision is purely down to him and what he would rather do.

END OF PAPER

Mock Paper E Answers

Section A: Verbal Reasoning
Passage 1

1. **D** The passage states that 'There were no chairs to be seen—the places of these useful articles being supplied by empty nail-kegs and blocks of wood'
2. **B** The passage states that 'of all the dinners that ever a white man sot down to' which would suggest that Godfrey is of Caucasian descent
3. **C** Based on the information given in the passage, the most likely option is that Godfrey is unemployed. Being a doctor, lawyer or university professor would mean that Godfrey would not live in poverty, as he does. He might be a farmer, but there is nothing in the passage to suggest so, hence the most likely option is unemployed.
4. **D** Based on the passage, one can infer that it is not set either in modern times, based on the state of the housing, nor is it set in the future. This leaves only option D as the plausible answer.

Passage 2

5. **A** The first line of the passage says that William Allen was a chemist, which is a scientist.
6. **B** It says in the passage that William Allen worked in Guy's Hospital, so option B is correct.
7. **C** William Allen discovered the proportion of carbon in carbonic acid; not the acid itself
8. **A** The only thing which can be properly inferred from the passage is that William Allen made a significant contribution to science, since he is quoted as an 'eminent scientist' and that the passage lists some of the achievements he had in the field of chemistry.

Passage 3

9. **B** Chaos is the name given to the mass of earth and sea and heaven before they were separated, not the name of a god.
10. **A** The passage states that 'The fiery part, being the lightest, sprang up, and formed the skies' so the skies are the lightest of the options
11. **A** The passage states that Prometheus 'made man in the image of the gods'
12. **C** The passage states that 'God and Nature at last interposed, and put an end to this discord, separating earth from sea, and heaven from both' which suggests that God and Nature together helped in the creation of the Earth from Chaos.

Passage 4

13. **B** The passage states that Merlin's mother was a woman
14. **A** The passage states that 'Merlin was the son of no mortal father' which would suggest that Merlin's father is immortal.
15. **D** The passage states that Merlin 'retained many marks of his unearthly origin', suggesting that he does have special abilities.
16. **D** Based on the information in the passage, that Vortigern is fearful for the return of the rightful heirs, one would suspect that Vortigern is a fearful character.

Passage 5

17. **A** The first line states that the author is born in Indiana, which is in the USA.
18. **C** The passage states that the author's father was James. P Mills, the grandfather was James Mills II and the great-grandfather was James Mills I
19. **B** The passage states that 'With his inheritance of $250, he and his brother Frank started West in a Dearborn wagon, crossing the Alleghenies.'
20. **C** There is no indication that the author is male or female based on the passage.

Passage 6

21. **C** The passage makes no mention of any siblings
22. **A** The passage states that Frank's face 'flushes with anger' when his friend suggests that Mr. Craven wishes to marry his mother, and refuses to think of it any more, suggesting that he is not comfortable with the idea of his mother marrying.
23. **A** Considering Frank is sitting outside on the lawn when Mr. Craven gets his attention, the most likely season would be summer.
24. **C** Considering Frank is worried about his mother getting married to Mr. Craven, the only plausible option is that his father is absent. Frank's mother may well be unmarried, but there is nothing in the text to distinguish whether she was ever married or not, so this option is not plausible.

Passage 7

25. **B** The passage states that 'no one in London who had a larger and more festive post than she', suggesting that she too lives in London
26. **C** The passage states that 'Even in her fiftieth year she retained with her youthful zest for life' but this does not give us any indication as to what age she currently is.
27. **A** This option correctly summarises the information in the passage. Although answer D seems to be appropriate, the passage focuses on Cynthia and her desires more than the benefits of sour milk injection.
28. **D** The passage states that 'but time was gradually lightening the heaviness of feature that had once formed so remarkable an ugliness' suggesting that Cynthia was ugly in youth, not good-looking

Passage 8

29. **A** The passage states that 'that other "Long Island"—the group of the Outer Hebrides—which, for an equal distance, extends along the Scottish coast from Butt of Lewis to Barra Head' so there is a Long Island in Scotland
30. **A** The passage does provide an account of the history of Long Island
31. **D** The passage states that 'the group of the Outer Hebrides—which, for an equal distance, extends along the Scottish coast from Butt of Lewis to Barra Head' so the Outer Hebrides are in Scotland
32. **D** The passage makes mention of all those animals, save for tigers

Passage 9

33. **A** The passage is set in the year 2126, which is in the future
34. **C** The passage talks about how the government and religion was a product of human behaviour, which would suggest that the passage is about human nature
35. **D** The passage states that England is 'under the absolute dominion of a female sovereign' so option D is correct
36. **C** The passage states nothing to suggest admiration for human compassion, however it also doesn't oppose this statement so the answer is C.

Passage 10

37. **A** The passage states that 'Moreover, he possessed only one eye, which was large and telescopic looking' which is proof of his one eye
38. **D** The protagonist describes the ghost as a 'horrid brute' which clearly demonstrates his lack of fondness for the ghost
39. **D** The description in the passage clearly brings out feelings of pity for the reader.
40. **A** The passage states that Ashton is interested in the story of the 'strange, dwarfish old man' and he 'resolved to look for him and see what his game really was' so clearly shows an interest in ghosts

Passage 11

41. **D** The passage states that they are based in Lytton Springs, India
42. **B** The passage states that the faith 'was a mixture of Catholicism and Hinduism' so cannot be labelled as either Hinduism or Catholicism
43. **B** The passage states that the Princes 'were all great Psychics', which would suggest that they had special abilities
44. **C** The passage makes no reference to Sita being the veiled princess, so the correct answer is can't tell.

END OF SECTION

Section B: Decision Making

1. A To calculate this one needs to find the lowest common multiple of both 73 and 104, and then add that value to 2007. The lowest common multiple of 73 and 104 is 7592, which when added to 2007 gives 9559 AD

2. A

A. This is the most feasible option
B. The ability to buy alcohol should have no semblance as to whether one can vote or not
C. In a democracy, the more people that vote, the fairer the voting system becomes
D. This is false. There will be plenty of people below the age of 18 who can still understand policies and the pros and cons of each

3. E When drawing out the whole arrangement as shown below we can clearly see that Caitlyn is directly opposite David.

Caitlyn
James Simon
Adam Ben
Joe David

4. C 8 is the only common code amongst all 3 codes, as is the word 'you' so 8 must mean 'you' in this code.

5. A

A. This provides the most sensible option as to why smoking should be condemned
B. Though this is true, there is an element of free choice which must also be considered and therefore does not form a strong enough argument as to why smoking should be condemned
C. The healthcare system being private does not form a coherent argument to this statement
D. Though most people that smoke do also drink, there is no strict causation so this statement does not form a reasonable argument

6. B Jason is older than Peter and John, so let's assume Jason is the oldest. If Alan is younger than John, and Peter is older than John, this means that Peter is the next oldest, followed by John, followed by Alan.

7. C Based on the given information, S=Y, OILE can be derived from 'TOILET' as 'DJEB' and D=L, so option C is correct

8. B Assuming the public are proactive about their healthcare and have easy access to the information then by publishing mortality rates the public can have a more active role in their healthcare. This is especially relevant in the current era of medicine seeing a transition away from more paternalistic views to patient autonomy.

9. B If the number of girls is 40 more than the number of boys, and the boys make up 40% of the total number of students, then the discrepancy of 40 between boys and girls must represent 20%. Therefore, 1%=2 students and therefore the total number of students is 200.

10. A If Anna and May are in the same school year, and Isaac is May's younger brother, then Anna must be older than Isaac.

11. E If French is the third lesson of the day then maths has to be fourth so that there is a lesson between French and history and so that Maths is neither second nor fifth. The complete subject order can be seen below.

1 – Science
2 – English
3 – French
4 – Maths
5 – Geography
6 – History

12. A This statement is true-one of the main concerns about legalising euthanasia is that it provides a way by which families push their elderly family members into euthanasia to relieve themselves of the burden.

13. A Days pass at 2/5 of the speed on Mars so the gap between Olympic games would be 2.5x longer so 4 years x 2.5 = 10 years.

14. B

A. This statement is **false**. There is no reason as to why the illiterate members of society should be segregated from schoolchildren
B. This statement is **true**- such a scheme should not come at the expense of a household income for the illiterate members of society
C. This statement is **false**- providing unnecessary hardship benefits neither the schoolteachers nor the illiterate members of society
D. This statement is **false**- there does not appear to be any correlation between literacy and how crowded the streets are at night time.

15. A The probability that Jay will be late is the probability that Jay will walk (30%) multiplied by the probability that Jay will be late when he walks (60%), added to the probability that Jay will take the bus (70%) multiplied by the probability that Jay will be late taking the bus (20%), which gives 32%.

16. C 273546 rearranged would give 234567, which means that 2 and 5 retain their position within the original number, so the correct number is 2

17. D Based on the given information, a Venn diagram can be drawn as follows: (top circle = English; right = PhDs)

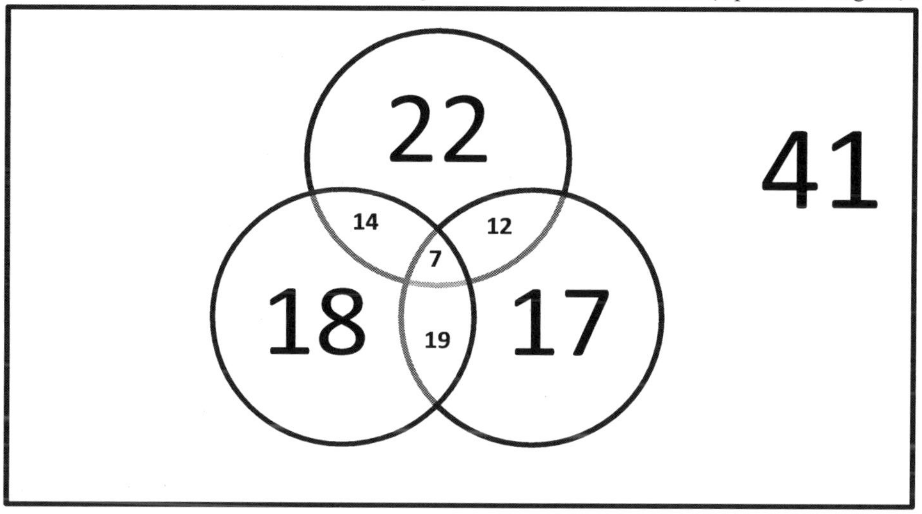

This means that the number of employees without any of the specifications is 41.

18. D The information provided states that motor vehicles include trucks, therefore it is fair for one to assume that all trucks are motor vehicles

19. C The information provided states that sharks are fish, and fish are aquatic animals. Therefore in turn sharks must be aquatic animals.

20. D If Alex starts off walking towards the sunrise, he is walking towards the east. If he then turns 90 degrees clockwise, he will be walking south. If he turns 180 degrees after this he will be walking north. Finally, by turning 90 degrees anticlockwise after this, he will be walking West for the last 4km.

21. A

A. This statement provides the strongest argument-if less people can possess a gun, then naturally there will be reduced murders because of gun crime
B. Although this argument is valid, it is not providing a strong case. Knife possession carries its own risks so carrying a knife instead of a gun does not really solve the issue
C. This statement is false-the point of black market sales is that it is already illegal-this will not really be affected whether possession is made illegal or not
D. This statement is false-using a gun in a public place is a crime anyway so people who are willing to use a gun in public are already not afraid of the consequences of possessing a gun.

22. E The Arabian Sea is a sea, which means that is must be a body of water partially enclosed by land.

23. A If 56% of the 300 students are boys, then 44% of the students are girls which =132 students. If 25% of these are Chinese that equates to 132 divided by 4 which = 33 students.

24. A

A. This option provides the strongest argument-the worst diets are often the cheapest and therefore tend to form a large proportion of the daily nutrition for the poorest of society. As a result, the poorest of society tend to be the most predisposed to obesity.
B. This option is false-obesity is associated with several co-morbidities and therefore is a very expensive morbidity
C. This option is false-contribution to the national health system is based on income, not weight
D. This option is false-although there is a genetic component to obesity and certain people are predisposed, unless one has a very rare mutation this is only a predisposition and can be controlled for.

25. C Karl is David's uncle.

26. C Based on the information, the school bus will get her to school at 09:01. The public bus arrives at 08:21, which she will miss, and the next bus will arrive at 08:38, which will take 18 minutes to arrive, meaning she will at school at 08:56, so the public bus at 08:38 will get her to school first

27. A Based on the information provided the seating arrangement can be drawn as shown below. Therefore, Neil must be sitting opposite Karen in the circle.

Neil

Richard Opie

Jason Mason

Pari Liam

Karen

1992 = Neil; 1996 = Liam; 1997 = Karen; 2000 = Obie; 2001 = Jason; 204 = Pari; 2005 = Richard; 2010 = Mason

28. C

A. This statement is not a good enough excuse for the continued legalisation of zoos
B. This statement is false-there are plenty of methods by which children can learn about animals without using zoos
C. This statement provides the best argument for zoos-animals such as the giant panda are no longer endangered due to the conservation efforts made by zoos and other conservation organisations
D. Although this is true, this does not provide a good enough excuse for zoos. Animals should not be held in captivity so that humans can make a living, the same way animals should not be held in captivity for the sake of human entertainment

29. A We are told that all humans are apes and secondly that all apes are mammals. Therefore it follows that all humans are mammals.

END OF SECTION

Section C: Quantitative Reasoning

Data Set 1

1. **E** The mode is the most frequent group within the data set. Both 5 and 4 people are in the shop twice, making the made the average of these two so 4.5.
2. **D** The best time to visit the shop would be when there are the least number of people in the shop, which would be at 10am
3. **C** The range is the maximum value subtract the minimum value, which would give a value of 20
4. **D** The number of people who visit the shop throughout the day is 70. If each person spends £5, then the total income for the day is £350

Data Set 2

5. **B** If £1=1.8595 CAD, then 500 multiplied by 1.8595=$929.75
6. **A** The conversion table shows that 1 CAD=£0.5364, so 150 multiplied by 0.5364=£80.46
7. **C** One can see that 1 CAD=£0.5364, so $150 will only get Sally £80.46. However, if Sally received the same rate as when she was exchanging from pounds to Canadian dollars, she would've received £80.67 for $150 (150 divided by 1.8595), so she loses £0.21 in this exchange
8. **C** using the rate given in the table, for USD 700 Shoko can get JPY 82425. Using the rate given by the travel agency, Shoko can get JPY 83041. She therefore can get JPY 616 more using the travel agency as compared to the table.

Data Set 3

9. **B** The temperature today is 22.6°C which corresponds to a temperature anomaly of 1.3°C. Therefore the baseline is 21.3°C. In 1940, the temperature anomaly was 0.3°C, so the surface temperature must have been 21.6°C
10. **A** as mentioned above, the baseline is 21.3°C, which is taken as the normal surface temperature
11. **E** One can see that the gradient of the line of the graph is greatest in the period from 2010 onwards
12. **B** the temperature anomaly increases from 0.4 to 0.8°C in this period of 20 years, which gives a rate of 0.2°C per year.

Data Set 4

13. **A** Out of all of the students, Muskan had the highest overall average of 77.5%
14. **C** Rohit scored 60% in his Computer Science exam, which has a maximum of 40 marks, so Rohit got 24 out of 40.
15. **A** Out of all of the subjects, Maths had the highest average score at 82%
16. **D** Sajal scored 90% on his Maths exam, which is scored out of 150, giving him a mark of 135

Data Set 5

17. **C** The graph shows that the rainfall in 2010 was 45 inches
18. **A** The graph shows that the rainfall in 2009 was the most of any year
19. **C** the graph shows that the rainfall in 2007 was 32 inches, whilst the rainfall in 2009 was 70 inches. The difference between the two is therefore 38 inches
20. **A** The total rainfall over these 5 years was 259 inches, giving an average of 52 inches a year.

Data Set 6

21. **B** If the train travels 5km in 10 minutes, then in one hour the train will travel 30km, so the speed is 30km/h
22. **A** if the train travels at 30km/h, then in 2 minutes the train will travel 1km
23. **D** If Jamie misses the 08:33 train by 7 minutes, then he will be at the station at 08:40, so he must wait 8 minutes until the 08:48 train
24. **E** If he has to be at work by 9am, then he needs to reach Forest Road by 08:48, which means he has to take the 07:48 train from Central park, which means he has to set off from his house at 07:40

Data Set 7

25. **B** The surface area of a cylinder is defined as $2\pi r^2+2\pi rh$ where r=radius of the circle and h=the perpendicular height. This calculation gives, to the nearest centimetre, 1232cm^2
26. **A** The volume of a cylinder is defined as πr^2h where r=radius of the circle and h=the perpendicular height. This calculation gives, to the nearest centimetre, 3233cm^3
27. **C** the circumference of a cross-section is defined as $2\pi r$ where r=radius of the circle. This calculation gives, to the nearest centimetre, 44cm
28. **B** As the volume is defined as πr^2h, an increase in the radius by a factor of 2 will cause an increase in the volume by a factor of $2^2=4$

Data Set 8

29. **A** If the value depreciates by 15% each year, then the value after 1 year will be 0.85 of 9000. After three years hence, the value of the car will be 9000 multiplied by 0.85^3, which gives £5527

30. **D** If the value depreciates by 15% each year, then after 6 years the value is £3394

31. **C** The runner in the lead will take 12 minutes to complete a lap; the runner in the back will take 18 minutes to complete a lap. If one takes the lowest common multiple of these two values, then the answer is 36 minutes. This is the time where the lead runner will complete 3 laps whilst the runner in the back will complete 2 laps, so at 36 minutes the lead runner will lap the runner at the back

32. **A** In order to find this, one needs to find the highest common factor of 32 and 78, which is 2.

Data Set 9

33. **C** If the red represents 44% of the survey, this equates to 132 people

34. **A** If the green represents 6% of the survey, the angle this makes on the pie chart is 6% of 360° which to the nearest degree is 22°

Data Set10

35. **A** 10% of 9.325 + 15% of 28624 + 25% of 53949 of 28% of 84099 = £41461

36. **C** If he gets married, he goes from being in the 33% tax bracket to being in the 28% tax bracket, so this is a 5% tax reduction

END OF SECTION

Section D: Abstract Reasoning

Rules:

Set 1: Acute angles in Set A= Even; in Set B = Odd.

Set 2: The shape on the inside has more sides than the shape on the outside in Set A; the shape on the outside has more sides than the shape on the inside in Set B

Set 3: Number of lines in set A=1, number of lines in Set B>1.

Set 4: Set A has an odd number of right-pointing arrows and an even number of left-pointing arrows; Set B has an even number of right-pointing arrows and an odd number of left-pointing arrows

Set 5: Shapes in Set A only have straight edges; Shapes in Set B have at least 1 curved edge

Set 6: The arrow is pointing towards the shaded corner in Set A; the arrow is pointing away from the shaded corner in Set B.

Set 7: The number of corners in Set A is an even number; odd in Set B

Set 8: Set A has a vertical line of symmetry; Set B has a horizontal line of symmetry.

Set 9: Set A has less than half the circle shaded; Set B has more than half the circle shaded

Set 10: In increasing order from 1, the correct shape is highlighted

Set 11: The line crosses the shape by an increasing number of times in the sequence

Set 12: The shapes at the top have a horizontal line of symmetry, the shapes at the bottom have a vertical line of symmetry

Set 13: The shapes at the top have an even number of circles and an odd number of sides on the large shape; the shapes at the bottom have an odd number of circles and an even number of sides on the large shape

Set 14: To get from the left to the right, one must reverse the shading of the shapes and the shapes on the top must go to the bottom

Set 15: The number of vertical lines in Set A are greater than the number of horizontal lines; in Set B the number of vertical lines is less than the number of horizontal lines

END OF SECTION

Section E: Situational Judgement Test

Scenario 1

1. **Inappropriate but not awful.** This would not be an awful decision, because what James is doing is technically cheating. However, being James's friend, this is not the best way to approach the situation given the ramifications of cheating, and a solution in which James is not litigated by the medical school should be explored if possible.
2. **Very inappropriate.** The question bank is against the rules and undermines the validity of the end of year exams. Utilising the question bank is still cheating regardless of whether you were involved in the making of the question bank or not.
3. **Very appropriate.** This is the best way to explore the situation, such that James is not punished by the medical school but is not cheating.
4. **Appropriate, but not ideal.** This is a possibility and would be appropriate, but if James is at university this may be inconvenient for the parents, and is delegating responsibility which, if you were a good friend, you should take on yourself.
5. **Very inappropriate.** This option not only does not give James the opportunity to rethink his options about making the question bank, but also publicly exposes him and ruins your friendship with him. This is a highly inappropriate action.

Scenario 2

6. **Very inappropriate.** This would call into account Rashid's personal professionalism and if Rashid's plan was found out by the clinical school, it would certainly call into consideration Rashid's fitness to practice and whether he should continue with medical school or not.
7. **Very appropriate.** This would be the best response to the situation. Informing the clinical school means that Rashid is maintaining transparency as much as possible, and means that he can travel without worry of repercussions.
8. **Inappropriate, but not awful.** If Rashid does enough work on the placement before the holiday that he can afford to take the 2 weeks off and his supervisor is happy with it, it is not the worst decision. However, it would still be inappropriate as the placement is specified as 6 weeks and the supervisor would have to be dishonest with the clinical school by signing Rashid off early.
9. **Appropriate, but not ideal.** This would be an appropriate response, because taking a holiday during the clinical year is not technically allowed. However, if his parents have already pad significant amounts for his ticket, which they will not get back if the tickets are cancelled, then this is not the best way to handle the situation.
10. **Very inappropriate.** This would be very inappropriate. By asking the clinical school and then openly disregarding their decision would call into account Rashid's professionalism and make the clinical school more likely to take drastic measures with regards to repercussions.

Scenario 3

11. **Very inappropriate.** Taking the questions still qualifies as cheating-this would be a very inappropriate action.
12. **Very inappropriate.** It qualifies as cheating, regardless of how many questions he takes
13. **Very appropriate.** This would be the best course of action, as it is not cheating and prevents Jamie's friend from getting in trouble as well.
14. **Inappropriate, but not awful.** This would be justified-Jamie's friend is cheating and reporting a cheater to the exam board is the right thing to do. However, taking into consideration that it is Jamie's friend and she is trying to help him, reporting her without at least consulting her and exploring other options is inappropriate.
15. **Very inappropriate.** Although this may equalise the proportions within the classroom, the classroom still gains an unfair advantage compared to everyone else in the country writing the exam, so this still is cheating and is inappropriate.

Scenario 4

16. **Appropriate, but not ideal.** This is true, and HIV is a disease which you do need to inform your patients about if they have a risk of developing it. However, this is not really the time or the place to reveal this to the wife after she has received such news; a more sensitive approach is required.
17. **Very appropriate.** This is probably the best response to the situation. This way, you can maintain trust with the wife, as well as making sure that the husband is aware of the risk of HIV infection.
18. **Very inappropriate.** This abuses the trust that the wife has placed in you and such large news is not really your place to reveal as a professional unless you absolutely must.
19. **Very inappropriate.** This pressurises the wife into revealing the news in a position when she is not comfortable and is an abuse of the trust she has placed in you.
20. **Inappropriate, but not awful.** This is inappropriate, as it is involving yourself as a professional in the personal lives of your patients. However, if it means that the husband is aware of the risk of developing HIV, then it is not awful.

Scenario 5

21. **Very appropriate.** This is the most appropriate response to the situation. The registrar is the senior-most member of the team and will know the best way to proceed.
22. **Very inappropriate.** This puts patients at risk if the doctor goes into theatre and reflects very badly on the profession if a drunk doctor is doing the ward round
23. **Inappropriate, but not awful.** This would be a sensible response. If the doctor is at risk of endangering patients, then he should be reported to the board. However, reporting the doctor without consulting anyone would be an inappropriate thing to do.
24. **Appropriate, but not ideal.** This is an appropriate action, and is a perfectly sensible option. However, as the junior doctor, it is not ideal to send the consultant in charge home without consulting anyone senior.
25. **Very inappropriate.** This would result in massive distrust between that consultant's patients and the consultant, and bring the profession into disrepute.

Scenario 6

26. **Appropriate, but not ideal.** This is an appropriate response. Maybe the pastoral care can help Neil with regards to his drug use before finals. However, consulting the pastoral care before speaking to Neil is not ideal.
27. **Very inappropriate.** The drug use may underlie a more serious problem, which you are not solving by reporting Neil to the medical school. In addition, Neil has trusted you with this information as his friend. Telling the clinical school is an abuse of this trust.
28. **Very appropriate.** This is the best way forward. Perhaps the reason Neil's drug taking has increased is because of a more serious underlying problem, and by speaking to you he can address it and move forward into finals without drugs, which is the best outcome in this situation.
29. **Very inappropriate.** Stealing from Neil is a crime, regardless of whether it is in good intentions, and is hence always inappropriate.
30. **Very inappropriate.** This is an abuse of Neil's trust, may result in criminal charges against Neil and the end of his medical career, and does not solve the underlying problem of why Neil is taking drugs if there is one.

Scenario 7

31. **Very important.** If the teaching is likely to come up in her end of year exams, it is important that she gets good notes on it which she can consolidate closer to the exam.
32. **Fairly important.** If transplant surgery is something Janice is interested in, and this is a rare opportunity that she might get, then she should try her best to utilise it. Clinical experience is invaluable in addition.
33. **Of minor importance.** Although she is interested in transplant surgery, she still must pass the exams sufficiently such that she is able to become a transplant surgeon. It is important to have interests, but it is more important to know the basics.
34. **Of no importance whatsoever.** Whether the teaching is small-group or large-group should have no effect on Janice's decision, as she has a legitimate decision as to why she could not attend the teaching.
35. **Fairly important.** If Janice knows that she will pursue transplant surgery, then it is important to get as much experience as possible. However, if it is at the expense of priceless teaching which is guaranteed to come up in the end of year exams, then one should prioritise the teaching. Once Janice has passed her finals, then she can try and explore opportunities in transplant surgery.

Scenario 8

36. **Very important.** This is a very important factor to consider. If Johnathan does not achieve a suitable work-life balance, he may not be able to carry on with his medical career.
37. **Of no importance whatsoever.** Although a prize would be nice, it should not be an important factor in deciding what he should do in this situation. There are more important factors to consider than how much prize money he can get.
38. **Fairly important.** His father clearly is enthusiastic for him to join the university cricket team and has invested a lot into making sure he gets there; completely disregarding this would be unfair to the father. However, he must also consider the importance of these exams and the importance of balancing work with his hobbies to attain maximum reward.
39. **Of minor importance.** This is important to consider, Johnathan wants to make a good impression with his new teammates, but compared to whether he is competent enough to progress with his studies, this is a minor factor.
40. **Of no importance whatsoever.** Like the prize consideration; who wins the bet should have no influence on Johnathan's decision.

Scenario 9

41. **Of minor importance.** This is slightly important, as it may be difficult for Hayley to rearrange the meeting if her director of studies is on a tight schedule. However, simply the fact that her director of studies should not have that large an influence on whether Hayley goes on the conference or not.
42. **Very important.** The elective is a wonderful opportunity for the medical student to gain experience in something that they are interested in, and offers a different perspective before they become junior doctors. As such, consideration of the elective is very important.
43. **Of no importance whatsoever.** Which city the conference is in and whether it is an attractive tourist prospect or not should have little influence in Hayley's decision-making process.
44. **Of minor importance.** This is at least a little bit important, as the consultant has chosen Hayley because she believes that Hayley has the responsibility to carry out the task. This should be given some consideration, but is not of paramount importance.
45. **Fairly important.** Getting a publication adds a point to Hayley's foundation programme application, and in the long-run may give her an advantage over other applicants for training jobs, registrar jobs and even consultant posts. Getting a publication at this stage is hence important to the extent that it will affect your future, but not as important as gaining valuable experience from the medical elective. There will always be opportunities to get publications, but the medical elective is really the last chance you get to explore another healthcare system without repercussion.

Scenario 10

46. **Fairly important.** Latisha's reputation with the doctors is an important point to consider. All professionals, including the medical students, on the ward are a team and work together to deliver safe and effective care. If one member of the team is not working well with the other members then the efficiency of the team decreases. As such, Latisha's reputation within the team is important to consider.
47. **Very important.** If the consultant on the ward round is determining whether they pass or fail the placement, it is important for Tim to ensure that Latisha is doing all that she can to pass, as her friend and her project partner.
48. **Very important.** As professionals in the healthcare industry, the public place their trust in doctors that they will provide them with optimum treatment. As such, it is the duty of doctors to remain professional in the public eye. Latisha is no exception, and Tim should make her aware of that.
49. **Of minor importance.** Yes, Tim's friendship with Latisha is important because as clinical partners it is likely that they will spend a lot of time together on the wards. However, it is more important for Tim to make Latisha realise that she is compromising her position as a medical student in this current situation.
50. **Of no importance whatsoever.** That is a personal issue and this is a professional one. It is important for Tim to distinguish between the two and leave the personal side of things out of the workplace.

Scenario 11

51. **Of no importance whatsoever.** This shouldn't matter that much. This is a professional issue here and is very serious; Javad's friendship should not influence the action in this scenario.
52. **This is very important.** If Javad does choose to tell the clinical school, it would ruin his friend's career as a doctor, from which he cannot recover.
53. **This is very important.** The hospital will have to face the consequences of his friend's blunder.
54. **Of no importance whatsoever.** The history does not excuse the actions now, nor should it influence Javad's decision, especially when it comes to a situation this serious.
55. **Of no importance whatsoever.** The friends struggle does not excuse such as breach in confidentiality so this is of no importance.

Scenario 12

56. **Fairly important.** If Ross is working on the night, and the hospital depends on Alex for working the following day, then it is important that Alex is in a fit enough state to do so.
57. **Very important.** If there is already a shortage of beds in the emergency department, then Alex is placing more strain on it by admitting himself.
58. **Very important.** If the consultant is doing the ward round the following morning, then the consultant will see Alex in the Emergency Department, and Ross will have to explain himself.
59. **Very important.** If IV fluids require inpatient admission, then Ross as the admitting doctor takes full responsibility for Alex as a patient and will have to answer for his decisions.
60. **Of no importance whatsoever.** Hopefully Ross should never be in this situation, given the position of the Emergency Department in this situation, so this should not play a role.
61. **Of no importance whatsoever.** This could affect Ross's professional career if he decides to admit Alex-he cannot be allowing personal entertainment to be driving his decision making in this situation

Scenario 13

62. **Very important.** If MRSA requires strict isolation, then unless the medical students know how to approach the situation, they should not go in to see the patient.
63. **Very important.** If the nurses have told them not to go inside, and they disregard the nurses' warnings, then if something happens to the patient the medical students will be responsible.
64. **Not important at all.** The medical students have been notified that they should not enter the room unless necessary by the nurses, so the knowledge of the ward should not play a part in their decision.
65. **Of minor importance.** If they must present the findings back to the junior doctor, they may feel less comfortable in going against his wishes, should they choose not to see the patient.
66. **Very important.** If the patient is clearly unwell, then it makes even less sense for the medical students to see them, as it could clearly compromise the patient's health further if they go and see him/her.
67. **Of no importance whatsoever.** Opportunities to learn in hospital are governed by the state of the patient, not the other way around. Patient safety should never be compromised with the goal of a better learning experience for medical students.
68. **Very important.** There is a significant risk to the students in entering the side room, and if it is not essential for the students to examine the patient then they should question whether it is worth the risk.
69. **Important.** MRSA not only poses a risk to themselves but also those they interact with since it is a highly infectious disease. A party obviously presents significant opportunity for MRSA transmission but it is no more important than the risk of transmission to others they meet on a bus or train.

END OF PAPER

Mock Paper F Answers

Section A: Verbal Reasoning

Passage 1

1. **A** The passages states the English Sparrow 'wages war upon song birds, destroying their young' making **A** correct. It was 'first introduced into the United States' in the mid 19th century, not discovered then, so **B** is incorrect, and song birds sing soul-inspiring songs, making **C** incorrect. **D** is incorrect as 'with the change of climate, came a change of taste for insects'.
2. **B** The good English Sparrows accomplish is 'nullified' according to the passage. The other statements are verified in the text.
3. **C** English Sparrows are described as devouring the common white butterfly, and 'seed and vegetable eaters'. They are described as 'great insect eaters' but never as preferring insects to grains so **A** is incorrect. Song birds are described as singing 'soul-inspiring songs' and English Sparrows as 'inharmonious' but this does not necessarily mean that song-birds are more harmonious than English Sparrows, so **B** is incorrect. It says that English Sparrows devour white butterflies, whose caterpillars wreak havoc, but does not directly say they eat them, so **D** is incorrect.
4. **B** The Sparrows were observed to convey 'no less than 40 grubs per hour' not more than 40 grubs per hour, so **A** is incorrect and **B** is correct. They were only observed for a day, so **C** and **D** are both incorrect.

Passage 2

5. **D** 'The mental qualifications of their gods were of a much higher order than those of men'. **A** is incorrect as the passage states that they have sometimes 'earnestly prayed to be deprived of their privilege of immortality'. **B** is incorrect as it says that gods and goddesses become attached to mortals 'not infrequently', and **C** is incorrect as it states that they do need daily nourishment and refreshing sleep.
6. **D** All the other qualities are stated to be different in gods and humans except emotions or 'passions' as stated in the text.
7. **C** This is stated when the offspring of gods and humans are described as 'heroes or demi-gods'. Although demi-gods are renowned for their courage, it doesn't explicitly say they are more courageous than gods so **A** is incorrect. Hercules isn't mentioned in the passage which makes **B** incorrect, and **D** is wrong because the passage does not talk about the life expectancy of demi-gods versus humans.
8. **C** Gods are 'more commanding in stature, height being considered by the Greeks an attribute of beauty in a man or woman'. The other statements are stated as true in the passage.

Passage 3

9. **B** The passage states that digestion is unappreciated because 'few of us are aware of its happening in the same way we are aware of making efforts to use our voluntary muscles'. The other statements are not stated as a reason for digestion being under appreciated.
10. **C** The aspects of digestion described as hard work/effort are: chewing, making saliva, churning in the stomach, and manufacturing bile and pancreatic enzyme.
11. **A** It states that 'a large portion of the blood supply is redirected from the muscles in the extremities to the stomach and intestines' to aid digestion. Bile, which aids digestion, is produced in the gall bladder but digestion doesn't take place there (**D**) and although this is true, amylase is not mentioned in the passage (**C**). **B** is incorrect as the cabbage and carrots were just used as an analogy to explain how much effort digestion requires.
12. **D** Although the passage states that pancreatin solubilises proteins, this may not be the only thing it does. The other facts are stated/implied in the text.

Passage 4

13. **D** It is stated that princess Victoria and her governess where devoted to each other before the governess died in 1870 (**C** is incorrect). It says that she would have excelled in music and drawing if she had devoted more time to them (**B**) and that she started lessons at age 5 (**A**).
14. **C** Tea was only allowed in later years as a treat. The other options are stated in the passage.
15. **A** It states that Princess Victoria did not know 'that she was likely at any future time to be Queen'. **B** is wrong because she states that she always slept in her mother's room before becoming Queen, **C** is wrong because she said that she read books about history recommended by her uncle, the King of the Belgians, but this does not mean that it is Belgian history. **D** is incorrect because although the passage states she is 'especially fond of music' it does not directly compare music to reading.
16. **D** It says that her education was 'chiefly' but not solely with a governess. The other statements are stated in the passage.

Passage 5

17. **A** 'the limit of endurance is reached more quickly towards the end of pregnancy'
18. **C** The passage states that exertion may need to be prohibited to prevent miscarriage. However, this does not mean that exhaustion is the cause of miscarriage.
19. **B** The passage states that sometimes women find it necessary to stop exercise a week or two before delivery.
20. **B** The passage states that women who have laborious household duties may need to exercise less than women with sedentary lives, but not that they don't need to exercise at all.

Passage 6

21. **C** the passage states that it is the simplest form in which spaghetti is served, but does not generalize to pasta as a whole.

22. **C** the passage states that Italians eat macaroni unbroken, but their ability to do this 'is not the privilege of everybody'. However it does not explicitly state whether any people of other nationalities are able to eat macaroni this way or not.

23. **B** The passage states that macaroni must be cooked for 12-15 minutes, not spaghetti. The other statements are in the passage as truths.

24. **C** The passage states that macaroni should be drained in a colander which means that pasta can be drained in a colander and **C** is correct. Spaghetti (but not pasta as a generalization) should be but in the water at boiling point (**B**) and both macaroni and spaghetti (but not pasta as a generalization) should be cooked in salted boiling water (**A**). Mezzani is the preferable kind of macaroni, but again not generalized to all pasta, for butter and cheese (**D**).

Passage 7

25. **D**

A. The passage states that penguins cannot fly, so this statement is incorrect

B. The text states that penguins 'have been termed the true inhabitants of that country' – this is not synonymous with being 'the first land inhabitants of the Antarctic region' – to see this you must think about how they qualify their statement and you will see that it due to penguins being best adapted rather than the first animals to evolve to this environment.

C. They would but the text clearly states that 'they never do this'.

D. By exclusion and by default after reading the phrase 'there is no food of any description to be had inland.'

26. **C** The passage states that bears and foxes live in the North Polar regions, so penguins in the Antarctic are safe, but it makes no statement as to whether penguins live in the North Polar regions, so one can't tell.

27. **B** Penguins do appear to be safe on land according to the text BUT there is no food for them on land – if both parts of the statement are not true it cannot be classed as true hence FALSE.

28. **C** The passage states that 'their four legs, in course of time, gave place to wide paddles or "flippers,"', so their legs did not evolve into fins; they evolved into flippers.

Passage 8

29. **D** The passage states that 'The breeding season of these birds begins in October or November', so this statement is incorrect.

30. **A** The passage states that 'Bonelli's eagles (Hieraetus fasciatus)' so one can imply that the Latin name for Bonelli's eagles is Hieraetus fasciatus

31. **C** The passage states that the pellets of the Benelli's eagle contains squirrels' skulls, but reveals no information about the kite's nest, so one cannot tell.

32. **C** The passage states that 'In India winter is the time of year at which the larger birds of prey, both diurnal and nocturnal, rear up their broods.', so one can imply that the larger birds of prey breed in winter.

Passage 9

33. **C** The passage states that 'it was 1896 and 1897 which were very serious years for the country' which suggests that these are the worst years for the country, not 1889

34. **C** The passage states that foreign capitalists were pouring in, and in this time there was a boom in land, so one can imply that foreign input influenced the boom in land.

35. **B** The passage states that 'The province of Buenos Aires, the largest in the country', so this statement is false.

36. **C** The passage makes no reference to when the monsoon in Buenos Aires is.

Passage 10

37. **B** 'Mosquito eggs are laid in water or in places where water is apt to accumulate, otherwise they will not hatch.' Hence the true statement would be that water is required for eggs to hatch rather than to be laid.

38. **B** 'Some of the eggs may remain over winter, but usually those laid in the summer hatch in thirty-six to forty-eight hours or longer according to the temperature.' This just requires some delicate reading of the phrase to understand that eggs generally hatch 36/48 hours after being laid, so you cannot directly compare the hatching times of summer eggs to winter eggs, as whichever were laid first will be hatched first, apart from the rare example where some eggs stay over Winter.

39. **C** There is no mention of whether the eyes can see or not when first hatched, so this answer is false.

40. **C** The feeding habits described are far too diverse to be summarised in one blanket statement – one point in exception to this statement is that 'Some mosquito larva are predaceous, feeding on the young of other species or on other insects'. Answer C however is mentioned directly in the text.

Passage 11

41. **A** The passage states that mites can transmit diseases from 'man to man' so this statement is correct

42. **B** The passage states that 'they may possibly aid in the dissemination of leprosy.', which is evidently more serious than blackheads, so this statement is false

43. **C** One would think this might be true considering that domestic animals are worse affected but there is no direct comparison, nor can it be inferred, so the answer is Can't Tell

44. **D** The passage states that 'The young have six legs, the adult eight' so one can infer that the mites develop two more legs as they mature

Section B: Decision Making

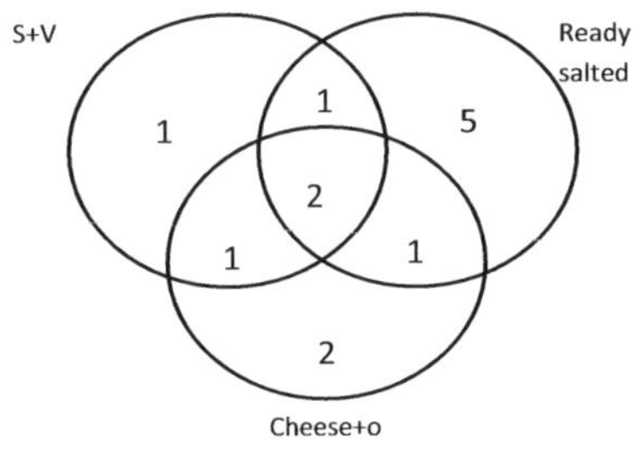

1. **B** Express the information in the following Venn diagram 5+1+1+1+1+2+2=13

2. **D** The statements can be written as: S<T, T< J<L, L<A. Therefore, Sam is the shortest.

3. **C** We do not know whether Alexandra and Katie are dancers, so **A** and **B** are wrong. We do not know whether any dancers are ugly, so **D** is wrong.

4. **D** 1 – 1/6 = 5/6 → 5/6 x 3/4 = 15/24 → 15/24 x 1/3 = 5/24

5. **B** 50 pieces minus 5 spares = 45. Half the meat eaters want 2 pieces and half want 1 piece splitting the remainder into 30 pieces for half and 15 for the other half. This means there are 30 meat eaters in total, and 40 total guests (1/4 are vegetarian).

6. **C** If he travels north, then turns to his right, he will be facing east. If he turns right after that, he will be facing south. If he travels 5km and 5km south, he is due east of his starting point.

7. **B** The pattern is squares of even numbers starting at 12, so 18 squared = 324

8. **E** A takes 10 days and B takes 15 days. Calculating the LCM of these we get 30 days – think of this as the 'total work'. If we then look at A in terms of 30/10 = 3 units of work. Similarly B is 30/15 = 2 units of work. So, finally 30/(3+2) = 6 days in total!

9. **E** Let the age of a = 2x and the age of b = 3x -> 2x=20 -> X=10
   Then present age of b is 3 * x= 3*10=30 years
   After 5 years, age of b = 30+5= 35 years

10. **C** 11+4=15 → 15+22=37 → 37-3=34

11. **C** 'Southampton is bigger than only Romsey.' -> therefore 4th- Southampton, 5th - Romsey
    Hence: London>Oxford>Cambridge>Southampton>Romsey

12. **C** If V is shorter only than R, R is the tallest and V is the 2nd tallest.
    J < M must mean that M is in the middle, followed by J and D therefore must be the shortest.
    R>V=160>M>J=135>D. Hence M must lie between 135 and 160 > can only be C

13. **C**
    A. All chemistry teachers are professionals-This cannot be determined based on the text and therefore cannot be assumed
    B. All professionals require a chemistry degree-This would imply that chemistry is the only university degree available which cannot be inferred from the questions
    C. All lawyers have a degree-This is true, considering that all lawyers are professionals and all professional jobs require a university degree
    D. All lawyers have a chemistry degree-there is no information in the text linking lawyers with chemistry
    E. All universities offer law as a degree course-this cannot be inferred from the information provided

14. **C** Joseph is a man and no man is a lion i.e. all men are NOT lions hence Joseph is not a lion.
    The statement is '1 to many' connection i.e. it puts Joseph in the bigger group of men BUT does not state that all men are or are not Joseph hence can't tell.

15. **B** Radius of circle = C and Side of Square = S
    C= 2/3(S)
    S2=441 therefore S=21
    Hence C=14
    Perimeter=2*pi*14

16. **D** a+b=3430 and 0.12a=0.28b
    Rearrange the second equation to a=7/3 b and substitute this into the first equation to get 10/3b=3430
    Hence b=1029 and a = 2401

17. **C** Son age now= S and Father age now= F
    F- 4 = 4(S-4) -> F = 4S -12
    F+6/S+6 =5/2 -> 2F +12 = 5S+ 30
    8S -12 = 5S +30
    S=14 and F=44

18. **D** Since the narrator has no brother, his father's son is he himself.
So, the man who is talking is the father of the man in the photograph.
Thus, the man in the photograph is his son

19. **C** Total of 12 = 73*12=876
E + A + O = (73.6*15) – 876 = 228
68 +A + (A+6) =228
2A = 154 -> A=77

20. **E** For this we need to know the area of a curved face of a cone is radius pi x radius x length (i.e. diagonal)
Diameter = 40m therefore radius = 40/2=20m
H=21m
l=$\sqrt{}$ (20^2+21^2) = $\sqrt{}$(400+441) = $\sqrt{841}$ =29m
Surface area of curved face = 29x20 pi
Total surface area = 480pi + 100pi therefore ratio = 480pi : 580pi = 24:29

21. **D** All the women have left for dinner so A and B cannot be correct and the sons went out to play so C is incorrect hence D is correct.

22. **B** Build up the order as you read the statements:
If A is placed below E -> E, A
C is placed above D -> C, D
B is placed below A -> E, A, B
and D is placed above E -> C, D, E, A, B

23. **B** Distance = 2/3S
distance=1-2/3S=1/3S
21/15 hr=2/3 S/4 + 1/3s /5
84=14/3S * 3 therefore S= 6km

24. **E** The relative speed of the boys = 5.5kmph – 5kmph = 0.5 kmph
Distance between them is 8.5 km
Time= 8.5km / 0.5 kmph = 17 hrs

25. **C** 34*8*9 = 2448
This is 2/5 of the total work, so multiplying this by 3/2 gives us 3/5 = 3672
3672 / (6*9) = 68. The question asks for how many more men should be employed so we need an additional 34.

26. **C** Jack is a human. Therefore, Jack is not a machine-If Jack is a human, and machines are not human, then one can infer that Jack is not a machine
All machines are robots-Just because all robots are machines does not mean that all machines are robots, one cannot tell this based on the information

27. **B**
A. 'Frustrated people are prone to be drug addicts' -> does not mean all are drug addicts hence A is false
B. 'Some artists are frustrated -> frustrated people are prone to be drug addicts' -> so Yes some artists may be drug addicts TRUE
C. Nothing is said about the relationship in this direction
D. The artists who are frustrated may also be whimsical but not ALL frustrated people.

28. **D** X is married to A who is a lawyer, so B and C are either a doctor or a lawyer respectively. Y is not married to an engineer, and C is not a doctor so Y must be married to B who is a doctor, and Z must be married to C who is an engineer, so the correct answer is D, as none of these options are available.

29. **A**
A. Vigorously learning the times tables in primary school provides an unnecessary level of stress. This is correct, primary school children have enough to worry about with 11+ exams at the end of year 6, forcing them to maintain high standards in the times tables will only add to this stress from an earlier age, and could lead to detrimental long-term effects.
B. Literacy is a more important skill than mathematics-This is false; both literacy and mathematics are equally important in terms of educational needs.
C. Knowing the times tables provides no benefit for children in later life-This is false; times tables forms an important part of mental arithmetic, which is an important life skill regardless of what career one goes in to.
D. There is no need for mental arithmetic when calculators are so readily available-This is false; as mentioned above mental arithmetic is still an important life skill to have at hand, and the availability of calculators should not affect this.

END OF SECTION

Section C: Quantitative Reasoning

Data Set 1

1. **D** 8.1g. A drink made of 18g of powder and 200ml of whole milk has 9.6g fat. 100g powder has 8.4g fat, therefore 18g powder has 18/100 x 8.4 = 1.512g. The amount of fat in 200ml whole milk is 9.6-1.512 = 8.1g.
2. **A** 56ml. The total fat content of 2.464g contains fat from the powder. Therefore, the milk/water mix contains 2.464-1.512 = 0.952g fat. Since there is no fat in water, this can only be from the semi skimmed milk. If 100ml semi skimmed milk contains 1.7g fat then to obtain 0.952, we need a volume of 0.952 x 100/1.7 is 56ml.
3. **C** 7.0 pints. The box contains 360g of powder. He therefore needs 20x200ml = 4000ml milk which is equivalent to 4000/570 = 7.0 pints.
4. **C** 164g. he box has 360g powder and therefore at 18g per drink there are 20 drinks in the box. For these 20 drinks John will need 20x200ml = 4 litres. The protein content of the whole box is 360/100 x 8.9g = 32.4g. The protein in the 4 litres of the semi skimmed milk is 40x3.3 = 132g. The total amount of protein is therefore 164g.
5. **C** 9kCal. (372 – 4x8.9 – 4x65.2)/8.4 = 9. OR (200-4x8..0-4x20.4)/9.6 = 9

Data Set 2

6. **E** £83.10. The Monday – Friday 9am-6pm stays will each cost:

- 9am-1pm: 4hrs x 6 periods x 20p = £4.80 and - 1pm-6pm: 5hrs x 6 periods x 30p = £9.00

Total cost = £13.80 per day.

Saturday and Sunday 9am-6pm stays will each cost: 9hrs x 3 periods x 15p = £4.05 per day.

6 overnight stays = £6.

Total cost = 5 days x £13.80 + 2 days x £4.05 + £6 overnight = £83.10

7. **E** £1.30. The first period of 5 mins (5:55-6:00pm) will be charged at 30p and the second part (6:00-6:15) will be charged at £1. Hence the total is £1.30.
8. **D** 80p. A 37-minute stay will be charged as 40 minutes and will therefore cost 4 x 20 = 80p.
9. **D** £20. The week-day cost from 9am-6pm is £13.80 (see previous). However he can use the ticket from 8:30-9:00am, which would normally be charged at £1. The total for the day is £14.80. Over 5 days, this costs £74, hence a saving of £20.
10. **E** 50p. He will be charged a full 20p for the first 2 minutes and a full 30p for the next 2 minutes,
11. **E** Saturday 1:40pm.

Cost of Friday 5pm to 6pm = 6 x 30 = £1.80.

Cost over overnight stay (Friday to Saturday) = £1. Cumulative total = £2.80.

This leaves £2.10 to spend on Saturday day time. The cost of 15p per period – he can spend 2:10/0.15 = 14 periods of 20 minutes. i.e. 4 hrs 40 mins in total. He must therefore have left the car ark by Saturday 1:40pm.

Data Set 3

12. **B** 1 850 000 Rupees. From the table it shows that the price of 10 grams of gold in 2010 is 18500 Rupees. There are 1000 grams in a kilogram, so the answer is 18500 multiplied by 100=1 850 000 Rupees.
13. **E** £21765. If there are 85 rupees to £1, then 1 850 000 rupees, which is the price of 1kg of gold in 2010, then this corresponds to 1 850 000 divided by 85, which gives 21765 to the nearest pound.
14. **B** 590kg. £25000 corresponds to 2125000 Rupees, which in 1940 would have bought you 58962 lots of 10 grams of gold, which corresponds to 590kg to the nearest kilogram
15. **C** 763kg. £25000 in 1940 would've corresponded to 2750000 Rupees, which in 1940, would have bought you 76304 lots of 10 grams of gold, which corresponds to 763kg to the nearest kilogram
16. **A** 2. To calculate this, one must find the highest common factor between 38 and 46, which is 2. 2 is therefore the highest number of each coloured pen that can go into each pencil case without leaving a remainder.

Data Set 4

17. **C** December 2013. This is when the peak of the graph is.
18. **A** $1020. One can see reading off from the graph that the maximum value that Bitcoin reaches is $1020
19. **D** Between July 2013 and December 2013, the value of bitcoin rose from $100 to $1020, over the period of 5 months. If we simplify such that the rise is uniform over the 5 months, then the rise is (1020-100) divided by 6 = $184 per month
20. **B** $1 600 000. Jamil bought $1000 of Bitcoin shares when it was 50 cents a share. He would've been able to buy 2000 shares with this amount. He sold it in March 2013, when the value was $220 a share, meaning that Jamil turned over a revenue of $440 000, with an overall profit of $439 000. However, had he sold it in December 2013, when the value was $1020 a share, then he would've made a revenue of $2 040 000, with a net profit of $2 039 000. This means that had he sold it in December 2013, he would've made $1 600 000 more.

Data set 5

21. **C** The volume of a cone is defined is one-third of the height multiplied by the radius cubed multiplied by pi. As a result, the correct answer is 1 400 632 cm^3, which is equivalent to 1.4m^3

22. **E** The surface area of a cone is defined as $\pi r^2 + \pi rs$. As a result, the correct answer is 5850 cm^2, which is equivalent to 0.58m^2

23. **B** If the angle between h and s=34°, and a right-angled triangle is formed between h, s and r, then the angle between s and r=180-(90+34) =56°

Data Set 6

24. **A** One can see that the data set with the highest number of deaths is ovary cancer

25. **A** 46250. The mean is the sum of all the groups divided by the number of groups there are. This gives a value of 46250 deaths

26. **D** 140 000. The range is taken as the largest value subtracted by the smallest value, which in this case gives a value of 140 000

Data Set 7

27. **C**1.2 billion. Based on the graph, one can estimate the population to have been 1.2 billion in 1900.

28. **E** 80 million per year. One can see that the population in 1960 was 3 billion, and the population in 2010 was 7 billion. This is a rate of 4 billion over 50 years, which equates to a rate of increase of 80 million per year.

29. **C**16.2 billion. If the population is 7 billion in 2010, and there is an increase in 80 million per year, then the population in 2125 will be 7 billion+(80 multiplied by 115) =16.2 billion

Data set 8

30. **A**37.5%. There is a drop of 1350 accounts, which out of 3600 represents a 37.5% drop

31. **D** $202.5 million. If each client contributes $150 000 to the firm, then the firm would have lost 1350 multiplied by $150 000 which equals $202.5 million

32. **E**2025. The minimum number of employees that must be fired would be if all the employees had the maximum salary of $100 000, so $202.5 million divided by 100000, which gives 2025.

Data Set 9

33. **D** 6 miles. If the bus takes 7 minutes to travel between these two stops, and the bus is travelling at 40 miles per hour, then the distance between the 2 stops is 40 multiplied by (7 divided by 60) which equals 4.66 miles

34. **C** 66mph. The bus takes 31 minutes to travel the 34 miles, which means that the average speed of the bus is 34 divided by (31 divided by 60) which = 66 miles per hour

35. **C** 5.3 miles per hour. If she misses the bus by 2 minutes, then she will be at the Weeping Cross Lane at 0735. If she needs to be at the station by 0752, then she has 17 minutes to walk 1.5 miles, which means she must walk at 5.3 miles per hour

36. **D** 0.264. If skittles only come in one of these 4 colours, then the probability that they draw a purple skittle will be (53-(12+13+14))/53, which equals 0.264.

END OF SECTION

Section D: Abstract Reasoning

Rules:

Set 1: In Set A, all objects with a right angle are striped. All objects with no right angle are black. The number of white circles is equal to the number of right angles present within the striped objects within the shape. In Set B, all objects with a right angle are black and all objects with no right angle are striped. The number of white circles is equal to the number of angles which are not right angles within the shapes.

Set 2: The number of sides in increasing by 1 in order, with even-sided shapes being shaded and odd-sided shapes being clear.

Set 3: The black circle is moving around the corners of the square, with the arrow being in the opposite corner to the black circle

Set 4: The letter on the right is 16 letters of the alphabet after the letter on the left.

Set 5: The shape on the right is the mirror image of the shape on the left, with a vertical line of symmetry.

Set 6: The shape on the right has 3 times the number of sides as the shape on the left

Set 7: The number of acute angles is odd and the number of obtuse angles is even in Set A; The number of acute angles is even and the number of obtuse angles is odd in Set B

Set 8: In Set A, if there is an upwards pointing arrow then there is an even number of circles. In Set B, if there is an upwards pointing arrow then there is an odd number of circles.

Set 9: In Set A, the number of edges adds up to a multiple of 3. In set B, the number of edges = 8.

Set 10: In Set A, arrows point towards rectangles and away from circles. In Set B, arrows point towards triangles and away from rectangles.

Set 11: In Set A, there are twice as many hexagons as triangles. In Set B, there are twice as many triangles as hexagons.

Set 12: In Set A, there is always a rectangle cut by one circle. In Set B, there is always a rectangle cut by two circles.

Set 13: In Set A, all shapes contain 9 arrowheads. In Set B, all shapes contain 8 arrowheads.

Set 14: In Set A, there are four curved edges. In Set B, there are 3 curved edges.

Set 15: In Set A, there are 10 shapes if white shapes count as two. In Set B, there are 8 shapes if black shapes count as two

END OF SECTION.

Section E: Situational Judgement Test

Scenario 1

1. **Very inappropriate.** It is highly inappropriate for a medical student to be drunk on a ward. As a fellow medical student, it John's professional duty to act in this situation.
2. **Very inappropriate.** Although he should act in this situation, the head of the medical school is not his first port of call.
3. **Very appropriate.** It would be most appropriate to speak to Tom first and see what is going on and advise him to go home. As John doesn't know what the context of the situation is, it is best to speak directly to Tom first.
4. **Inappropriate but not awful.** It would be more suitable to speak to a medical supervisor or to Tom first than to fellow medical students as a first port of call.
5. **Appropriate but not ideal.** Speaking to his supervisor would be a good thing to do but ideally, he should have spoken to Tom about it first.

Scenario 2

6. **Very inappropriate.** Jacob has a very legitimate reason for not attending the session but if nobody is aware of it then they will think he is missing the session because he can't be bothered to go (when the opposite is the case)
7. **Very inappropriate.** Jacob's mother was recently diagnosed with cancer so putting himself through a session like this would be unnecessary and unhelpful for him, especially as he thinks it would be too challenging. He shouldn't put himself through it just for the sake of it.
8. **Very appropriate.** The doctor will be extremely understanding if Jacob explains why he doesn't want to attend the session.
9. **Appropriate but not ideal.** It would be ideal to inform the doctor running the session directly about why he cannot come, but is understandable if he would rather his friend explained the situation to the doctor.
10. **Appropriate but not ideal.** Jacob shouldn't have felt the need to attend given his circumstances. But it was good that he left when he found it too overwhelming.

Scenario 3

11. **Very inappropriate.** As team captain, Lucy has a responsibility to the team and cannot abandon them a week before the match.
12. **Inappropriate but not awful.** As it is a week before the match, the team has probably practiced a lot with Lucy playing for the whole game. Changing this a week before the match is not ideal.
13. **Very appropriate.** This way Lucy is not letting down her team in any way and is attending as much of the conference as she can.
14. **Appropriate but not ideal.** Lucy's current priority is her responsibility for her hockey team and as a third year, there is plenty of time to attend conferences and build up medical interests. However, attending this conference in some capacity may have benefitted Lucy.
15. **Very inappropriate.** Lying to and abandoning her team members, especially as she is team captain, would be wrong.

Scenario 4

16. **Inappropriate but not awful.** It would be inappropriate to escalate a situation like this straight to the medical school director. However, Tara is distressed by the situation and at least in this scenario she is responding to the situation.
17. **Very appropriate.** A situation like this should be discussed with Tara's supervisor, as they can provide her with practical information and advice as to how to proceed.
18. **Inappropriate but not awful.** Although it is good that Tara did not passively accept the situation at hand, speaking directly to the consultant is difficult because of the power dynamic. It would be better to approach this situation from a different angle.
19. **Very inappropriate.** If Tara is finding the consultant distressing, she should definitely act in this situation as this should not be the experience that she is having.
20. **Very inappropriate.** Many things can be done in this situation, including changing wards, but stopping attending altogether compromises Tara's medical education.

Scenario 5

21. **Very inappropriate.** Revision cannot take place in two days even if she didn't fail by much and it is important to try not to fail the retake.
22. **Very appropriate.** This is ideal as she can be as involved in the wedding as is feasible whilst giving herself time to focus on the retake.
23. **Inappropriate but not awful.** Planning for a wedding is close to a full-time job and realistically does not leave time for much revision. However, at least she is planning on revising before the wedding unlike in scenario 1.
24. **Very inappropriate.** The wedding date has probably been in place for months and the venue hired etc. – this is not feasible.
25. **Appropriate but not ideal.** The wedding can still go ahead and Alice can revise for her retake. However, Alice's sister probably envisioned Alice as her maid of honour so changing this would not be the ideal situation for her sister.

Scenario 6

26. **Inappropriate but not awful.** Luke should speak to the student first before reporting him. This may be more appropriate if he found him doing the same thing a second time.
27. **Very inappropriate.** The student is breaking confidentiality and it is your responsibility as a medical professional to act in this situation.
28. **Very appropriate.** Speaking to a senior such as his supervisor is appropriate, especially if he is unsure of the most appropriate course of action in this situation.
29. **Very appropriate.** I is appropriate to speak directly to the student and explaining that what he did is breaking confidentiality.
30. **Very inappropriate.** The problem is not that he is in the hospital, it is that he is in the hospital lift and therefore a public place. The student should not be speaking about patients in any public place.

Scenario 7

31. **Fairly important.** This is a very good opportunity to practice on real patients and have a shot at the exam. However there are other ways to practice on real patients.
32. **Very important.** Some patients may have a compromised immune system and it is not worth risking their health.
33. **Very important.** This is Eva's only opportunity for a mock exam before finals.
34. **Of minor importance.** Although this is true it is still irresponsible to risk the health of patients who have medical conditions. Also they may have a serious condition that is stable at the moment.
35. **Very important.** Eva should obey the rules given by the medical school.
36. **Very important.** Eva has opportunities to practice for the exam, so even though the mock will be useful, she can still do well in her exam without it.

Scenario 8

37. **Very important.** It would not be fair for Lucy if she was not reimbursed, as it would cost her more in petrol to go to the further GP placement.
38. **Fairly important.** It would be kind to prevent Alice from making a long commute when it is much quicker and easier for Lucy by car.
39. **Very important.** She would be getting something equally valuable in return for swapping with Alice.
40. **Of minor importance.** Lucy would have to leave 20 minutes earlier than she would have originally left, which is not a big compromise.
41. **Of minor importance.** Alice may have already asked the other students who can drive and they may have refused, may not have their cars at university etc. Lucy does not know what the circumstances of the other students are.
42. **Of no importance.** Lucy chose her placement based on length of commute, not quality of placement/teaching. Therefore, by swapping with Alice, there is no reason to think that the quality of her placement would be decreased.

Scenario 9

43. **Fairly important.** If he learns better by reading a textbook, it is not as bad that he is missing some lectures. However, even if he learns better by reading a textbook, the lectures may be a helpful addition to his learning.
44. **Very important.** It would be worse to be tired all day and unable to concentrate in all the lectures, then to miss half of the lectures and have full concentration for the other half of the lectures.
45. **Of minor importance.** Even if the other students do not find the lectures useful, he may find them of use.
46. **Very important.** If the lectures are available online, Nick can catch up easily.
47. **Very important.** Again, if the lectures are available online, Nick will not have a problem catching up.
48. **Very important.** Insomnia is a medical condition and it is impacting Nick's studies. The medical student may be able to help him find a solution e.g. recording the lectures.

Scenario 10

49. **Very important.** If the consultant has other availabilities, Lorna need not compromise on either hockey or the teaching.
50. **Of no importance.** As Lorna is interested in paediatrics and likes her consultant, she is keen on the teaching for reasons unrelated to exams.
51. **Very important.** Again, if hockey practice were on for more than one evening a week, she could miss Thursday evenings but still have full attendance on other days in the week.
52. **Very important.** As Lorna is considering paediatrics, this teaching is extremely valuable for her.
53. **Fairly important.** It would not be good to let down the hockey team if she has made commitments. However, as she isn't captain, if she wants to prioritise the teaching over her extra-curricular activity, that would be valid.
54. **Fairly important.** It is healthy to have interests outside of studies and without hockey, Lorna wouldn't have this. However if she is committed to the teaching, Lorna can find a different extracurricular activity that does not take place on a Thursday evening.

Scenario 11

55. **Of minor importance.** Chris's friendship with Joe will undoubtedly have an effect on how Chris decides to act in this situation. However, plagiarism is wrong and Chris should not feel guilty about wanting to do act in this situation.
56. **Very important.** Plagiarism is wrong, and if it is directly stated that it is against university rules, Chris should act in this situation.
57. **Very important.** The medical student in the year above may have put a lot of effort into this essay and sent it to Joe and Chris to help them, but not for it to be replicated without any work on their part.
58. **Of no importance.** Whether or not the essay was good, what Joe did was wrong.
59. **Of no importance.** Again, what Joe did was wrong, even though the essay only counts for 5% of the grade.
60. **Of no importance.** Whether or not plagiarism is inevitable, if Chris has caught Joe doing it, he should act on this.

Scenario 12

61. **Very important.** By helping the surgeon, Chen may be assisting in saving this girl's life.
62. **Fairly important.** The procedure may be psychologically traumatic, but Chen is likely to be more traumatised if he does not assist and the girl subsequently dies. However, it is a lot to ask of a medical student.
63. **Very important.** Even though this wouldn't be a situation that ever occurred in the UK, the circumstances are different in Swaziland and so Chen should not feel guilty in helping the surgeon.
64. **Very important.** As the only person available to help, this increases Chen's responsibility and guilt if he doesn't.
65. **Of minor importance.** As previously stated, the UK and Swaziland are very different countries so Chen should feel justified in helping the surgeon.

Scenario 13

66. **Very important.** Although this publication could be useful, Jasmine should not compromise her exam results which are ultimately more important for her medical career.
67. **Fairly important.** A publication is useful for job application and CV, but as previously stated, it is not worth compromising exam results for.
68. **Of minor importance.** In this situation Jasmine's studies need to take priority since a manuscript can be submitted for publication at any time, her exam dates cannot be moved.
69. **Very important.** With further extracurricular activities to juggle her time for revision will be even more limited. Jasmine needs to prioritise and therefore knowing all of her possible commitments to make a reasoned decision.

END OF PAPER

Final Advice

Arrive well rested, well fed and well hydrated

UCAT is an intensive test, so make sure you're ready for it! Unfortunately you can't take water into the test, so be well hydrated before you go in. Make sure you're well rested and fed in order to be at your best!

Ask for extra whiteboards

If you're running short of whiteboard space and need another, **plan ahead and put up your hand in good time**. You don't want to be stuck with nowhere to write, waiting for someone to notice and come to help you! Act early.

Move On

If you're struggling, move on. Every question has equal weighting and there is no negative marking. **In the time it takes to answer on hard question, you could gain three times the marks** by answering the easier ones. Be smart to score points

Using your UCAT Score

Different medical schools use UCAT in different ways – so use this to your advantage! If you score well on UCAT, you may help your chances of success by choosing medical schools which use it as a major component of the application process. On the other hand, if your score isn't so good, you may prefer to opt for universities that don't look at your UCAT score, or ones that use it as a more minor consideration.

By making choices <u>after</u> finding out your score, you can increase your chance of getting a place.

Afterword

Remember that the route to a high score is your approach and practice. Don't fall into the trap that "*you can't prepare for the UCAT*"– this COULD NOT be further from the truth. With knowledge of the test, some useful time-saving techniques and plenty of practice you can dramatically boost your score.

Work hard, be persistent and do yourself justice.

Good luck!

About Us

Infinity Books is the publishing division of *Infinity Education*. We currently publish over 85 titles across a range of subject areas – covering specialised admissions tests, examination techniques, personal statement guides, plus everything else you need to improve your chances of getting on to competitive courses such as medicine and law, as well as into universities such as Oxford and Cambridge.

Outside of publishing we also operate a highly successful tuition division, called UniAdmissions. This company was founded in 2013 by Dr Rohan Agarwal and Dr David Salt, both Cambridge Medical graduates with several years of tutoring experience. Since then, every year, hundreds of applicants and schools work with us on our programmes. Through the programmes we offer, we deliver expert tuition, exclusive course places, online courses, best-selling textbooks and much more.

With a team of over 1,000 Oxbridge tutors and a proven track record, UniAdmissions have quickly become the UK's number one admissions company.

Visit and engage with us at:
Website (Infinity Books): www.infinitybooks.co.uk
Website (UniAdmissions): www.uniadmissions.co.uk
Facebook: www.facebook.com/uniadmissionsuk
Twitter: @infinitybooks7

Your Free Book

Thanks for purchasing this Ultimate Book. Readers like you have the power to make or break a book –hopefully you found this one useful and informative. *UniAdmissions* would love to hear about your experiences with this book. As thanks for your time we'll send you another ebook from our Ultimate Guide series absolutely FREE!

How to Redeem Your Free Ebook

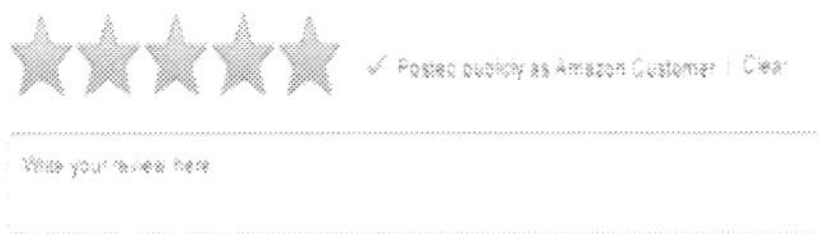

1) Either scan the QR code or find the book you have on your Amazon purchase history or your email receipt to help find the book on Amazon.

2) On the product page at the Customer Reviews area, click 'Write a customer review'. Write your review and post it! Copy the review page or take a screen shot of the review you have left.

3) Head over to www.uniadmissions.co.uk/free-book and select your chosen free ebook!

Your ebook will then be emailed to you – it's as simple as that!
Alternatively, you can buy all the titles at

www.uniadmissions.co.uk/our-books

Printed in Great Britain
by Amazon

58455835R00334